Gastrointestinal Malignancies

New Innovative Diagnostics and Treatment

Gastrointestinal Malignancies

New Innovative Diagnostics and Treatment

Editor

Qiang Cai
Emory University, USA

Co-Editors

Bassel F El-Rayes
Emory University, USA

Jinghua Hao
Shandong Provincial Hospital, affiliated to Shandong University, China

David A Kooby
Emory University, USA

Jerome Carl Landry
Emory University, USA

Virginia Oliva Shaffer
Emory University, USA

Hong Xu
The First Affiliated Hospital of Jilin University, China

World Scientific

NEW JERSEY • LONDON • SINGAPORE • BEIJING • SHANGHAI • HONG KONG • TAIPEI • CHENNAI

Published by

World Scientific Publishing Co. Pte. Ltd.
5 Toh Tuck Link, Singapore 596224
USA office: 27 Warren Street, Suite 401-402, Hackensack, NJ 07601
UK office: 57 Shelton Street, Covent Garden, London WC2H 9HE

Library of Congress Cataloging-in-Publication Data
Gastrointestinal malignancies (Cai)
Gastrointestinal malignancies : new innovative diagnostics and treatment / [edited by] Qiang Cai [and six others].
p. ; cm.
Includes bibliographical references and index.
ISBN 978-9814618984 (hardcover : alk. paper)
I. Cai, Qiang, editor. II. Title.
[DNLM: 1. Digestive System Neoplasms--diagnosis. 2. Digestive System Neoplasms--therapy. WI 149]
RC280.D5
616.99'43--dc23
2015004081

British Library Cataloguing-in-Publication Data
A catalogue record for this book is available from the British Library.

Typeset by Stallion Press
Email: enquiries@stallionpress.com

Printed in Singapore

Contents

Preface ix
Editors' Biography xi
List of Authors xxi

Chapter 1 The Descriptive Epidemiology of Gastrointestinal Malignancies 1
Anthony Gamboa, Qi Lin, Peng Jin, Yifeng Zhou, Qiang Liu, Jinghua Hao, Qiang Cai and Roberd M. Bostick

Chapter 2 Biomarkers and the Quest for Personalized Cancer Care 41
Sameer H. Patel and Shishir K. Maithel

Chapter 3 Prevention of Gastrointestinal Malignancy 55
Heval Mohamed Kelli, Jinghua Hao, Qing Shu, Endian Zheng, Kevin Woods and Qiang Cai

Chapter 4 Imaging in Gastrointestinal Malignancies 71
Iva Petkovska, Bobby Kalb and Diego R. Martin

Chapter 5 Nutritional Supports for Patients with Gastrointestinal Malignancies 123
Shadi S. Yarandi, Jinghua Hao, Qingwei Jiang, Zhuo Yang and Qiang Cai

Chapter 6 Palliative Care for Patients with Advanced Gastrointestinal Malignancies 141
Tilak U. Shah and Steven Keilin

Chapter 7 Endoscopic Diagnosis and Treatment of Esophageal Malignancies 171
Fan Zhang, Virginia O. Shaffer, Qiang Cai and Hong Xu

Chapter 8 Multimodality Management of Esophageal Malignancies beyond Endoscopy 199
Liza Stapleford and Nabil F. Saba

Chapter 9 Endoscopic Diagnosis and Treatment of Gastric Malignancies 241
Ke Tao, Virginia O. Shaffer, Qiang Cai and Hong Xu

Chapter 10 Management of Gastric and Gastroesophageal Junction Adenocarcinoma beyond Endoscopy 253
Gopi K. Prithviraj, Amit Mahipal and Richard Kim

Chapter 11 Endoscopic Diagnosis and Treatment of Colorectal Malignancies 279
Shuang Wu, Virginia O. Shaffer, Qiang Cai and Hong Xu

Chapter 12 Multimodality Management of Colorectal Malignancies Beyond Endoscopy 291
John D. Lyons and Virginia O. Shaffer

Chapter 13 Multimodality Management of Oligometastatic Colorectal Cancer 311
Teviah E. Sachs and Timothy M. Pawlik

Chapter 14 Diagnosis and Staging of Pancreatic Malignancies 351
Saurabh Chawla, Parit Mekaroonkamol and Field F. Willingham

Chapter 15 Borderline Resectable Adenocarcinoma of the Pancreas 415
Sarah B. Fisher, Michael C. Lowe and David A. Kooby

Chapter 16 Treatment of Advanced Pancreatic Cancer 451
Hemchandra Mahaseth, Bassel El-Rayes and Philip A. Philip

Chapter 17 Diagnosis of Hepatobiliary Malignancies 471
Xu Shu, Xu Guo, Viginia O. Shaffer, Jinghua Hao and Qiang Cai

Chapter 18 Non-Surgical Management of Hepatobiliary Malignancies 503
Anne M. Noonan and Tanios Bekaii-Saab

Chapter 19 Surgical Treatment of Hepatobiliary Malignancies and Liver Transplantation 527
Jean-Sébastien Pelletier and David A. Geller

Chapter 20 Image-Guided Therapy of Liver Malignancy 551
Samdeep K. Mouli, Riad Salem and Robert J. Lewandowski

Chapter 21 Rare Gastrointestinal Malignancies 589
Walid Shaib, Daniel Goldstein, Vinicus Ernani, Maria C. Russell and Kenneth Cardona

Chapter 22 The Essentials of the Gastrointestinal and Pancreaticobiliary Malignancies Pathology 625
Yue Xue

Chapter 23 Proton Therapy: A New Dawn for Gastrointestinal Cancer Treatment 637
Gary Y. Yang and Jerome C. Landry

Chapter 24 Radiotherapy for Rectal Cancer 647
Jordan Torok, Manisha Palta, Christopher Willett and Brian Czito

Chapter 25 Radiotheraphy for Pancreatic Cancer 661
Lauren Colbert, Richard J. Cassidy and David Marcus

Index 673

Preface

The most common types of gastrointestinal cancers are colorectal, pancreatic, liver, gastric, and esophageal cancers — which have high mortality rates. Many other gastrointestinal malignancies, such as cholangiocarcinoma, are responsible for high mortality rates as well. Although gastric cancer is declining worldwide and colorectal cancer is declining in the United States, esophageal adenocarcinoma and carcinoid tumor incidence rates continue to increase remarkably. Liver cancer incidence also continues to rise, though some predict that it will decline in the coming years as hepatitis B is addressed with vaccination and novel therapies for hepatitis C become available. Mortality trends for pancreatic cancer have shifted, with declining rates among African Americans and increasing rates among Caucasians, which is a reversal from a decade earlier.

Despite those changes over the last decade or so, gastrointestinal malignancies still account for approximately one-third of all cancers and almost 40% of cancer-related mortality worldwide. In other words, gastrointestinal malignancies are still the major killer of the human body.

Over the last decade, there are many new innovative diagnostics and treatment for gastrointestinal malignancies, such as positron emission tomography-computed tomography, cryotherapy, endoscopic submucosal dissection, etc. We believe it is time to write such a book to summarize new diagnostic and therapeutic modalities and provide these information to care givers of patients with gastrointestinal malignancies, such as oncologists, surgeons, and gastroenterologists.

To achieve this goal, many of the finest experts from varieties specialties, including gastroenterology, oncology and surgery, from China and United

States have written this book. Each chapter is prepared by an authority who is actively engaged in advancing our knowledge of the subject matter of the chapter. The editors really appreciate all authors' effort in the process of writing this book and believe that the expertise of this group of physicians has ensured that the book will achieve its aims.

The editors also wish to express their gratitude to the staff at World Scientific Press for their commitment to quality, integrity and excellence. The editors sincerely thank Ms. Ching Ting, for her initial invitation to write this book on behalf of the publisher and Ms. Darilyn Yap, our desk editor, for her patience and expertise in editing this book. Without the dedication and extraordinary talent of our colleagues and the staff, the edition of this book would not been possible.

Qiang Cai, M.D., Ph.D.

Editors' Biography

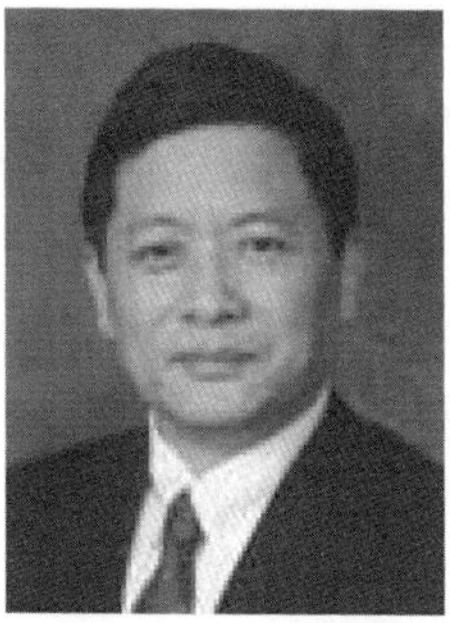

Qiang Cai, M.D., Ph.D., F.A.S.G.E.
Professor of Medicine
Director, Advanced Endoscopy Fellowship
Emory University School of Medicine

Mailing address:
1365 Clifton Road, B1262
Atlanta, GA 30322

Tel: 404-778-2714
Fax: 404-778-2578
Email: qcai@emory.edu

Dr. Qiang Cai is a therapeutic endoscopist at Emory University, Director of Advanced Endoscopy Fellowship, and Professor of Medicine at the Division of Digestive Diseases at the School of Medicine.

Dr. Qiang Cai is a graduate of Nanchang University School of Medicine in China. After graduating from the medical school in 1982, he attended Peking Union Medical College Hospital, one of the best hospitals in China, where he began his career in Gastroenterology under the tutorship of Drs. Xiao-Qian Zhang, Min-Zhang Chen, Shou-Po Chen and Yuan-Fang Chen. There, he obtained his master degree in gastrointestinal physiology and served as a gastroenterologist and faculty member before moving to the United States in 1987. In 1992, Dr. Cai obtained his Ph.D in gastrointestinal physiology from Cornell University, where he studied intestinal calcium absorption under the guidance of Dr. Robert H. Wasserman, the father of intestinal calcium binding protein. He completed his second internal medicine residency training at Marshfield Clinic, one of the training facilities of the University of Wisconsin, and his second gastroenterology fellowship at Emory University. Dr. Cai joined the faculty team at the Division of Digestive Diseases, Department of Medicine, Emory University School of Medicine in July 2001.

Dr. Cai's main research interests are pancreatobiliary diseases, including diseases in the pancreas, gallbladder and bile duct, as well as diagnostic and therapeutic endoscocpy for gastrointestinal malignancies. Dr. Cai can perform all endoscopic procedures. He is one of the few gastroenterologists in the United States who can perform endoscopic submucosal dissection to remove early gastrointestinal malignancies.

Dr. Cai is a member of many committees of the American College of Gastroenterology, American Society of Gastrointestinal Endoscopy and serves on the editorial boards of various medical publications, including *American Journal of Gastroenterology*, *Chinese Medical Journal*, *Chinese Journal of Digestive Diseases* etc.

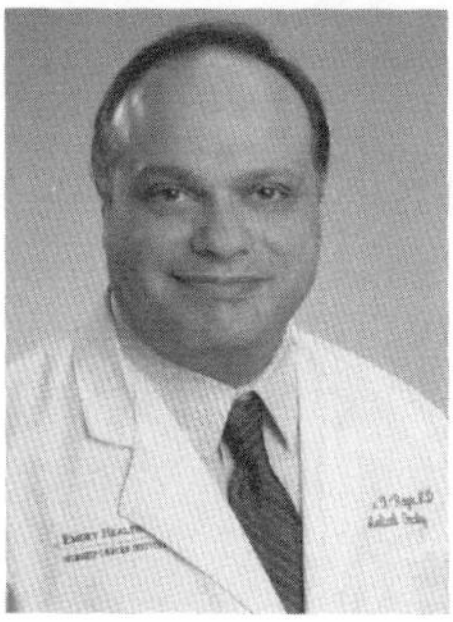

Bassel F. El-Rayes, M.D.
Professor of Hematology and Oncology
Director of GI Oncology Program
Associate Director of Clinical Research
Winship Cancer Institute

Mailing address:
1365C Clifton Rd NE, 2nd floor
Atlanta, GA 30322

Tel: 404-778-1900
Email: belraye@emory.edu

Dr. El-Rayes specializes in treatment of GI cancers as well as early phase translational research in GI oncology. His particular area of interest is multimodality management of colorectal and pancreatic cancer as well as treatment of neuroendocrine tumors. He has led several innovative trials including investigator initiated clinical trials. Dr. El-Rayes has also done preclinical research that has been the basis of his early phase clinical trials. He received his M.D. at the American University of Beirut, Beirut, Lebanon, in 1996; completed his internal medicine residency at Wayne State University in Detroit, where he was selected to serve as a chief medical resident. He completed his clinical fellowships in Hematology and Medical Oncology at Karmanos Cancer Institute, Wayne State University. He was recruited to stay as faculty member in GI Oncology at Karmanos Cancer Institute where he stayed until 2009. During this time, he chaired the Data Safety and Monitoring Committee and was the Medical Director of the outpatient clinic. Dr. El-Rayes then joined Emory University as Director of GI oncology program in 2009.

Dr. El-Rayes has received numerous honors and awards, including being selected as teacher of the year at Karmanos Cancer Institute, receiving the teacher of the year award at Emory University, Georgia Cancer Coalition Scholar award in 2010, Physician of the Year award for Hematology Oncology in 2014 etc. He serves on the editorial boards for several journals including *Cancer*. He serves on several national committees including the NCI task force for neuroendocrine tumors. He is a leader in multicenter clinical research.

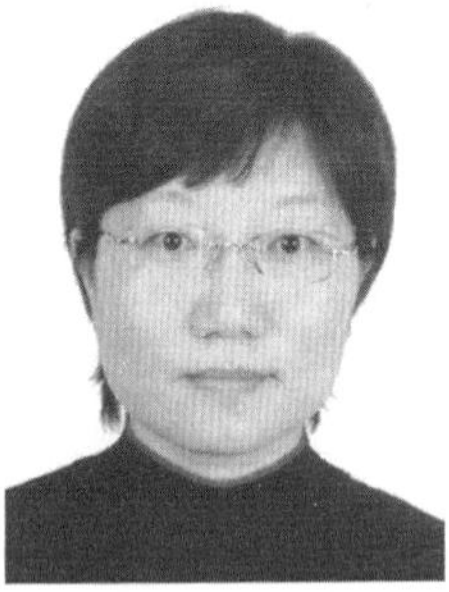

Jinghua Hao, M.D.
Professor of Medicine
Department of Digestive Diseases
Provincial Hospital
Affiliated to Shandong University

Mailing address:
324 Jingwu Road
Ji'nan, Shandong, China 250021

Tel: 86-531-68776350
Email: jinghua_hao@hotmail.com

Dr. Jinghua Hao is a Chinese gastroenterologist and hepatologist.

Dr. Hao attended Shandong Medical University, where she earned a bachelor's degree in 1995. She went on to earn her M.D. and Ph.D. from the same university in 2000.

Dr. Hao completed her internal medicine residency training at Shandong Provincial Hospital and Affiliated Hospital, Qingdao University. Dr. Hao was then recruited by Shandong Provincial Hospital in 2001. During 2006–2008, as a research fellow, she went to Nanyang Technological University, Singapore, and focused on biomedical engineering studies. Dr. Hao was promoted to a professor in 2013 as a result of her remarkable contributions on clinical works and scientific researches, especially on chronic liver diseases and gastrointestinal tract malignancies.

Dr. Hao has expertise in chronic hepatitis, liver cirrhosis, and also gastrointestinal tract malignancies. She organized emergent rescue of patients with gastrointestinal tract hemorrhage, acute pancreatitis, and so on. Dr. Hao can perform most GI endoscopy on patients with digestive diseases. As principal investigator, she has tutored postgraduates on conducting ongoing research projects aimed at developing new therapeutic strategies for alcoholic liver disease and non-alcoholic fatty liver disease. Dr. Hao has published more than 40 papers in peer-review science journals, and compiled eight academic works. Her doctorate thesis was awarded by Shandong University for excellent doctorate thesis in the year 2002. In addition, she was awarded three times by Shandong Province Science & Technology Department for the studies of hepatic microcirculation, liver fibrosis, and gastric carcinoma, respectively.

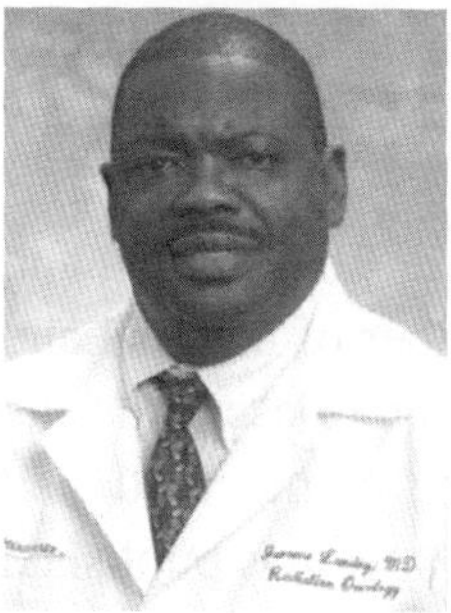

Jerome C. Landry, M.D., M.B.A.
Professor of Radiation Oncology
Emory University School of Medicine
Winship Cancer Institute
Chief of Service
Edward Loughlin Oncology Center
Grady Health System

Mailing address:
1365 Clifton Rd NE, Suite A1305
Atlanta, GA 30322

Tel: 404-778-3473 Emory
404-616-3947 Grady
Fax: 404-616-6380
Email: jland01@emory.edu

Dr. Jerome Landry specializes in the evaluation and treatment of patients with pancreas, anus, colorectal and esophagus, bile duct and stomach cancers. He treats patients with advanced radiation techniques such as IMRT and SBRT. He also has expertise in Sarcoma, a rare soft tissue and bone tumors that frequently pose significant diagnostic and therapeutic challenges. He has taught many national courses on advanced radiation techniques and treatment of the liver, pancreas, and colon, and is frequently invited to speak at national conferences. He was the first to use Varian's Trilogy On-Board Imaging system for gastrointestinal tumors. Dr. Landry has performed on-site IMRT training in more than 40 radiation oncology centers in the US and abroad. His research focus is on translational research in gastrointestinal oncology. This entails collaborating with molecular and radiobiology scientists to test new chemotherapy and molecular agents in combination with radiation.

Dr. Landry is a graduate of Harvard Medical School in 1983. He completed his internship at Emory University Hospital and his residency in radiation medicine at Harvard's Massachusetts General Hospital, where he served as chief resident in his final year. He has served as Chief of

Service of the Edward Loughlin Radiation Oncology Center of Grady Health Systems since 1987. Dr. Landry also holds a MBA from Kennesaw State University obtained in 1998.

He has published extensively on IMRT for gastrointestinal tumors and soft tissue sarcomas, been an invited speaker at a number of medical and academic conferences, and is the lead editor for a chapter describing the use of IMRT in the treatment of pancreatic cancer in the textbook, *Intensity Modulated Radiation Therapy: A Clinical Perspective*, published by BC Decker in 2005. Dr. Landry has won numerous awards and grants and has been ranked one of the best doctors in America by a number of publications including *Atlanta Magazine* (1995, 1997–1998, 2000–2014), *Red Book Magazine* (2001) and *Ladies Home Journal* (2002).

Dr. Landry is a recipient of the Whalley Foundation GI Oncology Fund Award, a Winship philanthropic pilot fund, in 2012 and 2013. He received the American Board of Radiation Oncology (ABR) Distinguished Service Award in 2010. Dr. Landry is a member of the NRG Colorectal Cancer Radiotherapy Working Group and the Grady Hospital Research Oversight Committee (ROC).

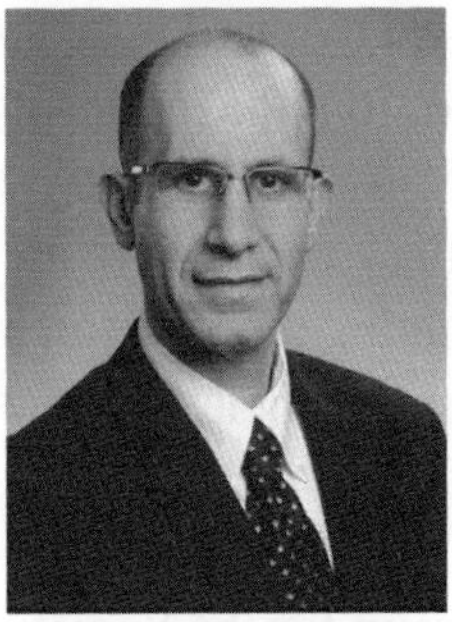

David A. Kooby, M.D., F.A.C.S.
Professor of Surgery
Director of Surgical Oncology,
Emory/Saint Joseph's Hospital
Director of Minimally Invasive GI Surgical Oncology
Emory University School of Medicine
Winship Cancer Institute

Mailing address:
1365C Clifton Rd NE, 2nd floor
Atlanta, GA 30322

O: 404-778-3805
F: 404-778-4255
Email: dkooby@emory.edu

Dr. David Kooby specializes in laparoscopic/robotic and open surgical treatment of liver, bile duct, pancreas, stomach, and colon tumors/cancers. He also has expertise in tumors and diseases of the spleen, adrenal glands, and retroperitoneum. He has taught many national courses on laparoscopic resection of the liver, pancreas, and colon, and is frequently invited to speak at national conferences. He received his M.D. at the State University of New York, Downstate Medical College, Brooklyn, NY, in 1994; completed his surgical residency at Vanderbilt University, where he won medical student and resident teaching awards. He completed both bench research and clinical fellowships at Memorial Sloan-Kettering Cancer Center, New York, NY. He was recruited by Emory in 2003, and is currently an Associate Professor of Surgery in the Division of Surgical Oncology, Director of Surgical Oncology at Emory/Saint Joseph's Hospital, and Director of Minimally Invasive GI Surgical Oncology. He is a recipient of a Cancer Scholar Stipend from the Georgia Cancer Coalition in 2004, was named as an Honored Clinical Professor by the Emory University School of Medicine Class of 2007, and inducted into the Alpha Omega Alpha medical honor society at Emory in 2008. He is the recipient of the Ann & Paul Hastings Scholar for Excellence in Surgical Oncology and Patient Care Award in 2012 and the Faculty Excellence Award in 2014 at Emory University School of Medicine. He serves on the editorial boards for *Annals of Surgical Oncology* and *Journal of Surgical Oncology*, for which he is an associated editor for the hepatobiliary and pancreatic section. He serves on several national committees including the task force charged with updating the staging of hepatobiliary malignancies for the American Joint Committee on Cancer's Cancer Staging Manual, the research and education committee for the American Hepato-Pancreato-Biliary Association, and the Hepatobiliary Working Group for the Society of Surgical Oncology. He is a leader in multicenter clinical research and a national leader in minimally invasive pancreatic surgery.

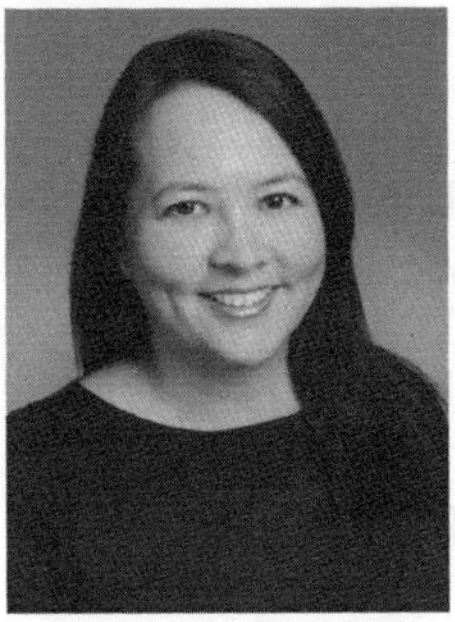

Virginia Oliva Shaffer, M.D., F.A.C.S.
Assistant Professor of Surgery
Colorectal Surgery
Co-Director Surgical Grand Rounds
Emory University Hospital/The Emory Clinic

Mailing address:
1365 Clifton Road, Building A, Suite 3300
Atlanta, GA 30322

Tel: 404-778-5809
Fax: 404-778-5033
Email: virginia.o.shaffer@emory.edu

Dr. Virginia Shaffer is an Assistant Professor of Surgery at Emory University and specializes in laparoscopic and open surgical treatment of diseases of the colon and rectum.

She received her M.D. at the University of Texas Health Science Center San Antonio, and completed general surgery residency at Emory University in Atlanta, GA.

Dr. Shaffer did a research fellowship in Transplant Immunology and subsequently did a fellowship in Colon and Rectal Surgery at Cleveland Clinic Florida. She is board certified in both General Surgery and Colon and Rectal Surgery. Her research interests include health outcomes research and translational research. She currently holds an IND for fecal microbiota transplantation in post-surgical patients.

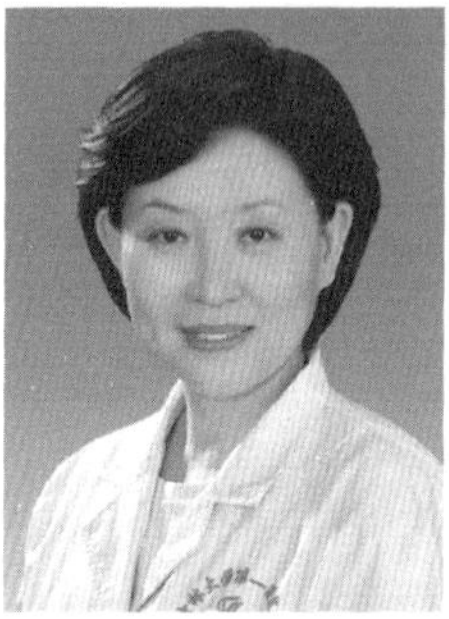

Hong Xu, M.D., Ph.D.
Director, Professor
Department of Endoscopy & Gastroenterology
First Hospital of Jilin University

Mailing address:
71 Xinmin Street
Changchun, Jilin, China, 130000

Tel: 86-431-8878-2821
Mobile phone: 86-13756661648
Email: chxuhong@163.com

Dr. Hong Xu is a Professor of Medicine at Jilin University, Changchun China. She is Director of the Department of Gastroenterology and the Gastrointestinal Endoscopy Center at the First Affiliated Hospital of Jilin University. She is also an Associate Dean of the Bethune Medical School of the university.

Dr. Xu completed her medical school training and also her mast and doctoral graduate studies in Jilin University. She then became a faculty member in the First Affiliated Hospital of Jilin University.

Despite having a very busy administration schedule, Dr. Xu still sees patients and performs gastrointestinal endoscopy on a weekly basis. She is especially interested in endoscopic diagnosis and treatment for early gastrointestinal cancers and has an excellent national reputation. She is a member of Chinese Gastrointestinal Endoscopy Society and President of Gastrointestinal Endoscopy Society of Jilin Province.

List of Authors

Tanios Bekaii-Saab, M.D.
Section Chief , Gastrointestinal Oncology
Chair , OSUCCC Gastrointestinal Disease Research Group
Associate Professor of Medicine and Pharmacy
The Ohio State University — James Cancer Hospital
Columbus, OH, USA

Roberd M. Bostick, M.D., M.P.H.
Professor, Department of Epidemiology
Professor (Joint), Department of Hematology & Medical Oncology
Program Leader, Cancer Prevention & Control, Winship Cancer Institute
Georgia Cancer Coalition Distinguished Scholar
Rollins School of Public Health
Emory University
Atlanta, GA, USA

Qiang Cai, M.D., Ph.D., F.A.S.G.E.
Professor of Medicine
Director, Advanced Endoscopy Fellowship
Emory University School of Medicine
Atlanta, GA, USA

Richard J. Cassidy, M.D.
Resident
Department of Radiation Oncology

Emory University
Atlanta, GA, USA

Kenneth Cardona, M.D.
Assistant Professor of Surgery
Division of Surgical Oncology
Emory University
Atlanta, GA, USA

Saurabh Chawla, M.D.
Director of Interventional Endoscopy
Grady Memorial Hospital
Assistant Professor of Medicine
Digestive Diseases
Emory University School of Medicine
Atlanta, GA, USA

Lauren Colbert, M.D.
Resident
Department of Radiation Oncology
Memorial Sloan Kettering Cancer Center
New York, NY, USA

Brian Czito, M.D.
Assistant Professor
Department of Radiation Oncology
Duke University
Durham, NC, USA

Bassel F. El-Rayes, M.D.
Professor
Director, GI Oncology Program
Associate Cancer Center Director for Clinical Research
Georgia Research Alliance Cancer Scientist
Winship Cancer Institute
Emory University
Atlanta, GA, USA

Vinicus Ernani, M.D.
Fellow, Hematology/Oncology Department
Winship Cancer Institute
Emory University School of Medicine
Atlanta, GA, USA

Sarah B. Fisher, M.D., M.S.C.R.
Resident, Department of General Surgery
Emory University
Atlanta, GA, USA

Anthony Gamboa, M.D.
Chief Fellow
Department of Medicine, Division of Digestive Diseases
Emory University
Atlanta, GA, USA

David A. Geller, M.D.
Richard L. Simmons Professor of Surgery
Chief, Division of Hepatobiliary and Pancreatic Surgery
Director, UPMC Liver Cancer Center
University of Pittsburgh
Pittsburgh, PA, USA

Daniel Goldstein, M.D.
Fellow, Hematology/Oncology Department
Winship Cancer Institute
Emory University School of Medicine
Atlanta, GA, USA

Xu Guo, M.D.
Attending Physician
Department of Gastroenterology and Hepatology
General Hosptial of PLA
Beijing, China

Jinghua Hao, M.D.
Professor, Department of Digestive Diseases
Provincial Hospital, Affiliated to Shandong University
Ji'nan, Shandong, China

Qingwei Jiang, M.D.
Attending Physician
Department of Gastroenterology
Peking Union Medical College Hospital
Chinese Academy of Medical Sciences
Beijing, China

Peng Jin, M.D.
Associate Professor
Department of Gastroenterology & GI Endoscopy Center
Beijing Military General Hospital
Beijing, China

Bobby Kalb, M.D.
Associate Professor of Medical Imaging, Department of Medical Imaging
University of Arizona
Tucson, Arizona, USA

Steven Keilin, M.D.
Assistant Professor of Medicine
Director Pancreaticobiliary Service
Associate Director, Advanced Endoscopy Fellowship
Division of Gastroenterology
Emory University Hospital/The Emory Clinic
Atlanta, GA, USA

Heval Mohamed Kelli, M.D.
Internal Medicine Resident
Emory School of Medicine
J. Willis Hurst Internal Medicine Residency Program
Atlanta, GA, USA

Richard Kim, M.D.
Associate Member, GI Oncology
Associate Professor, Department of Internal Medicine and Interdisciplinary Oncology
Moffitt Cancer Center
Tampa, FL, USA

David A. Kooby, M.D., F.A.C.S.
Professor of Surgery
Director of Surgical Oncology, Emory/Saint Joseph's Hospital
Director of Minimally Invasive GI Surgical Oncology
Emory University School of Medicine
Winship Cancer Institute
Atlanta, GA, USA

Jerome C. Landry, M.D., M.B.A.
Professor of Radiation Oncology
Emory University School of Medicine
Winship Cancer Institute
Chief of Service, Edward Loughlin Oncology Center, Grady Health System
Atlanta, GA, USA

Robert J. Lewandowski, M.D., F.S.I.R.
Associate Professor of Radiology
Director of Interventional Oncology
Section of Vascular and Interventional Radiology
Feinberg School of Medicine
Northwestern University
Chicago, IL,USA

Qiang Liu, M.D.
Associate Professor
Department of Gastroenterology
The First Affiliated Hospital of Suzhou University
Suzhou, Jiangsu, China

Qi Lin, M.D.
Director, Gastroenterology Department
Chief Physician
Yinzhou No. 2 Hospital
Ningbo, Zhejiang, China

Michael C. Lowe, M.D.
Surgical Fellow
Memorial Sloan-Kettering Cancer Center
New York, NY, USA

John D. Lyons, M.D.
Postdoctoral Research Fellow
Department of Surgery
Emory University
Atlanta, GA, USA

Hemchandra Mahaseth, M.D.
Assistant Professor of Oncology
Karmanos Cancer Institute
Wayne State University
Detroit, MI,USA

Amit Mahipal, M.D.
Assistant Member, GI Oncology
Assistant Professor
Department of Internal Medicine and Interdisciplinary Oncology
Moffitt Cancer Center
Tampa, FL, USA

Shishir K. Maithel, M.D., FACS
Associate Professor of Surgery
Winship Cancer Institute, Division of Surgical Oncology
Department of Surgery, Emory University
Atlanta, GA, USA

David Marcus, M.D.
Attending
Department of Radiation Oncology
Valley View Hospital
Glenwood Springs, CO, USA

Diego R. Martin, M.D., Ph.D., F.R.C.P.C.
Chair and Cosden Endowed Professor
Department of Medical Imaging
College of Medicine
University of Arizona
Tucson, Arizona, USA

Parit Mekaroonkamol, M.D.
Gastroenterology Fellow
Emory University School of Medicine
Atlanta, GA, USA

Samdeep K. Mouli, M.D., M.S.
Fellow, Vascular and Interventional Radiology
Department of Radiology
Feinberg School of Medicine, Northwestern University
Chicago, IL, USA

Anne M. Noonan, M.B.B.Ch.B.A.O., M.Sc., M.R.C.P.I.
Assistant Professor Clinical
Department of Internal Medicine
Division of Medical Oncology
The Ohio State University
Columbus, OH, USA

Manisha Palta, M.D.
Assistant Professor
Department of Radiation Oncology
Duke University
Durham, NC, USA

Sameer H. Patel, M.D.
Resident, General Surgery
Emory University
Atlanta, GA, USA

Timothy M. Pawlik, M.D., M.P.H., Ph.D., F.A.C.S.
Professor of Surgery and Oncology
John L. Cameron M.D. Professor of Alimentary Tract Diseases
Chief, Division of Surgical Oncology
Johns Hopkins Hospital
Baltimore, MD, USA

Jean-Sébastien Pelletier, M.D.
HPB Surgery Fellow
Clinical Instructor of Surgery
University of Pittsburgh Medical Center
Pittsburgh, PA, USA

Iva Petkovska, M.D.
Assistant Professor of Medical Imaging, Department of Medical Imaging
University of Arizona
Tucson, Arizona, USA

Philip A. Philip, M.D., Ph.D.
Professor of Oncology
Karmanos Cancer Institute
Wayne State University
Detroit, MI, USA

Gopi K. Prithviraj, M.D.
Fellow
Department of Hematology and Oncology
Moffitt Cancer Center
Tampa, FL, USA

Maria C. Russell, M.D.
Assistant Professor of Surgery
Division of Surgical Oncology
Emory University
Atlanta, GA, USA

Nabil F. Saba, M.D.
Associate Professor of Oncology and Hemotology
Emory University School of Medicine
Atlanta, GA, USA

Teviah E. Sachs, M.D., M.P.H.
Assistant Professor of Surgery
Department of Surgical Oncology
Boston Medical Center
Boston, MA, USA

Riad Salem, M.D., M.B.A.
Professor of Radiology, Medicine and Surgery
Chief, Section of Vascular and Interventional Radiology
Vice-Chairman, Image-Guided Therapy
Department of Radiology
Feinberg School of Medicine, Northwestern University
Chicago, IL, USA

Virginia Oliva Shaffer, M.D., F.A.C.S.
Assistant Professor of Surgery
Colorectal Surgery
Co-Director Surgical Grand Rounds
Emory University Hospital/The Emory Clinic
Atlanta, GA, USA

Tilak U. Shah, M.D., M.H.S.
Assistant Professor of Medicine
Virginia Commonwealth University

Director of Interventional Endoscopy
Hunter Holmes Mcguire Veterans Affairs Medical Center
Richmond, Virginia, USA

Walid Shaib, M.D.
Assistant Professor, GI Oncology
Winship Cancer Institute
Emory University School of Medicine
Atlanta, GA, USA

Qing Shu, M.D.
Associate Professor
The Shenzhen Second Hosptial
Shenzhen, Guangdong, China

Xu Shu, M.D., Ph.D.
Associate Professor of Medcine
Associate Director, Department of Gastroenterology
First Affiliated Hospital of Nanchang University
Nanchang, Jiangxi, China

Liza Stapleford, M.D.
Assistant Professor
Radiation Oncology
Emory Midtown
Winship Cancer Center
Atlanta, GA, USA

Ke Tao, M.D.
Attending Doctor
Department of Endoscopy & Gastroenterology
First Hospital of Jilin University
Changchun, Jilin, China

Jordon Torok, M.D.
Resident
Department of Radiation Oncology
Duke University School of Medicine
Durham, North Carolina, USA

Christopher Willett, M.D.
Professor and Chairman
Department of Radiation Oncology
Duke University School of Medicine
Durham, North Carolina, USA

Field F. Willingham, M.D., M.P.H.
Director of Endoscopy
Assistant Professor of Medicine
Digestive Diseases
Emory University Healthcare
Atlanta, GA, USA

Kevin Woods, M.D., M.P.H.
Assistant Professor of Medicine
Director, Advanced Endoscopic Imaging, Informatics and Innovation
Digestive Diseases — Interventional Endoscopy
Emory University School of Medicine
Atlanta, GA, USA

Shuang Wu, M.D.
Attending Physician
Department of Gastroenterology & Endoscopy Center
First Hospital of Jilin University
Changchun, Jilin, China

Hong Xu, M.D., Ph.D.
Director, Professor
Department of Endoscopy & Gastroenterology
First Hospital of Jilin University
Changchun, Jilin, China

Yue Xue, M.D., Ph.D.
GI/Liver Pathology Fellow, Department of Pathology
Emory University Hospital
Atlanta, GA, USA

Gary Y. Yang, M.D.
Professor and Del E. Webb Chair
Residency Program Director
Director of Education and Development
Department of Radiation Medicine
Loma Linda University
Loma Linda, CA, USA

Zhuo Yang, M.D.
Deputy Director, Associate Professor
Department of Endoscopy,
General Hospital of Shenyang Military Command
Shenyang, Liaoning, China

Shadi S. Yarandi, M.D.
Gastroenterology Fellow
John Hopkins University School of Medicine
Baltimore, MD, USA

Fan Zhang, M.D.
Attending Doctor
First Hospital of Jilin University
Changchun, Jilin, China

Endian Zheng, M.D.
Associate Professor
Wenzhou People's Hospital
Wenzhou, Zhejiang, China

Yifeng Zhou, M.D., Ph.D.
Assistant Professor of Medicine
Digestive Department, Hangzhou First People's Hospital
Nanjing Medical University
Hangzhou, Zhejiang, China

Chapter 1

The Descriptive Epidemiology of Gastrointestinal Malignancies

Anthony Gamboa, Qi Lin, Peng Jin, Yifeng Zhou, Qiang Liu, Jinghua Hao, Qiang Cai and Roberd M. Bostick

What is New

- Esophageal adenocarcinoma and carcinoid tumor incidence rates continue to increase remarkably, while the rates for gastric cancer is declining worldwide, and that for colorectal cancer is declining in the United States.
- Liver cancer incidence continues to rise, though some predict that it will decline in the coming years as hepatitis B is addressed with vaccination and novel therapies for hepatitis C become available.
- Mortality trends for pancreatic cancer have shifted, with declining rates among African Americans and increasing rates among Caucasians, which is a reversal from a decade earlier.

Introduction

Examining the epidemiology of gastrointestinal malignancies reveals varying trends and evolving populations at risk. The most reliable data for determining incidence rates, mortality, and trends for various malignancies of the gastrointestinal system include those from large public data sets. Worldwide, the *GLOBOCAN* project of the World Health Organization (WHO) provides incidence and mortality data for many types of cancer. In the United States, the American Cancer Society annually collates data from the tumor registries of all 50 states and publishes incidence and mortality estimates for the various cancers. Finally, the National Cancer Institute's *Surveillance Epidemiology and End Results (SEER)* collects more in-depth data from selected regions of the United States; these data are readily accessed and frequently utilized by researchers who elucidate trends and updated data on cancer epidemiology. Epidemiological trends are key for investigators who address evolving threats in gastrointestinal malignancies, and awareness of these trends allows clinicians to maximize the application of current diagnostic and therapeutic tools for patient care.

The most common types of gastrointestinal cancers are colorectal, pancreatic, liver, gastric, and esophageal cancers, and many other gastrointestinal malignancies are responsible for high mortality rates as well.

Esophageal Cancer

The epidemiology of esophageal cancer continues to evolve rapidly. The incidence of adenocarcinoma of the esophagus has risen dramatically over the last four decades, and its incidence is surpassing that of squamous cell carcinoma of the esophagus in many Western countries, corresponding to increases in obesity and gastroesophageal reflux disease (GERD).

The most common histologic types of esophageal cancer are squamous cell carcinoma and adenocarcinoma. Typically, data are reported separately for the two types because their incidence rates and trends vary substantially.

Worldwide, the number of incident esophageal cancer cases was approximately 482,000 in 2008; there were 3–4 times more cases among males than among females;[1] and the age-standardized esophageal cancer incidence rate is 7.0 per 100,000 population, making esophageal cancer the sixth most common malignancy among men and the ninth most common among women worldwide. The annual number of deaths from esophageal cancer is approximately 406,000, or 5.8 per 100,000 population worldwide. It is the fifth most common cause of cancer-related deaths among men, eighth most common among women, and the sixth most common overall worldwide. Approximately 83% of individuals diagnosed with esophageal cancer and 86% of those who die from the disease are in developing countries.[2]

In the United States, the lifetime risk of an individual being diagnosed with esophageal cancer is less than 1%.[3] The American Cancer Society estimates that 18,170 new cases of esophageal cancer will be diagnosed in 2014. Among these, 14,660 are expected to be in men and 3,510 in women. There will be an estimated 15,450 deaths from esophageal cancer in 2014, 12,450 in men and 3,000 in women. Among men in the United States, esophageal cancer will be the seventh leading cause of death from cancer. Using data from SEER, during 2003–2009, at diagnosis, approximately 22% of new cases had localized disease, 30% had regional spread, 36% had distant metastasis, and the remainder did not have staging information available. During the same time, the five-year relative survival rates for esophageal cancer were 39% for those with localized cancer at diagnosis, 21% for those with regional nodal spread, and 4% for those with distant metastasis. Over the last several decades, the esophageal cancer relative survival rates have improved. During 1975–1977, the overall five-year relative survival rate in the United States was 5%; during 1987–1989 it was 9%; and during 2003–2009, 19%. There is no difference in survival between adenocarcinoma and squamous cell carcinoma in this data.[4]

There are important differences in the epidemiology of esophageal cancer by histologic type, geographic location, and race. Squamous cell carcinoma is more common worldwide than adenocarcinoma of the esophagus; however, the incidence of adenocarcinoma has surpassed that of squamous cell carcinoma in the United States, the United Kingdom, Australia, France, and some other Western European countries.[5] In the United States, the incidence of esophageal adenocarcinoma increased from 0.4 to 2.58 per 100,000 between 1975 and 2009.[6] The incidence increased 463% from 1975 to 2004 among white males and 335% among women, despite a declining rate of squamous cell carcinoma.[7] Similar trends are reported in Western Europe. These rate changes correspond to changes in rates of obesity and GERD, which can cause Barrett's esophagus. More than 90% of squamous cell carcinoma cases in the United States are attributed to alcohol and tobacco use. Declining rates of tobacco use may explain the decline in squamous cell carcinoma.[8]

The respective overall five-year relative survival rate among white and black patients in the United States diagnosed with esophageal cancer is 17% and 11%; for those with localized cancers, they are 41% and 20%; for those with regional spread, 21% and 15%; and for those with distant metastasis, 4% and 3%. The incidence of squamous cell carcinoma is higher among Blacks.[4,9]

Education has been inversely associated with esophageal cancer mortality rates. Among white males 25 to 64 years old, the mortality rate per 100,000 in 2007 was 7.92 among those with less than 12 years education compared to 2.93 among those with more than 16 years education. The mortality rates have also been increasing at a faster pace among those with less education; from 1993 to 2007, mortality annually increased 2.99% among those with less than 12 years education and 0.6% among those with more than 16 years education. In black males, mortality annually increased by 2.47% among those with less than 12 years education but *decreased* by 1.63% per year among those with more than 16 years education. These findings may be related to less or delayed access to medical care. They may also be related to different rates of smoking, alcohol consumption, and obesity between groups with different levels of education.[10]

In southern Africa, the incidence rate of esophageal cancer is more than 20 times higher than in northern, middle and western Africa. A particularly high incidence is found in the "Asian belt" or "esophageal cancer belt," which includes Turkey, northern Iran, central Asian republics, and northern and central China. The annual incidence in this region is more than 100/100,000, and of these cases, 90% are squamous cell carcinoma.[1] Risk factors contributing to these high rates are poorly understood but may include drinking beverages at high temperatures, tobacco, and chewing Betel and Areca nut.[11,12] There are wide variations in the incidence within these regions that remain unexplained. In China, the highest rates are found in the north-central provinces Shanxi and Henan. In central Asia, Turkmenistan and Kazakhstan have higher rates than their neighbors, and in within Iran, dry regions east of the Caspian Sea have a much higher incidence than the nearby humid regions to the west.[9] In Taiwan, the incidence rate of squamous cell carcinoma continues to rise while that for adenocarcinoma remains unchanged.[13]

Known risk factors for esophageal adenocarcinoma include higher body mass index, history of smoking, gastroesophageal reflux disease, and low fruit and vegetable consumption. Factors that contribute the development of esophageal squamous cell carcinoma include history of smoking, alcohol use, and low fruit and vegetable consumption.[8]

Gastric Cancer

Gastric cancer incidence continues to decline in most parts of the world, but cancers in the gastric cardia are increasing, as are noncardia gastric cancers among 25–39-year-olds in the United States.

Gastric adenocarcinoma is the most common form of cancer of the stomach, and herein it will be referred to as "gastric cancer." Gastric cancer is the fourth most common type of malignancy in the world after lung, breast, and colorectal cancer, accounting for 8% of all new cases (989,600 diagnoses) and 9.7% of all cancer-related deaths (738,000 deaths). It is the third most common cause of cancer death among men and fifth among women. The incidence is twice as high among males than females, and over 70% of cases occur in developing countries.[1,2,14]

Across the world, gastric cancer incidence varies considerably. The incidence among Korean males is 62/100,000 and among Guatemalan women 26/100,000, compared to less than 1/100,000 in Botswana. Incidence is highest in Korea, Japan, China, Brazil, much of South America, Eastern Europe, and Portugal and lowest in North America, India, and much of Africa.

In the United States, the American Cancer Society estimates that 22,220 new cases will be diagnosed in 2014, and that 13,730 will be males and 8,490 females. It is estimated that 10,990 deaths will occur in 2014, 6,720 among males and 4,270 among females. Over the last several decades in the United States, gastric cancer relative survival rates have improved. Between 1975–1977, the overall five-year relative survival rate in the United States was 15%; between 1987–1989 it was 20%, and between 2003–2009, 29%. Five-year survival rates are similar in Blacks (29%) and Whites (28%).[4] In SEER, 25% of cases are localized, 30% have regional nodal spread, 34%

have distant metastasis at diagnosis, and 11% are unstaged. The five-year relative survival is 63.2% among those with localized tumors, 28.4% among those with regional nodal spread, and 3.9% among cases with distant metastasis.[15,16]

Incidence rates among immigrants tend to be similar to those in the country to which they move rather than to those in their country of origin, especially as successive generations are born in their adopted country. Environmental factors are therefore thought to play a large role in the incidence rates. However, gastric cancer incidence among Japanese-born immigrants to the United States is three to six times higher than that among United States-born whites. Among Chinese male immigrants, the rate is the same as among United States-born white males, but among Chinese female immigrants, the rate is twice as high as among United States-born white females. These findings suggest that early environmental factors may play an important role in gastric carcinogenesis.[17]

In most parts of the world, gastric cancer incidence has decreased. In 1975, it was the leading cause of cancer worldwide.[1] The incidence rate has declined by more than 80% over the last 50 years in North America and many parts of Europe.[14] The relative risk in the United Kingdom declined throughout the 20th century.[18] More recently, rates have declined in China, Japan, Korea, and in parts of South America.[14]

The declining incidence worldwide is attributed to multiple factors. The introduction and widespread use of refrigerators may have corresponded to a decline in gastric cancer, presumably by reducing exposures to potentially harmful bacteria or fungi. Refrigerators also allow increasing amounts of fresh fruits and vegetables to be accessible to more people, and they reduce the need for highly salted or preserved foods. Other contributing factors include the identification and use of antibiotics for *Helicobacter pylori* (*H. pylori*) and the use of gastric cancer screening in Japan.[14,19]

However, gastric cancer incidence has not decreased uniformly. Declining rates are noted for cancers of the fundus, body, and distal stomach, but cancers of the cardia have not decreased. Cardia cancers, which share many histologic and epidemiologic features with esophageal adenocarcinoma,[20] are influenced by reflux disease and show less geographic variability.[21]

Proximal gastric cancers are relatively more common among young white males in the United States, while distal gastric cancers are more common in asian, black, and hispanic populations. Different risk factors are thought to relate to cardia versus noncardia gastric cancers. *H. pylori* is strongly associated with noncardia gastric cancers, but it is inversely associated with gastric cardia cancer.[22] In the United States between 1978 and 2005, the overall incidence of gastric cancer decreased by 34%, but the incidence of cardia cancers increased by 23%.[23]

Trends in incidence also vary by histologic type of gastric cancer. There are two distinct histologic patterns for gastric cancers, which differ in epidemiology and behavior. The intestinal type, which is more common, is associated with *H. pylori*, male sex, and increasing age, and is frequently noncardia. The incidence of the intestinal type decreased by 44% between 1978 and 2005 in the United States. The diffuse type, which can be seen anywhere in the stomach and occurs approximately equally in males and females, is more common in younger groups and has a worse prognosis. Its incidence in the US increased by 62% through 2000 then slightly declined through to 2005. Among cardia cancers, the diffuse type increased by 377%.[23,24]

While the overall incidence rate of gastric cancer is declining, data suggest that it may be rising again among the youngest cohorts. From 1977 to 2006, noncardia gastric cancer incidence declined in all age and race groups except Whites, ages 25–39 years. In this demographic, the incidence increased from 0.27 to 0.45 per 100,000. The importance of this finding, despite the low absolute incidence, is that it may be foreshadowing changes in incidence as this cohort ages. It also suggests the possibility of new environmental risk factors for the disease.[25]

Many risk factors, including smoking and first-degree relative with gastric cancer, have been associated with gastric cancer. Precursor lesions include adenomatous gastric polyps, chronic atrophic gastritis, dysplasia, intestinal metaplasia, and Menetrier disease.[3] More information is needed to outline risk factors associated with cardia cancers and each histologic type.

Biliary Cancers

Biliary cancers include gallbladder cancer, cholangiocarcinoma, and ampullary carcinoma. Taken together, biliary cancers comprise the sixth most common type of gastrointestinal malignancy in the United States after colorectal, pancreatic, liver, gastric, and esophageal cancers. While the different forms of biliary cancers share some risk factors, they all have distinct behaviors. Data for incidence and trends for these tumors are less clear than those for other cancers because of the different methods of classifying these tumors used in the various large databases. In some cases there is conflicting evidence regarding trends, and much about the epidemiology of these cancers remains to be clarified.[26]

Cholangiocarcinoma

Cholangiocarcinomas are subcategorized as intrahepatic and extrahepatic because of differences in their anatomy, epidemiology, behavior, and therapy. Intrahepatic lesions arise from small bile ducts or large ducts proximal to the bifurcation of the left and right hepatic ducts. Extrahepatic lesions include hilar lesions, also known as Klatskin tumors, and include those involving the bifurcation of the left and right hepatic ducts, as well as the distal bile duct, which begin where the bile duct begins to traverse the duodenum. The epidemiology of cholangiocarcinoma differs between these two categories. However, various large databases have accounted for cholangiocarcinoma differently. For example, the SEER database includes most Klatskin tumors as intrahepatic cholangiocarcinomas, despite their usual classification as extrahepatic. Frequently, extrahepatic cholangiocarcinoma is grouped with gallbladder cancer, while intrahepatic cholangiocarcinoma is grouped with primary liver cancers, including hepatocellular carcinoma.[27]

Data on cholangiocarcinomas are limited and mostly based on a decades-old series of autopsies and a few studies from Japan.[28] From these studies, cholangiocarcinomas were estimated to account for approximately 3% of all gastrointestinal malignancies, and among primary liver tumors, to be the second most common malignancy after hepatocellular carcinoma (HCC), accounting for approximately 10–20% of the total diagnoses.[29] Data on the worldwide incidence of cholangiocarcinoma are not readily available. Estimated incidence rates for intrahepatic cholangiocarcinoma have ranged from 96/100,000 in men and 38/100,000 in women in parts of Thailand to as low as 0.2/100,000 in men and

0.1/100,000 in women in Australia.[27] Males are more frequently affected than women, at a ratio of 1:1.2–1.5.[30]

In reports from the American Cancer Society, intrahepatic cholangiocarcinoma (ICC) is grouped with primary liver tumors and extrahepatic cholangiocarcinoma (ECC) is grouped with gallbladder cancer. Incidence rates for cholangiocarcinoma therefore are not well defined.

Some reports indicate that, in the United States, the incidence of ICC is increasing while that of ECC is decreasing. An analysis of SEER data revealed a 9.11% annual increase in ICC incidence and 9.44% annual increase in mortality from 1973 to 1997. In white persons, the age-adjusted mortality rate increased from 0.14 to 0.65/100,000, and in black persons 0.15 to 0.58/100,000 over the same time period.[31] From 1975 to 1999, there was a 165% increase in ICC incidence.[32] These studies were questioned because of misclassification of Klatskin tumors as ICC rather than as ECC. Correction for the misclassification yielded a more modest estimated 4% annual increase in ICC.[33] Other reports from SEER indicate that from 2000 to 2005, the trends have changed, with ICC rates down slightly and those for ECC increasing.[30] In summary, the true incidence and trends in ICC and ECC remain unclear and require further investigation.

Well-known risk factors for the development of cholangiocarcinoma include parasite infections, primary sclerosing cholangitis, choledochal cysts, gallstone disease, and toxins. Other risk factors include inflammatory bowel disease, hepatitis C or hepatitis B infection, cirrhosis, diabetes mellitus, obesity, alcohol use, and smoking.[30]

Gallbladder cancer

The incidence rate of gallbladder cancer is estimated to be 2.4/100,000 men in more developed areas, and 1.4/100,000 in less developed areas; in females, the corresponding rates are 2.1 and 2.2/100,000.[4] The overall incidence is estimated to be 2.0/100,000 worldwide.[2] The rates are generally higher in areas with a higher incidence of cholelithiasis. The overall mortality rates are greater than 90% at five years. The highest mortality rates for biliary tract cancers, which primarily consist of gallbladder cancer, have been observed in Chile, at up to 15.5/100,000.[34,35]

The incidence of gallbladder cancer differs according to various demographic, geographic, and other factors. The female to male ratio has been estimated to be 3:1. In general, the incidence is highest in India (it has been reported to be as high as 21.5 per 100,000 females in Delhi), Asia, South and Central America, and parts of Eastern Europe, and lowest in North America and Northern Europe. The strongest risk factor is a history of cholelithiasis, with an estimated relative risk of 4.9. Gallstones that are present for 20 or more years may promote epithelial dysplasia and, ultimately, adenocarcinoma by causing trauma and promoting inflammation and infection in the gallbladder. Despite the increased risk, less than 1% of people with cholelithiasis develop gallbladder cancer.[35] In Japan, gallstones were not found to be a risk factor.

Incidence rates in the United States are relatively low compared to worldwide rates and have been estimated at approximately 1.5/100,000.[36] Rates vary widely by sex and ethnicity or race. The highest rates are among American Indians/Alaska Natives at 5.4 and 3.9/100,000 in women and men, respectively. In North America, among women, incidence rates per 100,000 are 3.7 in Hispanics, 1.6 in Asians/Pacific Islanders, 1.6 in Blacks, and 1.2 in Whites; among men, the rates per 100,000 are 1.3 in Hispanics, 1.3 in Asians/Pacific Islanders, 0.9 in Blacks, and 0.7 in Whites. From 1974 to 2009, the incidence declined among Whites and remained stable among Blacks. From 1992 to 2009, the incidence declined slightly among all groups except Blacks, in whom they were stable. There is speculation that rates may be declining due to the increased availability of cholecystectomy for patients with symptomatic gallstones, despite the increase in obesity, which is a risk factor for gallbladder cancer.[26]

Ampullary tumors

Tumors of the Ampulla of Vater arise distal to the confluence of the pancreatic duct and common bile duct, proximal to the duodenum. These are relatively uncommon tumors, comprising 0.5% of all gastrointestinal cancers. Incidence rates vary from less than 0.1/100,000 in Finland to 1.2/100,000 in Colombia and 1.1/100,000 in Korea. In the United States, the incidence per 100,000 is approximately 0.3 in women and 0.4 in men.[34] There is a male predominance, with a ratio of 1.48 men for every woman.

Among periampullary tumors, which may cause biliary obstruction and include ampullary tumors, pancreatic, duodenal, and distal bile ducts tumors, ampullary tumors account for approximately 8% of the total.[37]

In the United States the incidence is higher among Whites than Blacks, with incidence rates of 0.48 and 0.40/100,000 respectively. As estimated from SEER data, from 1973 to 2005, the incidence among all races increased 0.9% annually and was increasing faster in men than in women. Most persons diagnosed with these carcinomas had well- or moderately-differentiated tumors, and had better survival rates than those with advanced histologic grade tumors. Five-year survival rates vary by the extent of the disease. Patients with localized tumors have a 45% five-year survival rate; those with regional nodal spread, 31%; and those with distant metastasis, 4%. Among those with new diagnoses, 22.7% have localized disease, 67.1% have regional nodal spread, and 10.2% have distant metastasis. The overall survival rate tends to be better for papillary carcinomas than for other adenocarcinomas of the ampulla, possibly because of their exophytic growth pattern, which may cause earlier biliary obstruction precipitating earlier detection.[38]

Various risk factors for ampullary carcinomas have been identified. Ampullary carcinoma is the second most common site of malignancy after colorectal cancer in persons with Familial Adenomatous Polyposis (FAP). The mean age of development of ampullary carcinoma in FAP patients is 45 years, compared to that in non-FAP patients who develop sporadic ampullary carcinoma, on average, in their seventh or eighth decade. There is an association between ampullary tumors and Neurofibromatosis Type I and Muir-Torre syndrome. Smoking and chronic liver fluke infection are also risk factors. Most ampullary cancers develop from adenomas, which tend to develop approximately eight years before a cancer.[37]

Liver Cancer

Liver cancers primarily include hepatocellular carcinoma (HCC) and intrahepatic cholangiocarcinoma (ICC). Many large databases, including the National Cancer Institute's SEER and the World Health Organization's GLOBOCAN, group these malignancies together for epidemiological analysis. HCC accounts for 70–85% of primary liver cancers.[1] For a specific discussion of ICC, please see the section above on cholangiocarcinoma.

The worldwide incidence of liver cancer is 10.8/100,000 population, and accounts for 5.9% of all cancer diagnoses. Among males, the incidence per 100,000 population is 8.1 in more developed areas, 18.9 in less developed areas, and 16 overall, making primary liver cancers the fifth most common cancer site among men. Among women, the rate per 100,000 population is 2.7 in more developed areas, 7.6 in less developed areas, and 6 overall, making primary liver cancers the seventh most common cancer site among women. Liver cancer is the second leading cause of cancer death worldwide. In total in 2008, there were approximately 748,300 new diagnoses and 695,900 deaths from liver cancer, 50% of which were in China. The highest rates are in East Asia, Southeast Asia, and Africa.[1,2]

In the United States, there will be an estimated 33,190 new diagnoses and 15,870 deaths from liver cancer in 2014. The male predominance is approximately 3:1 for diagnosis and 2:1 for death from liver cancer. Liver cancers are the tenth most common cancer diagnosis among men and the fifth leading cause of cancer death in the United States; in women, they are the ninth leading cause of cancer death. From 1992 to 2010, the annual increase in liver cancer diagnosis was 3.7% in men and 2.9% in women, with mortality increasing 2.3% per year in men and 1.4% per year in women. The five-year survival rate for localized cancers is 29%; for cancers with regional nodal spread, 10%; and for those with distant metastasis, 3%. A total of 22% of new diagnoses are localized, 30% have regional nodal spread, and 36% have distant metastasis. Overall five-year survival rates increased from 3% between 1975 and 1977 to 18% between 2003 and 2009. Survival among white patients from 2003 to 2009 was 17% at five years compared to 12% among black patients.[4]

Hepatocellular carcinoma

Hepatocellular carcinoma (HCC) is the most common primary malignancy of the liver. There is wide geographic and age-related variation in its incidence, which is largely related to the prevalence of the hepatitis B and C viruses. These viruses are strong risk factors for developing HCC.

In addition, incidence rates have been evolving as African and Asian populations migrate to North America and Europe. There is also variation across ethnic groups within a country. The broad epidemiological trends discussed above in regards to all primary liver cancers can be extrapolated to HCC, since HCC is the most common liver cancer in most countries.[39]

HCC incidence rates are highest in Asia and sub-Saharan Africa, where more than 80% of all HCC cases occur. The incidence rate in parts of China is higher than 30/100,000, though recent decreases in incidence have been reported in China.[40] In much of sub-Saharan Africa, where it is thought that HCC is under-diagnosed and reported, the published rates exceed 16/100,000. These rates reflect the high incidence of hepatitis B in these areas. In northern Europe and North America, incidence rates are less than 5/100,000. In southern Europe, where hepatitis C is more common than in northern Europe, rates are around 12/100,000. [41] While HCC incidence tends to increase with age, the mean age at diagnosis in Africa and East Asia, excluding Japan, is lower than in Western countries, presumably because of the high rates of hepatitis B vertical transmission in these areas. The mean age of diagnosis in China is approximately 55–59 years, and in Europe and North America, 63–65 years.

In Japan, the rates per 100,000 in 2003 were 24 in men and 7.3 in women, and have declined steadily since the mid-1990s. The declining rates in Japan may be related to a decreasing prevalence of hepatitis C among younger generations. The highest incidence of hepatitis C may have been related to blood transfusions in the mid-20th century and to intravenous amphetamine use during and after World War II. There were stiffer penalties in place for amphetamine use starting in 1954, and there was a change from paid to voluntary blood donations in late 1960s. These changes may have led to the declining rates of hepatitis C infection and, therefore, HCC seen in Japan.

In the United States, as estimated from SEER data, the incidence rates per 100,000 are approximately 7.9 in men and 2.3 in women; between 1975 and 2005 the overall age-adjusted incidence increased 4.9% annually, tripling from 1.6 to 4.9/100,000. The incidence increased in all birth cohorts between 1900 and 1959. Examining racial trends between 1992 and 2005 reveals that Asians/Pacific Islanders have the highest incidence of HCC. However, the incidence of HCC in this group increased only

1.0% annually, but increased faster in all other racial groups. The annual change was 5.0% in American Indians/Alaska Natives, 4.9% in Blacks, 4.6% in Whites, and 4.0% in Hispanics. The rates per 100,000 population were still highest among Asians/Pacific Islanders at 11.7, followed by Hispanics at 8.0, Blacks at 7.0, American Indians/Alaska Natives at 6.6, and Whites at 3.9. A total of 80% of the Asians/Pacific Islanders with HCC were born outside of the United States, as were 40% of Hispanics, 17% of Whites, 6% of Blacks, and 3% of American Indian/Native Alaskans.[42]

More recent incidence data from 2000 to 2005 revealed dramatic increases among black, white, and Hispanic men aged 50 to 59 years. In fact, Blacks aged 50 to 59 years had a higher overall incidence from 2003 to 2005 than did Asians/Pacific Islanders. The reasons for this shift in HCC incidence patterns among races is thought to relate to the high prevalence of hepatitis C among Blacks. Many of these individuals acquired hepatitis C in the 1960s, which led to increases in HCC incidence. Conversely, many Asians/Pacific Islanders with HCC were born outside of the United States in regions with a high hepatitis B prevalence. Asians/Pacific Islanders may not have been as affected by the hepatitis C epidemic as were other racial groups, as indicated by their relatively slower increase in HCC incidence among the 50 to 59 years age cohort. Hispanics born inside the United States tend to have higher incidence rates of HCC than do Hispanics born outside the United States, indicating that hepatitis B is less likely the principal risk factor in this group, and more likely that hepatitis C and other risk factors for cirrhosis in the United States, including hepatitis C, alcohol, and non-alcoholic fatty liver disease, may be contributing to HCC risk.[42]

The overall age-adjusted mortality rates from HCC are increasing 1.6% per year as incidence rates continue to rise. However, the cause-specific one-year survival rates in patients with HCC have almost doubled in the United States, from 25% in the early 1990s to 47% in the mid-2000s. Increased survival has been documented across all racial groups except American Indians/Alaska Natives, who had an annual 0.6% decrease in one-year survival. Five-year survival increased between 1992 and 1999 from 8% to 13%. These increased survival rates are correlated with diagnosing HCC at earlier stages. Between 1992 and 1993, at diagnosis, 28% of HCC cases had localized disease, 22% had regional spread, and 22% had distant metastasis; and between 2003 and 2004, 44% had localized disease, 29%

had regional spread, and 17% had distant metastasis. This trend may be related to increased screening efforts with imaging and alpha-fetoprotein levels. Increased survival may also be related to the more widespread utilization of surgery or liver transplant and to advances in medical and radiologic therapies for HCC. The cause-specific survival rates for patients with localized disease who received surgery were 91% at one-year.[42]

Certain populations are at increased risk for HCC, and identification of these groups is relevant because it allows for targeted screening and earlier identification of HCC. Patients with compensated cirrhosis have a HCC incidence rate of approximately 3% per year.[43] HCC incidence is highest in patients with decompensated cirrhosis and those with hepatitis C cirrhosis.[40] While the male-to-female ratio of HCC is around 3.7:1, the rates in men and women are almost equal in Western countries among those who do not have cirrhosis.[9] An increased survival rate has been found in cirrhotic patients who have HCC diagnosed during screening.[44]

Hepatitis B, hepatitis C, non-alcoholic fatty liver disease, alcohol, and smoking are considered risk factors for HCC.[45,46] Viral hepatitis, either hepatitis B or C, causes approximately 80% of HCC cases worldwide. Hepatitis B virus (HBV) is the leading cause of HCC worldwide, accounting for approximately half of all cases, and almost all cases in children.[40] While HBV can lead to HCC in the absence of cirrhosis, approximately 85% of patients with HBV and HCC also have cirrhosis.[47] Hepatitis B is transmitted by sexual contact, blood products, or vertically from mother to child. The risk for HCC among patients with HBV relative to those without is 10- to 100-fold higher. HBV accounts for a large proportion of HCC cases worldwide, including up to two-thirds in East Asia and Africa and one-fifth in Western countries. In patients with HBV, a family history of HCC confers a higher risk for HCC.[48] Having a positive HBV surface antigen or e-antigen confers a higher risk for HCC. In Asia, the incidence of HCC per 100 person-years in inactive carriers of HBV is 0.2-100 person-years, 0.6 in patients with chronic infection but no cirrhosis, and 3.7 in those with compensated cirrhosis.[40] In addition, a strong correlation was found between HBV serum viral load and HCC risk.[49]

Patients infected with the hepatitis C virus (HCV) are also at higher risk for HCC. In the United States, hepatitis C may account for 21% of

HCC cases, and the incidence appears to be increasing.[50] In Taiwan, the lifetime incidence of HCC in patients with a positive hepatitis C serum antibody is 17% in women and 24% in men. In patients with both HBV surface antigen and HCV serum antibody, the HCC incidence rates are 27% and 39% for women and men, respectively. Risk increases with increasing HBV or HCV viral load.[51] Typically, annual HCC incidence rates in patients with HCV cirrhosis range from 1–3%. Not all studies have shown reduced risk of HCC in patients treated with interferon regimens,[52] but patients who have sustained virologic responses seem to have low rates of HCC, especially if there is no prior evidence of cirrhosis.[53] This finding may be relevant going forward as more effective treatments for HCV become widespread. Rates of HCC will likely begin to decline with widespread use of the HBV vaccine, and as the age cohorts affected by the hepatitis C epidemic become a smaller proportion of the population.

Education level has been associated with trends in liver cancer mortality. In the United States, among Whites with less than 12 years of education, liver cancer mortality is increasing 6.49% annually, compared to only 0.41% annually among those with more than 16 years of education. Among Black men, the annual increase in incidence among those with less than 12 years of education is 5.19%, compared to an annual 0.47% decrease among those with more than 16 years of education. These trends have been attributed to higher levels of alcohol use, obesity, and HBV and HCV among those who are less educated.[10] Coffee drinking has been associated with not only lower levels of inflammation and fibrosis, but with a lower risk for developing HCC.[40]

Pancreatic Cancer

Most (95%) pancreatic cancers are ductal adenocarcinomas. The overall annual incidence of pancreatic cancer is 3.9/100,000 worldwide; among men and women the incidence is 4.4 and 3.3/100,000, respectively. Pancreatic cancer accounts for 2.2% of all cancer diagnoses and for approximately 266,000 deaths annually, accounting for 3.5% of all cancer-related mortality worldwide. The cumulative risk of developing pancreatic cancer until age 74 is 0.5% in men and 0.3% in women.[2]

In more developed areas, the incidence per 100,000 population is 8.2 in men and 5.4 in women; in less developed areas, it is 2.7 in men and 2.1 in women.[1] In the United States, the incidence rate exceeds that found in many other developed parts of the world. During 2005–2009, the age-adjusted incidence in the United States was 13.6 and 10.5/100,000 in men and women, respectively.[54] The American Cancer Society estimates that there will be 46,420 new cases of pancreatic cancer and 39,590 deaths from the disease in 2014. Of the new cases, 23,530 will be males and 22,890 females. Despite being only the tenth leading incident cancer among men and ninth among women, because of its poor prognosis, pancreatic cancer is the fourth leading cause of cancer-related deaths among both males and females in the United States, accounting for approximately 7% of all cancer related deaths. The lifetime risk of developing pancreatic cancer is 1.48% in men and 1.45% in women in the United States.[4]

The five-year survival for pancreatic cancer varies by stage. For those with localized disease, the five-year survival is 24%; for those with regional spread it is 9%, and for those with distant metastasis, 2%. At diagnosis, only 9% of cases have localized disease, while 27% have regional spread and 58% have distant metastasis. Five-year overall survival has improved modestly but statistically significantly between 1975–1977 and 2003–2009, from 2% to 6%.[4]

The incidence of pancreatic cancer increases with age. Between 2005 and 2009, among 35–39 year-olds, the incidence per 100,000 in men was 1.2 and in women, 1.0. Among persons older than 85 years, the incidence per 100,000 in men was 100.5 and in women, 87.7. The median age at diagnosis was 71 years.[54]

Incidence and mortality rates also vary by race. During 2005 to 2009, the highest rates were in Blacks, with incidence and mortality rates of 15.2 and 13.8/100,000, respectively. The incidence and mortality rates per 100,000 among other groups were as follows: in Whites, the incidence was 11.7 and the mortality was 10.9; in Hispanics, they were 10.6 and 8.3; in American Indians/Alaska Natives, 9.9 and 8.8; and in Asians/Pacific Islanders, 8.8 and 7.5. Higher rates in African Americans have been associated with long-term diabetes, smoking, and family history of pancreatic cancer in men, and moderate-to-heavy alcohol consumption (more than seven drinks per week) and an elevated body mass index in women. In the absence of these risk factors, it has been postulated that there would be no Black-White disparity.[55]

While overall mortality rates from pancreatic cancer increased slightly during the 2000s, the trends were different for Whites and Blacks. From the early 1970s to the mid-1990s, mortality rates decreased in Whites but increased in Blacks. From the mid-1990s to 2009, those trends reversed, with mortality rates increasing in Whites and decreasing in Blacks. The reasons for the trends are unknown and not readily explained by any known risk factors.[56] From 2000 to 2009, there was a 0.5% annual increase in mortality in white men and women; in Asian/Pacific Islander men, there was an increase of 1.0% per year, while among other race groups, there was no change in mortality. The incidence of pancreatic cancer increased 0.7% annually in men and 1.1% in women.[54,57]

Education level has been associated with recent trends in pancreatic cancer, and increases in mortality rates have been limited to those with less education, while rates among persons with more than 16 years of education have not increased since the 1990s. An analysis of SEER data from 1993 to 2007 revealed that among white men aged 25 to 64 years, there was an average increase in mortality from pancreatic cancer of 1.43% per year, compared to a decrease of 0.4% among those with more than 16 years of education. Among white women, those with less than 12 years of education had a 1.57% increase in mortality from pancreatic cancer per year, compared to an annual decrease of 0.69% among those with more than 16 years of education. These trends may be related to differences in obesity, smoking and other risk factors.[10]

Certain groups of patients are at higher risk of developing pancreatic cancer, including those with chronic pancreatitis. A large, multinational study involving five countries in Europe plus the United States found a standardized incidence ratio of developing pancreatic cancer (ratio of observed to expected cases) of 26.3 in patients with chronic pancreatitis. In patients who were followed for 10 years, the cumulative risk of pancreatic cancer was 1.8%, and in those followed for 20 years, 4.0%. The increased risk was found in both men and women, patients with non-alcoholic and alcoholic pancreatitis, and in all six countries in the study.[58] However, the population attributable fraction from chronic pancreatitis was estimated at a modest 1.34%, suggesting that curtailing chronic pancreatitis prevalence would do little to reduce the overall incidence of pancreatic cancer.[59]

Heredity appears to play a role in the risk of developing pancreatic cancer. Patients with autosomal dominant hereditary pancreatitis, which is associated with mutations in the *HRSS1* gene, are at up to an 87-fold higher risk for pancreatic cancer. A French study found cumulative risks of pancreatic cancer in these patients at ages 50 and 75 years of 11% and 49% in men and 8% and 55% in women, respectively.

Between 4 and 16% of patients with pancreatic cancer have a family member who was also afflicted with this disease.[60] There is higher risk among relatives of an individual with pancreatic cancer, whether the pancreatic cancer case was considered sporadic or familial. Pancreatic cancer patients with a family history of the disease tend to develop the cancer at a younger age. Persons with a family history of pancreatic cancer have, on average, twice the risk of developing pancreatic cancer as those without a family history; in those with a first-degree relative with the disease, the risk is 7–9 times higher.[54] There also appears to be an increased age-related risk in having a family member who was diagnosed before age 50 in cases of familial pancreatic cancer, but not in sporadic pancreatic cancer.[61]

Specific gene mutations have been recognized as conferring higher risk for pancreatic cancer. Overall, these mutations are rare and account for 5 to 10% of pancreatic cancer cases. *BRCA2* mutations are thought to account for 6 to 19% of familial pancreatic cancer cases. It has been suggested that *BRCA2* should be included in genetic testing of patients with more than one first-degree relative with pancreatic cancer. Having the *BRCA2* mutation is associated with a 3- to 10-fold increase in pancreatic cancer risk.[54,62,63] Patients with the Familial Atypical Multiple Mole-Melanoma syndrome are at a higher risk of pancreatic cancer. This syndrome is associated with the *CDKN2A* gene, also called the *multiple tumor suppressor-1* gene. These patients have a 13- to 22-fold higher pancreatic cancer risk.[54] Patients with Peutz-Jeghers syndrome have up to a 132-fold relative risk of developing cancer and a cumulative risk of 36% of developing pancreatic cancer by the age of 64 years.[64] Patients with hereditary nonpolyposis colorectal cancer (Lynch syndrome) have a cumulative risk of 3.68% of developing pancreatic cancer by the age of

70 years and an 8.6-fold higher risk relative to those without Lynch syndrome. Patients with familial adenomatous polyposis may also be at higher risk for pancreatic cancer, although this is not as well-defined.[65]

Colorectal Cancer

Most colorectal cancers are adenocarcinomas. There were an estimated 1,233,000 new cases of colorectal cancer in 2008 worldwide, accounting for 9.7% of all cancer diagnoses. It is the third most common cancer in men and second in women. In 2008 the incidence per 100,000 population was 17.3 overall, 20.4 in men, and 14.6 in women. The cumulative risk of developing colorectal cancer to age 74 years is 2.0% overall, 2.3% in men, and 1.6% in women.[2]

In 2008, there were approximately 608,000 deaths worldwide related to colorectal cancer, accounting for 8.0% of all cancer-related deaths. The mortality per 100,000 population in 2008 was 8.2 overall, 9.7 in men, and 7.0 in women. The cumulative risk of dying from colorectal cancer to age 74 years is 0.9% overall, 1.1% in men, and 0.7% in women.[2]

Colorectal cancer is more common in developed countries: in more developed areas of the world, the incidence per 100,000 is 37.6 in men and 24.2 in women, and in less developed areas, it is 12.1 in men and 9.4 in women. The cumulative risk to age 74 years of developing colorectal cancer in developed areas is 4.4% in men and 2.7% in women, and in less developed areas, 1.4% in men and 1.1% in women. The highest incidence rates are in Australia, New Zealand, Europe and North America, and in Africa, South-central Asia, and Central America.[1] There is less variation in rectal cancer across different regions of the world. Most of the differences in colorectal cancer incidence are due to colon cancer, excluding rectal cancers. Higher ratios of colon-to-rectal cancer are seen in areas with higher incidence rates of colorectal cancer, such as in the United States.[9]

Incidence trends vary as well. Rates have declined in the United States, while in Eastern Europe, Spain, Italy, and parts of the United Kingdom, as well as China, Japan, India, rates increased from the early 1990s to the early 2000s. These differences are thought to be related to economic development and "Westernization" in Asia and parts of Europe, which have led to changes in diet and, possibly, smoking and physical activity.

Colorectal cancer screening in countries such as the United States, Canada, and New Zealand may also contribute to these differences, since screening practices can reduce colorectal cancer incidence rates by removing precancerous polyps.[66]

Colorectal cancer claims many more lives in developed countries than in less developed countries: the mortality per 100,000 population in more developed areas is 15.1 in men and 9.7 in women, and in less developed areas, it is 6.9 in men and 5.4 in women. The cumulative risk to age 74 years of dying from colorectal cancer in developed areas in 1.7% in men and 1.0% in women, and in less developed areas, 0.8% in men and 0.6% in women.[1]

In the United States, colorectal cancer is the second most common type of cancer overall, third among women and third among men.[59] The American Cancer Society estimates there will be 96,830 new cases of colon cancer and 40,000 of rectal cancer diagnosed in 2014. Almost equal numbers of incident colon cancer cases are predicted for men and women, but for rectal cancers, 23,380 are predicted in men and 16,620 in women. Colorectal cancer will account for 8% of the total cancer diagnoses in men and women. There will be an estimated 50,310 deaths from colorectal cancer in 2014, 26,270 in men and 24,040 in women, accounting for 8% of total cancer related deaths in men and 9% in women. Among men ages 40–59 and 60–79, colorectal cancer is the second most common type of cancer in the United States after lung cancer.[4]

Geographically, there is some variation within the United States. In general, the highest incidence is seen in southeastern states. The highest incidence of colorectal cancer is in Kentucky, where the incidence per 100,000 population is 63.9 in men and 46.0 in women, and the lowest is in Utah, where it is 39.4 in men and 31.2 in women. Among men, the mortality rate per 100,000 population is highest in Mississippi at 24.8 and lowest in Utah at 14.3. Among women, the highest mortality is in the District of Columbia at 18.9/100,000, and the lowest is in Utah at 10.7/100,000.[4]

The cumulative lifetime risk of developing colorectal cancer in the United States is 1 in 20 in men and 1 in 22 in women. The cumulative risk prior to age 50 years, when screening for cancer and precancerous polyps typically begins in average risk individuals, is 1 in 305 in men and 1 in 334 in women.[4]

There are racial disparities in the incidence and mortality of colorectal cancer within the United States. The highest incidence and mortality rates are among African Americans and the lowest is among Asian Americans. Per 100,000 population, the respective incidence rates for male and female Whites are 50.9 and 38.6; for Blacks, 62.5 and 46.7; for Asians/Pacific Islanders, 40.8 and 31.0; for American Indians/Alaska Natives, 51.7 and 42.7; and for Hispanics, 47.3 and 32.6. Mortality rates also reflect these disparities. Per 100,000, the respective mortality rates for male and female Whites are 19.2 and 13.6; for Blacks, 28.7 and 19.0; for Asians/Pacific Islanders, 13.1 and 9.7; for American Indians/Alaska Natives, 18.7 and 15.4; and for Hispanics, 16.1 and 10.2. Some of the racial disparities are thought to be related to access to colonoscopy for screening.[4]

Colorectal cancer survival rates in the United States vary widely by the stage at diagnosis. The five-year survival rate is 90% for those diagnosed with localized cancers, 70% for those with regional nodal spread, and 13% for those with distant metastasis. Fortunately, a minority of cases of colorectal cancer has distant metastasis at diagnosis. From 2003 to 2009, 40% of cases had localized disease, 38% had regional nodal spread, and 23% had distant metastasis at diagnosis. Overall, there has been an increase in five-year survival since the 1970s. In SEER data from 1975 to 1977, the five-year survival rate was 51%; from 1987 to 1989, it was 60%; and from 2003 to 2009, 65%. The most recent five-year survival rates were 67% in Caucasians and 56% in African Americans.[4]

In the United States, colorectal cancer incidence rates increased from the 1950s to the 1980s but have been declining over the last several decades. Between 2001 and 2010, the incidence decreased annually by an average of 3.0% in men and 2.6% in women, between 2006 and 2010, it decreased by an average of 3.6% in men and 3.3% women, and from 2008 to 2010, 4.7% in both men and women.[57]

Although colorectal cancer incidence is decreasing among all races and ethnicities, there are racial disparities in this trend. From 2001 to 2010, among White men the average decline in incidence was 4.0% per year; among Black men, 2.0%; among Asians/Pacific Islander men, 2.0%; among American Indian/Alaska Native men, 1.4%; and among Hispanic men, 2.9%. Trends in women were similar, although the disparity between Whites and Blacks was not as pronounced. The average annual decrease in incidence among women was 3.3% in Whites, 2.9% in Blacks, 2.2% in Asians/Pacific Islanders, 1.3% in American Indians/Alaska Natives, and 2.8% in Hispanics.[57]

Colorectal cancer mortality rates have also continued to decline. In men, from 1990 to 2002, the mortality rate declined by an average of 2.0% per year. From 2001 to 2010, the mortality rate declined even more rapidly at an average of 2.9% per year. Between 1984 and 2001, mortality rates in women declined by an average of 1.8% per year, and from 2001 to 2010, 2.9% per year. Mortality rates have declined in all races and ethnicities except among American Indian/Alaska Native women, in whom the mortality rates increased by an average of 0.4% per year from 2001 to 2010.[57] Declines in mortality and incidence have been attributed in part to colorectal cancer screening efforts, leading to both earlier diagnosis of cancers and removal of precancerous polyps. Polypectomy has been shown to reduce the development of colon cancer. Advances in treatment have also led to increases in mortality.[67]

Education and socioeconomic status are inversely associated with colorectal cancer incidence in the United States. In a large prospective cohort study of over 500,000 persons from various parts of the country, there was a significantly higher proportion of cancers of the right colon among study participants with postgraduate education than in those with less than 12 years of education. This relatively higher rate of cancers of the proximal colon was also seen in persons who live in neighborhoods in the top quintile of socioeconomic status relative to those in the bottom quintile. This study also found a 42% higher risk of colorectal cancer in those with less than 12 years of education compared to those with postgraduate education. Those in the bottom quintile in socioeconomic status had a 31% higher risk of colorectal cancer compared to those in the top quintile.[68] Much of the higher risk among people with less education and lower socioeconomic status was estimated to be related to lifestyle factors. Eating a poor diet, which was defined as a diet least similar to a Mediterranean diet, was associated with a 91% higher risk of colorectal cancer. Physical inactivity, compared to daily activity, was associated with a 44% higher risk. Body mass index (BMI) of 34 kg/m^2 relative to less than 20 kg/m^2 was associated with a 55% higher risk. Together, diet, physical activity level, smoking status, and BMI accounted for 43.9% of the estimated higher incidence of colorectal cancer in those with less education and 36.2% of the disparity based on socioeconomic status. Right-sided cancers were more frequently related to these lifestyle factors than were left-sided and rectal cancers. Some of the socioeconomic differences in incidence may also be related to access to colorectal cancer screening.[69,70]

There has been a relative increase in the number of right-sided colorectal cancers compared to the numbers of left colon and rectal cancers over the second half of the 20th century, both in the United States and internationally.[71,72] However, an analysis of SEER data from 1992 to 2008 revealed a slight increase in right-sided colon cancer rates in men until 1999, and then a decline in the incidence by an average of 2.6% per year. In women, the incidence of right-sided cancers was increasing slightly until 2000, and since then, it has annually decreased by an average of 2.3%. For late-stage right-sided tumors, the incidence rates from 2000–2008 annually declined 3.9% in men and 3.3% in women. Over this time period left-sided tumors also annually declined, 3.5% in men and 2.9% in women.[73]

There is some thought that this reversal in the trend of right-sided tumor incidence may be related to colonoscopy utilization. Colonoscopy use increased very gradually through the 1990s, and by 2000 the utilization rate was 20%. By 2008, largely due to Medicare coverage for screening colonoscopy, the utilization rate was 48%.[73]

Right-sided tumors are more common in women than in men; in an analysis of SEER data, they accounted for 47% of colorectal tumors in women and for 37% in men.[73]

Small Bowel Tumors

Most tumors of the small intestine are adenocarcinomas, carcinoids, lymphomas, and sarcomas, the latter of which are typically gastrointestinal stromal tumors (GISTs). In contrast to that for colon cancer, the incidence of small bowel cancer may be increasing. Despite accounting for 75% of the length of the gastrointestinal tract, small bowel tumors account for only 5% of gastrointestinal tract tumors.[74]

Worldwide incidence rates vary by region and are most common in the United States and Western Europe and least common in Asia. The incidence per 100,000 is typically reported to be near 2 in North America, where the highest incidence rates are seen, and less than 1 in China and India. Small bowel cancers tend to be more common in areas where colon cancer incidence is higher, but there is no correlation between small bowel and stomach cancer rates. In France, small bowel cancer incidence per 100,000 was estimated to be 1.2 in men and 0.8 in women.[74,75]

In the United States, the American Cancer estimates there will be 9,160 new cases of small intestinal cancer in 2014, with 4,880 in men and 4,280 in women. The estimated number of deaths from small bowel cancers in 2014 is 1,210, 640 of which are in men and 570 in women.[4] The SEER program of the National Cancer Institute estimates that there were 2.1 cases per 100,000 individuals in the US in 2013, and 0.4 deaths from small bowel cancer per 100,000 individuals from 2006–2010. The incidence per 100,000 population is 2.5 in men and 1.7 in women. The estimated cumulative lifetime risk of developing small bowel cancer in the United States is 0.2%. Small bowel tumors are the 24th most common cancer in the United States, accounting for 0.5% of all cancers and 0.2% of all cancer related deaths. The median age at diagnosis is 66 years. The overall five-year survival rate with malignancies of the small intestine was 64.5% from 2003–2009.[15]

Incidence varies by race in the United States, with the highest rates in African Americans and the lowest in Asians/Pacific Islanders, Hispanics, and American Indians/Alaska Natives. From 2006 to 2010, the incidence per 100,000 among African Americans was 3.9 in men and 2.8 in women, compared to 2.5 and 1.7 among male and female Whites, respectively. Rates among other populations were lower. Among men, the rates per 100,000 population were 1.6 in American Indians/Alaska Natives, 1.5 in Hispanics, and 1.2 in Asians/Pacific Islanders. Among women, the incidence per 100,000 was not reported for American Indians/Pacific Islanders because there were so few cases. In Hispanic women, the rate was 1.4, and in Asian/Pacific Islander women, it was 0.9 per 100,000.[15] The higher incidence among African Americans reflects higher rates of carcinomas and carcinoids, while Caucasians have a higher rate of small bowel lymphomas than do African Americans. The incidence of sarcomas is approximately the same in the two racial groups. The incidence differences are likely related to both environmental and genetic factors.[74]

The incidence of small bowel cancer is increasing in the United States. According to one estimate, in 1975 the incidence per 100,000 population was 1.1, whereas in 2010 it was 2.4. On average, the incidence rate has increased by 2.4% per year over the last ten years. Most of the increase has been in carcinomas, carcinoids, and lymphomas, whereas the increases in sarcomas have been more modest. The fastest rate of increases has been among African American men. Despite the increasing incidence, the number of deaths from small bowel cancer declined by 1.0% per year over the same time period. The five-year relative survival for those diagnosed with small bowel cancer increased from 32.8% in 1975 to 66.2% in 2005.[15] Other analyses have indicated that while small bowel carcinoids may have increased four-fold over the last several decades, increases in rates of other small bowel tumors were less pronounced.[76]

Survival with small bowel cancer varies by stage. The five-year relative survival of those with localized cases is 81.2% compared to 69.5% of those with regional nodal spread and 42.1% in those with distant metastasis. There are relatively similar numbers of localized, regional and distant cancers diagnosed. SEER estimates that 31% of cases have localized cancers, 36% have regional nodal spread, and 27% have distant metastasis, with the remainder being unstaged.[15]

The incidence of subtypes of small bowel tumors per 100,000 population were 0.59 for carcinomas, 0.55 for carcinoids, 0.3 for lymphomas, and 0.17 for sarcomas.[74]

Adenocarcinomas, carcinoids, lymphomas, and sarcomas each have a proclivity to certain parts of the small bowel. In general, adenocarcinomas occur most frequently in the duodenum and become less common moving distally through the small bowel. The opposite pattern is seen for carcinoids and lymphomas, which are much more common in the ileum than in the jejunum or duodenum.[76] A Canadian study reported that 54.7% of small bowel adenocarcinomas occurred in the duodenum, 29.9% in the jejunum, and 18% in the ileum; 3.9% of small bowel carcinoids occurred in the duodenum, 9.2% in the jejunum, and 86.7% in the ileum; 49.5% of lymphomas were in the ileum, 29.4% in the jejunum, and 21% in the ileum; and the highest frequency (46.7%) of small bowel sarcomas occurred in the jejunum.[77] In the United States, an analysis of SEER data revealed similar findings: 49% of carcinomas were found in the duodenum; 52% of carcinoids were in the ileum; lymphoma incidence increased moving distally, with approximately three times as many cases in the ileum than in the duodenum; and the incidence of sarcomas was similar throughout the small bowel.

Patients with small bowel cancer are at higher risk for cancers of the colon, rectum, pancreas, ampulla, and genitourinary system. This risk is most marked among patients with carcinoma of the small bowel, which is associated with an additional 68% higher risk for a second primary malignancy. Patients with Familial Adenomatous Polyposis, Hereditary Nonpolyposis Colorectal Cancer, and Peutz-Jeghers syndrome are at higher risk for both small and large bowel cancers. In general, patients with colon cancer are also at higher risk of small bowel cancer. It is speculated that this overlap in risk may be related to common genetic factors, including those related to DNA mismatch repair deficiencies, and environmental factors including diet.[78]

Gastrointestinal Lymphomas

The gastrointestinal (GI) tract is the most common extranodal site for Non-Hodgkin's lymphoma (NHL), while Hodgkin's lymphoma (HL) is extremely rare in the gastrointestinal tract. The GI tract is a common secondary location for lymphoma. From GLOBOCAN data, it was estimated that there were 355,000 new cases of NHL worldwide in 2008 with an incidence of 5.1/100,000. The American Cancer Society estimates that in the US, there will be 70,800 cases of NHL in 2014.[2,4]

Typically, lymphomas of the GI tract arise from the mucosa-associated lymphoid tissue of the GI tract (MALT) and are referred to as MALT lymphomas. Most are B-cell lymphomas, and most of these arise from the marginal zone B cells and therefore are classified as extranodal marginal zone B-cell lymphomas. T-cell lymphomas are rare but are seen in patients with celiac disease. Most GI lymphomas in developed countries arise from the stomach, whereas in the Middle East the small intestine is the predominant site.[9]

A population-based study from a cancer registry in France revealed an age-standardized incidence rate of GI lymphomas per 100,000 population of 0.94 in men and 0.54 in women (a 1.74 male:female incidence ratio). The mean age of diagnosis was 63 years. Gastrointestinal lymphomas accounted for 15.7% of all NHL diagnoses and 59% of extranodal NHL cases. Lymphomas accounted for 1.7% of all digestive tract malignancies overall, and for 6.5% of those in patients younger than 45 years.[79]

In the same study, the stomach was the most common site for gastrointestinal lymphomas, accounting for 54% of all cases, followed by the small bowel (17%), colon (15%), rectum (12%), and mesentery (3%). Many studies, however, estimate the incidence of gastric lymphomas to be relatively higher and the incidence of colon lymphomas to be relatively lower, closer to 3% of GI lymphomas.[83,84] Lymphomas accounted for 3.7% of all gastric, 18.8% of small bowel, 0.6% of colon, 0.7% of rectal, and 9.5% of mesenteric or peritoneal malignancies. Approximately half of the cases were low-grade and half were high-grade lymphomas. Overall five-year survival was 34%, and was higher for gastric and rectal lymphomas than for small bowel and colon lymphomas.[79]

Studies from Germany and Greece found relatively similar epidemiologic patterns. Approximately 16% of NHL cases were gastrointestinal. In these studies, 68 to 75% of gastrointestinal lymphomas occurred in the stomach. Up to 20% involved multiple sites in the gastrointestinal tract. Most cases, up to 90%, were stage I or II. Small intestinal lymphoma cases and cases with multiple gastrointestinal sites had the poorest survival rates.[80,81]

Gastric lymphoma is the most common primary GI lymphoma in developed countries. There is a strong direct association between *H. pylori* prevalence and gastric lymphoma incidence.[82] The incidence of GI lymphoma in *H. pylori* infected individuals ranges from 1/30,000 to 1/80,000. Some evidence suggests that *H. pylori* may be associated with higher risk for small bowel lymphomas.[83]

Other than those with *H. pylori*, populations potentially at risk for GI lymphomas include patients with celiac or inflammatory bowel disease (IBD), although the data are not entirely consistent. Although initial studies suggested that there may be higher risk for GI lymphomas among patients with IBD, most subsequent large population studies suggested that they may not be at higher risk. The initial findings may have been due to referral bias.[84,85]

Gastrointestinal Stromal Tumors (GISTs)

Gastrointestinal Stromal Tumors (GISTs) arise from submucosal tissue in the GI tract. The incidence of GISTs has been poorly elucidated because these tumors were not well-defined molecularly until around 2000, so the incidence rates derived from large data sets prior to 2000 are problematic. One study that used SEER data from 1992 to 2000 indicated that the incidence per 100,000 population was 0.74 overall, 0.86 in men, 0.66 in women, 1.24 in Blacks, and 0.64 in Whites. At diagnosis, 53% of cases had localized disease, 19% had regional nodal spread, and 23% had distant metastasis. The five-year survival rates were 64% for patients with localized tumors and 13% for those with distant metastasis.[86]

Other, newer studies with more reliable data on GISTs estimated higher incidences for the tumors. The incidence in Sweden was estimated to be 1.45/100,000 from 1983 to 2000,[87] in Iceland it was estimated to be 1.1/100,000,[88] and in Taiwan, 1.37/100,000.[89] The incidence of small GISTs in autopsy studies and analyses of whole stomachs was over 22%, primarily in the proximal stomach. The clinical significance of this is unknown.[90] The mean age at diagnosis for GISTs is around 60–65 years, and only 1% of cases are in persons less than 21 years of age.[91]

GISTs may be seen throughout the GI tract. Most, typically 60–70%, are found in the stomach, followed by 20–30% in the small intestine, 5% in the colon and rectum, and less than 5% in the esophagus.[92] From SEER data, the most common site for a GIST was found to be the stomach (51% of cases), followed by the small intestine (36%), the colon (7%), the rectum (5%), and the esophagus (1%).[86]

Neuroendocrine Tumors

Neuroendocrine tumors, which arise from cells of the neuroendocrine system, include those of the gastrointestinal tract, or carcinoid tumors, and the pancreas.

Gastrointestinal tract neuroendocrine tumors (carcinoid tumors)

Carcinoid tumors may arise anywhere within the gastrointestinal (GI) tract. They were originally termed carcinoid because they were noted to behave differently from gastrointestinal tract adenocarcinomas. It is thought that the incidence of these tumors may be increasing.[93]

A recent analysis of SEER data on GI carcinoid tumors found the average incidence of GI carcinoid in the United States from 2000 to 2009 to be 2.6/100,000, with the highest incidence among Blacks at 4.6/100,000. The incidence in men and women was found to be approximately equal, the mean age at diagnosis was 60 years, and 38% of tumors were in the small bowel and 34% in the rectum. The incidence from 1973 to 2009 increased 4.4% annually, faster than any other tumor type examined except esophageal adenocarcinoma. The increases in incidence were similar in men and women and among different races and ethnicities. Carcinoid tumors of the stomach increased 7.0% per year, those of the rectum increased 7.8% per year, and those of the appendix decreased 3.6% per year.[94] GI carcinoid accounts for 0.52% of all cancers diagnosed and 71% of all carcinoids, with most of the remainder being diagnosed in the lungs. Patients with carcinoid have substantially higher risk for developing a second primary malignancy, especially in the stomach or small bowel.[94]

Patients with GI carcinoid tumors have better survival rates than those with most other GI tumors. Using SEER data, the 5-, 10-, and 20-year disease specific survival rates for those with carcinoid were found to be 91%, 86%, and 77%, respectively. Most patients with GI carcinoid died from causes not related to their carcinoid, mainly cardiovascular causes. Those with tumors in the small bowel had a lower survival rates than did those with tumors located in other parts of the GI tract. Survival rates for localized carcinoids were 95.6%; for regional tumors, 86.5%; and for tumors with distant metastasis, 52.4%.[94]

The reasons that GI carcinoids are increasing rapidly are debated. Some suggest that the increasing use of endoscopy, especially colonoscopy, may lead to more of these tumors being identified. However, this does not explain the rise in incidence in the small bowel.

Although the incidence is increasing, the survival rates have not improved. Given the increasing incidence and lack of improvement in treatment, the National Institutes of Health placed neuroendocrine tumors and carcinoids as the second priority for funding after autism.[95]

Neuroendocrine tumors of the pancreas

Pancreatic neuroendocrine tumors (NETs), also referred to as islet cell tumors, include insulinomas, gastrinomas, glucagonomas, VIPomas, somatostatinomas, and others. According to SEER, they account for 1.3–3% of pancreatic tumors and have a better prognosis than do adenocarcinomas of the pancreas (median survival of 27 months vs. 4 months).[96,97] The most common types of pancreatic NETs are insulinomas and glucagonomas, which occur at similar rates of around 0.05–0.3 cases per 100,000, followed by VIPomas which are eight times less common, and glucagonomas, which are 17 times less common. Somatostatinomas and other pancreatic NETs are even less common.[9]

An analysis of SEER data from 1973 to 2003 revealed that the incidence of pancreatic endocrine tumors decreased from 0.16–0.12/100,000. Many cases are diagnosed at an advanced stage. Among the staged cases in SEER, 14% had localized disease, 23% had regional nodal spread, and 54% had distant metastasis. The median survival was 124 months for those with localized disease, 70 months for those with regional spread, and 23 months for those with distant metastasis. The incidence was similar in Whites and Blacks and in women and men. Those with NETs of the pancreatic head were less likely to have distant metastasis (48%) compared to those with tumors of the pancreatic body (57%) or tail (58%), but this was not associated with longer survival. Increasing age is associated with a worse prognosis. Over time, the overall survival from pancreatic NETs has improved.[97]

Anal Cancer

Cancers of the anus are rare but increasing in frequency. From SEER data, it was estimated that in the United States there were 7,060 new cases in 2013, accounting for 0.4% of all new malignancies. The American Cancer Society estimates there will be 7,210 new cases in 2014 with 2,660 being men and 4,550 women. The estimated number of deaths from anal cancer in 2013 was 880. The incidence rate from 2006 to 2010 was estimated to be 1.7/100,000 with 0.2 deaths per 100,000 population per year. The lifetime cumulative risk of developing anal cancer is 0.2%.[4,15] Among anal cancers, 80% are squamous cell carcinomas, 16% are adenocarcinomas, and 4% are other types.[9]

An analysis of SEER data indicates that the incidence of squamous cell carcinoma of the anus is increasing. The incidence per 100,000 from 1973 to 1996 was 1.0 in men and 1.4 in women, compared to 3.0 in men and

2.4 in women between 1997 and 2009. From 1997 to 2009, the annual average increase in incidence was 9.3% in men and 4.8% in women. Increases were seen in Whites and Blacks and across all age groups.[98]

Anal squamous cell carcinoma is linked to the human papilloma virus (HPV), and populations with a higher HPV prevalence are at higher risk for developing anal cancer.[99] HPV prevalence estimates range from 10 to 55% and varies by the population studied.[98]

Men who have sex with men (MSM) have higher risk for anal cancer.[100] AIDS is associated with higher risk for anal cancer, and it is estimated that the risk may be twice as high in MSM with AIDS as in MSM without AIDS.[101] In one study, other risk factors for anal cancer included receptive intercourse, especially among men for whom there was an estimated 33-fold higher risk (in women, it was estimated to be 1.8-fold higher, a finding that was also statistically insignificant). Among heterosexual men, a history of gonorrhea was associated with a 17-fold higher risk of anal cancer, being seropositive for Herpes simplex virus type 2 with a 4.1-fold higher risk, and Chlamydia with a 2.3-fold higher risk. Cigarette smoking was also found to be statistically significantly directly associated with risk.[102]

Take Home Messages

- Gastrointestinal malignancies account for approximately one-third of all cancers and almost 40% of cancer-related mortality worldwide.
- The most common malignancies of the gastrointestinal system include colorectal, gastric, liver, esophageal, and pancreatic cancers.
- Incidence and mortality rates are constantly evolving as risk factors change, populations move, and prevention efforts expand.

References

1. Jemal, A., Bray, F., Center, M.M., Ferlay, J., Ward, E., Forman, D., Global cancer statistics. *CA*, 2011. **61**: 69–90.
2. Ferlay, J., Shin, H.R., Bray, F., Forman, D., Mathers, C., Parkin, D.M., Estimates of worldwide burden of cancer in 2008: GLOBOCAN 2008. *Int J Cancer*, 2010. **127**: 2893–917.

3. DeVita, V.T.L., Theodore S.; Rosenberg, Steven A. eds. DeVita, Hellman, and Rosenberg's *Cancer: Principles & Practice of Oncology*, 9th ed. Lippincott Williams & Wilkins. 2011.
4. Siegel, R., Ma, J., Zou, Z., Jemal, A., Cancer statistics, 2014. *CA*, 2014. **64**: 9–29.
5. Pennathur, A., Gibson, M.K., Jobe, B.A., Luketich, J.D., Oesophageal carcinoma. *Lancet*, 2013. **381**: 400–12.
6. Hur, C., Miller, M., Kong, C.Y. *et al.*, Trends in esophageal adenocarcinoma incidence and mortality. *Cancer*, 2013. **119**: 1149–58.
7. Brown, L.M., Devesa, S.S., Chow, W.H., Incidence of adenocarcinoma of the esophagus among white Americans by sex, stage, and age. *J Natl Cancer Inst*, 2008. **100**: 1184–7.
8. Engel, L.S, Chow, W.H., Vaughan, T.L. *et al.*, Population attributable risks of esophageal and gastric cancers. *J Natl Cancer Inst*, 2003. **95**: 1404–13.
9. Feldman, M.F., L., Brandt, L. eds. Sleisenger and Fordtran's *Gastrointestinal and Liver Disease*. 9th. ed: Saunders Elsevier; 2010.
10. Jemal, A., Simard, E.P., Xu, J., Ma, J., Anderson, R.N., Selected cancers with increasing mortality rates by educational attainment in 26 states in the United States, 1993–2007. *CCC*, 2013. **24**: 559–65.
11. Islami, F., Boffetta, P., Ren, J.S., Pedoeim, L., Khatib, D., Kamangar, F., High-temperature beverages and foods and esophageal cancer risk — a systematic review. *Int J Cancer*, 2009. **125**: 491–524.
12. Akhtar, S., Areca nut chewing and esophageal squamous-cell carcinoma risk in Asians: a meta-analysis of case-control studies. *CCC*, 2013. **24**: 257–65.
13. Lu, C.L., Lang, H.C., Luo, J.C. *et al.*, Increasing trend of the incidence of esophageal squamous cell carcinoma, but not adenocarcinoma, in Taiwan. *CCC*, 2010. **21**: 269–74.
14. Society, A.C., *Global Cancer Facts & Figures* 2nd Edition. Atlanta: American Cancer Society, 2011.
15. Howlader, N.N.A., Krapcho, M., Garshell, J., Neyman, N., Altekruse, S.F., Kosary, C.L., Yu, M., Ruhl, J., Tatalovich, Z., Cho, H., Mariotto, A., Lewis, D.R., Chen, H.S., Feuer, E.J., Cronin, K.A. (eds)., *SEER Cancer Statistics Review*, 1975–2010, National Cancer Institute. Bethesda, MD, http://seer.cancer.gov/csr/1975_2010/, based on November 2012 SEER data submission, posted to the SEER web site, April 2013.

16. *SEER Cancer Statistics Factsheets: Stomach Cancer*. National Cancer Institute. Bethesda, MD. at http://seer.cancer.gov/statfacts/html/stomach.html.
17. Kamineni, A., Williams, M.A., Schwartz, S.M., Cook, L.S., Weiss, N.S., The incidence of gastric carcinoma in Asian migrants to the United States and their descendants. *CCC*, 1999. **10**: 77–83.
18. Fitzsimmons, D., Osmond, C., George, S., Johnson, C.D., Trends in stomach and pancreatic cancer incidence and mortality in England and Wales, 1951–2000. *Brit J Surgery*, 2007. **94**: 1162–71.
19. La Vecchia, C., Negri, E., D'Avanzo, B., Franceschi, S., Electric refrigerator use and gastric cancer risk. *Brit J Cancer*, 1990. **62**: 136–7.
20. Kalish, R.J., Clancy, P.E., Orringer, M.B., Appelman, H.D., Clinical, epidemiologic, and morphologic comparison between adenocarcinomas arising in Barrett's esophageal mucosa and in the gastric cardia. *Gastroenterology*, 1984. **86**: 461–7.
21. Bertuccio, P., Chatenoud, L., Levi, F. *et al.*, Recent patterns in gastric cancer: a global overview. *Int J Cancer*, 2009. **125**: 666–73.
22. Kamangar, F., Dawsey, S.M., Blaser, M.J. *et al.*, Opposing risks of gastric cardia and noncardia gastric adenocarcinomas associated with Helicobacter pylori seropositivity. *J Nat Cancer Inst*, 2006. **98**: 1445–52.
23. Wu, H., Rusiecki, J.A., Zhu, K., Potter, J., Devesa, S.S., Stomach carcinoma incidence patterns in the United States by histologic type and anatomic site. *Cancer Epidemiol Biomarkers Prev*, 2009. **18**: 1945–52.
24. Lauren, P., The two histological main types of gastric carcinoma: diffuse and so-called intestinal type carcinoma. An attempt at a histo-clinical classification. *APMS*, 1965. **64**: 31–49.
25. Anderson, W.F., Camargo, M.C., Fraumeni, Jr., J.F., Correa, P., Rosenberg, P.S., Rabkin, C.S., Age-specific trends in incidence of noncardia gastric cancer in US adults. *JAMA*, 2010. **303**: 1723–8.
26. Castro, F.A., Koshiol, J., Hsing, A.W., Devesa, S.S., Biliary tract cancer incidence in the United States-Demographic and temporal variations by anatomic site. *Int J Cancer*, 2013. **133**: 1664–71.
27. Shaib, Y., El-Serag, H.B., The epidemiology of cholangiocarcinoma. *Semin Liver Dis*, 2004. **24**: 115–25.
28. Patton, R.B., Horn, Jr., R.C., Primary Liver Carcinoma. Autopsy study of 60 cases. *Cancer*, 1964. **17**: 757–68.

29. Altaee, M.Y., Johnson, P.J., Farrant, J.M., Williams, R., Etiologic and clinical characteristics of peripheral and hilar cholangiocarcinoma. *Cancer*, 1991. **68**: 2051–5.
30. Tyson, G.L., El-Serag, H.B., Risk factors for cholangiocarcinoma. *Hepatology*, 2011. **54**: 173–84.
31. Patel, T., Increasing incidence and mortality of primary intrahepatic cholangiocarcinoma in the United States. *Hepatology*, 2001. **33**: 1353–7.
32. Shaib, Y.H., Davila, J.A., McGlynn, K., El-Serag, H.B., Rising incidence of intrahepatic cholangiocarcinoma in the United States: a true increase? *J Hepatology*, 2004. **40**: 472–7.
33. Welzel, T.M., McGlynn, K.A., Hsing, A.W., O'Brien, T.R., Pfeiffer, R.M., Impact of classification of hilar cholangiocarcinomas (Klatskin tumors) on the incidence of intra- and extrahepatic cholangiocarcinoma in the United States. *J Natl Cancer Inst*, 2006. **98**: 873–5.
34. Randi, G., Malvezzi, M., Levi, F. *et al.*, Epidemiology of biliary tract cancers: an update. *Ann Oncol*, 2009. **20**: 146–59.
35. Lazcano-Ponce, E.C., Miquel, J.F., Munoz, N. *et al.*, Epidemiology and molecular pathology of gallbladder cancer. *CA*, 2001. **51**: 349–64.
36. Randi, G., Franceschi, S., La Vecchia, C., Gallbladder cancer worldwide: geographical distribution and risk factors. *Int J Cancer*, 2006. **118**: 1591–602.
37. Fischer, H.P., Zhou H., Pathogenesis of carcinoma of the papilla of Vater. *J Hepato-Biliary-Pancreatic Surgery*, 2004. **11**: 301–9.
38. Albores-Saavedra, J., Schwartz, A.M., Batich, K., Henson, D.E., Cancers of the ampulla of vater: demographics, morphology, and survival based on 5,625 cases from the SEER program. *J Surg Oncol*, 2009. **100**: 598–605.
39. Venook, A.P., Papandreou, C., Furuse, J., de Guevara, L.L., The incidence and epidemiology of hepatocellular carcinoma: a global and regional perspective. *Oncologist*, 2010. **15**(Suppl 4): 5–13.
40. El-Serag, H.B., Epidemiology of viral hepatitis and hepatocellular carcinoma. *Gastroenterology*, 2012. **142**: 1264–73 e1.
41. Sherman, M., Epidemiology of hepatocellular carcinoma. *Oncology*, 2010. **78**(Suppl 1): 7–10.
42. Altekruse, S.F., McGlynn, K.A., Reichman, M.E., Hepatocellular carcinoma incidence, mortality, and survival trends in the United States from 1975 to 2005. *J Clin Oncol*, 2009. **27**: 1485–91.

43. Colombo, M., de Franchis, R., Del Ninno E. *et al.*, Hepatocellular carcinoma in Italian patients with cirrhosis. *New Eng J Medicine*, 1991. **325**: 675–80.
44. Sangiovanni, A., Del Ninno, E., Fasani, P. *et al.*, Increased survival of cirrhotic patients with a hepatocellular carcinoma detected during surveillance. *Gastroenterology*, 2004. **126**: 1005–14.
45. Tsukuma, H., Hiyama, T., Tanaka, S. *et al.*, Risk factors for hepatocellular carcinoma among patients with chronic liver disease. *New Eng J Medicine*, 1993. **328**: 1797–801.
46. Yang, J.D., Harmsen, W.S., Slettedahl, S.W. *et al.*, Factors that affect risk for hepatocellular carcinoma and effects of surveillance. *Clin Gastroenterol Hepatol*, 2011. **9**: 617–23 e1.
47. Beasley, R.P., Hepatitis B virus. The major etiology of hepatocellular carcinoma. *Cancer*, 1988. **61**: 1942–56.
48. Shlomai, A., de Jong, Y.P., Rice, C.M., Virus associated malignancies: the role of viral hepatitis in hepatocellular carcinoma. *Semin Cancer Biol*, 2014.
49. Chen, C.J., Yang, H.I., Su, J. *et al.*, Risk of hepatocellular carcinoma across a biological gradient of serum hepatitis B virus DNA level. *JAMA*, 2006. **295**: 65–73.
50. Davila, J.A., Morgan, R.O., Shaib, Y., McGlynn, K.A., El-Serag, H.B., Hepatitis C infection and the increasing incidence of hepatocellular carcinoma: A population-based study. *Gastroenterology*, 2004. **127**: 1372–80.
51. Huang, Y.T., Jen, C.L., Yang, H.I. *et al.*, Lifetime risk and sex difference of hepatocellular carcinoma among patients with chronic hepatitis B and C. *J Clin Oncol*, 2011. **29**: 3643–50.
52. Lok, A.S., Seeff, L.B., Morgan, T.R. *et al.*, Incidence of hepatocellular carcinoma and associated risk factors in hepatitis C-related advanced liver disease. *Gastroenterology*, 2009. **136**: 138–48.
53. George, S.L., Bacon, B.R., Brunt, E.M., Mihindukulasuriya, K.L., Hoffmann, J., Di Bisceglie, A.M., Clinical, virologic, histologic, and biochemical outcomes after successful HCV therapy: a 5-year follow-up of 150 patients. *Hepatology*, 2009. **49**: 729–38.
54. Society, A.C., *Cancer Facts & Figures 2013*. Atlanta: American Cancer Society. 2013.
55. Silverman, D.T., Hoover, R.N., Brown, L.M. *et al.*, Why do Black Americans have a higher risk of pancreatic cancer than White Americans? *Epidemiology*, 2003. **14**: 45–54.

56. Ma, J., Siegel, R., Jemal, A., Pancreatic cancer death rates by race among US men and women, 1970–2009. *J Natl Cancer Inst*, 2013. **105**: 1694–700.
57. Edwards, B.K., Noone, A.M., Mariotto, A.B. *et al.*, Annual Report to the Nation on the status of cancer, 1975–2010, featuring prevalence of comorbidity and impact on survival among persons with lung, colorectal, breast, or prostate cancer. *Cancer*, 2013.
58. Lowenfels, A.B., Maisonneuve, P., Cavallini, G. *et al.*, Pancreatitis and the risk of pancreatic cancer. International Pancreatitis Study Group. *N Eng J Med*, 1993. **328**: 1433–7.
59. Duell, E.J., Lucenteforte, E., Olson, S.H. *et al.*, Pancreatitis and pancreatic cancer risk: a pooled analysis in the International Pancreatic Cancer Case-Control Consortium (PanC4). *Ann Oncol*, 2012. **23**: 2964–70.
60. Klein, A.P., Hruban, R.H., Brune, K.A., Petersen, G.M., Goggins, M., Familial pancreatic cancer. *Cancer J*, 2001. **7**: 266–73.
61. Brune, K.A., Lau, B., Palmisano, E. *et al.*, Importance of age of onset in pancreatic cancer kindreds. *J Nat Cancer Inst*, 2010. **102**: 119–26.
62. Couch, F.J., Johnson, M.R., Rabe, K.G. *et al.*, The prevalence of BRCA2 mutations in familial pancreatic cancer. *Cancer Epidemiol, Biomarkers Prev*, 2007. **16**: 342–6.
63. White, K., Held, K.R., Weber, B.H., A BRCA2 germ-line mutation in familial pancreatic carcinoma. *Int J Cancer*, 2001. **91**: 742–4.
64. Giardiello, F.M., Brensinger, J.D., Tersmette, A.C. *et al.*, Very high risk of cancer in familial Peutz-Jeghers syndrome. *Gastroenterology*, 2000. **119**: 1447–53.
65. Giardiello, F.M., Offerhaus, G.J., Lee, D.H. *et al.*, Increased risk of thyroid and pancreatic carcinoma in familial adenomatous polyposis. *Gut*, 1993. **34**: 1394–6.
66. Center, M.M., Jemal, A., Ward, E., International trends in colorectal cancer incidence rates. *Cancer Epidemiol Biomarkers Prev*, 2009. **18**: 1688–94.
67. Winawer, S.J., Zauber, A.G., Ho, M.N. *et al.*, Prevention of colorectal cancer by colonoscopic polypectomy. The National Polyp Study Workgroup. *N Eng J Med*, 1993. **329**: 1977–81.
68. Doubeni, C.A., Laiyemo, A.O., Major, J.M. *et al.*, Socioeconomic status and the risk of colorectal cancer: an analysis of more than a half million adults in the National Institutes of Health-AARP Diet and Health Study. *Cancer*, 2012. **118**: 3636–44.

69. Doubeni, C.A., Major, J.M., Laiyemo, A.O. *et al.*, Contribution of behavioral risk factors and obesity to socioeconomic differences in colorectal cancer incidence. *J Natl Cancer Inst*, 2012. **104**: 1353–62.
70. Klabunde, C.N., Cronin, K.A., Breen, N., Waldron, W.R., Ambs, A.H., Nadel, M.R., Trends in colorectal cancer test use among vulnerable populations in the United States. *Cancer Epidemiol, Biomarkers Prev*, 2011. **20**: 1611–21.
71. Vukasin, A.P., Ballantyne, G.H., Flannery, J.T., Lerner, E., Modlin, I.M., Increasing incidence of cecal and sigmoid carcinoma. Data from the Connecticut Tumor Registry. *Cancer*, 1990. **66**: 2442–9.
72. Thorn, M., Bergstrom, R., Kressner, U., Sparen, P., Zack, M, Ekbom, A., Trends in colorectal cancer incidence in Sweden 1959–93 by gender, localization, time period, and birth cohort. *CCC*, 1998. **9**: 145–52.
73. Siegel, R.L., Ward, E.M., Jemal, A., Trends in colorectal cancer incidence rates in the United States by tumor location and stage, 1992-2008. *Cancer Epidemiol, Biomarkers Prev*, 2012. **21**: 411–6.
74. Haselkorn, T., Whittemore, A.S., Lilienfeld, D.E., Incidence of small bowel cancer in the United States and worldwide: geographic, temporal, and racial differences. *CCC*, 2005. **16**: 781–7.
75. Lepage, C., Bouvier, A.M., Manfredi, S., Dancourt, V., Faivre, J., Incidence and management of primary malignant small bowel cancers: a well-defined French population study. *Am J Gastroenterol*, 2006. **101**: 2826–32.
76. Bilimoria, K.Y., Bentrem, D.J., Wayne, J.D., Ko, C.Y., Bennett, C.L., Talamonti, M.S., Small bowel cancer in the United States: changes in epidemiology, treatment, and survival over the last 20 years. *Ann Surg*, 2009. **249**: 63–71.
77. Hatzaras, I., Palesty, J.A., Abir, F. *et al.*, Small-bowel tumors: epidemiologic and clinical characteristics of 1260 cases from the connecticut tumor registry. *Arch Surg (Chicago, Ill: 1960)*, 2007. **142**: 229–35.
78. Gabos, S., Berkel, J., Band, P., Robson, D., Whittaker, H., Small bowel cancer in western Canada. *Int J Epidemiol*, 1993. **22**: 198–206.
79. Ducreux, M., Boutron, M.C., Piard, F., Carli, P.M., Faivre, J., A 15-year series of gastrointestinal non-Hodgkin's lymphomas: a population-based study. *Brit J Cancer*, 1998. **77**: 511–4.
80. Koch, P., del Valle, F., Berdel, W.E. *et al.*, Primary gastrointestinal non-Hodgkin's lymphoma: I. Anatomic and histologic distribution, clinical

features, and survival data of 371 patients registered in the German Multicenter Study GIT NHL 01/92. *J Clin Oncol*, 2001. **19**: 3861–73.

81. Papaxoinis, G., Papageorgiou, S., Rontogianni, D. *et al.*, Primary gastrointestinal non-Hodgkin's lymphoma: a clinicopathologic study of 128 cases in Greece. A Hellenic Cooperative Oncology Group study (HeCOG). *Leukemia Lymphoma*, 2006. **47**: 2140–6.
82. Doglioni, C., Wotherspoon, A.C., Moschini, A., de Boni, M., Isaacson, P.G., High incidence of primary gastric lymphoma in northeastern Italy. *Lancet*, 1992. **339**: 834–5.
83. Zaki, M., Schubert, M.L., Helicobacter pylori and gastric lymphoma. *Gastroenterology*, 1995. **108**: 610–2.
84. Lewis, J.D., Bilker, W.B., Brensinger, C., Deren, J.J., Vaughn, D.J., Strom, B.L., Inflammatory bowel disease is not associated with an increased risk of lymphoma. *Gastroenterology*, 2001. **121**: 1080–7.
85. Verbeek, W.H., Van De Water, J.M., Al-Toma, A., Oudejans, J.J., Mulder, C.J., Coupe, V.M., Incidence of enteropathy — associated T-cell lymphoma: a nation-wide study of a population-based registry in The Netherlands. *Scand J Gastroenterol*, 2008. **43**: 1322–8.
86. Tran, T., Davila, J.A., El-Serag, H.B., The epidemiology of malignant gastrointestinal stromal tumors: an analysis of 1,458 cases from 1992 to 2000. *Am J Gastroenterol*, 2005. **100**: 162-8.
87. Nilsson, B., Bumming, P., Meis-Kindblom, J.M. *et al.*, Gastrointestinal stromal tumors: the incidence, prevalence, clinical course, and prognostication in the preimatinib mesylate era — a population-based study in western Sweden. *Cancer*, 2005. **103**: 821–9.
88. Tryggvason, G., Gislason, H.G., Magnusson, M.K., Jonasson, J.G., Gastrointestinal stromal tumors in Iceland, 1990-2003: the icelandic GIST study, a population-based incidence and pathologic risk stratification study. *Int J Cancer*, 2005. **117**: 289–93.
89. Tzen, C.Y., Wang, J.H., Huang, Y.J. *et al.* Incidence of gastrointestinal stromal tumor: a retrospective study based on immunohistochemical and mutational analyses. *Digest Dis Sci*, 2007. **52**: 792–7.
90. Agaimy, A., Wunsch, P.H., Hofstaedter, F. *et al.*, Minute gastric sclerosing stromal tumors (GIST tumorlets) are common in adults and frequently show c-KIT mutations. *Am J Surg Pathol*, 2007. **31**: 113–20.
91. Miettinen, M., Lasota, J., Gastrointestinal stromal tumors. *Gastroenterol Clin North Am*, 2013. **42**: 399–415.

92. Miettinen, M., Lasota, J., Gastrointestinal stromal tumors — definition, clinical, histological, immunohistochemical, and molecular genetic features and differential diagnosis. *Virchows Archiv*, 2001. **438**: 1–12.
93. Modlin, I.M., Lye, K.D., Kidd, M., A 5-decade analysis of 13,715 carcinoid tumors. *Cancer*, 2003. **97**: 934–59.
94. Mocellin, S., Nitti, D., Gastrointestinal carcinoid: epidemiological and survival evidence from a large population-based study (n = 25 531). *Ann Oncol*, 2013. **24**: 3040–4.
95. Modlin, I.M., Oberg, K., Chung, D.C. *et al.*, Gastroenteropancreatic neuroendocrine tumours. *Lancet Oncology*, 2008. **9**: 61–72.
96. Fesinmeyer, M.D., Austin, M.A., Li, C.I., De Roos, A.J., Bowen, D.J., Differences in survival by histologic type of pancreatic cancer. *Cancer Epidemiol Biomarkers Prev*, 2005. **14**: 1766–73.
97. Yao, J.C., Eisner, M.P., Leary, C. *et al.*, Population-based study of islet cell carcinoma. *Ann Surg Oncol*, 2007. **14**: 3492–500.
98. Nelson, R.A., Levine, A.M., Bernstein, L., Smith, D.D., Lai, L.L., Changing patterns of anal canal carcinoma in the United States. *J Clin Oncology*, 2013. **31**: 1569–75.
99. Melbye, M., Frisch, M., The role of human papillomaviruses in anogenital cancers. *Semin Cancer Biol*, 1998. **8**: 307–13.
100. Daling, J.R., Weiss, N.S., Klopfenstein, L.L., Cochran, L.E., Chow, W.H., Daifuku, R., Correlates of homosexual behavior and the incidence of anal cancer. *JAMA*, 1982. **247**: 1988–90.
101. Melbye, M., Cote, T.R., Kessler, L., Gail, M., Biggar, R.J., High incidence of anal cancer among AIDS patients. The AIDS/Cancer Working Group. *Lancet*, 1994. **343**: 636–9.
102. Daling, J.R., Weiss, N.S., Hislop, T.G. *et al.*, Sexual practices, sexually transmitted diseases, and the incidence of anal cancer. *N Eng J Med*, 1987. **317**: 973–7.

Chapter 2

Biomarkers and the Quest for Personalized Cancer Care

Sameer H. Patel and Shishir K. Maithel

What is New

- One of the paradigm shifts that has occurred in cancer therapy is an effort to move from a generalized blanket therapy of treating all patients with the same disease the same way to a more individualized approach with patient and/or tumor specific treatment strategies.
- One of the obstacles to provide this personalized cancer therapy involves determining what characteristics, or biomarkers, of the tumor to specifically target.

Introduction

Gastrointestinal (GI) malignancies are estimated to affect 289,610 individuals in the United States in 2014 with approximately half of those patients succumbing to their disease.[1] The quest for cure for most patients remains elusive, but for select individuals, it can become a reality. Currently, the approach to cancer therapy is disease-based while patients continue to exhibit differential responses to the same therapy.

Definitions

There are two features of biomarkers that need to be defined; those that are prognostic and those that are predictive. Prognostic value refers to a factor that is independently associated with patient outcome such as survival. In contrast, predictive value refers to a factor that is associated with response to a particular treatment.

Biomarkers can provide either prognostic or predictive value or both. An example is the tyrosine kinase transmembrane receptor human epidermal growth factor 2 (Her2) in breast cancer.[2] Studies have shown that Her2 overexpression is associated with poor overall survival and disease free survival, thereby providing prognostic information.[3] In addition, because the Her2 protein is the target of Herceptin, a monoclonal antibody against the receptor, it also provides predictive information; those patients with Her2 overexpression will respond to Herceptin. The ideal biomarker is one that provides both prognostic as well as predictive value.

Pathways and Progression to Cancer: Choosing the Right Target

The natural progression of cancer is thought to involve sequential alterations in genes causing changes in proteins that are involved in normal cellular processes. Although there is significant variability in these changes, not just between different GI malignancies but also between those of the same type, the major pathways involved are often the same. The order and rates of changes are variable and can explain the unpredictable nature of disease progression.[4]

The progression to carcinoma is thought to involve six fundamental alterations in several basic functions of normal cells (Fig. 1). These are the ability to become self-sufficient in growth signals, insensitivity to anti-growth signals, limitless replicative potential, tissue invasion, sustained angiogenesis, and evasion of apoptosis.[5] Through a variety of mechanisms and changes in different subtypes of genes, cells undergo malignant transformation.

There are several major classes of genes that are affected during the process of malignant transformation. The first is an oncogene, which is a

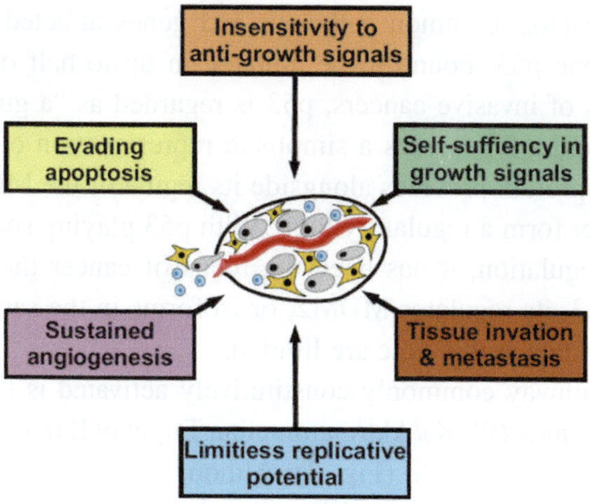

Fig. 1. The hallmarks of cancer involves the ability of malignant cells to develop self-sufficiency in growth signals, insensitivity to anti-growth signals, ability to invade tissues, develop limitless replicative potential, sustain angiogenesis, and evade apoptosis.

gene capable of inducing one or more aspects of the malignant phenotype.[6] This can occur through either promoting cell proliferation or by preventing programmed cell death. These genes are commonly considered to be dominant, in that a change in one copy of the gene will promote unregulated cell growth. Proto-oncogenes on the other hand are normal genes that become altered and turn into an oncogene.

In contrast to oncogenes which become activated with mutations, tumor suppressor genes become inactivated thereby promoting tumorigenesis. They can be thought of as normal "brakes" in cell proliferation that when released, allow for unregulated growth. Classic examples of tumor suppressor genes include the retinoblastoma (Rb) and p53 genes.

Finally, changes in gene expression can occur in the absence of mutations. These alterations are referred to as epigenetic changes. A classic example is the methylation of DNA which inhibits specific gene expression. Inactivation of the X chromosome during development occurs via this mechanism.[7] Regardless of the specific mechanism by which cells transform, there are multiple pathways that seem to be uniformly affected, ultimately resulting in the same end result, malignant transformation.

One of the most common pathways and genes affected is the tumor suppressor gene p53. Found to be mutated in up to half of tumors and three-quarters of invasive cancers, p53 is regarded as "a guardian of the genome." [8] Figure 2 provides a simplistic representation of the multiple functions the protein provides alongside its regulator the MDM2 protein, which together form a regulatory loop. With p53 playing such an integral role in cell regulation, it has been the focus of cancer therapy. Studies examining p53, its regulator MDM2, or isoforms in the same family are underway but data at this time are limited.

Another pathway commonly constitutively activated is the phosphatidylinositol 3-kinase (PI3K)/Akt/mammalian Target of Rapamycin (mTOR) signal transduction cascade (Fig. 3). Although not the initial targets of mutations, they can be activated by other important regulatory proteins such as G protein coupled receptors such as *Ras* or receptor tyrosine kinases. Like p53, because of the commonality of the pathway, they are the focus of anticancer therapeutics. One of specific drugs targeted against this pathway include the mTOR inhibitor, Everolimus, approved for use in renal cell carcinoma and pancreas neuroendocrine tumors. [9]

The search is still underway to identify effective agents capable of targeting multiple pathways and many of these drugs remain in clinical trials.

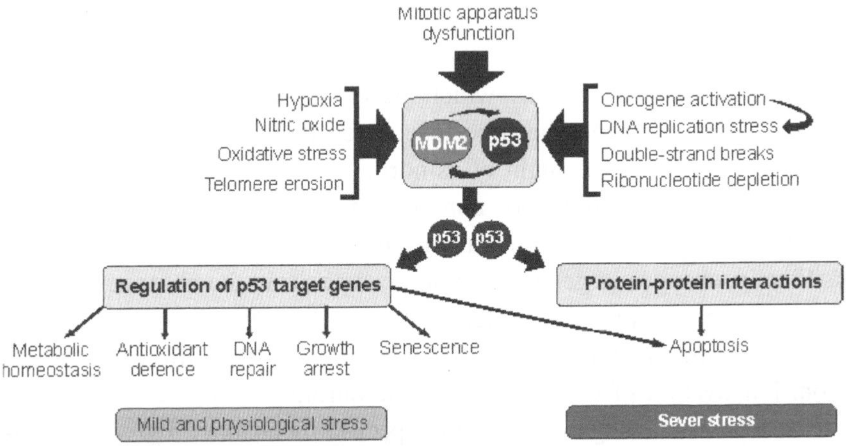

Fig. 2. The p53-MDM2 feedback loop regulate many tegral cellular activities. Varying degrees of stress can result in either transient or permanent responses.

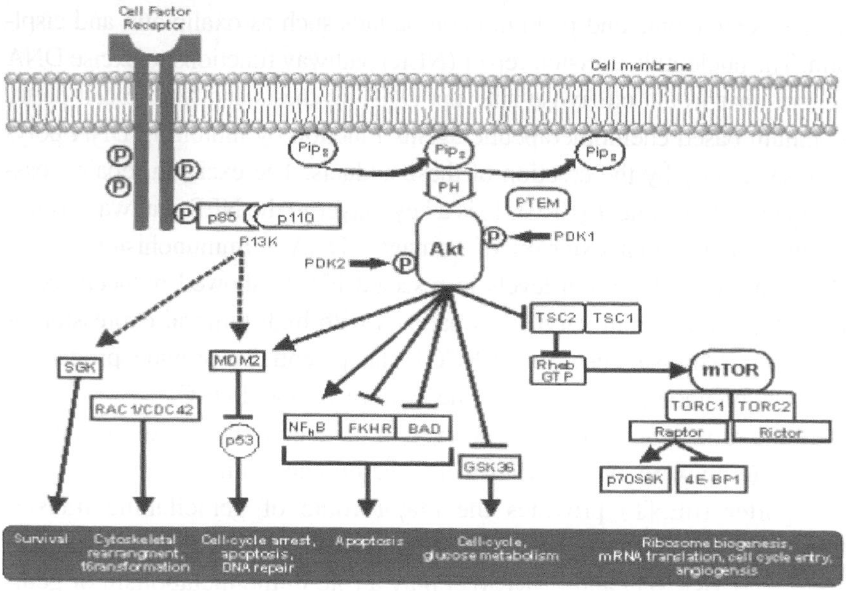

Fig. 3. Schematic representation of the PI3K/AKT/mTOR signal transduction pathway.

Regardless of the drug, proper patient/tumor selection will determine the best agent for the patient as no two tumors are the same.

Specific Malignancies

Pancreas cancer

Pancreas cancer is expected to affect 46,420 individuals in the United States in 2014.[1] It remains a unique organ composed of four different cell types: ductal, endocrine, acinar, and mesenchymal.[10] Of these cell types, malignancies of the ductal cells, or pancreas ductal adenocarcinomas (PDAC) account for more than 85% of all pancreas neoplasms.[11] One of the major oncogenes frequently mutated in PDAC and involved in the PI3K/AKT/mTOR pathway is the Ras protein.[12] Functioning as a guanosine triphosphatase that controls cell growth and proliferation, mutations result in a constant state of activation and unregulated cell growth.[10]

Several biomarkers that have been investigated for resectable PDAC are focused around current treatment strategies, primarily the chemotherapeutic agents gemcitabine and platinum compounds such as oxaliplatin and cisplatin. The nucleotide excision repair (NER) pathway functions to excise DNA adducts that would otherwise interrupt DNA synthesis and lead to cell death. Platinum-based chemotherapeutic agents function by inhibiting DNA polymerase activity by the creation of these adducts. The excision repair cross-complementing gene-1 (ERCC1) is a key player in the NER pathway, as it is integral to the final excision of damaged DNA.[13] Immunohistochemical (IHC) analysis of protein levels in resected PDAC showed reduced recurrence free and overall survival in patients with high tumoral expression of ERCC1.[13] This suggests that ERCC1 can potentially provide prognostic information about survival in patients with resectable PDAC.

In the same study, proteins involved in the metabolism and transport of Gemcitabine were evaluated as well. The human equilibrative nucleotide transporter (hENT) provides the major route of gemcitabine transfer through the cell. In addition, the ribonucleotide reductase (RR) protein complex 1 (RRM1) and 2 (RRM2) play a role in the metabolism of gemcitabine. Elevated RRM2 expression was found to be associated with reduced recurrence free survival as well as overall survival.[13] Authors suggested that ERCC1 and RRM2 can be used as biomarkers capable of providing prognostic value in resected PDAC. Given that these proteins are intimately linked with current treatment therapies, with additional research they may also provide predictive value as well, specifically for response to Gemcitabine and platinum-based therapy.

Cholangiocarcinoma

Cholangiocarcinoma (CCA) is a unique but lethal hepatobiliary malignancy that arises from epithelial cells known as cholangiocytes. This ominous diagnosis afflicts approximately 5,000 individuals in the United States per year.[1] The backbone of chemotherapy involves gemcitabine and cisplatin. In a similar protein (IHC) evaluation of the gemcitabine transporter hENT1 in resectable cholangiocarcinoma, high expression was associated with improved overall survival.[14] Unlike PDAC, overexpression of RRM2 in cholangiocarcinoma exhibited a trend towards improved overall survival.[14] The differences found between PDAC and cholangiocarcinoma illustrate that protein expression is not only variable between different malignancies, but can also carry different prognostic value.

Hepatocellular carcinoma (HCC)

One of the hallmarks to the progression to cancer is the ability to sustain angiogenesis. Hepatocellular carcinoma (HCC) is an extremely vascular malignancy of the liver notorious for its highly aggressive behavior, venous invasion, and early metastasis.[15] One of the most important mediators of angiogenesis is the vascular endothelial growth factor (VEGF). VEGF mediates its action through vascular endothelial growth factor receptors (VEGFR), including VEGFR2. Evaluation of VEGFR2 via IHC in resected HCC showed trends towards reduced overall survival with overexpression.[16] This may suggest that in the progression to cancer, those patients with tumors that have increased the amount of VEGFR2 expression do poorly because they have moved to a more aggressive phenotype.

In addition to angiogenesis, another unique feature of liver hepatocytes is their extraordinary capacity for regeneration. This is especially true after liver resection or damage and is mediated in part by the upregulation of growth factors, such as platelet derived growth factor (PDGFR) alpha and beta.[15] IHC evaluation of PDGFRα and PDGFRβ in resectable HCC showed that elevated expression was associated with reduced overall survival.[16]

Despite these early findings and limited sample sizes, additional data are required before these proteins can routinely be used for prognostic or predictive purposes in the clinical arena.

Colorectal cancer

No GI malignancy has been studied more extensively than colorectal cancer (CRC), affecting nearly 150,000 individuals in the United States in 2014.[1] The adenoma-carcinoma sequence of progression from normal colorectal epithelium to malignancy involves a series of mutations that progressively accumulate (Fig. 4). This results in dysplastic adenomatous polyps progressing into invasive malignant phenotypes. Among the oncogenes involved, the Ras G protein is found to be mutated in half of adenomas greater than 1 cm, leaving it constitutively activated, resulting in an unregulated pro-growth state.[17]

In addition to p53, the tumor suppressor gene APC gene is mutated in over three-quarters of patients with CRC.[17,18] Because it is a tumor suppressor

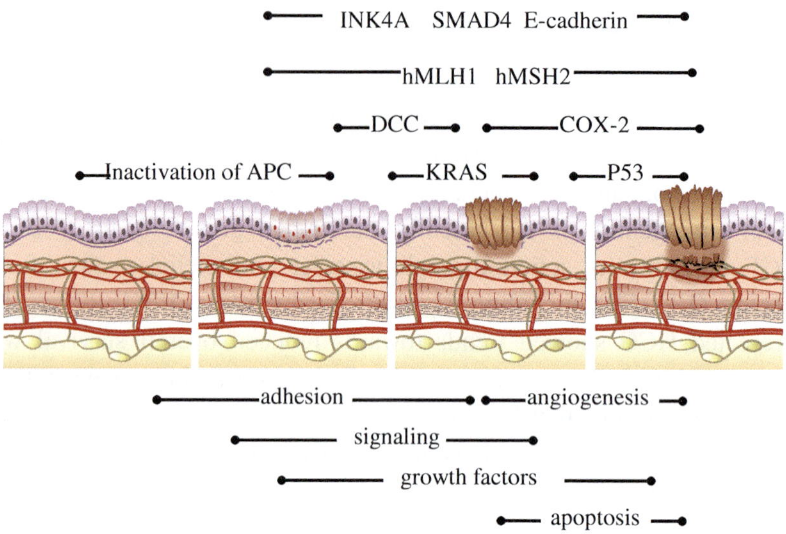

Fig. 4. The adenoma-carcinoma sequence and molecular alterations in colorectal cancer.

gene, mutations in both alleles are required to cause any phenotypic changes. Mutational activation also results in accumulation of the beta catenin protein leading to cell growth and resistance to apoptosis, two key hallmarks of cancer.[19] APC was studied in the Familial Adenomatous Polyposis (FAP) syndrome where germline mutations are inherited. As mentioned previously, a single gene mutation is not sufficient to progress to malignancy but rather, an accumulation of changes are required.

Like in APC, HNPCC or Lynch Syndrome is another hereditary syndrome arising from mutations in the microsatellite instability pathway. These genes include MLH1, MSH2, MSH6, PMS1, and PMS2.[20] Unlike patients with mutations associated with FAP, HNPCC CRCs are often located on the right side of the colon and carry a better prognosis.[20] MSI testing has shown to provide predictive information as low levels of instability are associated with improved outcomes with 5-FU based regimens.[21,22] In contrast, meta-analyses of patients with high degrees of microsatellite instability (MSI-H) were associated with improved overall survival regardless of tumor stage.[23] Therefore MSI status can provide both prognostic and predictive value for patients with CRC. Additional biomarkers are being explored but more investigation is required.

Gastric cancer

Gastric cancer (GC) is a unique but lethal malignancy whose incidence has slowly declined in most Western countries.[24] However, in Asia, GC remains the second most occurring cancer, following lung cancer, and is the second most common cause of cancer related deaths worldwide.[25] This ominous diagnosis is estimated to affect approximately 22,000 individuals in the United States in 2014 with about 13,730 of those succumbing to the disease.[1] The mainstay of therapy for gastric cancer is surgical resection either coupled with perioperative chemotherapy or followed by adjuvant chemoradiation. Current chemotherapy regimens are fluoropyrimidine and platinum-based with or without a third regimen (typically epirubicin or docetaxel).[25] A relatively recent adjunct to help stratify patients with advanced gastric cancer was determining the Her2 status.

One of the most innovative targets in human cancers involves the HER family of proteins. In humans, the HER family consists of four related members, Her1 (ErbB1 or EGFR), Her2 (ErbB2), Her3 (ErbB3), and Her4 (ErbB4). These proteins are transmembrane receptor tyrosine kinases that are activated by homo- or heterodimerization. This leads to the activation of various signal transduction pathways including Ras/Raf/MAPK and PI3K/Akt/mTOR involved in growth and survival.[26] Her2 is the most illustrious member of the family gaining fame from its involvement in breast cancer. Her2 overexpression and amplification is present in up to one-third of invasive breast cancers, is associated with poor prognosis, is a negative predictor of response to cytotoxic and endocrine therapy, and is a positive predictor of response to anti-Her2 agents.[26] The importance of Her2 is not just limited to breast cancer. Expression was first reported in gastric cancer in 1986 by Sakai *et al.*[27] Since then many studies have associated Her2 expression with negative prognosis, however, results are still conflicting. Nevertheless, the importance of Her2 in gastric cancer was established in the ToGA trial. A phase 3, open label, randomized control trial that demonstrated the efficacy and survival benefit of an anti-Her2 monoclonal antibody, trastuzumab, in patients with advanced gastric or GE junction tumors that were Her2 positive. They found that 22% of patients had tumors that were Her2 positive, potentially providing prognostic and predictive value in advanced gastric cancer for a good number of patients.[25] In a series looking at Her2 status in patients with early stage resected gastric cancer, no association with survival was found.[28] This illustrates the point that potential biomarkers need to be evaluated in early and advanced stage disease separately, as they can carry different prognostic and predictive information.

Gastrointestinal stromal tumor

Gastrointestinal stromal tumors (GIST) remain one of the most common sarcomas overall.[29] Originally, five-year median overall survival remained a dismal 9 months due to the relative resistance to chemo or radiotherapy.[30] One of the biggest breakthroughs in the management of GISTs was the discovery of mutations in the receptor tyrosine kinase KIT (CD 117) gene. Activation of the receptor involves binding of the KIT ligand, dimerization of the receptor complexes, phosphorylation and subsequent activation of pro-growth/survival pathways.[31] Mutation results in constitutive activation of the receptor and consequent downstream pathways. Studies have shown that KIT is mutated in up to 80% of all GISTs with the majority occurring in the juxtamembrane domain of exon 11 followed by the extracellular domain of exon 9.[32,33] Although there is conflicting data on the prognostic value of specific exonal mutations for GISTs, determining exon mutation status plays an important predictive role.

For the approximately 20% of patients who are KIT negative, another receptor tyrosine kinase is often affected, the platelet derived growth factor receptor alpha (PDGFRα).[34] Like KIT, PDGFRα mutation results in constitutive activation and pro-growth signals.

The dismal outcomes of patients with GISTs largely ended with approval of the tyrosine kinase inhibitor imatinib (Gleevac) for these tumors. Randomized controlled trials found improvements in progression free and overall survival with imatinib therapy.[35,36,37] Furthermore, on mutational analysis, patients with exon 11 mutations were found to have improved prognosis over those patients with exon 9 mutations when patients were treated with imatinib.[38,39,40] Combined analyses also elucidated that patients with exon 9 mutations had improvement in progression free survival when the dose of imatinib was doubled.[41]

Another receptor tyrosine kinase inhibitor, sunitinib has also been used for GISTs not responsive to imatinib therapy. Exon mutational analysis also helps guide therapy as studies proved that response rates with sunitinib were higher in patients with exon 9 rather than exon 11 mutations.[33] The KIT gene serves as one of the most important molecular markers in GI malignancies as it helps guide therapy based on not just the presence but also the specific subtype of mutation.

Take Home Messages

- The treatments of GI malignancies are evolving to provide patients with more patient/tumor specific therapies.
- One of the key factors remains understanding the biology of the tumor as well as changes in the key genes that control the rate of malignant progression. These genes often control several of the fundamental pathways found in the hallmarks of cancer and can potentially be targets of specific therapies.
- As we look to the future, our understanding will improve only through the identification of biomarkers that can provide both prognostic and predictive value, tested through randomized clinical trials.

References

1. Siegel, R., Ma, J., Zou, Z., Jemal, A., Cancer statistics, 2014. *CA*, 2014; **64**: 9–29.
2. Cooke, T., Reeves, J., Lanigan, A., Stanton, P., HER2 as a prognostic and predictive marker for breast cancer. *Ann Oncol*, 2001; **12** (Suppl 1): S23–8.
3. Piccart, M., Lohrisch, C., Di Leo, A., Larsimont, D., The predictive value of HER2 in breast cancer. *Oncology,* 2001; **61** (Suppl 2): 73–82.
4. Fearon, E.R., Vogelstein BCINCS, Pmid., A genetic model for colorectal tumorigenesis. *Cell*, 1990; **61**: 759–67.
5. Hanahan, D., Weinberg, R.A., The hallmarks of cancer. *Cell*, 2000; **100**: 57–70.
6. Cooper, G.M., *Oncogenes*. Jones and Bartlett 1995.
7. Goto, T., Monk, M., Regulation of X-chromosome inactivation in development in mice and humans. *Microbiol Mol Biol Rev*, 1998; **62**: 362–78.

8. Golubovskaya, V.M., Cance, W.G., Targeting the p53 pathway. *Surg Oncol Clin North Am*, 2013; **22**: 747–64.
9. Pavel, M.E., Hainsworth, J.D., Baudin, E. *et al.*, Everolimus plus octreotide long-acting repeatable for the treatment of advanced neuroendocrine tumours associated with carcinoid syndrome (RADIANT-2): a randomised, placebo-controlled, phase 3 study. *Lancet*, 2011; **378**: 2005–12.
10. Reid, M.D., Saka, B., Balci, S. *et al.*, Molecular genetics of pancreatic neoplasms and their morphologic correlates: an update on recent advances and potential diagnostic applications. *Am J Clin Pathol*, 2014; **141**: 168–80.
11. Li, C., Heidt, D.G., Dalerba, P. *et al.*, Identification of pancreatic cancer stem cells. *Cancer Res*, 2007; **67**: 1030–7.
12. Almoguera, C., Shibata, D., Forrester, K. *et al.*, Most human carcinomas of the exocrine pancreas contain mutant c-K-ras *genes. Cell*, 1988; **53**: 549–54.
13. Fisher, S.B., Patel, S.H., Bagci, P. *et al.*, An analysis of human equilibrative nucleoside transporter-1, ribonucleoside reductase subunit M1, ribonucleoside reductase subunit M2, and excision repair cross-complementing gene-1 expression in patients with resected pancreas adenocarcinoma: implications for adjuvant treatment. *Cancer*, 2013; **119**: 445–53.
14. Fisher, S.B., Fisher, K.E., Patel, S.H. *et al.*, Excision repair cross-complementing gene-1, ribonucleotide reductase subunit M1, ribonucleotide reductase subunit M2, and human equilibrative nucleoside transporter-1 expression and prognostic value in biliary tract malignancy. *Cancer*, 2013; **119**: 454–62.
15. Thomas, M.B., Abbruzzese, J.L., Opportunities for targeted therapies in hepatocellular carcinoma. *J Clin Oncol*, 2005; **23**: 8093–108.
16. Patel, S.H., Kneuertz, P.J., Delgado, M. *et al.*, Clinically relevant biomarkers to select patients for targeted inhibitor therapy after resection of hepatocellular carcinoma. *Ann Surg Oncol*, 2011; **18**: 3384–90.
17. Vogelstein, B., Fearon, E.R., Hamilton, S.R. *et al.*, Genetic alterations during colorectal-tumor development. *Eng J Med*, 1988; **319**: 525–32.
18. Meguerditchian, A.N., Bullard Dunn, K., Biomarkers and targeted therapeutics in colorectal cancer. *Surg Oncol Clin North Am*, 2013; **22**: 841–55.
19. Korinek, V., Barker, N., Morin, P.J. *et al.*, Constitutive transcriptional activation by a beta-catenin-Tcf complex in APC-/- colon carcinoma. *Science*, 1997; **275**: 1784–7.

20. Abdel-Rahman, W.M., Mecklin, J.P., Peltomaki, P., The genetics of HNPCC: application to diagnosis and screening. *Crit Rev Oncol Hematol,* 2006; **58**: 208–20.
21. Kim, G.P., Colangelo, L.H., Wieand, H.S. *et al.*, Prognostic and predictive roles of high-degree microsatellite instability in colon cancer: a National Cancer Institute-National Surgical Adjuvant Breast and Bowel Project Collaborative Study. *J Clin Oncol*, 2007; **25**: 767–72.
22. Ribic, C.M., Sargent, D.J., Moore, M.J. *et al.*, Tumor microsatellite-instability status as a predictor of benefit from fluorouracil-based adjuvant chemotherapy for colon cancer. *Eng J Medi*, 2003; **349**: 247–57.
23. Popat, S., Hubner, R., Houlston, R.S., Systematic review of microsatellite instability and colorectal cancer prognosis. *J Clin Oncol*, 2005; **23**: 609–18.
24. Sasako, M., Inoue, M., Lin, J.T. *et al.*, Gastric Cancer Working Group report. *Jap J Clin Oncol*, 2010; 40 Suppl 1: i28–37.
25. Bang, Y.J., Van Cutsem, E., Feyereislova, A. *et al.*, Trastuzumab in combination with chemotherapy versus chemotherapy alone for treatment of HER2-positive advanced gastric or gastro-oesophageal junction cancer (ToGA): a phase 3, open-label, randomised controlled trial. *Lancet*, 2010; **376**: 687–97.
26. De Vita, F., Giuliani, F., Silvestris, N. *et al.*, Human epidermal growth factor receptor 2 (HER2) in gastric cancer: a new therapeutic target. *Cancer Treatment Rev*, 2010; **36S3**: S11–5.
27. Sakai, K., Mori, S., Kawamoto, T. *et al.*, Expression of epidermal growth factor receptors on normal human gastric epithelia and gastric carcinomas. *J Nat Cancer Inst*, 1986; **77**: 1047–52.
28. Fisher, S.B., Fisher, K.E., Squires, M.H. 3rd *et al.*, HER2 in resected gastric cancer: is there prognostic value? *J Surg Oncol,* 2014; **109**: 61–6.
29. Ducimetiere, F., Lurkin, A., Ranchere-Vince, D. *et al.*, Incidence of sarcoma histotypes and molecular subtypes in a prospective epidemiological study with central pathology review and molecular testing. *Plos One*, 2011; **6**: e20294.
30. DeMatteo, R.P., Lewis, J.J., Leung, D. *et al.*, Two hundred gastrointestinal stromal tumors: recurrence patterns and prognostic factors for survival. *Ann Surgery*, 2000; **231**: 51–8.
31. Balachandran, V.P., Dematteo, R.P., Targeted therapy for cancer: the gastrointestinal stromal tumor model. *Surg Oncol Clin North Am*, 2013; **22**: 805–21.

32. Rubin, B.P., Singer, S., Tsao, C. *et al.*, KIT activation is a ubiquitous feature of gastrointestinal stromal tumors. *Cancer Res*, 2001; **61**: 8118–21.
33. Demetri, G.D., von Mehren, M., Antonescu, C.R. *et al.*, NCCN Task Force report: update on the management of patients with gastrointestinal stromal tumors. *J Nat Comprehensive Cancer Network*, 2010; **8**(Suppl 2): S1–41; quiz S42–44.
34. Hirota, S., Ohashi, A., Nishida, T. *et al.*, Gain-of-function mutations of platelet-derived growth factor receptor alpha gene in gastrointestinal stromal tumors. *Gastroenterology*, 2003; **125**: 660–7.
35. Demetri, G.D., von Mehren, M., Blanke, C.D. *et al.*, Efficacy and safety of imatinib mesylate in advanced gastrointestinal stromal tumors. *Eng J Med,* 2002; **347**: 472–80.
36. Verweij, J., Casali, P.G., Zalcberg, J. *et al.*, Progression-free survival in gastrointestinal stromal tumours with high-dose imatinib: randomised trial. *Lancet,* 2004, **364**: 1127–34.
37. Blanke, C.D., Rankin, C., Demetri, G.D. *et al.*, Phase III randomized, intergroup trial assessing imatinib mesylate at two dose levels in patients with unresectable or metastatic gastrointestinal stromal tumors expressing the kit receptor tyrosine kinase: S0033. *J Clin Oncol,* 2008, **26**: 626–32.
38. Debiec-Rychter, M., Sciot, R., Le Cesne, A. *et al.*, KIT mutations and dose selection for imatinib in patients with advanced gastrointestinal stromal tumours. *Eur J Cancer*, 2006; **42**: 1093–103.
39. Heinrich, M.C., Corless, C.L., Demetri, G.D. *et al.*, Kinase mutations and imatinib response in patients with metastatic gastrointestinal stromal tumor. *J Clin Oncol*, 2003; **21**: 4342–9.
40. Heinrich, M.C., Owzar, K., Corless, C.L. *et al.*, Correlation of kinase genotype and clinical outcome in the North American Intergroup Phase III Trial of imatinib mesylate for treatment of advanced gastrointestinal stromal tumor: CALGB 150105 Study by Cancer and Leukemia Group B and Southwest Oncology Group. *J Clin Oncol*, 2008; **26**: 5360–7.
41. Gastro intestinal Stromal Tumor Meta-Analysis Group (Meta GISI), Comparison of two doses of imatinib for the treatment of unresectable or metastatic gastrointestinal stromal tumors: a meta-analysis of 1,640 patients. *J Clin Oncol*, 2010; **28**: 1247–53.

Chapter 3

Prevention of Gastrointestinal Malignancy

Heval Mohamed Kelli, Jinghua Hao, Qing Shu, Endian Zheng, Kevin Woods and Qiang Cai

What is New

- The association of prevention and reduction of gastrointestinal malignancies have resulted in the formation of screening tools targeting specific and modifiable risk factors.
- In addition to development of advanced and cost-effective endoscopic screening, there is also focus on narrowing surveillance intervals on specific target groups.
- Chemoprevention of using NSAIDs and PPIs has been an evolving and new concept in the promotion of prevention.
- Vaccination and infection eradication play a major role while more studies have strengthened the link between healthy lifestyle and reduction of cancer incidence.

Introduction

Prevention is a most effective and cost-saving strategy to control cancer overtime. It is defined as decreasing cancer incidents resulting in reduction of cancer related mortality. Gastrointestinal malignancies, including colon, stomach, liver and esophageal cancer, are in the top ten new cases of cancer worldwide. It is noted that colorectal cancer is the third most common malignancy with over 1.2 million new cases in 2008.[1] At least one third of cancers are preventable and prevention is a tool that has multidimensional approach toward reducing cancer burden. Prevention can be achieved by altering cancer risk factors through healthy lifestyles and avoiding carcinogens. In addition to early detection, prevention positively impacts survival and control cancer. In keeping with the old saying that "prevention is better than cure," there has been more focus on screening and chemoprevention as an approach to reduce the rise of cancer.

Screening

Screening is a preventive process of detecting premalignant or malignant disease in general population. The screening tools have shared properties to assure effective results; the screened disease is common, the diagnostic test is reliable and affordable in addition to the presence of effective treatment for the screened disease. There is a focused screening on patients with premalignant upper GI tract disease while the lower GI tract endoscopic screening is based on age and high risk patients. For example, Barrett's esophagus (BE) is associated with esophageal cancer development. The primary purpose of endoscopic screening is identifying dysplastic progression or esophageal cancer. Once Barrett's esophagus is diagnosed then surveillance endoscopic screening is based on grade of dysplasia to prevent or initiate early treatment of esophageal adenocarcinoma (EAC). According to the American College of Gastroenterology (ACG), screening of BE cannot be recommended and remains controversial due to the lack of its impact on EAC. Although patients who are older Caucasian males with chronic reflux symptoms are at higher risk, there are a larger number of patients who lack reflux symptoms but develop BE. The challenges also include inability to predict BE, lack of screening criteria and the cost-effectiveness of endoscopy.[2] BE is graded based on histology in the following categories: nondysplastic (NDBE), low-grade dysplasia (LGD), high-grade dysplasia (HGD), intramucosal carcinoma (IMC).[3] Surveillance interval is determined by the degree of dysplasia because of its impact on progression to EAC and its purpose identification of dysplasia and early EAC. According to the American Society for Gastrointestinal Endoscopy

(ASGE), endoscopic surveillance including biopsies can be performed every 3–5 years. The ASGE and ACG also recommend biannual-annual surveillance for LGD following the Seattle protocol.[2,3] In the case of HGD, patients are recommended to undergo operative or ablative therapy and surveillance should be offered only if patients declined or are not appropriate candidates for invasive procedures.[3]

Colorectal cancer (CRC) is the third leading cause of cancer related death in the US.[4] Regular CRC screening has been one of the powerful tools in cancer prevention. Colonoscopy is the most common screening test and proved its ability in detecting early-stage and mostly treatable malignancies. Adenomatous polyps can give rise to cancer and its detection and removal can prevent cancer occurrence. The first randomized trial of endoscopic screening of CRC, Telemark Polyp Study, in 1996, demonstrated that screening reduced the incidence of CRC by 80%.[5] A further 26 year follow-up of the trial also showed that endoscopic screening does reduce the CRC incidence and mortality for individuals with polyps. A recent study by Nishihara also supported the evidence that screening (colonoscopy and sigmoidoscopy) is associated with reduced cancer incidence and death.[6] Several large randomized trials showed the reduction of CRC incidence by 18–23% and mortality by 22–31%.[7–9]

An important aspect of cancer screening is recognition of risk factors, importantly the family history. An estimated 20% of CRC cases have familial relation with more than two first-degree family members and 5–10% in setting of hereditary syndrome.[10,11] The CRC screening tests are divided into cancer prevention and cancer detection categories. Cancer prevention tests possess the ability to visualize polyps and cancers. Cancer detection tests have lower sensitivity in detecting polyps and malignancy. ACG supports both categories of screening methods and recommends colonoscopy every 10 years as a preferred cancer prevention test while also recommends annual fecal immunochemical test as a preferred cancer detection test.

Chemoprevention

The concept of chemoprevention was first described by Sporn and defined as utilization of non-toxic, natural or synthetic chemicals that delay or reverse carcinogenesis.[12] Chemoprevention has become a target of studies to decrease the cancer incidence and mortality. It is a strategy that focuses on the three phases of carcinogenesis — initiation, promotion and progression. There are agents that target inhibition of carcinogen activation while others initiate detoxification in addition to stopping or reversing the progression of premalignant cells to malignant ones. Other targets of prevention act on suppression of reflux disease, treatment of Helicobacter pylori and controlling metabolic risk factors. In GI malignancy, chemoprevention has become one of the most effective approach to control cancer.

Proton pump inhibitors

Proton pump inhibitors (PPIs) are a class of drugs which irreversibly block the hydrogen-potassium adenosine triphosphatase enzyme system with the main purpose of long-lasting gastric acid reduction.[13] Several trials supported that PPIs are superior agents in relief and control of acid reflux symptoms compared with H_2-receptor antagonists.[14] In addition to its symptomatic effect, it has been suggested that PPIs can decrease the risk of neoplastic development in Barrett's esophagus.[15] The persistent exposure of metaplastic region to acid decreases cell differentiation and increases cell proliferation. In theory, effective intraesophageal acid suppression induces differentiation and decreases proliferation; therefore PPIs can play a role in slowing metaplastic transformation.[16] However, there has not been a definite long term study of PPI therapy in Barrett esophagus that had effect on slowing dysplastic progression. One study showed the protective effect of Rabeprazole against the development of esophageal cancer in a surgical rat reflux model.[17] The main concern of long term PPI therapy is development of hypergastrinemia and its association with colorectal cancer and gastric carcinoids which has been observed in *in vitro* studies. However recent studies opposed the hypothesis by showing that long-term application of proton pump inhibitors is not associated with a significantly increased risk of colorectal cancer in addition to low risk of gastric cancer.[18,19] On the other hand, PPIs play an essential part of the combination therapy in eradication of *H. pylori* which may be the main cause of gastric adenocarcinoma.[20,21] Overall, more studies are needed to show the long term use of PPI in cancer prevention. However, the effect of PPI in reducing dysplastic progression may play a role in GI chemoprevention.

NSAIDs

Various studies have shown the association of chronic use of nonsteroidal anti-inflammatory drugs (NSAIDs) with the reduction of GI malignancies, specifically in colorectal cancer.[22] Multiple epidemiological studies investigated the significant reduction of colorectal cancer in patients who are regular consumer of NSAIDs.[23–25] Baron *et al.* demonstrated in a randomized placebo-controlled study that patients with recent history of histologically documented adenoma who received low dose aspirin had significant reduction of risk of adenoma formation compared with a placebo group.[26] Another recent trial studied the regular use of aspirin in reduction of polyp formation and disease progression in patients with high risk of familial adenomatous polyposis.[27] In prospective study of a cohort of 350 people with Barrett's esophagus followed for 20,770 person-months, NSAID use had an effective chemopreventive effect in decreasing the risk of neoplastic progression in Barrett's esophagus.[28]

Several potential pathways were studied that can explain the chemopreventive effect of NSAIDs in malignancy. Aspirin and NSAIDs inhibit the enzyme cyclo-oxygenase (COX) which is involved in the production of prostaglandins and metabolism of arachidonic acid. There are two isoforms of COX with increased COX-2 activity that has been linked to carcinogenesis.[22] There is growing evidence that COX-2 isoform is involved in early stages of intestinal polyp formation. Elevated cellular levels of COX-2 was found in a number of GI malignancies.[29–32] Arachidonic acid is a critical signal for apoptosis. One suggestion is that NSAIDs activates apoptosis by inhibiting the metabolism of arachidonic acid.[33] Another pathway can be the effect of COX-2 in mediating the production of prostaglandins which are involved in DNA synthesis and cell division. Inhibition of prostaglandins production can decrease cell proliferation and reduce cancer formation.[34]

Infections

H. pylori eradication

Helicobacter pylori (*H. pylori*) is a gram-negative, microaerophilic bacteria found in the mucus layer of the inner surface of the gastric epithelium.

It has an enzyme called urease that converts urea to ammonia to neutralize the stomach acid and create a favorable environment for its growth.[35–37] *H. pylori* infection is one of the main causes of peptic ulcer disease which also increases the risk of non-cardia gastric malignancy.[35–38] The International Agency for Research on Cancer has recognized *H. pylori* as a group I carcinogen. In 2008, gastric cancer was the second most common cause of cancer-related deaths in the world.[39] Several epidemiologic studies have shown that infection with *H. pylori* increased the risk of developing gastric adenocarcinoma.[40–42] A large study in Finland, the Alpha-Tocopherol Beta-Carotene cancer prevention study, demonstrated that patients with infected *H. pylori* had 8-fold increased risk of non-cardia gastric cancer.[43]

A toxin produced by the gene named cytoxin-associated gene A (cag A) in the *H. pylori* bacteria changes the gastric cells and provides stable attachment of the bacteria. Persistent exposure to the toxin leads to chronic inflammation. Various strains of *H. pylori* carry the cag A gene.[44] A meta-analysis showed that infection with the cag A-positive strain was associated with twice the risk of non-cardia gastric cancer than patients with the negative strain.[45]

Therefore eradication of *H. pylori* will have the benefit of decreasing the incident of gastric cancer. Two randomized clinical trials in China, a therapy of two weeks of antibiotic treatment for *H. pylori* decreased the prevalence of precancerous gastric lesions.[46,47] Early elimination of the bacteria in patients with peptic ulcer disease decreased the risk of gastric cancer.[48] Although it may not completely eliminate the risk but early treatment in high risk patients can reduce the prevalence.[49] Currently, eight different *H. pylori* treatment regimens are approved by the Food and Drug Administration. The therapy consists of 10 days to 2 weeks of two effective antibiotics, such as amoxicillin, tetracycline, metronidazole, or clarithromycin, plus either ranitidine bismuth citrate, bismuth subsalicylate, or a proton pump inhibitor.

Hepatitis B vaccination

Chronic infection of hepatitis B virus (HBV) and hepatitis C virus (HCV) have become the most significant risk factor for Hepatocellular carcinoma

(HCC) worldwide. In 2010, around 24,000 new cases of HCC and more than 19,000 people died from HCC in the United States.[50] It is one of the lethal malignancies that can be preventable by controlling its risk factor such as hepatitis infection, alcohol intake and metabolic diseases. It is estimated that 380 million people are chronically infected with hepatitis B which is more observed in developing countries.[51] According to the WHO, it is estimated that 500,000 to 700,000 deaths worldwide are caused by chronic disease from HBV infection in 2004.[52]

Fortunately, there is a vaccine for hepatitis B that has been available since 1982. It is recommended that all children and adults at high risk should be vaccinated according to the US Centers for Disease Control and Prevention (CDC). Early vaccination is beneficial as chronic infection rates are as high as 90% in infancy compared to less than 5% in HBV infection acquired in adulthood.[53,54] Several observational studies in Taiwan, Thailand, China and South Africa reviewed the implementation of universal infant vaccination program and its long-term effect. The data demonstrated that HBV vaccine can be considered as a primary prevention of liver cancer.[55–58] The follow-up data from the Taiwan vaccination programs have shown a decrease in the incidence of HCC in children. The average annual incidence of HCC in children 6–14 years of age reduced from 0.70 per 100,000 children between 1981 and 1986 to 0.57 between 1986 and 1990, and drastically to 0.36 per 100,000 between 1990 and 1994.[59] These initiatives of infant vaccination against HBV reveal the significant protection against infection and development of cancer. While vaccination provides a primary prevention, there is also a need to focus on screening of high risk individuals. According to the CDC, high risk people include unprotected sex, multiple sexual partners, having sexually transmitted disease, IV drug user, blood products exposure and on long-term hemodialysis.

Lifestyle Modification

Tobacco use

Smoking is a risk factor for at least 15 different cancer types with risk of progression to cancer about 2.24 times greater for smokers than nonsmokers. The content of tobacco smoke contains several carcinogenic substances such as polycyclic carbohydrates and nicotine. These compounds play a role in formation of carcinogen metabolism that place patients with defective DNA repair and at risk for developing GI malignancies.[60] A study by the American Cancer Society of nearly 185,000 men and women in the CPS II Nutrient Cohort demonstrated increased risk of colorectal cancer in a setting of long-term smoking. Individuals who smoked for 40 years or longer or who did not quit before age 40 had a 30–50% increased risk of developing colorectal cancer.[61] A meta-analysis of 106 observational studies concluded that smoking was associated with an absolute risk increase of 10.8 cases per 100,000 person-years in addition to 6.0 deaths per 100,000 person-years.[62] The estimated proportion of stomach cancer deaths attributable to tobacco use would be 28% in United States men and 14% in women according to the Cancer Prevention Study II.[63] Tobacco is projected to be the most important and preventable cause of disease in the world by the 2020.[64] As it have been shown, it also has a strong association with various malignancies including GI cancers, it is important to promote and educate patients about smoking cessation and the danger of developing tobacco-related malignancies.

Dietary factors

The American Institute of Cancer Research and the World Cancer Research fund estimated that 30–40% of all malignancies are preventable by healthy diets and physical activity.[65] A retrospective study examining the population with attributable risks of esophageal and gastric cancers found that low fruit consumption accounted for 15.3% of esophageal cancer and 19.3% of gastric adenocarcinoma. On the other hand, several epidemiological studies showed that intake of fiber, fatty acids and vitamin D are linked to reduce risk of colon cancer.[66] Several hypotheses have been studied to examine the relationship of diet to progression of colon cancer. Fat digestion can be cytotoxic and become a promoter while fruits of vegetable can act as antioxidants and prevent carcinogenesis.[65,67] Another theory also examined link of insulin resistance and development of colon cancer. Hyperinsulinemia acts as a growth factor and tumor promoter and has been linked to colon cancer promotion. This is also supported by several cohort studies showing that patients with history of diabetes reported higher rate of colon cancer.[68–70] A meta-analysis of 37 studies revealed that increased level of physical activities is associated with 25% reduction in risk of colon cancer. This also supports that hyper-insulinemia can be a risk for cancer development which is less common in subjects who consume a healthy diet and active lifestyle. However, there is a need to study the biological and genetic response to dietary intake. The understanding of cellular process of food components and its molecular targets will help clarify benefit of specific dietary interventions.[71]

Take Home Messages

- The concept of cancer prevention is formulated from studies showing the associations between risk factors and development of cancer. Prevention can target the reduction of cancer incidence and mortality at several frontiers.
- Prevention can start as simple as education of promoting healthy life-style through diet, exercise and smoking cessation while assuring appropriate vaccination and eradication of certain disease associated with cancer progression.
- The application of chemoprevention and following screening and sur-veillance recommendations for high risk patients are essential and cost-effective.

References

1. Cancer, IAfRo, *Colorectal Cancer Estimated Incidence, Mortality and Prevalence Worldwide in 2012*. World Health Organization, 2012.
2. Wang, K.K., Sampliner, R.E., Updated guidelines 2008 for the diagnosis, surveillance and therapy of Barrett's esophagus. *Am J Gastroenterol*, 2008. **103**: 788–97.
3. Evans, J.A., Early, D.S., Fukami, N., Ben-Menachem, T., Chandrasekhara, V. *et al.,* The role of endoscopy in Barrett's esophagus and other premalignant conditions of the esophagus. *Gastrointest Endosc*, 2012. **76**: 1087–94.
4. Siegel, R., Naishadham, D., Jemal, A., Cancer statistics, 2013. *CA*, 2013. **63**: 11–30.

5. Thiis-Evensen, E., Hoff, G.S., Sauar, J., Langmark, F., Majak, B.M. *et al.*, Population-based surveillance by colonoscopy: effect on the incidence of colorectal cancer. Telemark Polyp Study I. *Scand J Gastroenterol*, 1999. **34**: 414–20.
6. Nishihara, R., Wu, K., Lochhead, P., Morikawa, T., Liao, X. *et al.*, Long-term colorectal-cancer incidence and mortality after lower endoscopy. *N Eng J Med*, 2013. **369**: 1095–105.
7. Atkin, W.S., Edwards, R., Kralj-Hans, I., Wooldrage, K., Hart, A.R. *et al.*, Once-only flexible sigmoidoscopy screening in prevention of colorectal cancer: a multicentre randomised controlled trial. *Lancet*, 2010. **375**: 1624–33.
8. Schoen, R.E., Pinsky, P.F., Weissfeld, J.L., Yokochi, L.A., Church, T. *et al.*, Colorectal-cancer incidence and mortality with screening flexible sigmoidoscopy. *N Eng J Med*, 2012. **366**: 2345–57.
9. Segnan, N., Armaroli, P., Bonelli, L., Risio, M., Sciallero, S. *et al.*, Once-only sigmoidoscopy in colorectal cancer screening: follow-up findings of the Italian Randomized Controlled Trial--SCORE. *J Nat Cancer Inst*, 2011. **103**: 1310–22.
10. Lynch, H.T., de la Chapelle, A., Hereditary colorectal cancer. *N Eng J Med*, 2003. **348**: 919–32.
11. Watson, P., Narod, S.A., Fodde, R., Wagner, A., Lynch, J.F. *et al.*, Carrier risk status changes resulting from mutation testing in hereditary non-polyposis colorectal cancer and hereditary breast-ovarian cancer. *J med genet*, 2003. **40**: 591–6.
12. Sporn, M.B., Approaches to prevention of epithelial cancer during the preneoplastic period. *Cancer res*, 1976. **36**: 2699–702.
13. Sachs, G., Shin, J.M., Howden, C.W., Review article: the clinical pharmacology of proton pump inhibitors. *Aliment Pharmacol Ther*, 2006. **23** (Suppl 2): 2–8.
14. Chiba, N., De Gara, C.J., Wilkinson, J.M., Hunt, R.H., Speed of healing and symptom relief in grade, II to IV gastroesophageal reflux disease: a meta-analysis. *Gastroenterology*, 1997. **112**: 1798–810.
15. Hillman, L.C., Chiragakis, L., Shadbolt, B., Kaye, G.L., Clarke, A.C., Effect of proton pump inhibitors on markers of risk for high-grade dysplasia and oesophageal cancer in Barrett's oesophagus. *Aliment Pharmacol Ther*, 2008. **27**: 321–6.
16. Ouatu-Lascar, R., Fitzgerald, R.C., Triadafilopoulos, G., Differentiation and proliferation in Barrett's esophagus and the effects of acid suppression. *Gastroenterology*, 1999. **117**: 327–35.

17. Miyashita, T., Shah, F.A., Marti, G.P., Wang, J., Bonde, P. *et al.,* Rabeprazole impedes the development of reflux-induced esophageal cancer in a surgical rat model. *Digest Dis Sci*, 2011. **56**: 1309–14.
18. Yang, Y.X., Hennessy, S., Propert, K., Hwang, W.T., Sedarat, A. *et al.,* Chronic proton pump inhibitor therapy and the risk of colorectal cancer. *Gastroenterology,* 2007. **133**: 748–54.
19. Genta, R.M., Rindi, G., Fiocca, R., Magner, D.J., D'Amico, D. *et al.,* Effects of 6–12 months of esomeprazole treatment on the gastric mucosa. *Am J Gastroentero,* 2003. **98**: 1257–65.
20. Uemura, N., Okamoto, S., Yamamoto, S., Matsumura, N., Yamaguchi, S. *et al.,* Helicobacter pylori infection and the development of gastric cancer. *N Eng J Med*, 2001. **345**: 784–9.
21. Atherton, J.C., The pathogenesis of Helicobacter pylori-induced gastroduodenal diseases. *Ann Rev Pathol*, 2006. **1**: 63–96.
22. Shaheen, N.J., Straus, W.L., Sandler, R.S., Chemoprevention of gastrointestinal malignancies with nonsteroidal antiinflammatory drugs. *Cancer*, 2002. **94**: 950–63.
23. Giovannucci, E., Rimm, E.B., Stampfer, M.J., Colditz, G.A., Ascherio, A. *et al.,* Aspirin use and the risk for colorectal cancer and adenoma in male health professionals. *Ann Internal Med*, 1994. **121**: 241–6.
24. Thun, M.J., Namboodiri, M.M., Heath, C.W., Jr., Aspirin use and reduced risk of fatal colon cancer. *N Eng J Med*, 1991. **325**: 1593–6.
25. Janne, P.A., Mayer, R.J., Chemoprevention of colorectal cancer. *N Eng J Med*, 2000. **342**: 1960–8.
26. Baron, J.A., Cole, B.F., Sandler, R.S., Haile, R.W., Ahnen, D. *et al.,* A randomized trial of aspirin to prevent colorectal adenomas. *N Eng J Med*, 2003. **348**: 891–9.
27. Burn, J., Bishop, D.T., Chapman, P.D., Elliott, F., Bertario, L. *et al.,* A randomized placebo-controlled prevention trial of aspirin and/or resistant starch in young people with familial adenomatous polyposis. *Cancer preven Res*, 2011. **4**: 655–65.
28. Vaughan, T.L., Dong, L.M., Blount, P.L., Ayub, K., Odze, R.D. *et al.,* Nonsteroidal anti-inflammatory drugs and risk of neoplastic progression in Barrett's oesophagus: a prospective study. *Lancet Oncol*, 2005. **6**: 945–52.
29. Ota, S., Bamba, H., Kato, A., Kawamoto, C., Yoshida, Y. *et al.,* Review article: COX-2, prostanoids and colon cancer. *Aliment Pharmacol Ther,* 2002. **16** (Suppl 2): 102–6.

30. Sano, H., Kawahito, Y., Wilder, R.L., Hashiramoto, A., Mukai, S. *et al.*, Expression of cyclooxygenase-1 and -2 in human colorectal cancer. *Cancer Res*, 1995. **55**: 3785–89.
31. Zimmermann, K.C., Sarbia, M., Weber, A.A., Borchard, F., Gabbert, H.E. *et al.,* Cyclooxygenase-2 expression in human esophageal carcinoma. *Cancer Res*, 1999. **59**: 198–204.
32. Kase, S., Osaki, M., Honjo, S., Hashimoto, K., Adachi, H. *et al.,* Expression of cyclooxygenase-1 and cyclooxygenase-2 in human esophageal mucosa, dysplasia and carcinoma. *Pathobio J Immunopathol Mol Cell Biol*, 2004. **71**: 84–92.
33. Cao, Y., Pearman, A.T., Zimmerman, G.A., McIntyre, T.M., Prescott, S.M., Intracellular unesterified arachidonic acid signals apoptosis. *Proc Nat Acad Sci USA*, 2000. **97**: 11280–5.
34. Fosslien, E., Biochemistry of cyclooxygenase (COX)-2 inhibitors and molecular pathology of, COX-2 in neoplasia. *Crit Rev Clin Lab Sci*, 2000. **37**: 431–502.
35. Hansson, L.E., Nyren, O., Hsing, A.W., Bergstrom, R., Josefsson, S. *et al.,* The risk of stomach cancer in patients with gastric or duodenal ulcer disease. *N Eng J Med*, 1996. **335**: 242–9.
36. Fox, J.G., Wang, T.C., Inflammation, atrophy, and gastric cancer. *J Clini Invest*, 2007. **117**: 60–9.
37. Bourke, B., Sherman, P., Drumm, B., Peptic ulcer disease: what is the role for Helicobacter pylori? *Semin Gastrointestinal Dis*, 1994. **5**: 24–31.
38. Parsonnet, J., Friedman, G.D., Vandersteen, D.P., Chang, Y., Vogelman, J.H. *et al.,* Helicobacter pylori infection and the risk of gastric carcinoma. *N Eng J Med*, 1991. **325**: 1127–31.
39. Ferlay, J., Shin, H.R., Bray, F., Forman, D., Mathers, C. *et al.,* Estimates of worldwide burden of cancer in 2008: GLOBOCAN 2008. *Int J Cancer*, 2010. **127**: 2893–917.
40. de Martel, C., Forman, D., Plummer, M., Gastric cancer: epidemiology and risk factors. *Gastroenterol Clin North Am*, 2013. **42**: 219–40.
41. Walker, A.R., Madden, M.V., Dent, D.M., Gastric cancer. Some aspects of epidemiology, risk factors, treatment and survival. *South African Medi J*, 1987. **72**: 30–3.
42. Brenner, H., Rothenbacher, D., Arndt, V., Epidemiology of stomach cancer. *Meth Mol Biol*, 2009. **472**: 467–77.

43. Kamangar, F., Dawsey, S.M., Blaser, M.J., Perez-Perez, G.I., Pietinen, P. *et al.,* Opposing risks of gastric cardia and noncardia gastric adenocarcinomas associated with Helicobacter pylori seropositivity. *J Nat Cancer Inst*, 2006. **98**: 1445–52.
44. Wen, S., Moss, S.F., Helicobacter pylori virulence factors in gastric carcinogenesis. *Cancer Lett*, 2009. **282**: 1–8.
45. Huang, J.Q., Zheng, G.F., Sumanac, K., Irvine, E.J., Hunt, R.H., Meta-analysis of the relationship between cagA seropositivity and gastric cancer. *Gastroenterology*, 2003. **125**: 1636–44.
46. You, W.C., Brown, L.M., Zhang, L., Li, J.Y., Jin, M.L. *et al.,* Randomized double-blind factorial trial of three treatments to reduce the prevalence of precancerous gastric lesions. *J Nat Cancer Instit*, 2006. **98**: 974–83.
47. Wong, B.C., Lam, S.K., Wong, W.M., Chen, J.S., Zheng, T.T. *et al.,* Helicobacter pylori eradication to prevent gastric cancer in a high-risk region of China: a randomized controlled trial. *JAMA*, 2004. **291**: 187–94.
48. Wu, C.Y., Kuo, K.N., Wu, M.S., Chen, Y.J., Wang, C.B. *et al.,* Early Helicobacter pylori eradication decreases risk of gastric cancer in patients with peptic ulcer disease. *Gastroenterology*, 2009. **137**: 1641–1648 e1641–2.
49. Kabir, S., Effect of Helicobacter pylori eradication on incidence of gastric cancer in human and animal models: underlying biochemical and molecular events. *Helicobacter*, 2009. **14**: 159–71.
50. Jemal, A., Siegel, R., Xu, J., Ward, E., Cancer statistics, 2010. *CA*, 2010. **60**: 277–300.
51. Plymoth, A., Viviani, S., Hainaut, P., Control of hepatocellular carcinoma through hepatitis B vaccination in areas of high endemicity: perspectives for global liver cancer prevention. *Cancer Lett*, 2009. **286**: 15–21.
52. WHO, Hepatitis B vaccines. *Wkly Epidemiol Rec*, 2004. **79**: 255–63.
53. Blum, H.E., Hepatocellular carcinoma: therapy and prevention. World journal of *Gastroenterol*, 2005. **11**: 7391–400.
54. Kudo, M., Management of hepatocellular carcinoma: from prevention to molecular targeted therapy. *Oncology*, 2010. **78** (Suppl 1): 1–6.
55. Chen, D.S., Hsu, N.H., Sung, J.L., Hsu, T.C., Hsu, S.T. *et al.,* A mass vaccination program in Taiwan against hepatitis B virus infection in infants of hepatitis B surface antigen-carrier mothers. *JAMA*, 1987. **257**: 2597–603.

56. Poovorawan, Y., Sanpavat, S., Chumdermpadetsuk, S., Safary, A., Long-term hepatitis B vaccine in infants born to hepatitis B e antigen positive mothers. *Arch Dis Childhood Fetal Neonatal Ed*, 1997. **77**: F47–51.
57. Sun, Z., Zhu, Y., Stjernsward, J., Hilleman, M., Collins, R. *et al.,* Design and compliance of HBV vaccination trial on newborns to prevent hepatocellular carcinoma and 5-year results of its pilot study. *Cancer Detect Prevent*, 1991. **15**: 313–8.
58. Hino, K., Katoh, Y., Vardas, E., Sim, J., Okita, K. *et al.,* The effect of introduction of universal childhood hepatitis B immunization in South Africa on the prevalence of serologically negative hepatitis B virus infection and the selection of immune escape variants. *Vaccine*, 2001. **19**: 3912–8.
59. Chang, M.H., Shau, W.Y., Chen, C.J., Wu, T.C., Kong, M.S. *et al.,* Hepatitis B vaccination and hepatocellular carcinoma rates in boys and girls. *JAMA*, 2000. **284**: 3040–2.
60. Das, S.K., Harmful health effects of cigarette smoking. *Mol Cell Biochem*, 2003. **253**: 159–65.
61. Hannan, L.M., Jacobs, E.J., Thun, M.J., The association between cigarette smoking and risk of colorectal cancer in a large prospective cohort from the United States. *Cancer Epidemio Biomarkers Prevent*, 2009. **18**: 3362–7.
62. Botteri, E., Iodice, S., Bagnardi, V., Raimondi, S., Lowenfels, A.B. *et al.,* Smoking and colorectal cancer: a meta-analysis. *JAMA*, 2008. **300**: 2765–78.
63. Chao, A., Thun, M.J., Jacobs, E.J., Henley, S.J., Rodriguez, C. *et al.,* Cigarette smoking and colorectal cancer mortality in the cancer prevention study, II. *J Nat Cancer Inst*, 2000. **92**: 1888–96.
64. Murray, C.J., Lopez, A.D., Alternative projections of mortality and disability by cause 1990–2020: Global Burden of Disease Study. *Lancet*, 1997. **349**: 1498–504.
65. Glade, M.J., Food, nutrition, and the prevention of cancer: a global perspective. American Institute for Cancer Research/World Cancer Research Fund, American Institute for Cancer Research, 1997. *Nutrition*, 1999. **15**: 523–6.
66. Kim, Y.S., Milner, J.A., Dietary modulation of colon cancer risk. *J Nutrition*, 2007. **137**: 2576S–9S.
67. de Kok, T.M., van Faassen, A., Glinghammar, B., Pachen, D.M., Eng, M.Z. *et al.,* Bile acid concentrations, cytotoxicity, and pH of fecal water from patients with colorectal adenomas. *Digest Dis Sci*, 1999. **44**: 2218–25.

68. Yamada, K., Araki, S., Tamura, M., Sakai, I., Takahashi, Y. *et al.,* Relation of serum total cholesterol, serum triglycerides and fasting plasma glucose to colorectal carcinoma in situ. *Int J Epidemiol*, 1998. **27**: 794–8.
69. Schoen, R.E., Tangen, C.M., Kuller, L.H., Burke, G.L., Cushman, M. *et al.,* Increased blood glucose and insulin, body size, and incident colorectal cancer. *J Nat Cancer Inst*, 1999. **91**: 1147–1154.
70. Kono, S., Honjo, S., Todoroki, I., Nishiwaki, M., Hamada, H. *et al.,* Glucose intolerance and adenomas of the sigmoid colon in Japanese men (Japan). *CCC*, 1998. **9**: 441–6.
71. Wolin, K.Y., Tuchman, H., Physical activity and gastrointestinal cancer prevention. *Recent Results Cancer Res*, 2011. **186**: 73–100.

Chapter 4

Imaging in Gastrointestinal Malignancies

Iva Petkovska, Bobby Kalb and Diego R. Martin

What is New

- Recent advances in medical imaging have allowed for more accurate, noninvasive methods of diagnosis for patients with gastrointestinal malignancies. Magnetic resonance imaging (MRI) in particular has specific strengths with respect to accuracy in initial diagnosis and staging, in comparison with other imaging methods.
- New advances in hardware design and sequence development have allowed MRI to produce high quality imaging even in freely breathing patients, and coverage of large anatomic regions is easily achievable with current technology.

Imaging Modalities

Medical imaging has become essential in the care of patients with gastrointestinal (GI) malignancies, assuming a central role in the diagnosis, staging and therapeutic decision-making for these patients. There has been an impressive evolution of diagnostic imaging methods in recent years, expanding the array of imaging techniques that can be used to analyse GI malignancies. Imaging modalities range from conventional fluoroscopic studies to nuclear medicine techniques to cross-sectional methods based upon ultrasound, computed tomography (CT) or magnetic resonance imaging (MRI). Optimum patient care depends upon an understanding of potential imaging applications and the benefits and risks related to these diagnostic imaging techniques; this is a task made more challenging due to continuing changes in imaging technology.

Ultrasound

Ultrasonography (US) is a non-ionizing technique which produces images in real time. Strengths of US include its safety profile, non-invasive nature, portability and widespread availability, with a lower initial test cost compared to CT or MRI. Additionally, US may be performed in patients with renal failure, as iodinated contrast is not required. However, ultrasound is inherently limited by a lack of sufficient soft tissue contrast to provide reliable sensitivity and specificity for lesion detection and characterization. In addition, image quality is often limited by a patient's body habitus and operator skills. Compared with the latest generation CT and MRI techniques, accurate tumor diagnosis and full body staging (essential components of workup for patients with GI malignancies) cannot be adequately performed with US.

Despite limitations that preclude the use of US as a primary method for imaging-based diagnosis and staging, several selected clinical scenarios remain where US is extremely useful and plays a vital role in the work-up of patients with GI malignancy. Endoscopic ultrasound (EUS) is frequently used for local staging of esophageal, gastric and pancreatic neoplasms. The advantage of EUS is the ability to reliably distinguish the different layers of the upper gastrointestinal (GI) tract and provide a guide for tissue sampling of the primary tumor or adjacent lymph nodes. Endorectal ultrasound may be used for local staging of the depth of bowel wall invasion by rectal carcinoma, again utilizing the ability of US to reliably distinguish different layers within the rectum for assessment of tumor penetration and perirectal spread.[1] However, with both endoscopic and endorectal ultrasound, subsequent cross-sectional imaging is required for a comprehensive assessment of any distant metastases.

Ultrasound is currently the mainstay of surveillance imaging for HCC in CLD at many centers, primarily due to ease of access, lack of ionizing radiation and a relative lower cost compared to CT and MRI. However, reports indicate highly variable sensitivity for the detection of HCC with ultrasound, ranging from 33–96%.[2] Multiple studies have shown a lower detection rate of HCC by ultrasound when compared with CT and MRI.[3] In addition, the sensitivity for the detection of dysplastic nodules and small HCC is poor; regenerative nodules, dysplastic nodules and small HCC may be indistinguishable with sonography. The use of contrast-enhanced ultrasound with microbubbles improves the diagnostic performance of ultrasound for HCC screening, however the use of ultrasound contrast adds both time and cost to the test, and is not yet approved for use in all countries, including the United States.

Computed tomography

In the last several decades, CT has played a pivotal role in the diagnosis and staging of GI malignancies. CT provides excellent spatial resolution imaging, with detailed anatomy of vasculature structures and organ morphology in the abdomen and pelvis. The introduction of multidetector CT systems allows for 0.5 mm resolution imaging that may be acquired in seconds.[4] Dual-energy computed tomography (DECT) is a recent advancement in CT hardware that provides information about how substances behave at different photon energies. The ability to generate virtual unenhanced datasets and the improved detection of iodine-containing substances on low-energy images are promising grounds for continued research and development in DECT. These newer generation CT systems also have the capability to deliver marked reduction in radiation dose to the patient, with maintenance of image quality and speed.

Despite the advantages of CT with regard to imaging speed and spatial resolution, the main limitation inherent to the technology is a relative deficiency of soft tissue contrast in comparison to MRI. CT may reliably differentiate soft tissue, calcium, simple lipid and air; however, differentiation between different soft tissues (such as between liver parenchyma and a tumor) may be challenging, and requires multiphase imaging after the administration of iodinated intravenous contrast to optimize diagnostic sensitivity. Administration of iodinated contrast introduces risks of contrast-induced nephropathy and renal dysfunction, and most patients with background Stage III to Stage V chronic kidney disease are not candidates for iodinated contrast administration. Even with optimized multiphase pre- and post-contrast CT, multiple studies have demonstrated reduced rates of lesion detection and characterization when compared with MRI for many organ systems involved in GI malignancies, especially the liver, bile ducts, prostate, and cystic neoplasms. Moreover, repeated use of CT for follow-up in patients that have received curative therapy raises safety concerns with regard to cumulative X-ray dose effects. The diagnostic benefits of CT should always be weighed against the cancer induction risk of ionizing radiation.

Positron emission tomography-CT

Positron emission tomography (PET)-CT is an imaging methodology that combines metabolic information from ^{18}F-labelled fluorodeoxyglucose (FDG) and the anatomic capabilities of computed tomography. A key feature of many GI malignancies is an increased rate of glucose utilization, which manifests on PET as increased uptake of the FDG tracer. Combining PET imaging with a cross-sectional imaging modality allows for more accurate anatomic localization of the regions of increased FDG uptake. Currently, this anatomic localization is most frequently accomplished with CT, though PET-MRI systems have been recently introduced into clinical use at some centers.

Advantages of PET-CT include a rapid ability to screen the entire body for FDG-avid tumors.[5] There is excellent soft tissue contrast between FDG-avid tumors and non-avid background tissues such as fat and muscle. In addition, a decrease in FDG activity between studies may be considered a biomarker for tumor response to therapy.[6] Disadvantages to PET-CT include reduced sensitivity for tumors that arise in organs that show baseline FDG avidity, such as the liver, kidney and brain. Inflammatory tissues are typically FDG-avid, and this is a common source of false positives for PET-CT. In addition, while PET-CT is excellent for whole body staging and identification of distant sites of disease, it is generally limited in its ability to provide a specific diagnosis of the tumor type.

Magnetic resonance imaging

MRI plays an important role in the diagnosis and staging of many GI malignancies. The primary strength of MRI is its superb soft tissue contrast which allows for reliable detection of tumor, sometimes possible even without the aid of intravenous contrast, relying instead on the intrinsic signal differences between normal soft tissues and tumor. The soft tissue resolution of MRI also allows for more reliable characterization of focal lesions, allowing more accurate distinction of benign from malignant disease, impacting therapeutic decision making with a potential reduced need for invasive tissue sampling/biopsy. A limitation of MRI has been the relative complexity of the image acquisition and decreased availability compared to CT and US; however, newer advances in technology have allowed for more robust imaging with reliable image quality even in sick and freely breathing patients, and an increasing number of tertiary cancer centers rely heavily on MRI to guide management in GI malignancies. For this reason, tumors will be depicted with MRI throughout this chapter to highlight the varied imaging appearance of different GI tumors and to demonstrate the ability of imaging to reliably differentiate between the different malignancies that present in the abdomen and pelvis.

While MR imaging protocols have the potential to be complex and widely varied, we have advocated a simplified, uniform protocol that may be applied to multiple indications, including tumor assessment and staging of the liver, pancreas and bowel. This protocol consists of dynamic contrast-enhanced T1-weighted (T1W) multiphase imaging which allows for assessment of tumor perfusion patterns that may be indicative of certain tumor histologies. Arterial phase images are acquired at an 8–10 s delay from the bolus trigger point, venous phase imaging is initiated at 70 s and delayed phase imaging at 180 s after the trigger point. Motion insensitive T2-weighted (T2W) sequences are the second major component of this simplified imaging protocol, providing an alternate method of tissue interrogation which helps drive up specificity of diagnosis, especially to more reliably differentiate metastases from benign entities such as cysts and hemangiomas. Magnetic resonance cholangiopancreatography (MRCP) techniques are T2W sequences that provide excellent visibility of the bile duct morphology, and are helpful in tumor diagnosis and presurgical planning of tumors involving the bile ducts. Finally, diffusion weighted imaging (DWI) is an additional noncontrast technique that has the potential to improve sensitivity for small malignant lesions in certain tumor subtypes, especially related to pancreatic neoplasms.

Liver

Hepatocellular carcinoma

Hepatocellular carcinoma (HCC) is the most common primary malignant tumor of the liver and most frequently occurs in the setting of background chronic liver disease. Multiple studies have demonstrated the superior sensitivity and specificity of MRI to either CT or US for detection and characterization of HCC,[7] particularly for smaller (1–2 cm in size) tumors (84% with MRI vs. 47% with CT).[8,9] Our own recent analysis of liver explant pathology versus prospective MRI staging of HCC demonstrated 97% sensitivity and 100% specificity for the detection of HCC.[10] HCC may manifest as a single focal tumor, as multifocal tumor, or with a poorly defined infiltrative growth pattern. MR imaging is a highly accurate diagnostic method for the pretransplant evaluation of HCC, and the United Network for Organ Sharing no longer requires biopsy confirmation and accepts MRI for staging disease in patients listed for liver transplantation.[11]

Imaging: HCC has a varied appearance on pre-contrast T1W images, and may present as hypointense, isointense or hyperintense to background liver parenchyma. On dynamic postcontrast imaging, HCC displays a characteristic pattern of arterial-phase enhancement with subsequent washout on delayed contrast-enhanced phases, with development of a peripheral capsule on delayed phase images (Fig. 1).[12] DWI is of questionable utility for HCC and may be normal or show only slightly elevated signal in many cases.

HCC may also present as a diffuse, infiltrative pattern of disease that may not form a focal lesion despite an extensive burden of tumor.[13] This aggressive form of HCC has a special propensity to invade the portal and hepatic veins, and the presence of tumor thrombus may be assessed on both contrast-enhanced and noncontrast images. Other distinct

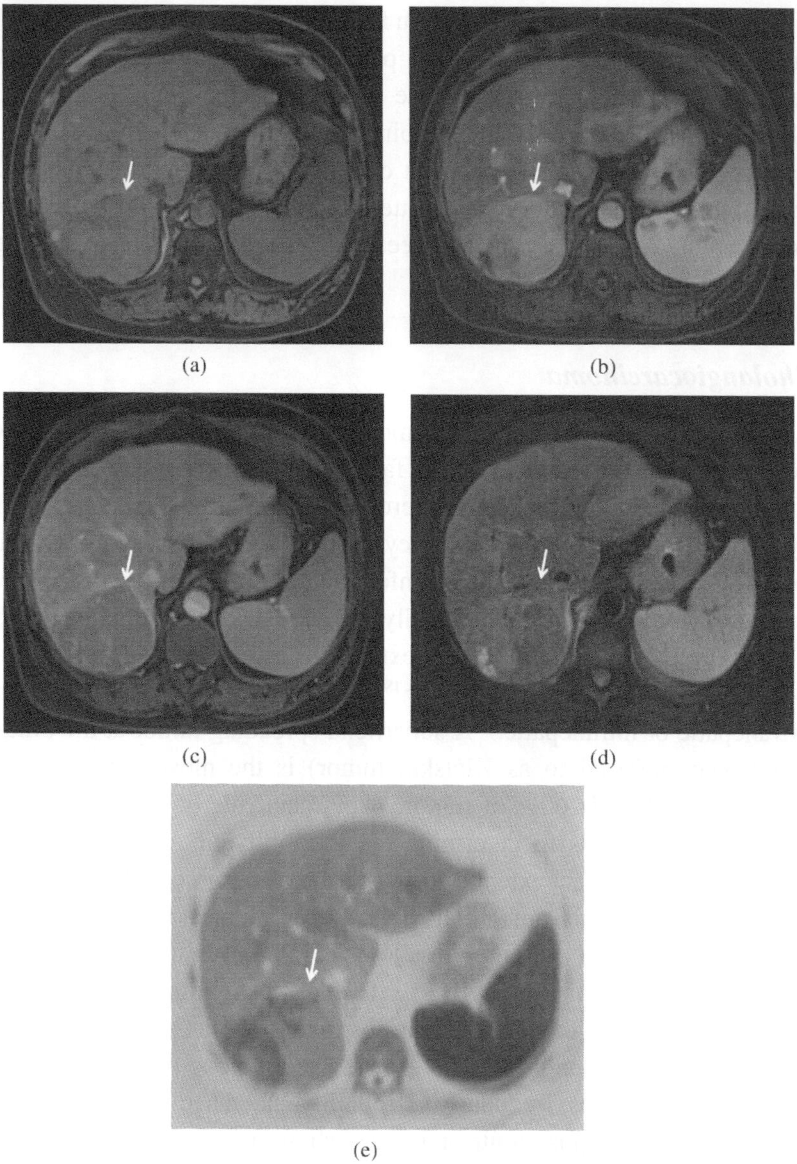

Fig. 1. 52-year-old male with hepatocellular carcinoma. Precontrast (a) and postcontrast T1-weighted (T1W) arterial phase (b) and delayed phase (c) images show an arterial enhancing tumor with washout (arrows, a–c), features that are characteristic of HCC. There is variable signal intensity on T2-weighted (T2W) (d) and diffusion-weighted (DWI) (e) sequences, which are less reliable than dynamic, T1W postcontrast sequences for detection of focal HCC.

enhancement patterns may be seen in HCC, including rare cases of rapidly progressive HCC that may occur in patients with underlying hepatitis C, and may show characteristic intense ring enhancement on initial MRI.[14] There are reported cases of combined HCC and cholangiocarcinoma (cholangiocellular tumor) that most commonly present as a single mass with high T2 signal and a mixed pattern of enhancement, with regions of tumor that show varying degrees of arterial and also delayed enhancement.[15]

Cholangiocarcinoma

Cholangiocarcinoma (CCA) is the most common primary malignancy of the biliary tree.[16,17] A number of risk factors are associated with cholangiocarcinoma, including primary sclerosing cholangitis (PSC), recurrent pyogenic cholangitis, choledochal cysts, Caroli's disease, clonorchiasis, toxins such as thorotrast, and viral infections, although most patients have no known risk factors.[18] Histologically, CCA is an adenocarcinoma arising from the bile duct epithelium, and extensive desmoplastic fibrous stroma is a defining feature of this tumor.[18,19] CCA are classified as perihilar, extrahepatic or intrahepatic.[15] A superficial spreading tumor at the biliary confluence (referred to as Klatskin tumor) is the most common form and accounts for 50–60% of tumors. The main role of imaging beyond accurate diagnosis is to determine the feasibility of resection through assessment of the local extent of disease, and also for staging.

Imaging: Superficial spreading cholangiocarcinomas (whether perihilar or extrahepatic) may present with a low volume of tumor, but are readily identified by the typical pattern of bile duct obstruction on MRCP and T2W sequences. At the site of duct obstruction, soft tissue is identified which demonstrates an infiltrative growth pattern along the bile ducts and into periductal tissues, frequently surrounding and narrowing hepatic vasculature. Dynamic post-contrast images show a progressive pattern of delayed contrast enhancement, and T2W images show the tumor to be variably hypointense, features that are reflective of the fibrotic component of the tumor (Fig. 2). MRCP sequences aid in global assessment of the biliary tree, demonstrating the length of biliary stricture and also the severity of bile duct dilatation. In the preoperative evaluation of hilar

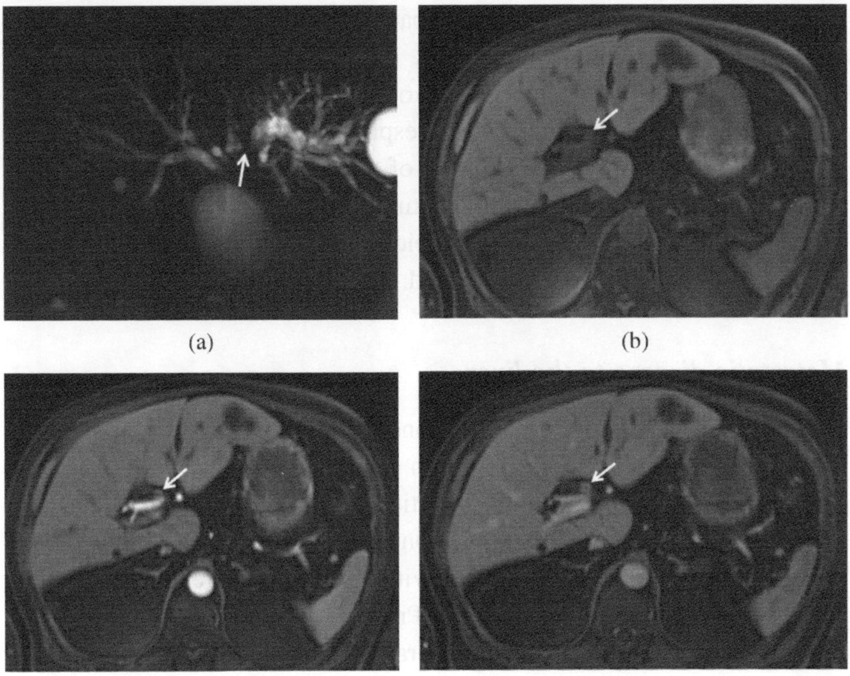

(a) (b) (c) (d)

Fig. 2. 69-year-old male with superficial spreading hilar cholangiocarcinoma. Magnetic resonance cholangiopancreatography (MRCP) image (a) demonstrates dilated intrahepatic ducts with stricture in the region of the liver hilum (arrow). Precontrast (b), arterial (c) and delayed phase (d) postcontrast T1W images demonstrate progressive, delayed enhancement of the obstructing soft tissue (arrows, b–d), a feature typical of adenocarcinomas.

cholangiocarcinoma, the addition of DWI may improve sensitivity in the evaluation of tumor extent.[20] Associated imaging findings of cholangiocarcinoma are hepatic lobar or segmental atrophy, encasement of hepatic vessels and capsular retraction. Criteria for unresectability include: (1) infiltration of tumor beyond the second-order bile duct branches in both lobes of the liver; (2) invasion into major vessels; (3) lymph node metastases beyond regional nodes; and (4) distant metastases.[21]

In distinction from the superficial spreading type, intrahepatic cholangiocarcinoma typically presents as a large intrahepatic tumor. On precontrast T1W sequences, intrahepatic cholangiocarcinoma is hypointense to the liver parenchyma, and on dynamic post-contrast images demonstrates a heterogeneous pattern of delayed enhancement that is typical of adenocarcinomas (Fig. 3).[18,19] Despite the intrahepatic location, these tumors typically show some degree of segmental bile duct obstruction, which is a potential distinguishing feature from metastatic adenocarcinoma to the liver. These tumors do not typically cause duct obstruction unless they are very large or centrally located.

Metastatic disease to the liver

Evaluation of hepatic metastases is one of the most common indications for liver MRI. The liver is a common site for metastatic disease because of its dual blood supply from the hepatic artery and portal vein. Metastases are the most common malignant lesion seen in the liver.[22] Accurate detection and diagnosis of metastases is vital for staging, treatment planning and monitoring of GI malignancies. Primarily due to its strengths in soft tissue resolution, MRI has been generally found to be superior to CT for the detection and characterization of metastatic disease.[23]

Imaging: Metastases from GI malignancies are typically hypointense on precontrast T1W images compared to background liver parenchyma, secondary to replacement of hepatic tissue with malignant cells. Some metastases may demonstrate intrinsically elevated T1 signal due to the presence of substances such as blood products, proteinaceous material and/or melanin.[24,25] Hemorrhagic metastases may be seen with colon, thyroid, breast, lung, renal, testicular and choriocarcinoma.[26] The dynamic enhancement pattern of hepatic metastases depends on the primary tumor, and may exhibit either hypervascular or hypovascular patterns of enhancement.[27–30] Hypervascular metastases will exhibit arterial enhancement with variable degrees of washout on delayed phase images;[30,31] this is a pattern frequently seen with carcinoid, melanoma, thyroid, renal, and breast carcinomas.[30] Hypovascular metastases will demonstrate a heterogeneous pattern of progressive, delayed enhancement, which is seen with the majority of GI adenocarcinomas including colon, pancreas and stomach.[30] Poorly vascularized metastases will also demonstrate a rim of perilesional enhancement, a typical feature of these malignancies.[29,32] Tumors demonstrating post-treatment changes will have alterations in this perfusion pattern with

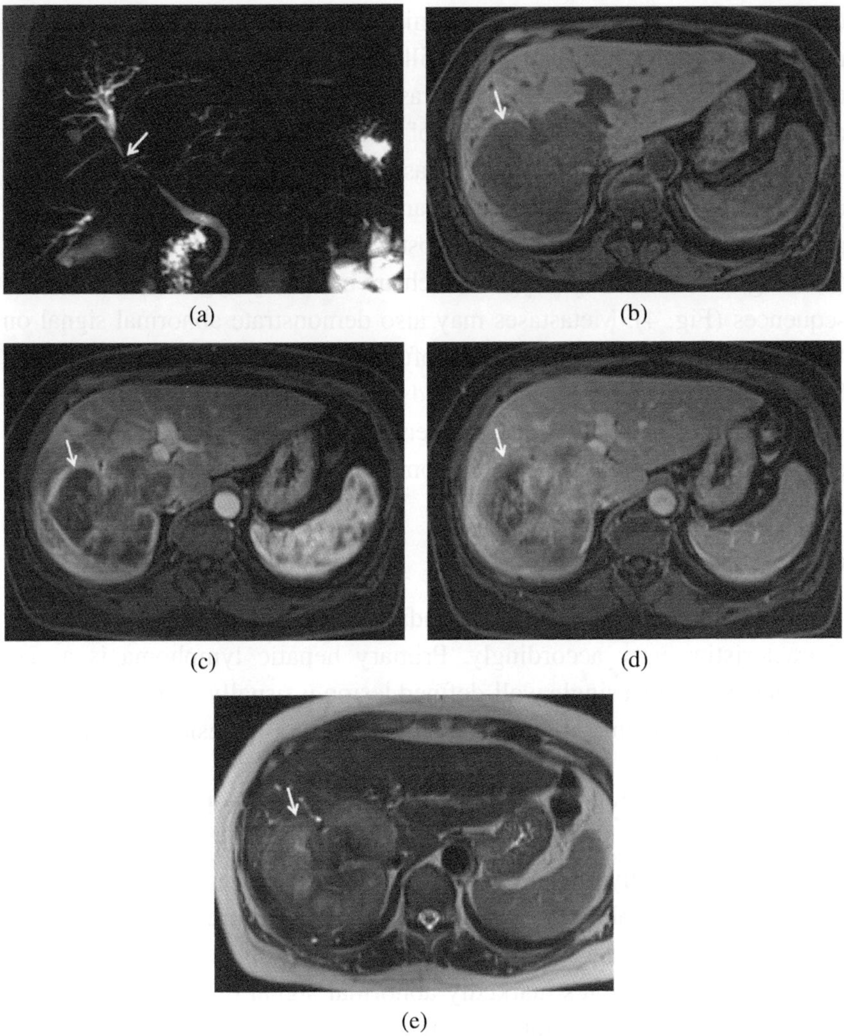

Fig. 3. 64-year-old male with intrahepatic cholangiocarcinoma. MRCP image (a) demonstrates long segment narrowing of an intrahepatic bile duct in the right hepatic lobe (arrow), with more peripherally dilated intrahepatic ducts. Precontrast T1W image (arrow, b) demonstrates tumor to be hypointense to background liver parenchyma. Arterial (c) and delayed phase (d) images show heterogeneous delayed enhancement in the tumor (arrows, c–d), a pattern typical for adenocarcinoma. Variable, heterogeneous signal intensity is noted on T2W image (e).

decreased enhancement on dynamic post-contrast imaging, though residual microscopic disease may still be identified at the time of resection.[33] New, liver specific, MRI contrast agents have been used in the preoperative setting for the assessment of small colorectal liver metastases.[34]

On T2W sequences, hepatic metastases are heterogeneous and show only mildly increased signal compared to background normal hepatic parenchyma, in contrast to the most common benign hepatic lesions (hemangiomas and simple cysts) which are markedly hyperintense on T2W sequences (Fig. 4). Metastases may also demonstrate abnormal signal on DWI sequences, which may be helpful for optimized detection of small lesions. However, any lesion identified on DWI must be fully characterized in terms of its dynamic perfusion pattern and T2 signal to provide a specific diagnosis and differentiate benign from malignant lesions.

Hepatic lymphoma

The liver may be a primary or secondary site of lymphoma, and imaging characteristics vary accordingly. Primary hepatic lymphoma is a rare malignancy,[35] and a single well-defined lesion is usually seen.[36] In secondary hepatic lymphoma, multiple or diffuse infiltrating lesions are typically present.[36]

Imaging: Focal lymphomatous involvement of the liver demonstrates hypointense signal on pre-contrast T1W images relative to the liver. Lymphoma typically demonstrates a uniform pattern of delayed enhancement, though variable areas of heterogeneity may be present. T2W images show mildly elevated T2 signal (similar to normal splenic tissue). Of note, lymphoma demonstrates markedly abnormal signal on DWI, which may be helpful for characterization of these lesions[35–38] (Fig. 5). Secondary hepatic involvement with lymphoma is typically associated with lymphadenopathy.[39]

Hemagioendothelioma

Hepatic epithelioid hemangioendothelioma (HEH) is a rare, low-grade malignant tumor arising from the vascular endothelial cells of the liver.[40–42] HEH has variable patterns of presentation, and may demonstrate diffuse, multifocal, or solitary nodular forms.

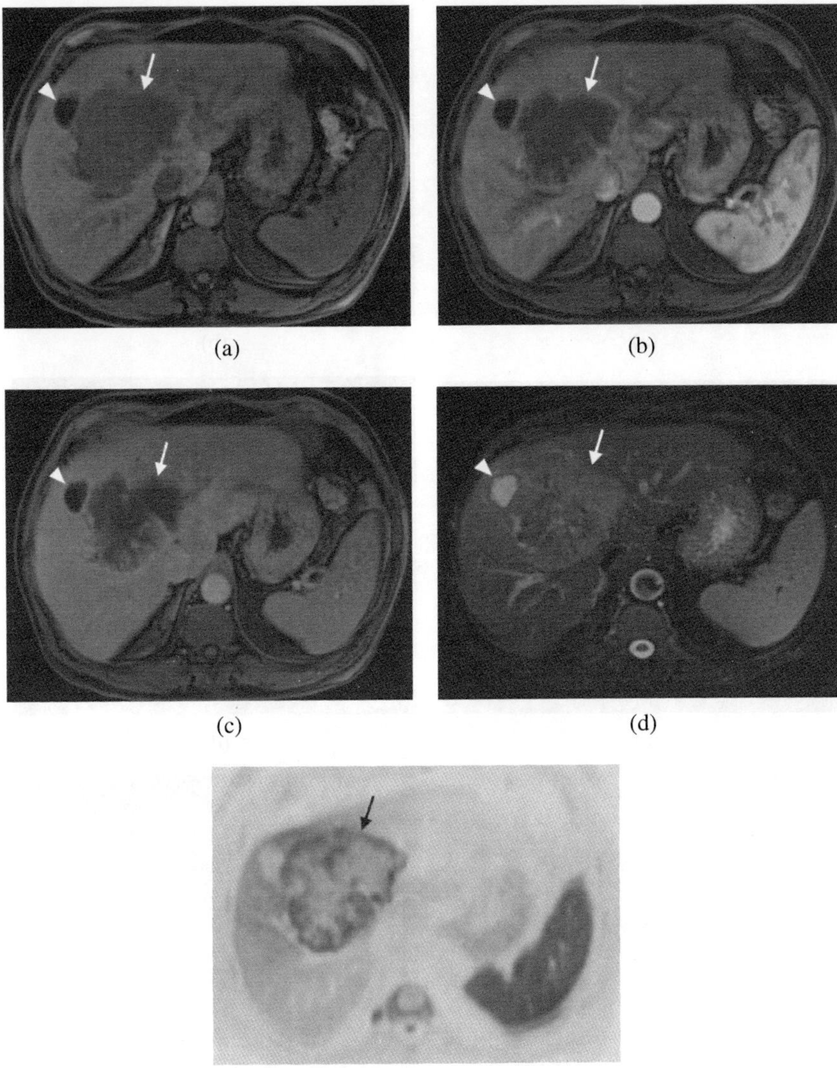

(a) (b) (c) (d) (e)

Fig. 4. 70-year-old male with metastatic colonic adenocarcinoma to the liver. The metastasis is hypointense on precontrast T1W image (arrow, a), while arterial (b) and delayed phase (c) postcontrast images show heterogeneous, delayed enhancement (arrows, b–c). Fat saturated T2W image (d) shows heterogeneous signal and ill-defined margins (arrow). Metastases demonstrate restricted diffusion on DWI images (arrow, e). Note in this case the adjacent, simple benign hepatic cyst/bile duct hamartoma, which shows well-defined borders, no internal enhancement and markedly elevated signal on T2W images (arrowheads, a–d).

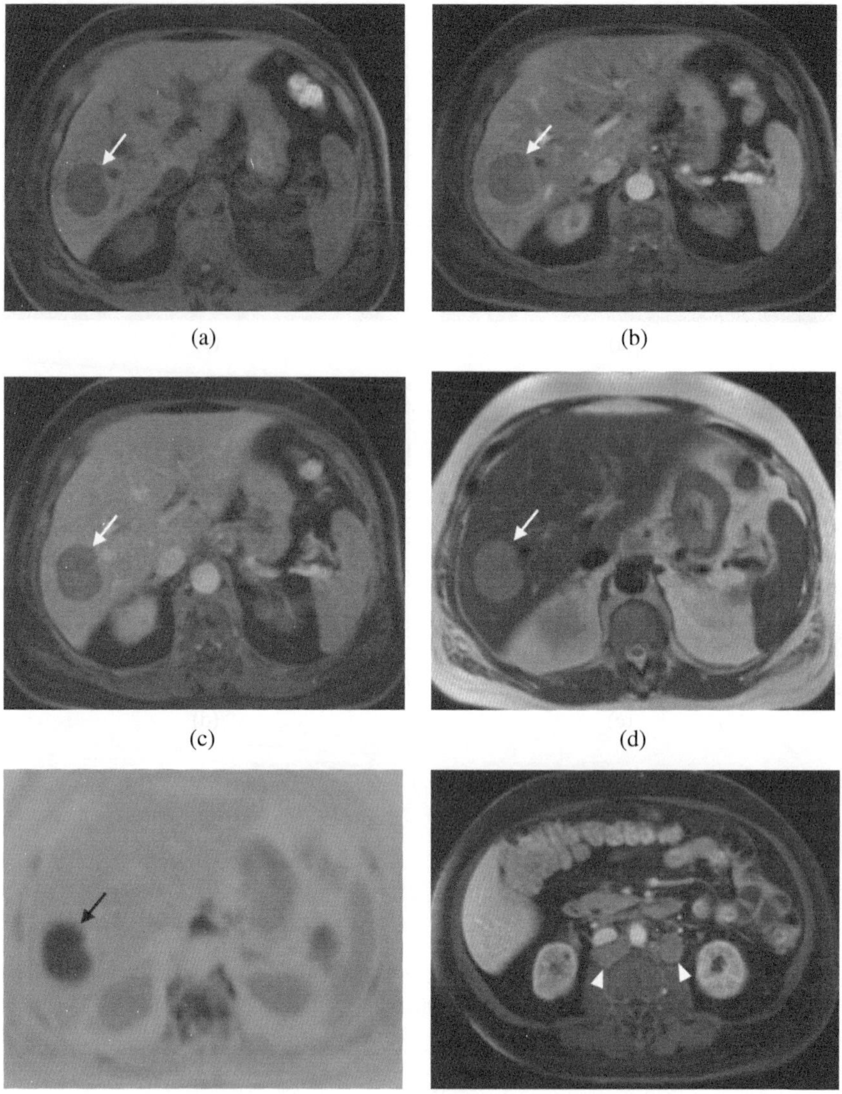

Fig. 5. 67-year-old female with hepatic lymphoma. Focal hepatic lymphoma (arrows, a–e) demonstrates hypointense signal on T1W precontrast images (a) relative to the liver. The tumor demonstrates uniform delayed enhancement on arterial (b) and delayed (c) phase postcontrast images. Lymphoma is hyperintense on T2W images (d) compared to normal background liver and shows restricted diffusion on DWI images (e). Note associated lymphadenopathy in the retroperitoneum on postcontrast images (arrowheads, f).

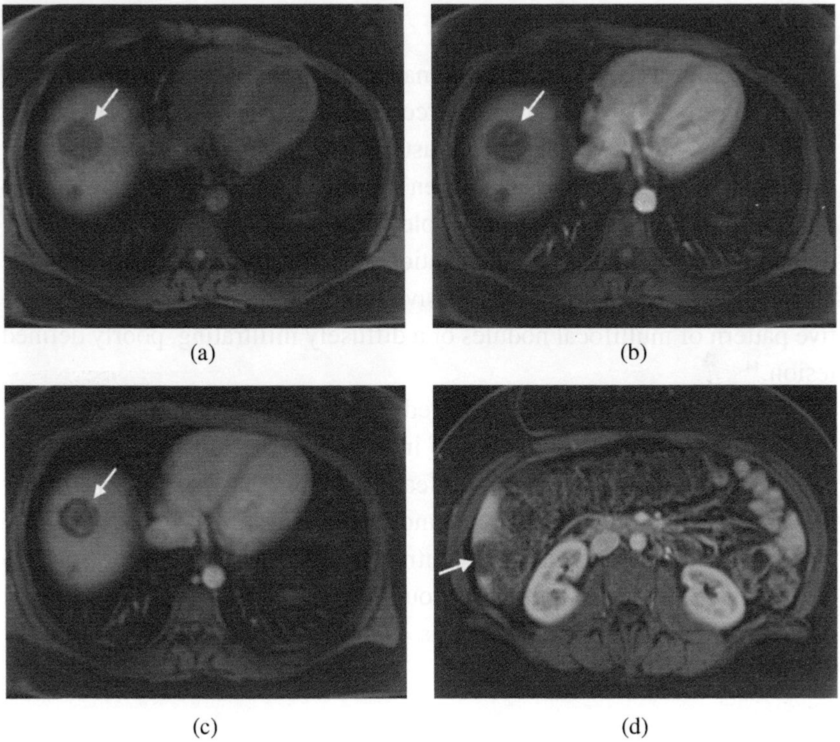

Fig. 6. 26-year-old female with hepatic hemangioendothelioma (HEH). Pre-contrast T1W image (a) demonstrates a focal hepatic lesion hypointense to the background liver (arrow). Arterial (b) and delayed (c) phase postcontrast images demonstrate a "target" appearance (arrows, b-c) that is frequently described with HEH. Capsular retraction (arrow, d) is an additional characteristic feature of this lesion.

Imaging: The most common presentation of HEH is multifocal nodular lesions with a predilection for peripheral subcapsular growth.[40–42] Each tumor is hypointense on T1W sequences, and heterogeneously hyperintense to the liver on T2W images. A potential distinguishing feature of HEH is a prominent, target-like appearance of some lesions.[40–42] Dynamic post-contrast sequences demonstrate this "target appearance," with a thick peripheral rim showing gradual enhancement on delayed phase images, reported as a "halo sign."[40] Nodular confluence of lesions and capsular retraction are characteristic imaging features frequently reported[40–42] (Fig. 6).

Hepatic angiosarcoma

Angiosarcoma is a very rare malignant tumor of the liver, and the most common primary mesenchymal sarcoma of the liver.[43] Angiosarcoma is associated with exposure to thorotrast, arsenic, radiation, hemochromatosis and also with von Recklinghausen's disease.[43] Clinical features associated with angiosarcoma include splenic metastases, thrombocytopenia, disseminated intravascular coagulation (DIC), and hemolytic anemia.[44] Hepatic angiosarcoma is an aggressive tumor, and presents as an infiltrative pattern of multifocal nodules or a diffusely infiltrating, poorly defined lesion.[44]

Imaging: Angiosarcoma is predominately hypointense on T1W images, though with focal areas of increased signal due to intratumoral haemorrhage, which is a common feature of this malignancy. The tumor is markedly heterogeneous with moderately elevated signal on T2W sequences.[44] On dynamic, post-contrast imaging, the enhancement pattern is markedly heterogeneous, though avidly enhancing tumor will be present on arterial-phase images as a marker of the vascular nature of this tumor (Fig. 7).[44]

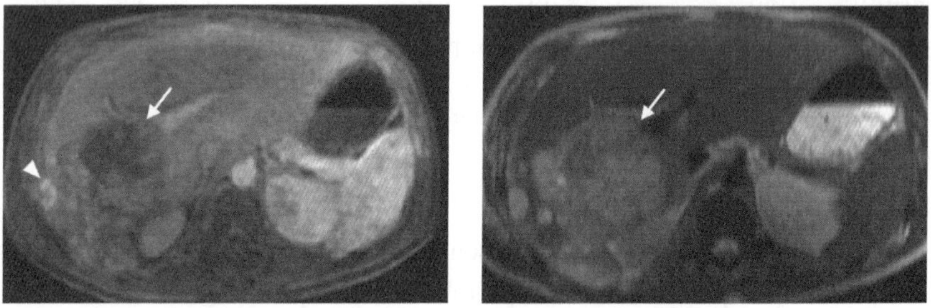

(a) (b)

Fig. 7. 27-year-old male with hepatic angiosarcoma. While the images are degraded by breathing motion artifact, there is a large, heterogeneous tumor present in the right hepatic lobe (arrows, a–b). Arterial phase images (a) show nodular, well-vascularized foci of tumor (arrowhead, a) in keeping with a vascular malignancy. T2W image again shows the heterogeneous appearance of the tumor (arrow, b) and an aggressive growth pattern, with multiple smaller satellite nodules.

Biliary cystadenoma/Cystadenocarcinoma

Biliary cystadenoma (BCA) is a rare cystic hepatic neoplasm with premalignant potential that originates from the biliary system and has a characteristic pattern of surrounding ovarian stroma on histologic analysis.[45–48] BCAs are classified as mucinous cystic neoplasms in the World Health Organization classification of biliary tumors,[49] and these neoplasms are seen almost exclusively in female patients.

Imaging: T2W imaging is the mainstay of diagnosis for BCA, and demonstrates a characteristic pattern of neoplastic septations (Fig. 8). The

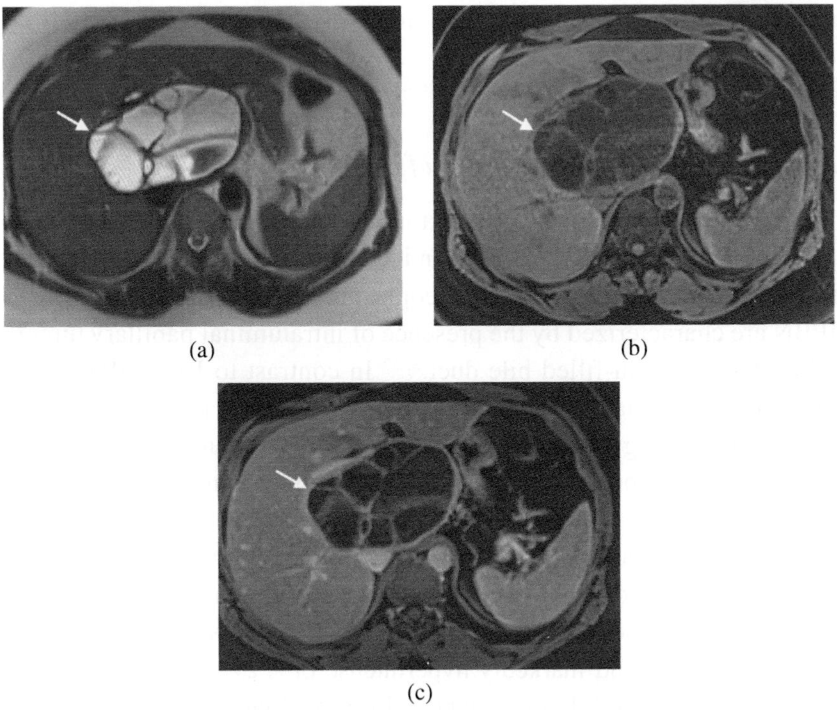

Fig. 8. 35-year-old female with biliary cystadenoma. T2W image (a) demonstrates a markedly complex hepatic cyst with multiple internal septations (arrow, a). Precontrast (b) and postcontrast (c) T1W images show enhancement of the thickened septations (arrows, b–c), but no mural nodularity is identified. Surgical resection demonstrated a biliary cystadenoma.

fluid within BCA is typically hypointense on T1W sequences, and the thickened septations will enhance on dynamic, post-contrast images. Any nodular enhancement associated with these lesions will then categorize the cyst as a biliary cystadenocarcinoma (BCCA).[45–48] While imaging may not reliably differentiate BCA from BCCA with small volume of carcinoma (especially carcinoma *in situ*), BCA is a surgical lesion due to its malignant potential. MRI is the best test to reliably differentiate BCA/BCCA from other benign hepatic cystic entities such as biliary hamartomas (BDH),[46] which may bleed, become quite complex and form a confusing picture on clinical presentation and even pathologic analysis. Given the difference in surgical management between BDH (which may be treated with laparoscopic fenestration) and BCA (which requires hepatic resection), accurate preoperative diagnosis is critical to optimized management.

Intraductal papillary neoplasm of the bile duct

Intraductal papillary neoplasms of the bile ducts (IPNB) are an uncommon variant of bile duct cancer, and share histologic and clinical features with intraductal papillary neoplasms (IPMN) of the pancreas.[50] IPBN are characterized by the presence of intraluminal papillary tumors in a dilated, mucin-filled bile duct.[51,52] In contrast to BCA, IPNB may present in both male and female patients. However, like BCA, IPBNs carry risk of progression to invasive carcinoma (if not present at the time of initial presentation) and should be treated with surgical resection.[50]

Imaging: Similar to BCA, the internal cystic architecture of IPNB is best characterized on MRI with T2W sequences, and the cystic lesion will show communication with an adjacent bile duct.[51,52] IPNB are hypointense on T1W images, and markedly hyperintense on T2W images due to the fluid component. Solid components with a papillary growth pattern are common and show delayed enhancement on dynamic, contrast-enhanced sequences[51,52] (Fig. 9).

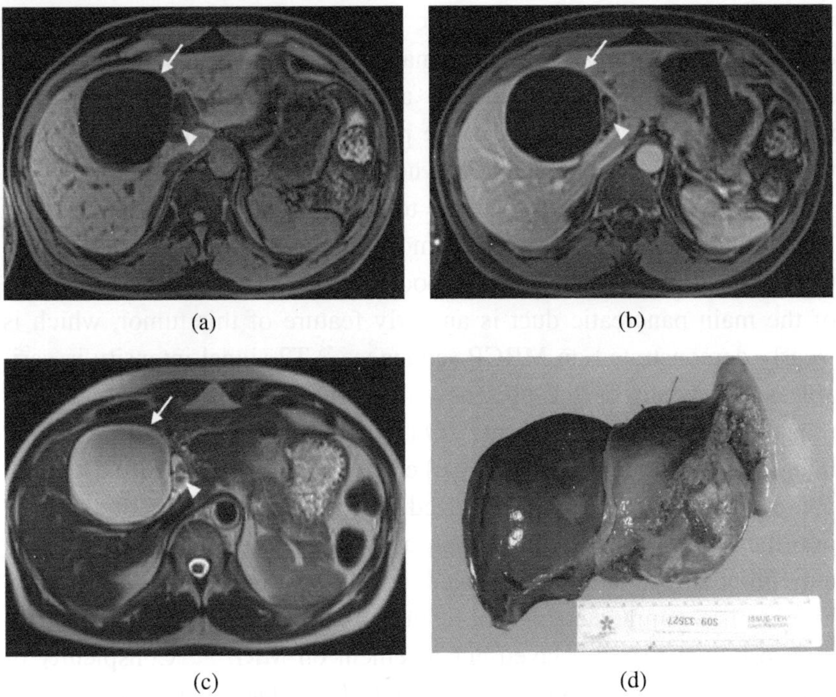

Fig. 9. 56-year-old male with intraductal papillary neoplasm of the bile duct (IPNB). Pre (a) and postcontrast T1W images (b) and T2W image (c) demonstrate a complex cystic lesion (arrows, a–c) with an enhancing nodule (arrowheads, a–c) along the medial margin. The lack of multiple internal septations on T2W imaging and the male sex of the patient is more in keeping with IPNB as opposed to BCA. Surgical pathology specimen (d) demonstrated the large complex cyst along the undersurface of the left hepatic lobe, and final pathology was in keeping with IPNB.

Pancreas

Pancreatic duct adenocarcinoma

Pancreatic duct adenocarcinoma (PDCA) is the most common form of pancreatic malignancy. Most PDCA occur in the head of the pancreas (75%), while a minority are found in the body (15%) and tail (10%). Mortality from PDCA is exceedingly high, with a five-year survival rate of approximately 6%.[53] Surgical resection is the only therapy with a potential for curative intent in non-metastatic disease, thus accurate preoperative diagnosis and staging is key to management of these patients. MRI has high sensitivity for the detection and characterization of pancreatic tumors,[54] and is a useful tool in the preoperative imaging of PDCA and triaging patients into resectable and nonresectable disease.[54]

Imaging: PDCA is hypointense to background normal pancreas on T1W imaging. PDCA typically demonstrates an infiltrative growth pattern, presenting as an ill-defined, poorly marginated tumor. Obstruction of the main pancreatic duct is an early feature of this tumor, which is clearly demonstrated on MRCP sequences.[55] T2 signal intensity is variable and depends on the presence of potential tumor necrosis, hemorrhage, inflammation and fibrosis. On dynamic post-contrast T1 dynamic imaging, PDCA demonstrates marked hypoenhancement in the arterial phase due to its poorly vascularized nature. Intravenous contrast leaks into the tumor interstitium through a disorganized tumor capillary system, producing a pattern of delayed, progressive enhancement (Fig. 10). Fibrosis is a common coexistent feature of this tumor which also contributes to its pattern of delayed enhancement on MRI.[54–57] Conspicuity of PDCA is often optimum in the arterial phase due to the hypovascular nature of the tumor contrasting with the well-vascularized background pancreatic parenchyma.[56] We have also shown that small, well-differentiated pancreatic adenocarcinomas enhance more than poorly differentiated tumors on early-phase contrast-enhanced images.[58] DWI may also be helpful to aid in the detection of small tumors or small hepatic metastases.

Pancreaticoduodenectomy (Whipple procedure) is the only potential cure for malignant tumors involving the head of the pancreas. MRI provides accurate distinction between resectable and unresectable disease,[54,56,57,59] and routine use of preoperative MRI for PDCA staging has been shown to obviate the need for routine staging laparoscopy.[59] Detection of metastases and nodal involvement is crucial for proper staging and treatment planning. MRI is particularly strong in assessment of peritoneal tumor involvement, showing improved sensitivity relative to CT in detection of subcentimeter peritoneal implants;[60] the addition of DWI to routine MRI protocols may improve the sensitivity of detection of nodal and peritoneal involvement.[61–63]

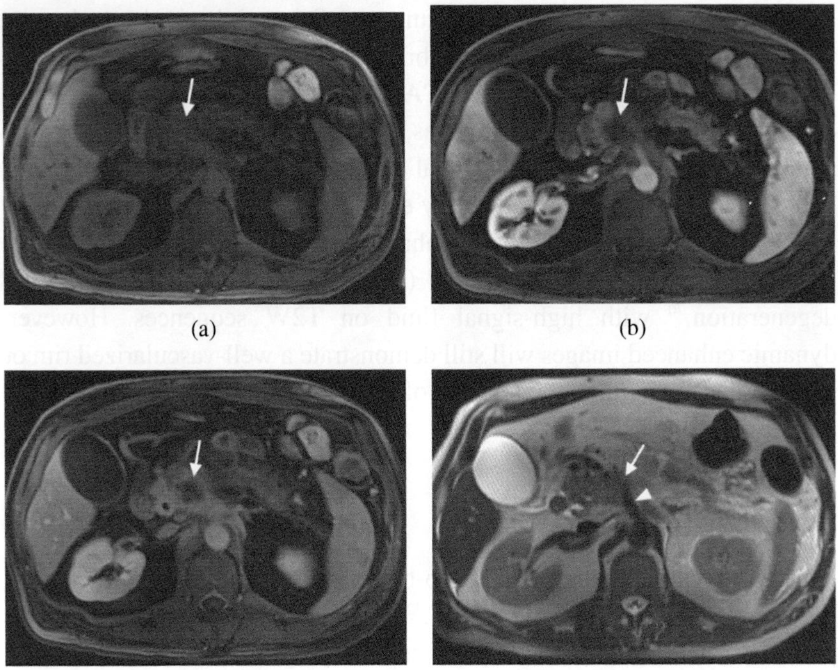

(a) (b)

(c) (d)

Fig. 10. 52-year-old male with pancreatic adenocarcinoma. Pre-contrast (a), arterial (b) and delayed (c) postcontrast T1W images demonstrate a poorly vascularized, ill-defined pancreatic tumor (arrows, a–c) with a pattern of heterogeneous, delayed enhancement. T2W image (d) demonstrates infiltrative tissue (arrow) surrounding the superior mesenteric artery (arrowhead), excluding this patient from surgical resection.

Neuroendocrine tumor of the pancreas

Neuroendocrine tumors (NET) are the second most common primary malignancy of the pancreas,[64,65] and imaging plays an important role in localization and staging.[66–69] NETs may be functional (associated with varying hormone secreting syndromes), or nonfunctional;[64,65] when nonfunctional, NET will usually present as a large tumor.[66–69] The most common functional NET of the pancreas is insulinoma,[65] followed by gastrinoma.[64,65] NET may also be seen in a variety of genetic conditions, such as multiple endocrine neoplasia type 1 (MEN-1), which is usually associated with nonfunctioning tumors. Other inherited syndromes include Von-Hippel Lindau, neurofibromatosis and tuberous sclerosis.[65]

Imaging: In distinction from PDCA, NETs of the pancreas are well circumscribed tumors. On T1W images, NETs are hypointense, contrasting well with the background high signal pancreatic parenchyma. T2 signal is variable, and is typically moderately elevated.[66–69] Dynamic, post-contrast images demonstrate intense early enhancement which may be homogeneous, ring-like or heterogeneous.[66–69] (Fig. 11). NET may undergo cystic degeneration,[70] with high-signal fluid on T2W sequences. However, dynamic enhanced images will still demonstrate a well-vascularized rim or internal nodularity that is indicative of a neoplastic process. DWI may aid in detection of NET.[71]

Pancreatic lymphoma

Pancreatic lymphoma is a B-cell sub-type of non-Hodgkin lymphoma and may be either primary or secondary.[72,73] Isolated primary pancreatic lymphoma is rare, while secondary pancreatic lymphoma is associated with extensive lymphadenopathy. Chemotherapy is effective in long-term disease regression or remission, and surgery is not required in most cases.[72,73] Imaging is an important biomarker to assess extent of disease and response to therapy.

Imaging: Similar to other solid pancreatic tumors, pancreatic lymphoma is hypointense on T1W sequences. T2 signal is moderately elevated, homogeneous and appears similar to normal splenic tissue.[72,73] Dynamic post-contrast images show a homogeneous pattern of delayed enhancement.[72,73] Lymphoma may cause obstruction of the main pancreatic duct, however typically to a lesser extent than PDCA.[74] As with other examples of lymphomatous infiltration, DWI is highly sensitive to nodal tissue and may aid in evaluation of tumor extent in the pancreas[75] (Fig. 12).

Acinar cell carcinoma of the pancreas

Acinar cell carcinoma is a rare pancreatic neoplasm, representing 1% of exocrine tumors. While malignant, acinar cell tumors have improved survival rates compared to PDCA.[76–78] Acinar cell carcinomas may show tumor-associated secretion of lipase, which produces a tumor specific

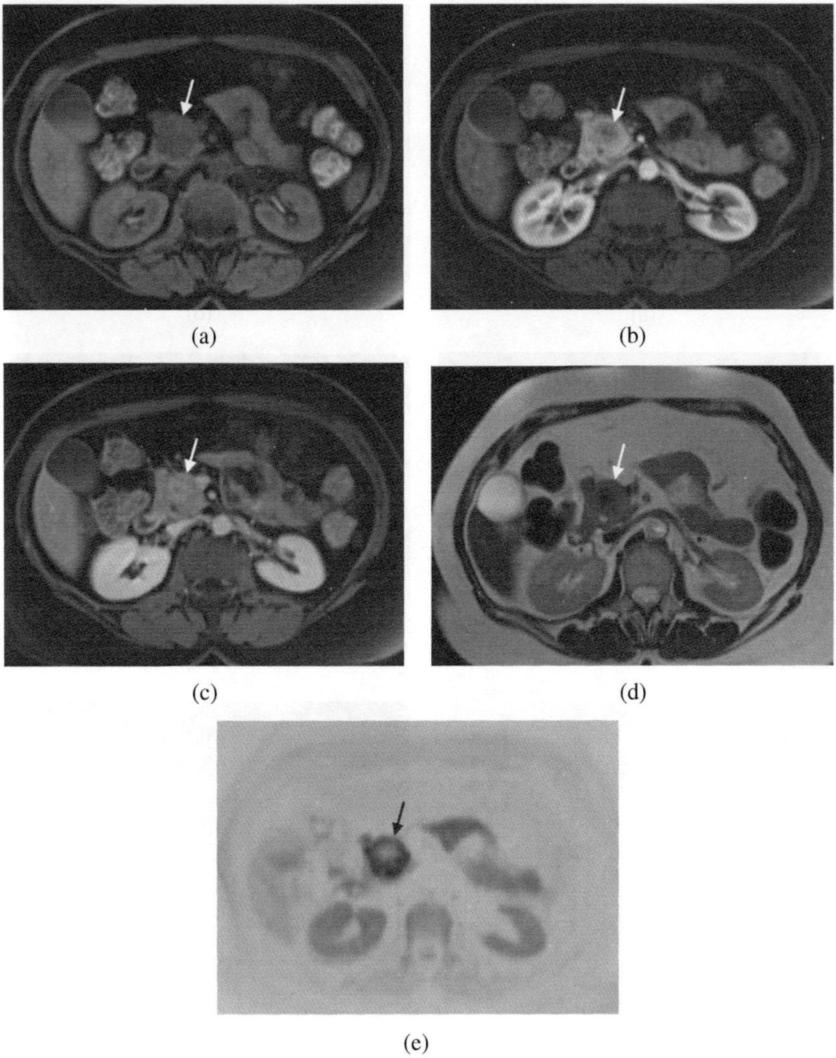

Fig. 11. 60-year-old female with pancreatic neuroendocrine tumor (NET). The tumor (arrows) demonstrates hypointense signal on precontrast images (a) compared to the background pancreatic parenchyma. Postcontrast arterial (b) and delayed (c) phase images show an arterial enhancement pattern of the lesion (arrows, b–c), while T2W images demonstrate variable signal features (arrow, d), DWI shows markedly abnormal signal in the tumor (arrow, e), and this sequence may hold utility in identification of small NET.

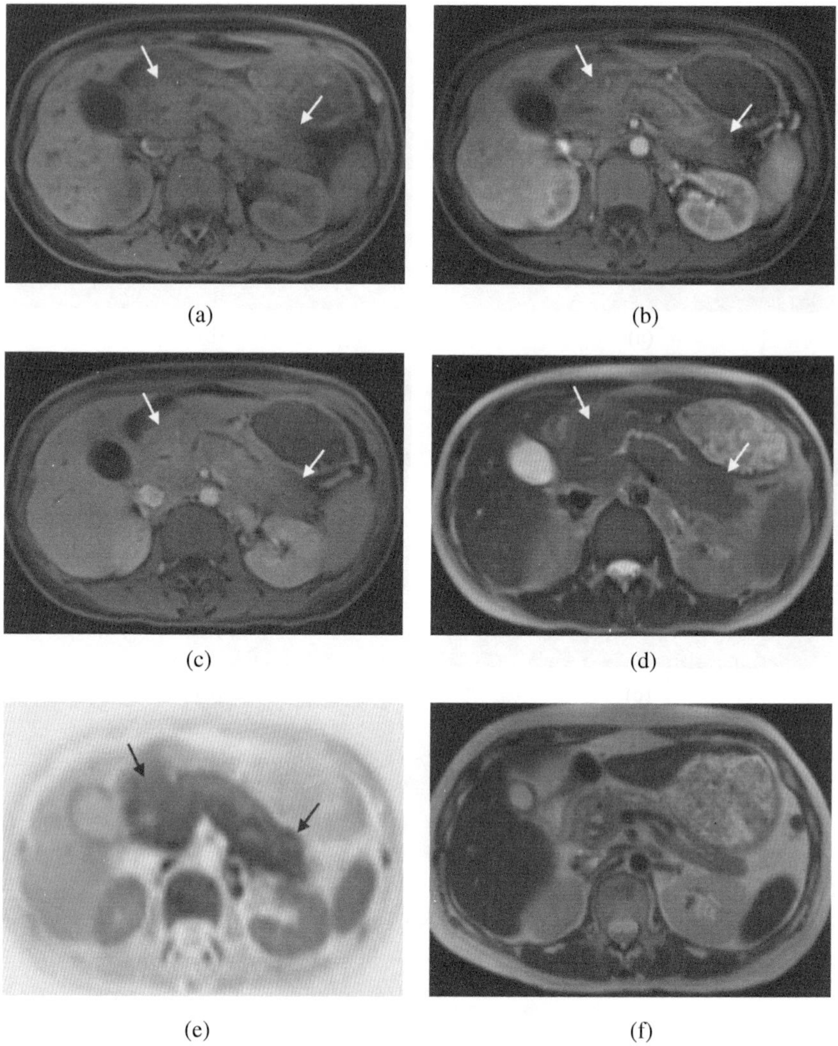

Fig. 12. 44-year-old female with pancreatic lymphoma. Pre-contrast (a), arterial (b) and delayed postcontrast (c) T1W images show infiltration of the entire pancreas by poorly defined tissue that demonstrates relatively uniform, delayed enhancement (arrows, a–c). T2W image (d) shows mildly elevated signal of the tissue (arrows) with some mass effect on the pancreatic duct. DWI image (e) shows highly restricted diffusion of the tissue infiltrating the pancreas (arrows), which is a feature of lymphoid tissue. Following chemotherapy, repeat imaging demonstrates marked reduction in the volume of tumor on T2W imaging (f).

syndrome of subcutaneous fat necrosis, panniculitis, polyarthralgia and blood eosinophilia.[78] When present, metastases are most commonly identified in the liver and lymph nodes.[78,79]

Imaging: Acinar cell tumors are mildly hypointense on T1W images and demonstrate a floccular morphology that is reflective of the acinar differentiation of this tumor. T2W images show moderately elevated signal; however this tumor may undergo cystic change which produces markedly elevated T2 signal in the cystic components (Fig. 13). The dynamic contrast-enhancement pattern is heterogeneous and typical of malignancy, demonstrating a pattern of heterogeneous, delayed enhancement.[80]

Intraductal papillary mucinous neoplasm

Intraductal papillary mucinous neoplasm (IPMN) of the pancreas is a tumor that arises from the main pancreatic duct or side branches. There is replacement of the normal duct epithelium by a mucinous lining with characteristic papillary projections, distending the duct with mucin.[81] Categorization of IPMN is based on the pattern of duct involvement: main duct, side branch or a combined pattern.[81] IPMN are the most common cystic tumors of the pancreas, and are more commonly seen in elderly male patients. While the vast majority of IPMN are benign,[82] a small percentage of IPMN demonstrate variable levels of aggressive biological behavior with a potential for malignant transformation. Main duct IPMNs are more at risk than side branch IPMN for this malignant change, and the five-year risk of malignancy in main duct IPMN has been reported to be 63%.[83–88]

Imaging: Side branch IPMN demonstrate a tubular configuration, reflective of the duct origin of this tumor. IPMN demonstrate simple fluid characteristics on MRI, with hypointense T1 signal and markedly hyperintense T2 signal.[84–88] Small IPMN are frequently best seen on heavily T2W MRCP sequences, which demonstrate a direct communication with the main duct. Main duct IPMN present as focal or diffuse distension of the main pancreatic duct, with similar imaging and signal features to side branch IPMN.[84–88]

Concerning imaging features for malignant transformation of the IPMN include: an internal mural enhancing nodule, size > than 3.5 cm, main pancreatic duct diameter of more than 10 mm, and the presence of a thickened, enhancing wall and/or septations[84–88] (Fig. 14). The addition of

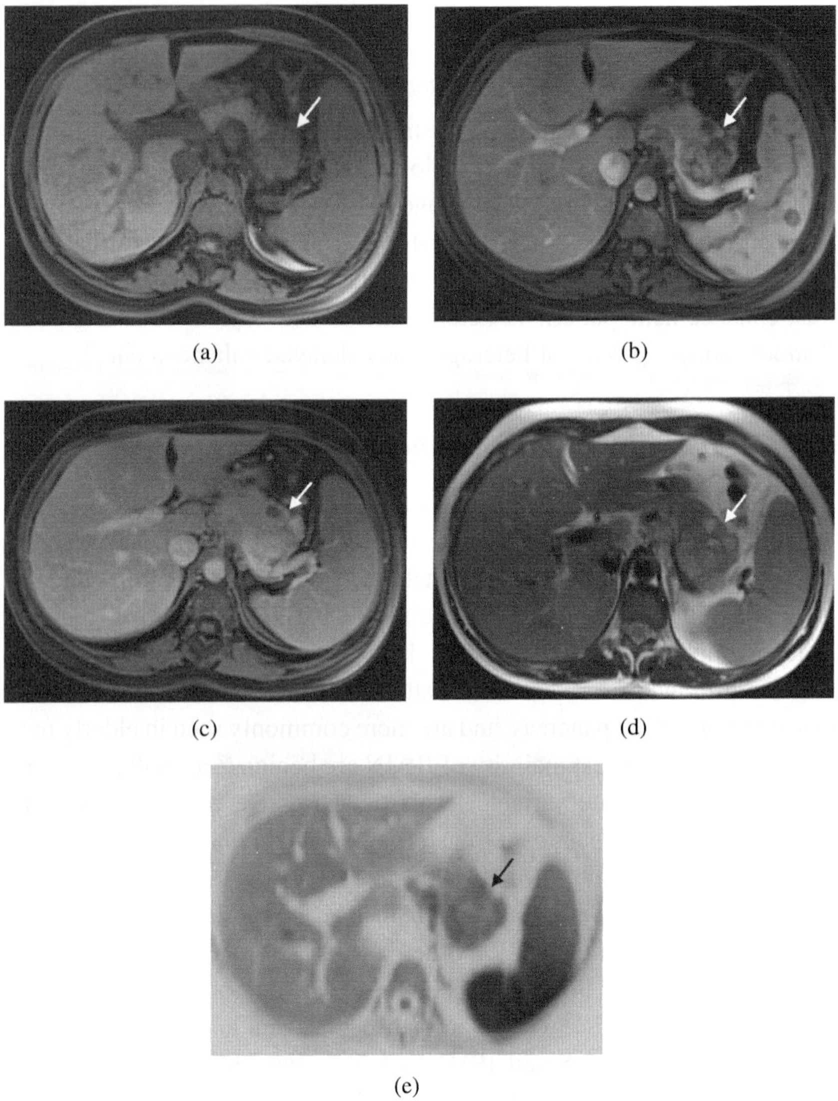

Fig. 13. 35-year-old female with acinar cell carcinoma of the pancreas. There is low signal intensity in the lesion on precontrast T1W imaging (arrow, a). Arterial (b) and delayed phase (c) postcontrast imaging shows heterogeneous delayed enhancement of the lesion (arrows, b–c). T2W imaging shows cystic change in the tumor (arrow, d). DWI (e) shows only mildly restricted diffusion (arrow). Surgical resection demonstrated acinar cell carcinoma of the pancreas.

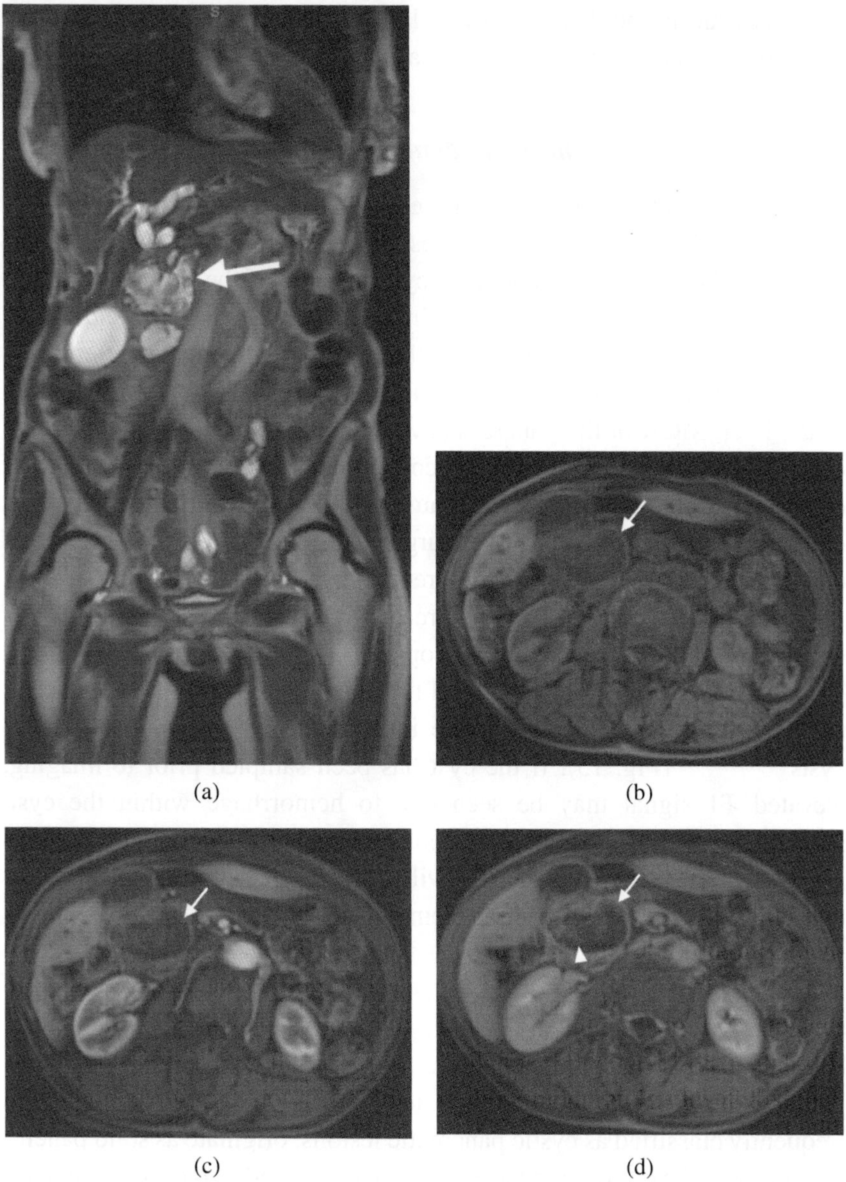

Fig. 14. 88-year-old female with malignant intraductal papillary mucinous neoplasm (IPMN). Coronal T2W image (a) shows a tubular, cystic structure in the pancreatic head (arrow) which involves the main pancreatic duct. Pre-contrast (b), arterial (c) and delayed (d) postcontrast T1W images show heterogeneously enhancing tissue (b–d, arrowheads) within the cystic lesion (b–d, arrows), in keeping with carcinomatous elements.

DWI may aid in the diagnosis of malignant transformation of IPMN and may hold utility for prediction of invasive carcinoma.[89–91]

Mucinous cystadenoma/Cystadenocarcinoma of the pancreas

Mucinous cystadenoma (MCA) of the pancreas occurs almost exclusively in women, with a mean age of diagnosis of approximately 50 years.[92,93] On histological examination, mucinous cystadenoma of the pancreas and biliary cystadenoma of the liver show similar features and a surrounding rim of ovarian stroma is a key feature to the histologic diagnosis, differentiating this lesion from other cystic lesions of the pancreas.[84] Similar to BCA of the liver, MCA of the pancreas have malignant potential, and the presence of carcinomatous elements converts the diagnosis to mucinous cystadenocarcinoma (MCCA). Because of this malignant potential, MCA of the pancreas is regarded as a surgical lesion even in the absence of enhancing soft tissue elements on preoperative imaging.[84,86–87,92–93]

Imaging: The internal architecture of MCA is depicted well on T2W sequences, which demonstrate a neoplastic pattern of internal sepations. These lesions are hypointense on T1W imaging and markedly hyperintense on T2W imaging due to the internal fluid composition of these cysts[84,86–87,92–93] (Fig. 15). If the cyst has been sampled prior to imaging, elevated T1 signal may be seen due to hemorrhage within the cyst. Dynamic post-contrast images demonstrate enhancement of the septations and wall of the cyst, while MCCA will show nodular foci of enhancement that represent the carcinomatous elements.[84,86–87,92–93]

Solid pseudopapillary tumor

Solid pseudopapillary tumors of the pancreas have low-grade malignant potential and occur predominantly in young women.[84] SPTs, although frequently classified as cystic pancreatic lesions, originate as solid pancreatic tumors.[84] These tumors have a propensity to undergo cystic degeneration, and the appearance on imaging will be reflective of the stage of cystic degeneration.

Imaging: SPT are well circumscribed, encapsulated lesions with variable internal cystic components.[84,86–87] T2 signal intensity is variable and depends on the level of tumor degeneration, and may range from

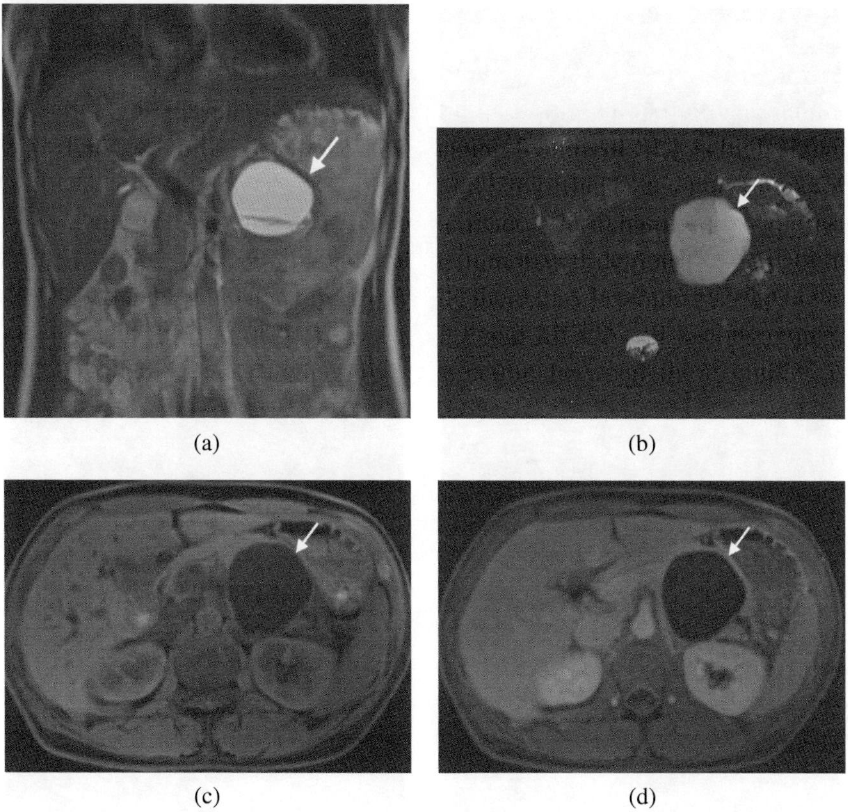

Fig. 15. 41-year-old female with mucinous cystadenoma of the pancreas. Coronal T2W (a) and MRCP (b) images show complex septations within a cyst in the pancreatic tail (arrows, a–b). Precontrast (c) and postcontrast (d) T1W images demonstrate the cystic lesion in the pancreas (arrows, c–d) but no nodular, internal enhancing elements. Surgical resection confirmed mucinous cystadenoma.

moderately hyperintense (mostly solid tumors) to markedly hyperintense (mostly cystic tumors).[84,86–87] A key imaging feature of SPT is high signal on T1W images secondary to intratumoral hemorrhage, and may allow for a more specific diagnosis of SPT to be made. On dynamic post-contrast sequences, the solid components of the tumor will demonstrate a pattern of delayed enhancement (Fig. 16). While there may be some overlap in the imaging appearance of SPT, cystic NET and MCCA, all lesions require surgical therapy and preoperative distinction between these entities is

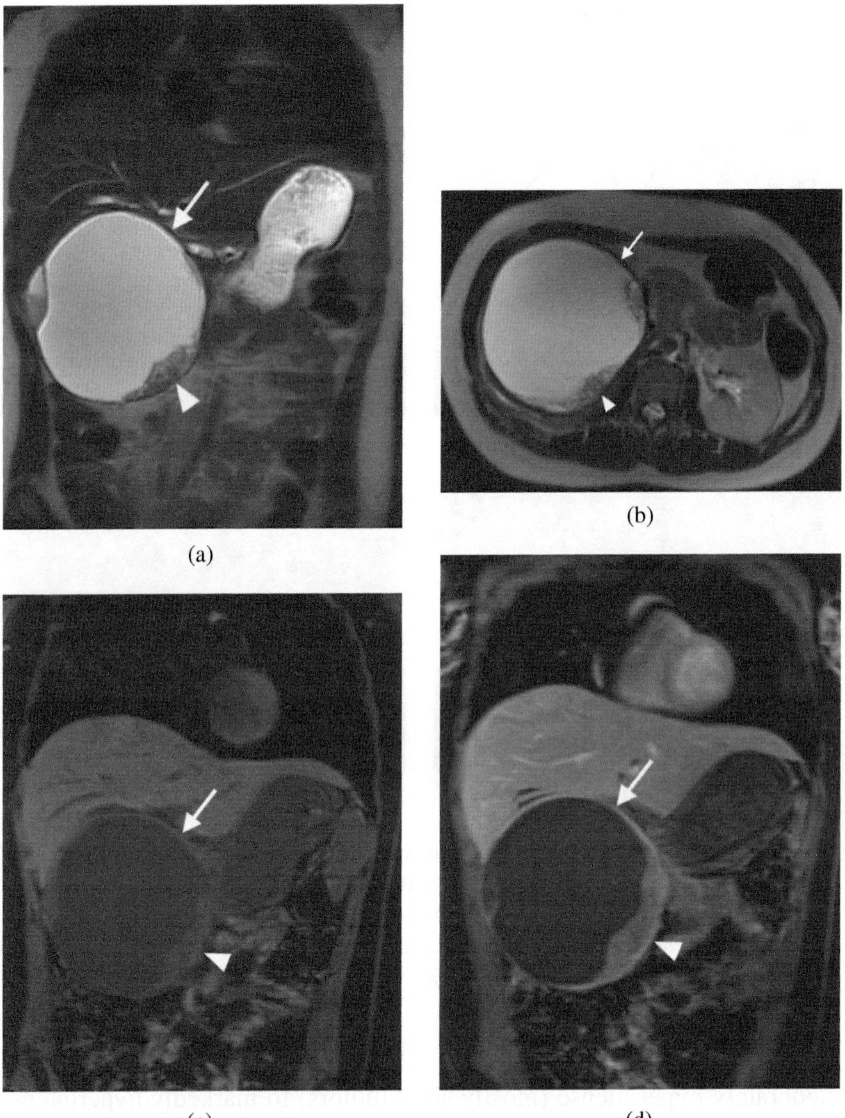

Fig. 16. 15-year-old female with solitary pseudopapillary tumor (SPT) of the pancreas. Coronal (a) and axial (b) T2W show a large, complex cyst (arrows, a–b) in the pancreatic head. While much of the cyst shows simple internal fluid, mural nodularity is present (arrowheads, a–b). Coronal precontrast (c) and postcontrast (d) T1W images show delayed enhancement of the regions of mural nodularity, in keeping with vascularized soft tissue components in the cyst.

typically not required. The role of preoperative imaging should be to classify the cystic lesion as one that requires surgical resection and to properly stage the patient with respect to vascular involvement, local growth patterns and the presence or absence of metastatic disease.[84,86–87]

Metastatic disease to the pancreas

Metastases to the pancreas are uncommon, and when present, are typically secondary to renal cell, lung or breast cancer.[94–96] Imaging features resemble that of the primary tumor, and MRI provides a sensitive method for detection.

Imaging: Metastases are typically well-circumscribed, rounded lesions that are hypointense on T1W imaging. T2 signal is variable, but is usually mildly elevated. Dynamic enhancement patterns are dependent on the primary tumor. Renal cell carcinoma metastases demonstrate avid arterial enhancement,[94–96] similar to that of a NET (Fig. 17). Breast and lung carcinoma metastases typically demonstrate a delayed enhancement pattern. Pancreatic metastases from bronchogenic carcinoma are typically multiple and may replace a majority of the pancreatic parenchyma. A clinical history of primary tumors known to metastasize to the pancreas is a key for accurate diagnostics.

Bowel

Rectal cancer

MRI plays a fundamental role in the pre-surgical planning and staging of primary rectal cancer.[97–103] The soft tissue resolution of MRI allows for accurate preoperative assessment of depth of invasion (T stage) and nodal involvement (N stage). A main advantage of MRI compared to endorectal ultrasound is the ability to provide concurrent assessment of metastatic disease (M stage) in the abdomen and pelvis.

Imaging: The most valuable sequence for the evaluation of primary rectal carcinoma is a high-resolution, T2W sequence with thin section slices which provide detailed analysis of the tumor and depth of rectal wall involvement.[97–103] On T2W images, the submucosa in the rectal wall

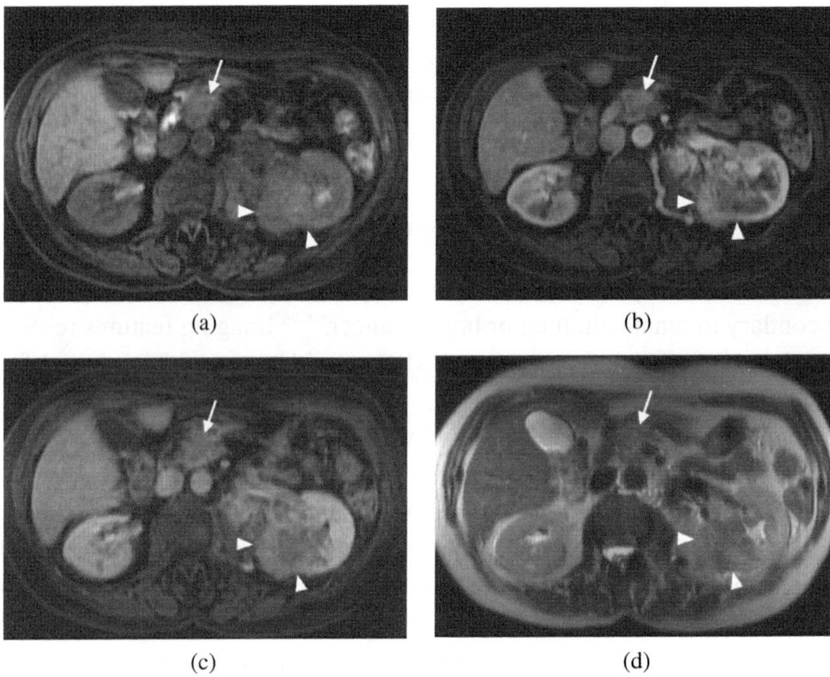

Fig. 17. 69-year-old female with metastatic renal cell carcinoma (RCC) to the pancreas. Precontrast (a), arterial (b) and delayed phase (c) postcontrast T1W images show a focal lesion in the pancreatic head (arrows, a–c) which shows avid arterial enhancement. T2W image (d) shows mildly elevated signal in the lesion (d, arrow), in keeping with malignancy. Note the patient's primary tumor in the left kidney (d, arrowheads).

is hyperintense, while the muscularis propria is hypointense. When tumor is confined to submucosa, it is staged as T1. In stage T2 disease, tumor is confined within the rectal wall, while in stage T3 tumor, it is noted to extend beyond the muscularis propria into the mesorectal fat[97–103] (Fig. 18). MRI has been shown to provide accurate assessment of the relationship of the tumor to the mesorectal fascia and the peritoneal reflection.[97–103] Invasion through the peritoneal reflection indicates stage T4a disease, while invasion into adjacent pelvic organs is classified as stage T4b. Evaluation of the relationship of the tumor to the anal sphincter will determine whether sphincter-sparing resection is feasible, and is well-demonstrated with MRI.

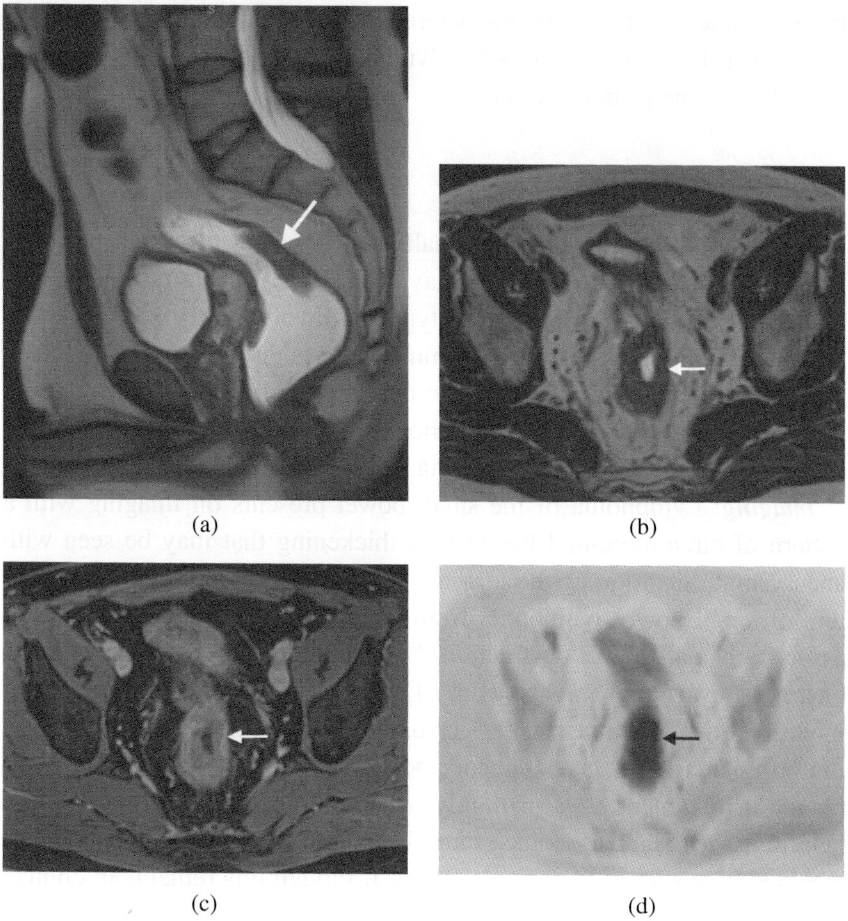

Fig. 18. 51-year-old male with rectal carcinoma. Sagittal T2W (a) and axial, high-resolution T2W images show an apple-core type lesion in the rectum (arrows, a–b). Axial, high resolution postcontrast T1W image (c) shows tumor extending outside the rectal wall just into the perirectal soft tissues (arrow, c), in keeping with stage T3 disease. DWI (d) shows marked restricted diffusion within the patient's rectal tumor (arrow, d).

High-resolution T2-weighted images also allow for assessment of pelvic lymph nodes, including the perirectal/mesorectal, superior rectal, inferior mesenteric, iliac, retroperitoneal, and inguinal stations.[104,105] Concerning features on T2 weighted images are nodal size > 5 mm, irregular spiculated margin, and heterogeneous signal intensity.[104,105] DWI is excellent for depiction of pelvic lymph nodes and also helps delineate the extent of the primary tumor.

Small bowel lymphoma

Lymphoma is the most common malignant tumor of the small bowel.[106] Primary or secondary lymphoma may occur in any portion of the gastrointestinal tract. Primary lymphoma typically involves only one site, while secondary lymphoma manifests at multiple sites throughout the abdomen and pelvis, commonly originating in mesenteric or retroperitoneal lymph nodes.[106] Advanced primary lymphomas may disseminate and mimic secondary gastrointestinal lymphoma.[106–116]

Imaging: Lymphoma of the small bowel presents on imaging with a pattern of circumferential bowel wall thickening that may be seen with aneurysmal dilatation of the lumen[107–116] (Fig. 19). A differentiating feature of small bowel lymphoma from adenocarcinoma is the absence of associated small bowel obstruction. Lymphoma of the small bowel demonstrates low signal intensity on T1W images and intermediate signal intensity on T2W images.[111–116] Dynamic post-contrast images show a uniform pattern of delayed enhancement.[111–116] As with other sites of lymphoma involvement, DWI is highly sensitive to nodal tissue and is often helpful in the diagnosis; some groups have used whole-body MRI-DWI as an alternative staging strategy to PET-CT, though this remains in clinical development.[116]

Carcinoid

Carcinoids are slowly growing, well-vascularized neuroendocrine tumors that arise from primitive stem cells in the gut wall. The most common location in the small bowel is the terminal ileum.[112] The majority of small bowel carcinoids are serotonin-producing tumors that manifest with carcinoid syndrome (cutaneous flushing, diarrhea, wheezing) when liver or retroperitoneal nodal metastases are present.[112]

Imaging: The primary carcinoid tumor in the bowel wall is frequently small and may not be identifiable on imaging. When present, the tumor

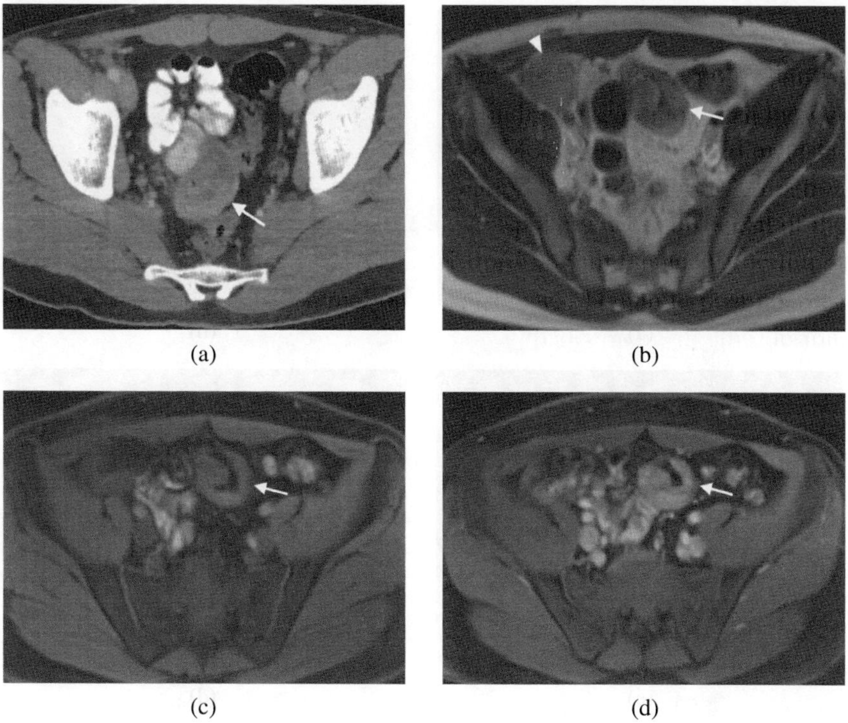

Fig. 19. 30-year-old male with small bowel lymphoma. The small bowel tumor is not well-demonstrated on CT (arrow, a). T2W image (b) shows marked abnormal thickening of the same small bowel loop in the pelvis (arrow); note the enlarged nodal conglomerate along the right external iliac chain (arrowhead, b). Precontrast (c) and postcontrast (d) T1W images show delayed enhancement of the thickened bowel wall (arrows, c–d); in the absence of bowel obstruction, lymphoma is the primary consideration, confirmed in this case with tissue sampling.

demonstrates avid arterial enhancement on dynamic, post-contrast images.[117,118] The most common imaging finding in carcinoid is a mesenteric metastasis in the right lower quadrant. Mesenteric carcinoid metastases are often spiculated with irregular margins and mesenteric retraction secondary to fibrosis, which may create a "spoke-wheel" dispersal of the mesenteric vessels[117–119] (Fig. 20). This fibrotic component of the tumor manifests as hypointense signal on T2W images. Dynamic post-contrast images again demonstrate avid arterial enhancement of the lesion,

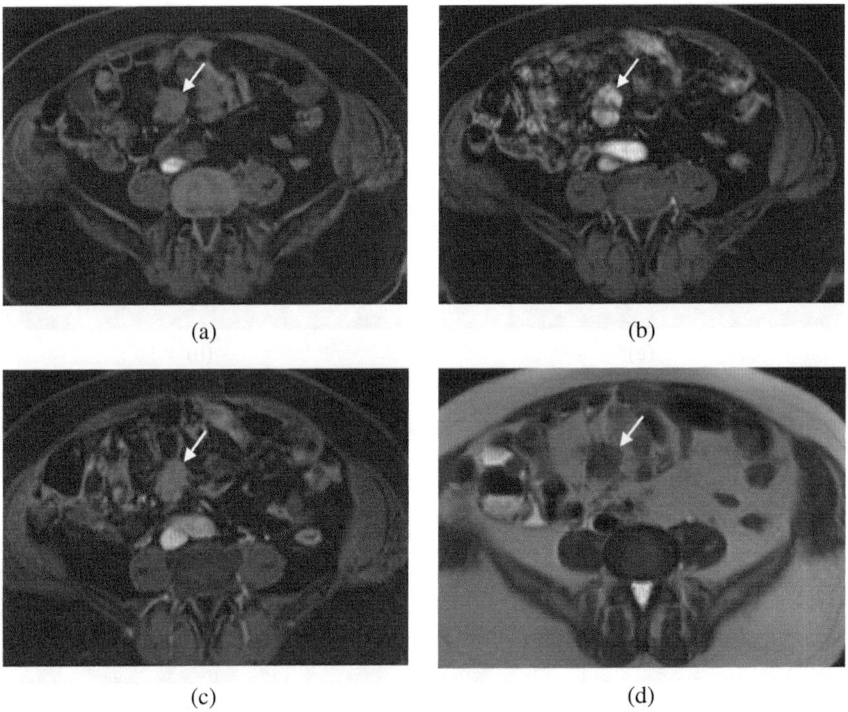

Fig. 20. 73-year-old male with carcinoid metastasis in the right lower quadrant. Precontrast (a), arterial (b) and delayed (c) phase T1W images show a mesenteric mass with avid arterial enhancement (arrows, a–c). T2W image (d) shows surrounding spiculation and adjacent fibrotic tethering (arrow, d), in keeping with carcinoid nodal metastases.

reflective of its vascular nature. Other common sites of metastases are the liver, lung, peritoneum, and omentum.[112]

Mucinous appendiceal carcinoma

Mucinous appendiceal adenocarcinoma is a rare neoplasm, and may present with peritoneal spread on initial presentation, known as "pseudomyxoma peritonei."

Imaging: On T2W sequences, mucinous appendiceal carcinoma demonstrates heterogeneous, markedly elevated signal; this pattern of elevated T2 signal in a solid neoplasm has been shown to be a reliable imaging feature of mucinous neoplasms.[120] On T1W sequences, mucinous tumors show variable signal. Dynamic post-contrast sequences show mucinous tumors to be poorly vascularized, with heterogeneous, delayed enhancement. The enhancement in mucinous lesions may be subtle, but careful comparison of pre-contrast and post-contrast sequences will reveal the enhancing components.[121]

Diagnosis and staging of peritoneal involvement from mucinous tumors is a relative strength of MRI compared to CT.[58–60] Mucinous peritoneal carcinomatosis will manifest as heterogeneous, high signal soft tissue implants on T2W imaging. Peritoneal involvement is best assessed on dynamic, post-contrast images, which demonstrate diffuse peritoneal thickening and enhancement, often with areas of nodularity (Fig. 21). Scalloping of the liver surface by peritoneal metastases is a common finding.[121]

Stomach

Gastric adenocarcinoma

Gastric adenocarcinoma originates from the epithelium of the stomach, and endoscopy is the primary method of diagnosis. The role of imaging is complementary to endoscopy and is primarily for local and distant tumor staging. Overall, gastric adenocarcinoma is a poorly defined, infiltrative tumor, and several growth patterns may be seen: (1) an exophytic lesion projecting into the lumen; (2) ulcerated growth pattern; or (3) diffusely infiltrative disease known as linitis plastic.[122] Metastases are frequently seen in regional lymph nodes, liver, peritoneum and lungs.[122]

Imaging: With respect to local T staging, MRI has been shown to be superior to CT.[123,124] T2W images demonstrate replacement of the normal gastric rugal fold pattern with infiltrative tissue that demonstrates heterogeneously elevated T2 signal. Dynamic post-contrast sequences show a heterogeneous pattern of delayed enhancement, similar to that seen in other adenocarcinomas (Fig. 22). DWI may be helpful is assessing the

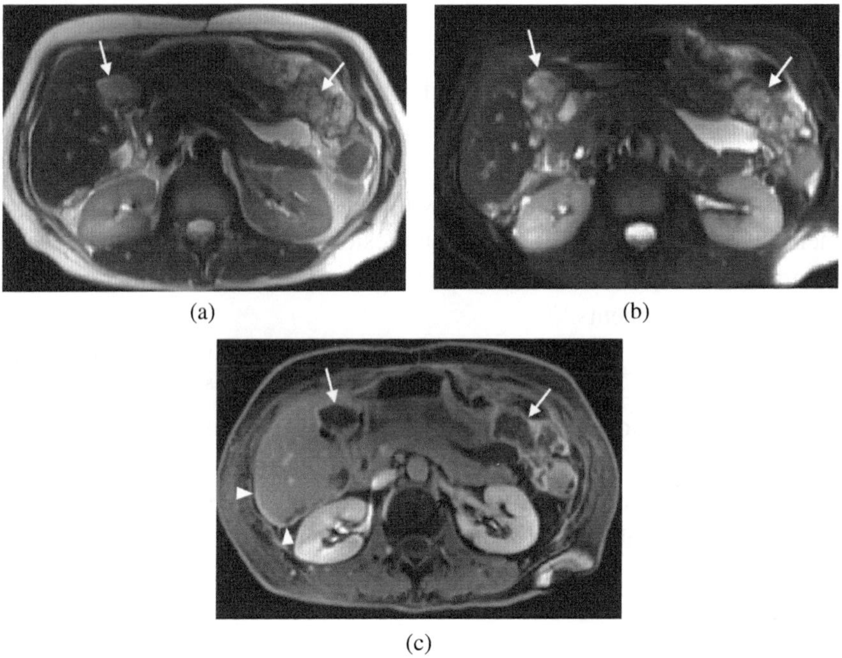

Fig. 21. 54-year-old female with metastatic mucinous appendiceal cancer. T2W images without (a) and with fat suppression (b) show high signal soft tissue implants along the gallbladder fossa and left anterior abdomen (arrows, a–b). The tumor implants show high signal on T2W imaging, which may serve as a biomarker for mucinous tumors. Postcontrast T1W image (c) shows heterogeneous enhancement of the peritoneal tumor implants (c, arrows). Note also the thickening and abnormal enhancement of the remainder of the peritoneal surfaces (arrowheads, c), in keeping with peritoneal carcinomatosis.

extent of disease in some patients[123,124] and also for identification of adjacent nodal disease.

Gastrointestinal stromal tumors

Gastrointestinal stromal tumors (GISTs) originate from the muscularis propria of the stomach or intestinal wall, and are the most common

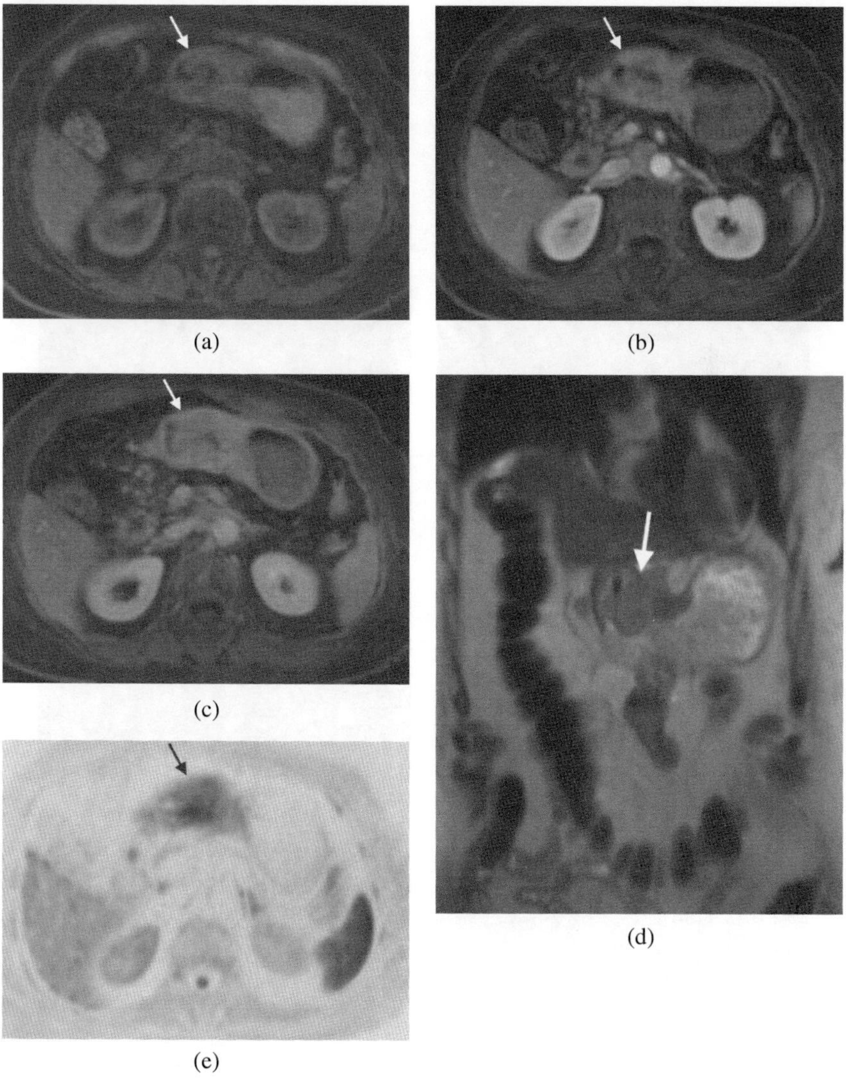

Fig. 22. 83-year-old female with gastric adenocarcinoma. Precontrast (a), arterial (b) and delayed (c) postcontrast T1W images show heterogeneous, delayed enhancing tissue replacing the gastric antrum (arrows, a–c). Coronal T2W image shows the tumor replacing the gastric antrum (arrow, d) with enlarged adjacent lymph nodes. DWI (e) shows marked restricted diffusion in the gastric carcinoma (arrow, e).

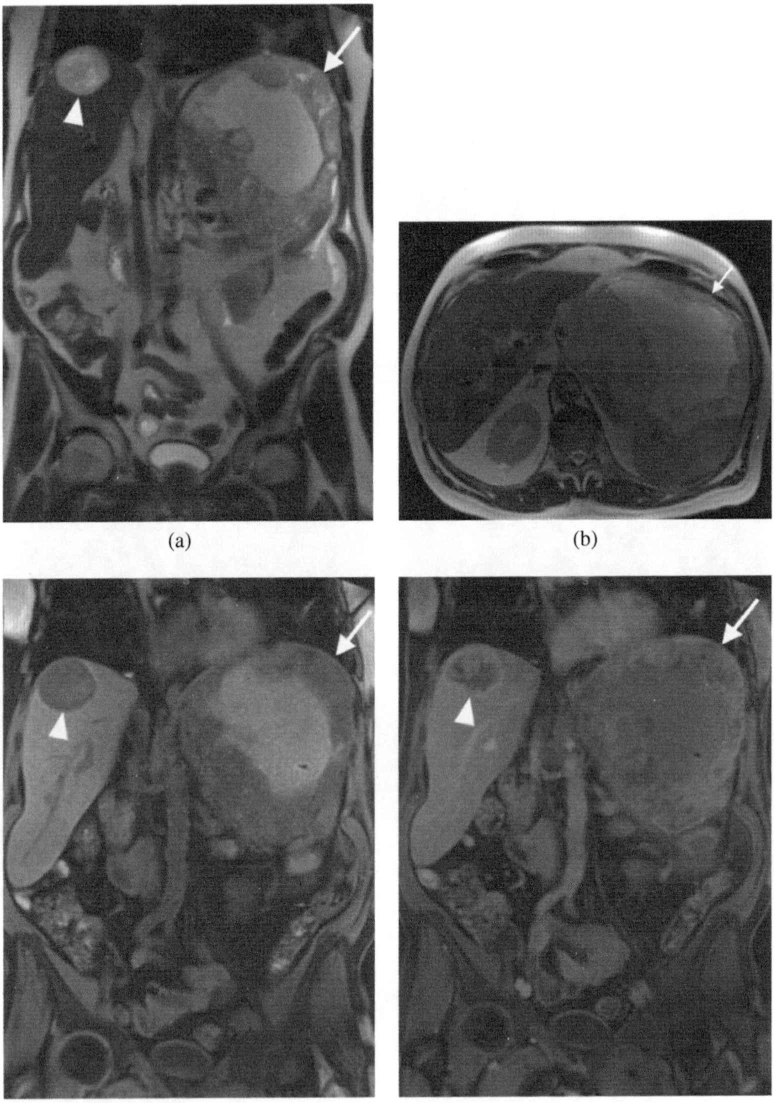

(a) (b) (c) (d)

Fig. 23. 66-year-old male with metastatic gastrointestinal stromal tumor (GIST) to the liver. Coronal (a) and axial (b) T2W images show the primary GIST in the left upper quadrant with internal cystic change (arrows, a–b); a metastasis is noted at the hepatic dome (arrowhead, a). Coronal precontrast T1W image (c) shows elevated T1 signal in the GIST, in keeping with hemorrhage (arrow, c), while coronal postcontrast T1W image (d) demonstrates heterogeneous enhancement of the mural soft tissue components in the primary GIST (arrow, c–d) and also the hepatic metastasis (arrowheads, c–d).

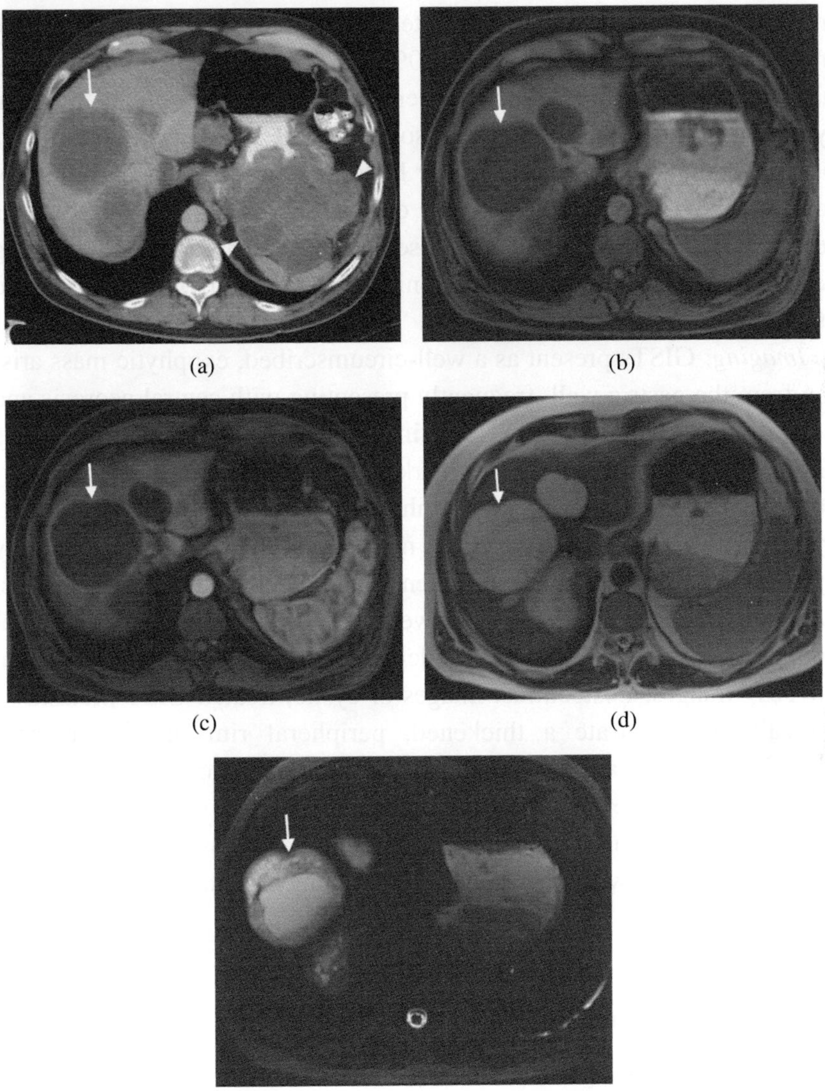

(a) (b) (c) (d) (e)

Fig. 24. 58-year-old with cystic GIST metastases after Gleevac therapy. Initial CT (a) shows a large gastric tumor (arrowhead, a) and metastasis in the liver (arrow, a). After Gleevac therapy, MRI was performed for restaging. Precontrast (b) and postcontrast arterial phase (c) T1W images (c) show no residual enhancement in the hepatic metastases (arrows, b–c), in keeping with an excellent response to therapy. T2W (d) and MRCP (e) images show complex, internal cystic changes that are markedly accentuated after Gleevac therapy.

mesenchymal tumor of the gastrointestinal system.[125] The stomach is the most common site of occurrence (60%). GISTs may be benign or malignant,[125] and metastases, when present, are frequently seen in regional lymph nodes, liver and lungs. An isolated GIST is not easily defined as benign or malignant on imaging or histologic assessment, and the biological behavior of each tumor may only be assessed over time. For this reason, GISTs are resected on presentation, and preoperative imaging serves to provide an accurate, noninvasive method of diagnosis and staging.

Imaging: GISTs present as a well-circumscribed, exophytic mass arising from the gastric wall, frequently presenting with central necrosis and hemorrhage[125] (Fig. 23). On T2W imaging, the solid components of a GIST range from moderate to markedly hyperintense. Dynamic postcontrast sequences show delayed enhancement of the tumor. After treatment with Gleevac, hepatic GIST metastases demonstrate a markedly cystic apperance that may be mistaken for simple hepatic cysts or bile duct hamartomas, especially on CT. However, MRI demonstrates the internal complexity of the metastases, best demonstrated by heterogeneous signal on T2W images. Postcontrast images of cystic, treated GIST metastases typically demonstrate a thickened, peripheral rim of enhancement (Fig. 24), which is a differentiating feature from simple hepatic cysts that show only a thin peripheral rim of enhancement. With successful therapy, no enhancement will be seen within the metastatic lesions, though residual viable disease will show delayed enhancement, similar to the primary tumor.[126]

Take Home Messages

- Medical imaging has become essential to the care of patients with GI malignancies.
- With new advances in imaging technology (especially MRI), increased accuracy in diagnosis and staging through noninvasive methods has the potential to reduce invasive tissue sampling and to more accurately guide therapeutic decision-making in patients with GI malignancies.

References

1. ACR Appropriateness Criteria pretreatment staging of colorectal cancer. *J Am Coll Radiol*, 2012. **9**(11): 775–81.
2. Digumarthy, S.R., Sahani, D.V., Saini, S., MRI in detection of hepatocellular carcinoma (HCC). *Cancer Imaging*, 2005. **5**: 20–4.
3. Yu, N.C., Chaudhari, V., Raman, S.S. *et al.*, CT and MRI improve detection of hepatocellular carcinoma, compared with ultrasound alone, in patients with cirrhosis. *Clin Gastroenterol Hepatol,* 2011. **9**(2): 161–7.
4. Raman, S.P., Fishman, E.K., Advances in CT imaging of GI malignancies. *Gastrointest Cancer Res*, 2012. **5**(3 Suppl 1): S4–S9.
5. Hicks, R.J., Ware, R.E., Lau, E.W., PET/CT: will it change the way that we use CT in cancer imaging? *Cancer Imaging*, 2006. **6**: S52–62.
6. Weber, W.A., Assessing tumor response to therapy. *J Nucl Med*, 2009. **50**(Suppl 1): 1S–10S.
7. Pitton, M.B., Klockner, R., Herber, S. *et al.*, MRI versus 64-row MDCT for diagnosis of hepatocellular carcinoma. *World J Gastroenterol*, 2009. **15**(48): 6044–51.
8. Ayuso, C., Rimola, J., Garcia-Criado, A., Imaging of HCC. *Abdom Imaging*, 2012. **37**(2): 215–30.
9. Burrel, M., Llovet, J.M., Ayuso, C. *et al.*, MRI angiography is superior to helical CT for detection of HCC prior to liver transplantation: an explant correlation. *Hepatology*, 2003. **38**(4): 1034–42.
10. Becker-Weidman, D.J., Kalb, B., Sharma, P. *et al.*, Hepatocellular carcinoma lesion characterization. *Radiology*, 2011. **261**(3): 824–33.
11. *4 United Network for Organ Sharing*. http://www.unos.org/. Accessed August 1, 2010.
12. Elsayes, K.M., Narra, V.R., Yumin, Y. *et al.*, Focal hepatic lesions: diagnostic value of enhancement pattern approach with contrast-enhanced 3D gradient-echo MR imaging. *Radiographics*, 2005. **25**: 1299–1320.
13. Rosenkrantz, A.B., Lee, L., Matza, B.W. *et al.*, Infiltrative hepatocellular carcinoma: comparison of MRI sequences for lesion conspicuity. *Clin Radiol*, 2012. **67**(12): e105–11.
14. Kierans, A.S., Leonardou, P., Hayashi, P. e*t al.*, MRI findings of rapidly progressive hepatocellular carcinoma. *Magn Reson Imaging*, 2010. **28**(6): 790–6.

15. de Campos, R.O., Semelka, R.C., Azevedo, R.M. *et al.*, Combined hepatocellular carcinoma-cholangiocarcinoma: report of MR appearance in eleven patients. *J Magn Reson Imaging*, 2012. **36**(5): 1139–47.
16. Buetow, P.C., Midkiff, R.B., MR imaging of the liver. Primary malignant neoplasms in the adult. *Magn Reson Imaging Clin N Am*, 1997. **5**(2): 289–318.
17. Jarnagin, W.R., Cholangiocarcinoma of the extrahepatic bile ducts. *Semin Surg Oncol*, 2000. **19**(2): 156–76.
18. Sainani, N.I., Catalano, O.A., Holalkere, N.S. *et al.*, Cholangiocarcinoma: current and novel imaging techniques. *Radiographics*. 2008. **28**(5): 1263-87.
19. Vanderveen, K.A. and Hussain, H.K., Magnetic resonance imaging of cholangiocarcinoma. *Cancer Imaging*, 2004. **4**(2): 104–15.
20. Park, M.J., Kim, Y.K., Lim, S. *et al.*, Hilar cholangiocarcinoma: value of adding DW imaging to gadoxetic acid-enhanced MR imaging with MR cholangiopancreatography for preoperative evaluation. *Radiology*, 2014. **270**(3): 768–76.
21. Chung, Y.E., Kim, M.J., Park, Y.N. *et al.*, Staging of extrahepatic cholangiocarcinoma. *Eur Radiol*, 2008. **18**(10): 2182–95.
22. Craig, J.R., Peters, R.L., Edmondson, H.A, Tumors of the liver and intrahepatic bile ducts. *Atlas of Tumor Pathology*. Second series, fasc 26. Washington DC, 1989.
23. Semelka, R., Martin, D., Balci, C., Lance, T., Focal liver lesions: comparison of dual-phase CT and multisequence multiplanar MR imaging including dynamic gadolinium enhancement. *J Magn Reson Imaging*, 2001. **13**(3): 397–401.
24. Lee, M.J., Hahn, P.F., Saini, S., Mueller, P.R., Differential diagnosis of hyperintense liver lesions on T1-weighted MR images. *AJR Am J Roentgenol*, 1992. **159**(5): 1017–20.
25. Kelekis, N.L., Semelka, R.C., Woosley, J.T., Malignant lesions of the liver with high signal intensity on T1-weighted MR images. *J Magn Reson Imaging*, 1996. **6**(2): 291–4.
26. Casillas, V.J., Amendola, M.A., Gascue, A. *et al.*, Imaging of nontraumatic hemorrhagic hepatic lesions. *Radiographic*, 2000. **20**(2): 367–78.
27. Pedro, M.S., Semelka, R.C., Braga, L., MR imaging of hepatic metastases. *Magn Reson Imaging Clin N Am*, 2002. **10**(1): 15–29.

28. Low, R.N., MR imaging of the liver using gadolinium chelates. *Magn Reson Imaging Clin N Am*, 2001.
29. Danet, I.M., Semelka, R.C., Leonardou, P. *et al.*, Spectrum of MRI appearances of untreated metastases of the liver. *AJR Am J Roentgenol*, 2003. **181**(3): 809–17.
30. Namasivayam, S., Martin, D.R., Saini, S., Imaging of liver metastases: MRI. *Cancer Imaging*, 2007. **7**(1): 2–9.
31. Mahfouz, A.E., Hamm, B., Wolf, K.J., Peripheral washout: a sign of malignancy on dynamic gadolinium-enhanced MR images of focal liver lesions. *Radiology*, 1994. **190**(1): 49–52.
32. Yu, J.S., Rofsky, N.M., Hepatic metastases: perilesional enhancement on dynamic MRI. *AJR Am J Roentgenol*, 2006. **186**(4): 1051–8.
33. Bischof, D.A., Clary, B.M., Maithel, S.K. *et al.*, Surgical management of disappearing colorectal liver metastases. *Br J Surg*, 2013. **100**(11): 1414–20.
34. Scharitzer, M., Ba-Ssalamah, A., Ringl, H. *et al.*, Preoperative evaluation of colorectal liver metastases: comparison between gadoxetic acid-enhanced 3.0-T MRI and contrast-enhanced MDCT with histopathological correlation. *Eur Radiol*, 2013. **23**(8): 2187–96.
35. Resende, V., Oliveira, T.S., Gomes, R.T. e*t al.*, Primary hepatic lymphoma: a case report. *Int J Surg Case Rep*, 2013. **4**(12): 1165–8.
36. Gazelle, G.S., Lee, M.J., Hahn, P.F. e*t al.*, US, CT, and MRI of primary and secondary liver lymphoma. *J Comput Assist Tomogr*, 1994. **18**(3): 412–5.
37. Kelekis, N.L., Semelka, R.C., Siegelman, E.S. *et al.*, Focal hepatic lymphoma: magnetic resonance demonstration using current techniques including gadolinium enhancement. *Magn Reson Imaging*, 1997. **15**(6): 625–36.
38. Rizzi, E.B., Schina, V., Cristofaro, M. *et al.*, Non-hodgkin's lymphoma of the liver in patients with AIDS: sonographic, CT, and MRI findings. *J Clin Ultrasound*, 2001. **29**(3): 125–9.
39. Manzella, A., Borba-Filho, P., D'Ippolito, G. *et al.*, Abdominal manifestations of lymphoma: spectrum of imaging features. *ISRN Radiology*, 2003. **2013**, Article ID 483069.
40. LV, P., Lin, J., MRI findings of a hepatic epithelioid hemangioendothelioma. *Quant Imaging Med Surg*, 2012. **2**(3): 237–8.
41. Earnest, F. 4th, Johnson, C.D., Case 96: hepatic epithelioid hemangioendothelioma. *Radiology*, 2006. **240**: 295–8.

42. Dong, A., Dong, H., Wang, Y. *et al.*, MRI and FDG PET/CT findings of hepatic epithelioid hemangioendothelioma. *Clin Nucl Med*, 2013. **38**(2): e66–73.
43. Buetow, P.C., Maj, M.C., Buck, J.L., Ros, P.R., Goodman, Z.D., Malignant vascular tumors of the liver: radiologic-pathologic correlation. *Radiographics*, 1994; **14**: 153–66.
44. Koyama, T., Fletcher, J.G., Johnson, C.D., M.S. *et al.*, Primary hepatic angiosarcoma: findings at CT and MR imaging. *Radiology*, 2002. **222**(3): 667–673.
45. Levy, A.D., Murakata, L.A., Abbott, R.M. *et al.*, From the archives of the AFIP. Benign tumors and tumorlike lesions of the gallbladder and extrahepatic bile ducts: radiologic-pathologic correlation. Armed Forces Institute of Pathology. *Radiographics*, **22**(2): 387-413.
46. Martin, D.R., Kalb, B., Sarmiento, J.M. e*t al.*, Giant and complicated variants of cystic bile duct hamartomas of the liver: MRI findings and pathological correlations. *J Magn Reson Imaging*, 2010. **31**(4): 903–11.
47. Soares, K.C., Arnaoutakis, D.J., Kamel, I. e*t al.*, Cystic neoplasms of the liver: biliary cystadenoma and cystadenocarcinoma. *J Am Coll Surg*, 2014. **218**(1): 119–28.
48. Lewin, M., Mourra, N., Honigman, I. *et al.*, Assessment of MRI and MRCP in diagnosis of biliary cystadenoma and cystadenocarcinoma. *Eur Radiol*, 2006. **16**(2): 407–13.
49. Bosman, F.T., Carneiro, F., Hurban, R.H., Theise, N.D., (eds.), *WHO Classification of Tumours of Digestive System*. Lyon, France: international Agency for Research on Cancer Press, 2010: 222–224, 236–238.
50. Rocha, F.G., Lee, H., Katabi, N. *et al.*, Intraductal papillary neoplasm of the bile duct: a biliary equivalent to intraductal papillary mucinous neoplasm of the pancreas? *Hepatology*, 2012. **56**(4): 1352–60.
51. Yoon, H.J., Kim, Y.K., Jang, K.T. *et al.*, Intraductal papillary neoplasm of the bile ducts: description of MRI and added value of diffusion-weighted MRI. *Abdom Imaging*, 2013. **38**(5): 1082–90.
52. Lim, J.H., Zen, Y., Jang, K.T., Kim, Y.K., Nakanuma, Y., Cyst-forming intraductal papillary neoplasm of the bile ducts: description of imaging and pathologic aspects. *AJR Am J Roentgenol*, 2011. **197**: 1111–20.
53. Siegel, R., Naishadham, D., Jemal, A., Cancer statistics, 2013. *CA Cancer J Clin*, 2013. **63**(1): 11–30.

54. Tapper, E.B., Martin, D.R., Adsay, N.C. *et al.*, An MRI-driven practice: a new perspective on MRI for the evaluation of adenocarcinoma of the head of the pancreas. *J Gastrointest Surg*, 2010. **14**(8):1292–7.
55. Ichikawa, T., Sou, H., Araki, T., Arbab, A.S., Yoshikawa, T., Ishigame K. *et al.*, Duct-penetrating sign at MRCP: usefulness for differentiating inflammatory pancreatic mass from pancreatic carcinomas. *Radiology*, 2001. **221**: 107–16.
56. Miller, F.H., Rini, N.J., Keppke, A.L. *et al.*, MRI of adenocarcinoma of the pancreas. *AJR*, 2006. **187**(issue 4).
57. Obuz, F., Dicle, O., Coker, A. e*t al.*, Pancreatic adenocarcinoma: detection and staging with dynamic MR imaging. *Eur J Radiol*, 2001. **38**: 146–50.
58. Launstein, T.C., Martin, D.R., Darmiento, J.M. *et al.*, Pancreatic adenocarcinoma tumor grade determination using contrast-enhanced magnetic resonance imaging. *Pancreas*, 2010. **39**(1): 71–5.
59. Tapper, E., Kalb, B., Martin, D.R. *et al.*, Staging laparoscopy for proximal pancreatic cancer in a magnetic resonance imaging-driven practice: what's it worth? *HPB (Oxford)*, 2011. **13**(10): 732–7.
60. Low, R.N., Barone, R.M., Lacey, C., Sigeti, J.S., Alzate, G.D., Sebrechts, C.P., Peritoneal tumor: MR imaging with dilute oral barium and intravenous gadolinium containing contrast agents compared with unenhanced MR imaging and CT. *Radiology*, 1997. **204**: 513–20.
61. Low, R.N., MR imaging of the peritoneal spread of malignancy. *Abdom Imaging*, 2007. **32**(3): 267–83. Review.
62. Low, R.N., Gurney. J., Diffusion-weighted MRI (DWI) in the oncology patient: value of breathhold DWI compared to unenhanced and gadolinium-enhanced MRI. *J Magn Reson Imaging*, 2007. **25**(4): 848–58.
63. Low, R.N., Sebrechts, C.P., Barone, R.M. *et al.*, Diffusion-weighted MRI of peritoneal tumors: comparison with conventional MRI and surgical and histopathologic findings — a feasibility study. *AJR Am J Roentgenol*, 2009. **193**(2): 461–70.
64. Yao, J.C., Eisner, M.P., Leary, C. *et al.*, Population-based study of islet cell carcinoma. *Ann Surg Oncol*, 2007. **14**: 3492–500.
65. Asa, S.L., Pancreatic endocrine tumors. *Mod Pathol*, 2011. **24**(Suppl 2): S66–77.
66. Semelka, R.C., Custodio, C.M., Cem Balci, N., Woosley, J.T., Neuroendocrine tumors of the pancreas: spectrum of appearances on MRI. *J Magn Reson Imaging*, 2000. **11**: 141–8.

67. Owen, N.J., Sohaib, S.A., Peppercorn, P.D. *et al.*, MRI of pancreatic neuroendocrine tumours. *Br J Radiol*, 2001. **74**(886): 968–73.
68. Semelka, R.C., Custudio, C.M., Cen Balci, N. *et al.*, Neuroendocrine tumors of the pancreas: spectrum of appearances on MRI. *J Magn Reson Imaging*, 2000. **11**(2): 141–8.
69. Bhosale, P.R., Menias, C.O., Balachandran, A. *et al.*, Vascular pancreatic lesions: spectrum of imaging findings of malignant masses and mimics with pathologic correlation. *Abdom Imaging*, 2013. **38**(4): 802–17.
70. Bordeianou, L., Vagefi, P.A., Sahani, D. *et al.*, Cystic pancreatic endocrine neoplasms: a distinct tumor type? *J Am Coll Surg*, 2008. **206**: 1154–8.
71. Jang, K.M., Kim, S.H., Lee, S.J. *et al.*, The value of gadoxetic acid-enhanced and diffusion-weighted MRI for prediction of grading of pancreatic neuroendocrine tumors. *Acta Radiol*, 2014. **55**(2): 140–8.
72. Merkle, E.M., Bender, G.N., Brambs, H.J., Imaging findings in pancreatic lymphoma: differential aspects. *AJR Am J Roentgenol*, 2000. **174**(3): 671–5.
73. Low, G., Panu, A., Millo, N. *et al.*, Multimodality imaging of neoplastic and nonneoplastic solid lesions of the pancreas. *Radiographics*, **31**(4): 993–1015.
74. Van Beers, B., lalonde, L., Soyer, P. *et al.*, Dynamic CT in pancreatic lymphoma. *J Compu Assist Tomogr*, 1993. **17**: 94–97.
75. Fattahi, R., Cem Balci, N., Perman, W. *et al.*, Pancreatic diffusion-weighted imaging (DWI): comparison between mass-forming focal pancreatitis (FP), pancreatic cancer (PC), and normal pancreas. *J Magn Reson Imaging*, 2009. **29**(2): 350–6.
76. Chen, J., Baithun, S.I., Morphological study of 391 cases of exocrine pancreatic tumors with special reference to the classification of exocrine pancreatic carcinoma. *J Pathol*, 1985. **146**: 17–29.
77. Virlos, I.T., Papazachariou, I.M., Wiliamson, R.C.N., Acinar cell carcinoma of the pancreas with and without endocrine differentiation. *HPB (Oxford)*, 2002. **4**(2): 87–90.
78. Klimstra, D.S., Heffess, C.S., Oertel, J.E., Rosai, J., Acinar cell carcinoma of the pancreas: a clinicopathological study of 28 cases. *Am J Surg Pathol*, 1992. **16**: 815–37.
79. Hewan-Lowe, K.O., Acinar cell carcinoma of the pancreas: metastases from occult primary tumour. *Arch Pathol Lab Med*, 1983. **107**: 552–4.
80. Tatli, S., Mortele, K.J., Levy, A.D. *et al.*, CT and MRI features of pure acinar cell carcinoma of the pancreas in adults. *AJR Am J Roentgenol*, 2005. **184**(2): 511–9.

81. Katabi, N., Klimstra, D.S., Intraductal papillary mucinous neoplasms of the pancreas: clinical and pathological features and diagnostic approach. *J Clin Pathol*, **61** (2008), 1303–13.
82. Andrejevic-Blant, S., Kosmahl, M., Sipos, B. *et al.*, Papillary intraductal mucinous neoplasm: a new and evolving entity. *Virchows Arch*, **451** (2007), 863–9.
83. Kawamoto, S., Lawler, L.P., Horton, K.M. *et al.*, MDCT of intraductal papillary mucinous neoplasm of the pancreas: evaluation of features predictive of invasive carcinoma. *Am J Roentgenol*, 2006. **186**(3). 687–95.
84. Kalb, B., Sarmiento, J.M., Kooby, D.A. e*t al.*, MR imaging of cystic lesions of the pancreas. *Radiographics*, 2009. **29**(6): 1749–65.
85. Shin, S.S., Armao, D.M., Shah, M. *et al.*, Management of branch-duct intraductal papillary mucinous neoplasms of the pancreas: observation with MR imaging. *Magn Reson Imaging*, 2010. **28**(10): 1440–6.
86. Mortele, K.J., Cystic pancreatic neoplasms: imaging features and management strategy. *Semin Roentgenol*, 2013. **48**(3): 253–63.
87. Dewhurst, C.E., Mortele, K.J., Cystic tumor of the pancreas: imaging and management. *Radiol Clin North Am*, 2012. **50**(3): 467–86.
88. Irie, H., Honda, H., Aibe, H. *et al.*, MR cholangiopancreatographic differentiation of benign and malignant intraductal mucin-producing tumors of the pancreas. *AJR Am J Roentgenol*, **174** (2000), 1403–8.
89. Wang, Y., Miller, F.H., Chen, Z.E. *et al.*, Diffusion weighted MR imaging of solid and cystic lesions of the pancreas. *Radiographics*, 2011. **31**(3): E47–64.
90. Mottola, J.C., Sahni, V.A., Erturk, S.M. *et al.*, Diffusion-weighted MRI of focal cystic pancreatic lesions at 3.0-Tesla: preliminary results. *Abdom Imaging*, 2012. **37**(1): 110–7.
91. Kang, K.M., Lee, J.M., Shin, C.I. e*t al.*, Added value of diffusion-weighted imaging to MR cholangiopancreatography with unenhanced MR imaging for predicting malignancy or invasiveness of intraductal papillary mucinous neoplasm of the pancreas. *J Magn Reson Imaging*, 2013. **38**(3): 555–63.
92. Scott, J., Martin, I., Redhead, D. e*t al.*, Mucinous cystic neoplasms of the pancreas: imaging features and diagnostic difficulties. *Clin Radiol*, 2000. **55**: 187–92.
93. Goh, B.K., Tan, Y.M., Chung, Y.F. *et al.*, A review of mucinous cystic tumors of the pancreas defined by ovarian type stroma: clinicopathological features in 344 patients. *World J Surg*, 2006. **30**: 2236–45.

94. Scatarige, J.C., Horton, K.M., Sheth, S. *et al.*, Pancreatic parenchymal metastases: observations on helical CT. *AJR Am J Roentgenol*, 2001. **176**(3): 695–9.
95. Ng, C.S., Loyer, E.M., Iyer, R.B. *et al.*, Metastases to the pancreas from renal cell carcinoma: findings on three-phase contrast-enhanced helical CT. *AJR Am J Roentgenol*, 1999. **172**(6): 1555–9.
96. Klein, K.A., Stephens, D.H., Welch, T.J., CT characteristics of metastatic disease of the pancreas. *Radiographics*, **18**(2): 369–78.
97. Kaur, H., Choi, H., You, Y.N. *et al.*, MR imaging for preoperative evaluation of primary rectal cancer: practical considerations. *Radiographics*, 2012. **32**(2): 389–409.
98. Dewhurst, C.E., Mortele, K.J., Magnetic resonance imaging of rectal cancer. *Radiol Clin North Am*.
99. Low, R.N., McCue, M., Barone, R. *et al.*, MR staging of primary colorectal carcinoma: comparison with surgical and histopathologic findings. *Abdom Imaging*, 2003. **28**(6): 784–93.
100. Brown, G., Richards, C.J., Newcombe, R.G. *et al.*, Rectal carcinoma: thin-section MR imaging for staging in 28 patients. *Radiology*, 1999. **211**(1): 215–22.
101. MERCURY Study Group. Extramural depth of tumor invasion at thin-section MR in patients with rectal cancer: results of the MERCURY study. *Radiology* 2007. **243**(1): 132–9.
102. MERCURY Study Group. Diagnostic accuracy of preoperative magnetic resonance imaging in predicting curative resection of rectal cancer: prospective observational study. *BMJ*, 2006. **333**(7572): 779.
103. Beets-Tan, R.G., Beets, G.L., Vliegen, R.F. *et al.*, Accuracy of magnetic resonance imaging in prediction of tumour-free resection margin in rectal cancer surgery. *Lancet*, 2001. **357**(9255): 497–504.
104. Brown, G., Richards, C.J., Bourne, M.W. *et al.*, Morphologic predictors of lymph node status in rectal cancer with use of high-spatial-resolution MR imaging with histopathologic comparison. *Radiology*, 2003. **227**(2): 371–7.
105. Chun, H.K., Choi, D., Kim, M.J. *et al.*, Preoperative staging of rectal cancer: comparison of 3-T high-field MRI and endorectal sonography. *AJR Am J Roentgenol*, 2006. **187**(6): 1557–62.
106. Serour, F., Dona, G., Birkenfield, S., Balassiano, M., Krispin, M., Primary neoplasms of the small bowel. *J Surg Oncol*, 1992. **49**: 29–34.

107. Chou, C.K., Chen, L.T., Sheu, R.S. *et al.*, MRI manifestations of gastrointestinal lymphoma. *Abdom Imaging*, 1994. **19**: 495–500.
108. Ghai, S., Pattison, J., Ghai, S., O'Malley, M.E., Khalili, K., Stephens, M., Primary gastrointestinal lymphoma: spectrum of imaging findings with pathologic correlation. *Radiographics*, 2007. **27**: 1371–88.
109. Lee, W.K., Lau, E.F., Duddalwar, V.A. *et al.*, Abdominal manifestations of extranodal lymphoma: spectrum of imaging findings, *American Journal of Roentgenology*, 2008. **191**: 198–206.
110. Rubesin, S.E., Gilchrist, A.M., Bronner, M., Saul, S.H., Herlinger, H., Grumbach, K. *et al.*, Non-Hodgkin lymphoma of the small intestine. *Radiographics*, 1990. **10**: 985–98.
111. Lohan, D.G., Alhajeri, A.N., Cronin, C.G., Roche, C.J., Murphy, J.M., MR enterography of small-bowel lymphoma: potential for suggestion of histologic subtype and the presence of underlying celiac disease. *AJR Am J Roentgenol*, 2008. **190**: 287–293.
112. Kavaliauskiene, G., Ziech, M.L., Yung, Nio C. *et al.*, Small bowel MRI in adult patients: not just Crohn's disease — a tutorial. *Insights Imaging*, 2011; **2**(5): 501–13.
113. Lauenstein, T.C., Semelka, R.C., Emerging techniques: whole-body screeing and staging with MRI. *J Magn Reson Imaging,* 2006. **24**: 489–98.
114. Kwee, T.C., Kwee, R.M., Nievelstein., Imaging in staging of malignant lymphoma: a systematic review. *Blood*, 2008. **111**(2): 504–16.
115. Kwee, T.C., Vermoolen, M.A., Akkerman, E.A. *et al.*, Whole-body MRI, including diffusion-weighted imaging, for staging lymphoma: comparison with CT in a prospective multicenter study. *J Magn Reson Imaging*, 2013.
116. Littooij, A.S., Kwee, T.C., Barber, I. *et al.*, Whole-body MRI for initial staging of pediatric lymphoma: prospective comparison to an FDG-PET/CT-based reference standard. *Eur Radiol*, 2014.
117. Bader, T.R., Semelka, R.C., Chiu, V.C., Armao, D.M., Woosley, J.T., MRI of carcinoid tumors: spectrum of appearances in the gastrointestinal tract and liver. *J Magn Reson Imaging*, 2001. **14**: 261–9.
118. Levy, A.D., Sobin, L.H., From the archives of the AFIP: gastrointestinal carcinoids: Imaging features with clinicopathologic comparison. *Radiographics*, 2007. **27**: 237–57.
119. Chang, S., Choi, D., Lee, S.J., Lee, W.J., Park, M.H., Kim, S.W. *et al.*, Neuroendocrine neoplasms of the gastrointestinal tract: classification, pathologic basis, and imaging features. *Radiographics*, 2007. **27**: 1667–79.

120. Hussain, S.M., Outwater, E.K., Siegelman, E.S., Mucinous versus nonmucinous rectal carcinomas: differentiation with MR imaging. *Radiology*, 1999. **213**(1): 79–85.
121. Low, R.N., Barone, R.M., Gurney, J.M. *et al.*, Mucinous appendiceal neoplasms: preoperative MR staging and classification compared with surgical and histopathologic findings. *AJR Am J Roentgenol,* 2008. **190**(3): 656–65.
122. Gore, R.M., Gastric cancer. Clinical and pathologic features. *Radiol. Clin. North Am*, 1997. **35**(2): 295–310.
123. Kim, A.Y., Han, J.K., Seong, C.K. *et al.*, MRI in staging advanced gastric cancer: is it useful compared with spiral CT? *JCAT*, 2000. **24**(3): 389–94.
124. Kim, A.Y., Han, J.K., Kim, T.K. *et al.*, MR imaging of advanced gastric cancer: comparison of various MR pulse sequences using water and gadopentetate dimeglumine as oral contrast agents. *Abdom Imaging*, 2000. **25**(1): 7–13.
125. Levy, A.D., Remotti, H.E., Thompson, W.M. *et al.*, Gastrointestinal stromal tumors: radiologic features with pathologic correlation. *Radiographics*, **23**(2): 283–304, 456.
126. Warakaulle, D.R., Gleeson, F., MDCT appearance of gastrointestinal stromal tumors after therapy with imatinib mesylate. *AJR Am J Roentgenol*, 2006. **186**(2): 510–5.

Chapter 5

Nutritional Supports for Patients with Gastrointestinal Malignancies

Shadi S. Yarandi, Jinghua Hao, Qingwei Jiang, Zhuo Yang and Qiang Cai

What is New

- The prevalence of malnutrition in patients with gastrointestinal carcinoma is estimated to be 42–87%.
- Many reasons contribute to malnutrition in patients with gastrointestinal malignancies. Patients are often suffering from malnutrition even before any treatment. Therapeutic interventions for treating gastrointestinal malignancies can potentially worsen the situation.
- Some beneficial effects of nutritional support for patients with gastrointestinal malignancies have been reported. However, the effects of nutritional support remain controversial.

Definition and Prevalence of Malnutrition in Patients with Malignancies

Malnutrition is common in patients with gastrointestinal (GI) carcinoma. However, as for the exact definition of malnutrition, there are a few tools and questionnaires available for assessment of nutritional status in patients with malignancies. The European Society of Clinical Nutrition and Metabolism (ESPEN) guidelines have recommended use of two validated questionnaires in evaluation of nutritional status. One of these questionnaires is Nutritional Risk Screening 2002 (NRS2002) which consists of a pre-screening four questions module and final screening module. Another questionnaire is malnutrition universal screening tool (MUST) which is a five step screening questionnaire. Subjective global assessment (SGA) is a scoring system that includes physical exam findings, nutrition requirement, weight change, and GI symptoms and classifies nutritional status into well-nourished, at risk for malnutrition and malnourished based on the score.

The prevalence of malnutrition, defined as loss of more than 10% of weight over 6 months or 5% over 3 months or body mass index (BMI) of less than 18, in patients with GI malignancies has been estimated to be 42–87%.

Although several studies have examined the benefits of nutritional support in patients with GI malignancies and an apparent consensus among expert that oral peri-operative nutritional supplementation might reduce surgical complications, there is a significant amount of center to center variability in the approach to nutritional evaluation and therapeutic interventions. For example, one study performed in United Kingdom (UK) investigated the common practice in more than 60 centers treating patients with esophageal cancers. Among these centers, only 33% would perform routine nutritional assessment including measuring BMI, weight loss and serum albumin level. Pre-operative nutritional support was only provided in 17% of institutions routinely, and mostly for malnourished patients. Post-operative nutritional support was more common and was provided in 70% of practices.[1] Lack of widely accepted guidelines is one of the major reasons for lack of a common practice. Another study from UK reported that over a period of two years, from 517 patients with GI malignancies being treated at a cancer center who had experienced significant weight loss, only 299 were referred to a nutritionist and even most of these referrals happened after a significant delay.[2]

Factors Associated with Malnutrition

Many reasons contribute to malnutrition in patients with GI malignancies. Anorexia caused by malignancy can restrict nutritional input. Additionally, nausea, early satiety, dysphagia and altered intestinal motility are common in GI malignancies that can further limit the nutritional intake. On the other hand, cachexia caused by systemic release of tumor products leads to weight loss, fatigue and negative nitrogen balance. Therefore, patients with GI malignancies are often suffering from malnutrition even before any treatments.

Of note, therapeutic interventions for treating GI malignancies can potentially worsen the situation. Surgical interventions such as removing of esophagus and stomach can significantly affect route of nutritional intake and therefore amount of food being consumed by patients. Surgeries on small intestine and colon can also affect the food intake by altering intestinal motility and causing diarrhea. Furthermore, psychological and social factors might also add to the problem. Immediately after the surgery, patient may experience a hypermetabolic state that can exacerbate the imbalance between inadequate nutritional intake and calorie expenditure. Toxicities such as nausea, vomiting, diarrhea, anorexia or dysphagia can negatively affect nutritional status by decreasing food intake and/or absorption of nutrients, which may compound any pre-existing malnutrition.

Effects of Malnutrition on the Patients with GI Malignancies

Malnutrition and weight loss are associated with poor outcomes in patients with GI malignancies undergoing surgery and/or chemotherapy.[3,4] Weight loss before chemotherapy in 3,047 patients with cancer including GI malignancies reduces the survival of patients. A retrospective study of 143 patients with esophageal cancer using The Nutritional Risk Index (NRI) or Buzby Index [1.519 * serum albumin level (g/l) + 41.7 *(weight at the beginning of radiotherapy/baseline weight)] showed that low baseline pre-treatment NRI is a major predictor of reduced survival.[5,6] Another retrospective study of 268 patients with adenocarcinoma of pancreas undergoing Whipple procedure using serum albumin and Onodera's prognostic nutrition index (PNI) [10 × serum albumin (g/dl) + 0·005 × total lymphocyte count] showed that low pre-operative PNI is an independent predictive factor of poor survival.[7] Effects of weight loss on cancer prognosis are not limited to the immediate peri-operative timeframe. It has been shown that in patients with esophageal cancer, weight loss persists even one year after the treatment and can adversely affect long-term survival.[8]

Malnutrition and weight loss may also influence quality of life.[9] It has been shown that patients with <10% postoperative weight loss had a significantly better quality of life than those with more weight loss.[10] In a group of 73 patients with GI malignancies undergoing radiation therapy, a significant number of patients became malnourished during the treatment. These patients experienced a significantly higher prevalence of radiation therapy toxicity and poor clinical outcomes.[11] A prospective multicenter study reported that low NRI in patients with metastatic colon cancer is associated with increased chemotherapy related toxicity and reduced overall survival.[12] Furthermore, low NRI has also been shown to be associated with increased prevalence of wound infection after Whipple surgery in patients with pancreatic cancer.[13]

Another point is that the patients with poor nutritional status evident by low BMI, weight loss > 10% of the baseline, and low serum albumin level had higher odds of not responding to chemoradiation therapy.[14] In addition, study of 95 patients with colorectal or upper GI malignancies showed that pre-operative weight loss is associated with a significant increase in length of hospital stay.

Controversies on the Effects of Nutritional Supports

The beneficial effects of nutritional support before or immediately after initiation of treatment for GI malignancies have been investigated over the past several years and some beneficial effects have been reported. These effects have been attributed to several factors including the prevention of gastrointestinal mucosal atrophy, attenuation of the injury stress response, maintenance of immunocompetence, and the preservation of normal gut flora.

Oral nutritional support in the peri-operative time in patients undergoing elective gastrointestinal surgery or GI surgery in non-cancer patients has been shown to be beneficial.[15] In a large retrospective study, medical records of 1,410 patients who had surgery for GI malignancies were reviewed. It was found that pre-operative weight loss and low serum albumin level were associated with increased incidence of major and minor surgical complications while nutritional supplementation with either standard formula through parenteral or enteral route or with immune-enhancing formula had protective effects against post-operative complications. Amongst the formulas used, immune-enhancing formula had the most protective effects, followed by enteral supplementation of standard formula.[16] In patients who are malnourished before the surgery but not from cancer, same beneficial effect has been shown as well.[17] Even in well-nourished patients with GI malignancies, immune-enriched nutritional support peri-operatively has shown to reduce surgical complications, reduce length of hospital stay and cost of healthcare.[18] A prospective study of 67 well-nourished patients with colorectal cancer undergoing surgery showed that pre-operative supplementation with nutrition-enhancing diet reduced wound complications.[19]

A single-center randomized prospective study of 305 patients with gastrointestinal carcinoma examined the effect of an immune-enriched diet that contains arginine, glutamine and other immunonutrients peri-operatively on surgical outcomes. They excluded patients who had more than 10% weight loss before the surgery and divided the included patients to three groups. One group received only pre-operative oral supplementation, second group received both oral pre-operative supplementation as well as jejunal post-operative supplementation and third group received no supplementation. The results showed similar mortality in all groups, but reduction in infectious complication in both pre-operative only and peri-operative supplementation. Another study from Japan, randomized 60 patients with gastric carcinoma undergoing elective gastrectomy into two groups either receiving 750 ml/day of immune-enhanced formulas supplemented with arginine, RNA, and omega-3 PUFAs plus a conventional liquid diet or liquid diet alone for seven consecutive days until a day before the operation. Post-operatively, the duration of systemic inflammatory response (SIRS), need for antibiotic treatment, infectious complications and length of hospital stay were significantly lower in patients who received the supplemental immune-enhanced nutrition.[20] A study from China produced similar results by studying 60 patients with GI malignancy in a randomized fashion and reporting that pre-operative use of immune-enhancing nutritional supplement significantly reduces surgical complications and length of hospital stay.[21] Another small study compared the outcomes of 25 patients who received 5 days pre-operative immune-enhancing nutritional support with 13 control patients undergoing Whipple procedure and reported reduced risk of incisional infection.[22] A randomized clinical trial of patients with colorectal cancer divided 200 patients randomly to four groups: 1–5 days of oral immune-enhancing nutrition containing arginine and omega-3 fatty acids; 2–5 days of pre-op in addition to post-operative nutritional supplementation with same immune-enhancing formula; Pre-operative supplementation with standard nutritional formula; and Control group. Results showed significant decrease in surgical morbidity in the two groups who received immune-enhancing nutritional supplementation.[23] However, not all studies have produced positive results. A prospective, randomized, double-blind, placebo-controlled multicenter study of 108 well-nourished patients with GI adenocarcinoma undergoing major surgery receiving a immune-enriched diet vs. a regular diet for 3 days pre-operatively failed to show any benefit of nutritional supplementation on mortality, morbidity, surgical complications or length of hospital stay. A randomized clinical trial of 244 well-nourished patients with gastric cancer reported no benefit from pre-operative nutritional supplementation with an immune-enhancing formula. Another study of 221 patients with esophageal cancer treated with pre-operative immune-enhancing nutrition reported no effects on clinical outcome.

Preoperative use of this diet has shown to be well-tolerated by cancer patients and induces favorable structural changes in the white blood cell membranes and increased the body store of arginine and nucleotides.[24] Peri-operative use of immunonutrition reduces stress-induced immunosuppression after a major surgery, likely through the modulation of Th1/Th2 differentiation and interleukin-17 response.[25,26] A study of 60 patients undergoing surgery for GI malignancy receiving enteral immune-enhancing nutritional support showed increase in omega-3 fatty-acid concentration and decrease in prostaglandins along with reduced infectious/wound complications. Oral immune-enhancing nutritional supplementation has also shown to improve Th1/Th2 balance in patients with colorectal cancer.[27] Thirty-three patients with gastric cancer undergoing gastrectomy were randomized into a group receiving oral cystine (700 mg) and theanine (280 mg) or a placebo 4 days before to 5 days after surgery. The group treated with cystine and theanine had significantly lower IL-6 values, CRP levels, neutrophil counts and body temperatures.[28] The duration of required nutritional supplement in these patients has been estimated between 2–5 days, with change in immunological status has been shown as early as 2 days after the initiation of nutritional support. However, the optimal timing, duration and dosing of starting nutritional support, i.e pre-operatively vs. post-operatively, are not clear yet.

Efforts have been made to elucidate the optimal dose of oral immunonutrition before GI cancer surgeries. One prospective non-randomized study of patients with esophageal cancer undergoing esophagectomy examined 20 patients divided in two groups. One group received 500 ml/day and the other 1000 ml/day of a supplemental diet including arginine (12.8 g/l), n-3 fatty acids (4.1 g/l), and RNA (1.29 g/l) for 7 days before the operation. They measured the serum levels of interleukin-6 (IL-6), the C-reactive protein (CPR), and the total albumin and prealbumin one day before surgery and day 8 after surgery. They did not report any significant difference in biomarkers or outcomes between the two groups, concluding that administration of more than 500 ml/day of nutritional support is of no additional value.[29]

Early post-operation nutritional support via placement of a jejunal feeding tube has been studied but failed to prove any benefits. One study of 195 patients undergoing lapartomy for GI malignancy showed that starting nutritional supplementation rich in aminoacids and calories on post-op day 1 through a feeding tube did not affect mortality, morbidity or surgical complications. This finding was confirmed by other studies, even though some studies have shown beneficial effects of early enteral feeding after GI cancer surgery on net balance of nitrogen metabolism and aminoacid flux across the tissues.[30] A randomized clinical trial of 120 patients undergoing GI surgeries for malignancy showed no difference in infectious and non-infectious complications, mortality rate and length of hospital stay in patients who received immune-enhancing diet through a jejunostomy tube early after surgery. Additionally, more than 50% of patients experienced complications associated with jejunostomy tube.[31] In a randomized clinical trial of 58 patients with gastric cancer undergoing gastric surgery, not only no beneficial effects for early enteral nutrition was reported, but patients in the intervention group had lower quality of life due to increased incidence of nausea, vomiting and abdominal pain.[32] In a randomized clinical trial studying 167 malnourished patients with upper GI malignancies, pall patients received parenteral nutrition for 14 days before the surgery and were divided based on post-operative nutritional supplementation into four groups receiving either enteral or parenteral standard or immunoenhancing nutrition. The results showed no significant difference in clinical outcomes between the groups.[33] Study of 183 well-nourished patients who received immune-enhancing nutritional supplementation after the surgery showed no beneficial effects on clinical outcome.

Despite the negative result reported above, some studies have shown a positive effect for early post-operative enteral feeding, especially with immune-enhanced diet. Early oral feeding after gastric surgery for gastric cancer has been reported to be safe and feasible.[34] In a small randomized prospective study of 24 patients undergoing curative surgery for esophageal carcinoma, patients who received early enteral nutrition (post-operative day 1) showed significantly earlier recovery of the total lymphocyte count, lower serum levels of total bilirubin and C-reactive protein and tolerated the feeding well compared to those who were started on enteral feeding on post-operative day 5. However, there was no difference in clinical outcomes.[35] A randomized clinical trial of 48 patients with GI cancer undergoing surgery reported that starting immune-enhancing diet as early as 48 hours after the surgery can increase levels of nitric oxide, total lymphocytes, T lymphocytes, T-helper cells, and NK cells while reducing levels of IL-6 and TNF-α. In a study from Italy, 109 patients with gastric cancer undergoing gastrectomy were randomized into groups either receiving early post-operative immune-enhanced nutrition or an isocaloric–isonitrogenous control diet. The authors reported that incidence of infectious complications, anastomosis leak, and length of hospital stay were significantly lower in the early post-operative immune-enhance nutrition group.[36] Another study with positive results is from a group of researchers in Japan who studied 40 patients undergoing esophageal cancer surgery. They divided these patients into a group of 20 patients as control, 6 patients with only pre-operative immune-enhanced nutritional supplement and 14 patients with both pre- and post-operative nutritional supplement. They reported reduced length of SIRS and incidence of wound infection in the group who received post-operative nutritional supplementation.[37] A group from Spain reported that early post-operative enteral feeding with immune-enhancing diet would reduce wound complications in patients undergoing surgery for gastric cancer.[38] A meta-analysis of 15 randomized clinical trial including 1,240 patients undergoing GI surgeries showed reduction of surgical complications in patients undergoing early post-surgical enteral nutrition, but this was an all-inclusive meta-analysis that was not limited to surgeries for GI malignancies.

Prolonged nutritional supplementation has also been studied in patients with GI malignancies. A study of long-term nutritional supplementation in patients with colon and gastric malignancy showed improved quality of life and enhanced weight gain in patients undergoing the intervention.[39] A recent study investigated the effect of prolonged nutritionist-controlled intensive nutritional support before the surgery in 28 patients with esophageal cancer and reported an adjusted odds ratio of 0.23 (95% confidence interval: 0.053–0.97; $p = 0.045$) of developing serious complications after the surgery compared with a control group.[40]

Several meta-analysis have been performed to investigate the effects of peri-operative use of immunonutriton in patients undergoing gastrointestinal surgery. Cerantola *et al.*[41] published one of these meta-analysis in which they included 21 randomized clinical trials published between 1985 and 2009 consisting of 2,730 patients. They showed siginifcant heterogeneity in the trials and reported that use of immunonutrition before, after or both before and after the surgery can reduce surgical complications and length of hospital stay but does not have any effect on mortality.[41] However, they did not attempt to separate patients with GI malignancy from others. A meta-analysis performed by Carey *et al.* focusing on long-term nutritional support in patients undergoing GI surgery between 1980 and 2009 reported that long-term oral nutritional supplementation improves multiple clinical outcomes after surgery. Zhang *et al.* reviewed 19 randomized clinical trial performed between 1995 and 2011 investigating effects of immunonutriton on outcomes of surgery for GI malignancies. The analysis included 231 patients and showed the perioperative immnuonutrition reduces length of hospital stay, morbidity from infectious complications and morbidity from non-infectious complications.[42] Marimuthu *et al.* performed a meta-analysis of 26 randomized clinical trials performed between 1980 and 2011 consisting of 2,496 patients undergoing major gastrointestinal surgery and reported strong evidence in support of beneficial effects of immune-enhancing nutrition on reducing surgical complications and length of hospital stay. Heys *et al.* reported a meta-analysis of 11 randomized clinical trials of patients with critical illness and cancer receiving pre-operative immune-enhancing nutritional support and found strong evidence in support of role of immune-enhancing nutrition in reducing incidence of infectious complications, pneumonia, death, and length of hospital stay.[43]

The role of parenteral nutritional support in cancer patients undergoing major surgeries including those with GI malignancies is more controversial. Several studies have examined the effect of total parenteral nutrition (TPN) on reducing mortality and morbidity after surgery with conflicting results. While several studies failed to show any benefit on post-surgical complications, morbidity or length of hospital stay, some have shown some benefits.[44] A prospective study of 258 patients undergoing surgery for pancreatic malignancy treated with TPN pre- and post-operatively showed that the total rate of major complication after surgery was actually higher in patients receiving TPN. Therefore, routine use of TPN in patients undergoing surgery for GI malignancies is not recommended. In another prospective study of 68 patients undergoing hepatobilliary surgery and receiving TPN post-operatively, there was no significant difference in surgical outcomes and patients receiving TPN had higher incidence of septic complications. Forty-one patients with GI cancer were divided based on their nutritional status into malnourished and well-nourished and either received TPN or did not receive nutritional support. Regardless of baseline nutritional status, TPN did not change the clinical outcomes while it helped patients maintain weight.[45] A randomized study of 90 patients with gastric cancer, showed no benefit for two weeks of pre-operative TPN, while showing that loss of more than 10% weight before surgery can adversely affect the outcome. A multi-center randomized clinical trial of 317 malnourished patients undergoing surgery for GI malignancy compared the benefits of enteral vs. parenteral nutrition and found that patients who received enteral nutrition had less post-surgical complications and shorter length of hospital stay.[46] A meta-analysis of 29 clinical trials including 2,552 patients undergoing gastrointestinal surgery comparing enteral vs. parenteral nutrition peri-operativley showed that enteral nutrition is superior in reducing surgical complication and hospital stay.[47]

On the other hand, a randomized study of 124 patients with hepatocellular carcinoma showed that peri-operative intravenous supplementation with a diet consisting of branched chain aminoacids, dextrose, and lipid emulsion for 8 days reduced overall post-operative morbidity rate, weight loss, and deterioration of liver functions.[48] A study of 55 patients with carcinoma of stomach and esophagus undergoing surgery and receiving TPN pre-operatively showed reduction of wound infection, pneumonia and other major complications in the group receiving TPN. A randomized clinical trial of 90 malnourished patients with gastric and colorectal cancers suggested that use of TPN 10 days before the surgery and continued after the surgery might reduce non-infectious complications and improve survival.[49] There is an ongoing open label, controlled, prospective, randomized, multicentre phase IIIb trial to investigate the effect of parenteral nutritional support on the outcome of chemotherapy in patients with pancreatic cancer.[50] Outpatient use of TPN has been examined in patients with pancreatic adenocarcinoma. Out of 32 patients who received treatment for 18 months, 27 of them experienced some benefit in improving and stabilization of nutritional status.[51]

One important question is whether use of immune-enhancing nutritional support is cost-effective.[52] A recent study has addressed this question by using data from a meta-analysis of clinical trials investigating benefits of nutritional supplementation and calculating the costs of this intervention. The authors reported relative risk of complications with pre-, peri- and post-operative use of immune-modulating formula to be 0.69 (95%CI 0.58–0.83), 0.62 (95%CI 0.53–0.73) and 0.73 (95%CI 0.35–0.96) respectively. They also reported a significant reduction in cost of hospital care for patients receiving immune-enhancing nutritional support and concluded that this intervention is effective and cost-saving.[53] Another meta-analysis done showed that use of immunonutrition in patients who undergo elective surgeries for GI malignancies can result in reducing the cost of care per patient up to $3,300 with reduction in infectious complication rates or $6,000 based on length of hospital stay.[54]

Take Home Messages

- Malnutrition is common in patients with GI malignancies and adversely affects surgical and oncologic outcomes.
- Although there is evidence for benefit of pre-operative use of oral immune enhancing nutritional support, this is not routinely recommended or used in practice.
- Post-operative parenteral nutrition or oral nutrition remains controversial and should not be used routinely.

References

1. Murphy, P.M., Modi, P., Rahamim, J., Wheatley, T., and Lewis, S.J., An investigation into the current peri-operative nutritional management of oesophageal carcinoma patients in major carcinoma centres in England. *Ann R Coll Surg Engl*, 2006. **88**(4): 358–62.
2. Baldwin, C., McGough, C., Norman, A.R., Frost, G.S., Cunningham, D.C., and Andreyev, H.J., Failure of dietetic referral in patients with gastrointestinal cancer and weight loss. *Eur J Cancer*, 2006. **42**(15): 2504–9.
3. Mullen, J.L., Consequences of malnutrition in the surgical patient. *Surg Clin North Am*, 1981. **61**(3): 465–87.
4. Di Carlo, V., Gianotti, L., Balzano, G., Zerbi, A., and Braga, M., Complications of pancreatic surgery and the role of perioperative nutrition. *Dig Surg*, 1999. **16**(4): 320–6.
5. Clavier, J.B., Antoni, D., Atlani, D., Ben Abdelghani, M., Schumacher, C., Dufour, P., Kurtz, J.E., and Noel, G., Baseline nutritional status is prognostic factor after definitive radiochemotherapy for esophageal cancer. *Dis Esophagus*, 2012.

6. Bollschweiler, E., Herbold, T., Plum, P., and Holscher, A.H., Prognostic relevance of nutritional status in patients with advanced esophageal cancer. *Expert Rev Anticancer Ther*, 2013. **13**(3): 275–78.
7. Kanda, M., Fujii, T., Kodera, Y., Nagai, S., Takeda, S., and Nakao, A., Nutritional predictors of postoperative outcome in pancreatic cancer. *Br J Surg*, 2011. **98**(2): 268–74.
8. D'Journo, X.B., Ouattara, M., Loundou, A., Trousse, D., Dahan, L., Nathalie, T., Doddoli, C., Seitz, J.F., and Thomas, P.A., Prognostic impact of weight loss in 1-year survivors after transthoracic esophagectomy for cancer. *Dis Esophagus*, 2012. **25**(6): 527–34.
9. Gavazzi, C., Colatruglio, S., Sironi, A., Mazzaferro, V., and Miceli, R., Importance of early nutritional screening in patients with gastric cancer. *Br J Nutr*, 2011. **106**(12): 1773–8.
10. O'Gorman, P., McMillan, D.C., and McArdle, C.S., Impact of weight loss, appetite, and the inflammatory response on quality of life in gastrointestinal cancer patients. *Nutr Cancer*, 1998. **32**(2): 76–80.
11. Hill, A., Kiss, N., Hodgson, B., Crowe, T.C., and Walsh, A.D., Associations between nutritional status, weight loss, radiotherapy treatment toxicity and treatment outcomes in gastrointestinal cancer patients. *Clin Nutr*, 2011. **30**(1): 92–98.
12. Barret, M., Malka, D., Aparicio, T., Dalban, C., Locher, C., Sabate, J.M., Louafi, S., Mansourbakht, T., Bonnetain, F., Attar, A., and Taieb, J., Nutritional status affects treatment tolerability and survival in metastatic colorectal cancer patients: results of an AGEO prospective multicenter study. *Oncology*, 2011. **81**(5–6): 395–402.
13. Shinkawa, H., Takemura, S., Uenishi, T., Sakae, M., Ohata, K., Urata, Y., Kaneda, K., Nozawa, A., and Kubo, S., Nutritional risk index as an independent predictive factor for the development of surgical site infection after pancreaticoduodenectomy. *Surg Today*, 2013. **43**(3): 276–83.
14. Di Fiore, F., Lecleire, S., Pop, D., Rigal, O., Hamidou, H., Paillot, B., Ducrotte, P., Lerebours, E., and Michel, P., Baseline nutritional status is predictive of response to treatment and survival in patients treated by definitive chemoradiotherapy for a locally advanced esophageal cancer. *Am J Gastroenterol*, 2007. **102**(11): 2557–63.
15. Braga, M., Gianotti, L., Radaelli, G., Vignali, A., Mari, G., Gentilini, O., and Di Carlo, V., Perioperative immunonutrition in patients undergoing cancer

surgery: results of a randomized double-blind phase 3 trial. *Arch Surg*, 1999. **134**(4): 428–33.

16. Bozzetti, F., Gianotti, L., Braga, M., Di Carlo, V., and Mariani, L., Postoperative complications in gastrointestinal cancer patients: the joint role of the nutritional status and the nutritional support. *Clin Nutr*, 2007. **26**(6): 698–709.
17. Giger, U., Buchler, M., Farhadi, J., Berger, D., Husler, J., Schneider, H., Krahenbuhl, S., and Krahenbuhl, L., Preoperative immunonutrition suppresses perioperative inflammatory response in patients with major abdominal surgery-a randomized controlled pilot study. *Ann Surg Oncol*, 2007. **14**(10): 2798–806.
18. Helminen, H., Raitanen, M., and Kellosalo, J., Immunonutrition in elective gastrointestinal surgery patients. *Scand J Surg*, 2007. **96**(1): 46–50.
19. Horie, H., Okada, M., Kojima, M., and Nagai, H., Favorable effects of preoperative enteral immunonutrition on a surgical site infection in patients with colorectal cancer without malnutrition. *Surg Today*, 2006. **36**(12): 1063–8.
20. Okamoto, Y., Okano, K., Izuishi, K., Usuki, H., Wakabayashi, H., and Suzuki, Y., Attenuation of the systemic inflammatory response and infectious complications after gastrectomy with preoperative oral arginine and omega-3 fatty acids supplemented immunonutrition. *World J Surg*, 2009. **33**(9): 1815–21.
21. Xu, J., Zhong, Y., Jing, D., and Wu, Z., Preoperative enteral immunonutrition improves postoperative outcome in patients with gastrointestinal cancer. *World J Surg*, 2006. **30**(7): 1284–9.
22. Shirakawa, H., Kinoshita, T., Gotohda, N., Takahashi, S., Nakagohri, T., and Konishi, M., Compliance with and effects of preoperative immunonutrition in patients undergoing pancreaticoduodenectomy. *J Hepatobiliary Pancreat Sci*, 2012. **19**(3): 249–58.
23. Braga, M., Gianotti, L., Vignali, A., and Carlo, V.D., Preoperative oral arginine and n-3 fatty acid supplementation improves the immunometabolic host response and outcome after colorectal resection for cancer. *Surgery*, 2002. **132**(5): 805–14.
24. Tsujinaka, T., Hirao, M., Fujitani, K., Mishima, H., Ikenaga, M., Sawamura, T., and Kurata, M., Effect of preoperative immunonutrition on body composition in patients undergoing abdominal cancer surgery. *Surg Today*, 2007. **37**(2): 118–21.

25. Suzuki, D., Furukawa, K., Kimura, F., Shimizu, H., Yoshidome, H., Ohtsuka, M., Kato, A., Yoshitomi, H., and Miyazaki, M., Effects of perioperative immunonutrition on cell-mediated immunity, T helper type 1 (Th1)/Th2 differentiation, and Th17 response after pancreaticoduodenectomy. *Surgery*, 2010. **148**(3): 573–81.
26. Maruyama, T., Mimura, K., Izawa, S., Shiba, S., Watanabe, M., Kawaguchi, Y., Fujii, H., and Kono, K., Immunonutritional diet modulates natural killer cell activation and Th17 cell distribution in patients with gastric and esophageal cancer. *Nutrition*, 2011. **27**(2): 146–52.
27. Matsuda, A., Furukawa, K., Takasaki, H., Suzuki, H., Kan, H., Tsuruta, H., Shinji, S., and Tajiri, T., Preoperative oral immune-enhancing nutritional supplementation corrects TH1/TH2 imbalance in patients undergoing elective surgery for colorectal cancer. *Dis Colon Rectum*, 2006. **49**(4): 507–16.
28. Miyachi, T., Tsuchiya, T., Oyama, A., Tsuchiya, T., Abe, N., Sato, A., Chiba, Y., Kurihara, S., Shibakusa, T., and Mikami, T., Perioperative oral administration of cystine and theanine enhances recovery after distal gastrectomy: a prospective randomized trial. *JPEN J Parenter Enteral Nutr*, 2013. **37**(3): 384–91.
29. Nakamura, M., Iwahashi, M., Takifuji, K., Nakamori, M., Naka, T., Ishida, K., Ojima, T., Iida, T., Katsuda, M., Hayata, K., and Yamaue, H., Optimal dose of preoperative enteral immunonutrition for patients with esophageal cancer. *Surg Today*, 2009. **39**(10): 855–60.
30. Harrison, L., Hochwald, S., Heslin, M., Berman, R., Burt, M., and Brennan, M., Early postoperative enteral nutrition improves peripheral protein kinetics in upper gastrointestinal cancer patients undergoing complete resection: a randomized trial. *J Parenteral Enteral Nut*, 1997. **21**(4): 202–7.
31. Lobo, D.N., Williams, R.N., Welch, N.T., Aloysius, M.M., Nunes, Q.M., Padmanabhan, J., Crowe, J.R., Iftikhar, S.Y., Parsons, S.L., Neal, K.R., Allison, S.P., and Rowlands, B.J., Early postoperative jejunostomy feeding with an immune modulating diet in patients undergoing resectional surgery for upper gastrointestinal cancer: a prospective, randomized, controlled, double-blind study. *Clin Nutr*, 2006. **25**(5): 716–26.
32. Hur, H., Kim, S.G., Shim, J.H., Song, K.Y., Kim, W., Park, C.H., and Jeon, H.M., Effect of early oral feeding after gastric cancer surgery: a result of randomized clinical trial. *Surgery*, 2011. **149**(4): 561–8.

33. Klek, S., Sierzega, M., Szybinski, P., Szczepanek, K., Scislo, L., Walewska, E., and Kulig, J., Perioperative nutrition in malnourished surgical cancer patients — a prospective, randomized, controlled clinical trial. *Clin Nutr*, 2011. **30**(6): 708–13.
34. Jo, D.H., Jeong, O., Sun, J.W., Jeong, M.R., Ryu, S.Y., and Park, Y.K., Feasibility study of early oral intake after gastrectomy for gastric carcinoma. *J Gastric Cancer*, 2011. **11**(2): 101–8.
35. Aiko, S., Yoshizumi, Y., Sugiura, Y., Matsuyama, T., Naito, Y., Matsuzaki, J., and Maehara, T., Beneficial effects of immediate enteral nutrition after esophageal cancer surgery. *Surg Today*, 2001. **31**(11): 971–8.
36. Marano, L., Porfidia, R., Pezzella, M., Grassia, M., Petrillo, M., Esposito, G., Braccio, B., Gallo, P., Boccardi, V., Cosenza, A., Izzo, G., and Di Martino, N., Clinical and immunological impact of early postoperative enteral immunonutrition after total gastrectomy in gastric cancer patients: a prospective randomized study. *Ann Surg Oncol*, 2013. **20**(12): 3912–8.
37. Takeuchi, H., Ikeuchi, S., Kawaguchi, Y., Kitagawa, Y., Isobe, Y., Kubochi, K., Kitajima, M., and Matsumoto, S., Clinical significance of perioperative immunonutrition for patients with esophageal cancer. *World J Surg*, 2007. **31**(11): 2160–7.
38. Farreras, N., Artigas, V., Cardona, D., Rius, X., Trias, M., and Gonzalez, J.A., Effect of early postoperative enteral immunonutrition on wound healing in patients undergoing surgery for gastric cancer. *Clin Nutr*, 2005. **24**(1): 55–65.
39. Carey, S., Ferrie, S., Young, J., and Allman-Farinelli, M., Long-term nutrition support in gastrointestinal disease — a systematic review of the evidence. *Nutrition*, 2012. **28**(1): 4–8.
40. Ligthart-Melis, G.C., Weijs, P.J., te Boveldt, N.D., Buskermolen, S., Earthman, C.P., Verheul, H.M., de Lange-de Klerk, E.S., van Weyenberg, S.J., and van der Peet, D.L., Dietician-delivered intensive nutritional support is associated with a decrease in severe postoperative complications after surgery in patients with esophageal cancer. *Dis Esophagus,* 2013. **26**(6): 587–93.
41. Cerantola, Y., Hubner, M., Grass, F., Demartines, N., and Schafer, M., Immunonutrition in gastrointestinal surgery. *Br J Surg*, 2011. **98**(1): 37–48.
42. Zhang, Y., Gu, Y., Guo, T., Li, Y., and Cai, H., Perioperative immunonutrition for gastrointestinal cancer: a systematic review of randomized controlled trials. *Surg Oncol*, 2012. **21**(2): e87–95.

43. Heys, S.D., Walker, L.G., Smith, I., and Eremin, O., Enteral nutritional supplementation with key nutrients in patients with critical illness and cancer: a meta-analysis of randomized controlled clinical trials. *Ann Surg*, 1999. **229**(4): 467–77.
44. Muller, J.M., Brenner, U., Dienst, C., and Pichlmaier, H., Preoperative parenteral feeding in patients with gastrointestinal carcinoma. *Lancet*, 1982. **1**(8263): 68–71.
45. Thompson, B.R., Julian, T.B., and Stremple, J.F., Perioperative total parenteral nutrition in patients with gastrointestinal cancer. *J Surg Res*, 1981. **30**(5): 497–500.
46. Bozzetti, F., Braga, M., Gianotti, L., Gavazzi, C., and Mariani, L., Postoperative enteral versus parenteral nutrition in malnourished patients with gastrointestinal cancer: a randomised multicentre trial. *Lancet*, 2001. **358**(9292): 1487–92.
47. Mazaki, T., and Ebisawa, K., Enteral versus parenteral nutrition after gastrointestinal surgery: a systematic review and meta-analysis of randomized controlled trials in the English literature. *J Gastrointest Surg*, 2008. **12**(4): 739–55.
48. Fan, S.T., Lo, C.M., Lai, E.C., Chu, K.M., Liu, C.L., and Wong, J., Perioperative nutritional support in patients undergoing hepatectomy for hepatocellular carcinoma. *N Engl J Med*, 1994. **331**(23): 1547–52.
49. Bozzetti, F., Gavazzi, C., Miceli, R., Rossi, N., Mariani, L., Cozzaglio, L., Bonfanti, G., and Piacenza, S., Perioperative total parenteral nutrition in malnourished, gastrointestinal cancer patients: a randomized, clinical trial. *J Parenteral Enteral Nutr*, 2000. **24**(1): 7–14.
50. Marten, A., Wente, M. N., Ose, J., Buchler, M.W., Rotzer, I., Decker-Baumann, C., Karapanagiotou-Schenkel, I., Harig, S., Schmidt, J., and Jager, D., An open label randomized multicentre phase IIIb trial comparing parenteral substitution versus best supportive nutritional care in subjects with pancreatic adenocarcinoma receiving 5-FU plus oxaliplatin as 2nd or higher line chemotherapy regarding clinical benefit — PANUSCO. *BMC Cancer*, 2009. **9**: 412.
51. Pelzer, U., Arnold, D., Govercin, M., Stieler, J., Doerken, B., Riess, H., and Oettle, H., Parenteral nutrition support for patients with pancreatic cancer. Results of a phase II study. *BMC Cancer*, 2010. **10**: 86.

52. Gianotti, L., Braga, M., Frei, A., Greiner, R., and Di Carlo, V., Health care resources consumed to treat postoperative infections: cost saving by perioperative immunonutrition. *Shock*, 2000. **14**(3): 325–330.
53. Chevrou-Severac, H., Pinget, C., Cerantola, Y., Demartines, N., Wasserfallen, J.B., and Schafer, M., Cost-effectiveness analysis of immune-modulating nutritional support for gastrointestinal cancer patients. *Clin Nutr*, 2013.
54. Mauskopf, J.A., Candrilli, S.D., Chevrou-Severac, H., and Ochoa, J.B., Immunonutrition for patients undergoing elective surgery for gastrointestinal cancer: impact on hospital costs. *World J Surg Oncol*, 2012. **10**: 136.

Chapter 6

Palliative Care for Patients with Advanced Gastrointestinal Malignancies

Tilak U. Shah and Steven Keilin

What is New

- **Esophagus**
  - ♦ Until recently, available esophageal stents in the United States could not pass through the working channel of a gastroscope. A through the scope (TTS) esophageal metal stent has recently been approved for use in the United States.
  - ♦ Cryoablation is a promising new technique for palliating malignant dysphagia in advanced esophageal cancer.
- **Biliary**
  - ♦ Endoscopic ultrasound guided transpapillary or biliary drainage is an option when endoscopic retrograde transpapillary access is unsuccessful; EUS guided drainage is technically challenging and consequently not widely available.
  - ♦ Radiofrequency ablation is a promising adjunctive therapy for palliation of malignant obstructive jaundice.
  - ♦ Paclitaxel drug eluting covered metal biliary stents do not appear to increase stent patency compared to non-drug eluting

metal stents; gemcitabine drug eluting metal biliary stents are currently being evaluated as a means of increased metal stent patency.

- **Gastroduodenal**
  - Covered metal gastroduodenal stents have been developed, but their widespread use in clinical practice will likely be limited by the higher risk of migration compared to uncovered stents, and their potential for obstructing the biliary orifice.
- **Colorectal**
  - Emerging data suggest that bevacizumab is associated with increased risk of perforation after colonic stent placement for malignant colorectal obstruction. Colonic stenting is best avoided in patients who are receiving or will receive bevacizumab.

Palliation of Advanced Esophageal Cancer

Introduction

The most common primary malignancies arising from the esophagus are squamous cell carcinoma and adenocarcinoma. Lung cancers are the most common extra-esophageal malignancies associated with extrinsic esophageal compression and trachea-esophageal fistula, accounting for 30% to 50% of extra-esophageal malignant dysphagia.[1] Less frequent extra-esophageal cancers associated with malignant dysphagia include metastatic breast cancers, liposarcomas, and lymphomas.[1]

Approximately 50–60% of patients with esophageal cancer have locally advanced or metastatic disease at the time of diagnosis.[2] In these patients, palliation of dysphagia, nutritional support, and managing complications like trachea-esophageal fistula become the primary focus of therapy. Currently available methods of palliating dysphagia in patients with esophageal cancer include endoscopic therapies and radiation therapy. Palliative chemotherapy has a limited impact in this setting, and a marginal impact on survival. Palliative surgery is seldom performed in patients with advanced esophageal cancer because of its unacceptably high morbidity and mortality. Palliative esophagectomy is associated with 10–20% mortality, and 50% risk of major non-fatal complications.[3] Surgical bypass carries a 15–20% mortality risk, and a 75% risk of non-fatal complications.[4] Endoscopic approaches to manage dysphagia due to luminal obstruction by tumor include esophageal stenting, mechanical dilation, and endoscopic tumor ablation (e.g. laser, photodynamic therapy, and cryoablation). Among these options, esophageal stenting is the most frequently utilized endoscopic technique for management of malignant dysphagia.[5]

Esophageal stents

The initial stents described for palliation of esophageal obstruction were rigid prostheses made from polyvinyl plastic or rubber. These prostheses were difficult to place and required mechanical dilation before placement. Consequently, they were associated with high rates of bleeding and perforation, which limited their widespread use.[5,6] In the 1990s, self-expandable metal stents (SEMS) were introduced. These stents demonstrated equivalent or better palliation of dysphagia, shorter hospital stay, and reduced risk of complications when compared to the older endoprostheses.[7,8] Although plastic endoprostheses are cheaper, metal stents are more cost-effective because of their reduced rate of complications and decrease in length of hospitalization.[9] Esophageal SEMS in the United States range from 6 cm to 15 cm in length and 10 mm to 23 mm in diameter. Until recently, available esophageal metal stents in the United States (Figs. 1a, 1b) were all deployed over the wire (OTW). A through the scope (TTS) metal stent has recently been introduced in the United States.

Recurrent dysphagia due to tumor ingrowth between the stent interstices was an important limitation of the initial uncovered SEMS. Partially covered metal stents were subsequently developed to address this limitation. Prospective and retrospective studies have demonstrated significant decrease in need for re-intervention due to tumor ingrowth in patients receiving partially covered metal stents compared to uncovered metal stents.[9,10] Retrospective data suggested that stent migration was more common in patients receiving partially covered stents, although this difference was not observed in a multicenter prospective study.[9,10] There are several partially covered SEMS currently available. Randomized trials have not demonstrated any significant differences in technical success, relief of dysphagia, tumor ingrowth, or stent migration among

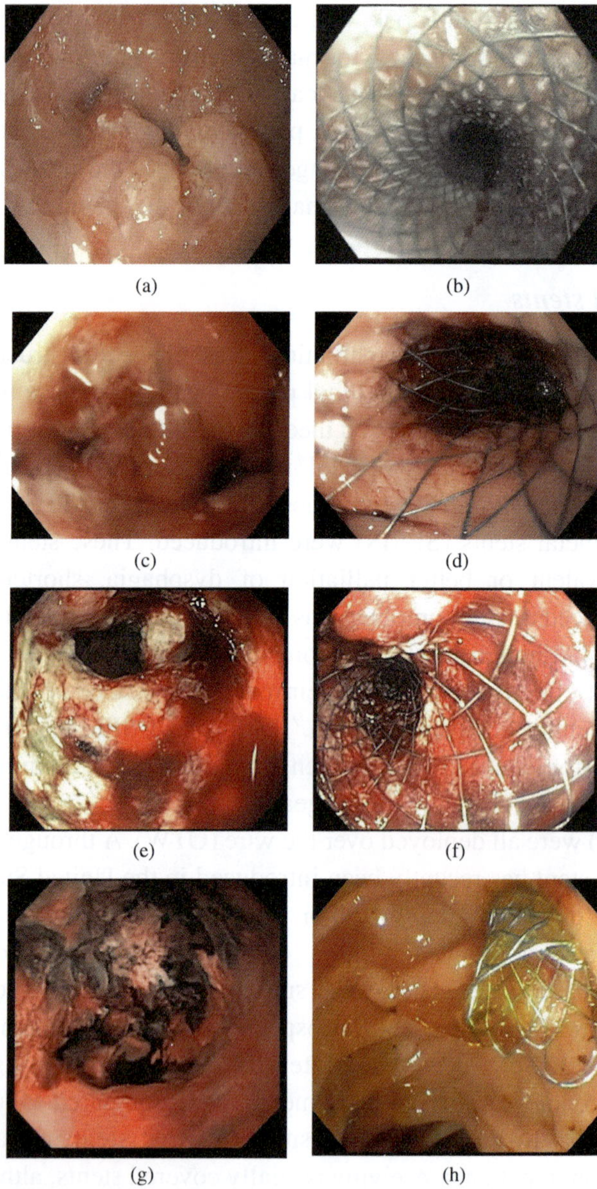

Fig. 1. (a) Middle esophageal adenocarcinoma; (b) Partially covered metal esophageal stent (23 mm × 12 cm); (c) Pancreatic adenocarcinoma with duodenal obstruction; (d) Uncovered metal duodenal stent (22 mm × 9 cm); (e) Sigmoid adenocarcinoma; (f) Uncovered metal colonic stent within a stent for tumor ingrowth (25 mm × 9 cm); (g) Cholangiocarcinoma seen on high definition cholangioscopy with narrow band imaging; (h) Covered metal biliary stent (10 mm × 6 cm).

different partially covered esophageal SEMS.[11,12] Fully covered metal stents that are potentially retrievable have recently been introduced, but available evidence suggests that they migrate more frequently than partially covered metal stents without any significant decrease in technical success, tumor ingrowth or complications.[13] A self-expandable plastic stent has also demonstrated safety and efficacy in palliation of malignant dysphagia. Comparative studies of SEMS versus plastic stents have shown similar dysphagia relief, but self-expandable plastic stents are more technically difficult to place and migrate more frequently.[14,15] Consequently, self-expandable plastic stents are less frequently used when compared to SEMS.

In addition to their utility in the palliation of malignant dysphagia, covered stents have emerged as an alternative to surgery in patients with malignant trachea-esophageal fistulas.[16] Fistulas can occur due to tumor infiltration into the respiratory tract or pressure necrosis from stents or radiation therapy. In a large case series of 60 patients, covered SEMS successfully sealed off the fistula in 80% of patients.[17] Thirty patients had recurrent fistulas, many of who were successfully re-treated with covered stents. Covered metal stents are therefore the first-line therapy in patients with malignant tracheo-esophageal fistula, particularly given the high morbidity of surgery and the poor overall median survival of three months.[5]

Esophageal stenting can lead to early complications (within first 2 to 4 weeks) as well as delayed complications (after 2 to 4 weeks). The most common early and late complication is stent migration. Other common early complications include chest pain, gastro-esophageal reflux disease, and globus sensation. Significant bleeding and perforation are uncommon early complications that occur in less than 1% of cases.[18] Delayed complications occur in up to 50%, and often require re-intervention. Common delayed complications include recurrent dysphagia (due to tumor ingrowth, stent migration or food impaction) and trachea-esophageal fistula.[19]

Several technical considerations may complicate the placement, effectiveness, or tolerability of an esophageal stent. High-grade strictures may require dilation prior to stent placement or placement of a smaller diameter stent. Stent placement across a large bulky tumor in the proximal or mid esophagus can cause tracheal compression. In these patients, placement of a tracheal stent prior to esophageal stenting should be considered.

In order to adequately palliate dysphagia, esophageal stents must not only bridge the stricture but also extend 2–4 cm beyond the proximal and distal end of the stricture. Strictures located close to the upper esophageal sphincter or lower esophageal sphincter may therefore be difficult to stent properly. Stenting across an upper esophageal stricture can cause intolerable pain and globus sensation. Attempting to place the proximal end of the stent at least 2 cm below the upper esophageal sphincter is generally advised to minimize these symptoms. Stenting across the gastro-esophageal junction increases risk of aspiration and reflux. Stents with anti-reflux valves have been designed to address these potential complications of stenting across the gastro-esophageal junction. In one randomized trial, reflux occurred in only 12% of patients who received an anti-reflux valve stent, compared to 96% of patients who received a standard metal stent.[20] Subsequent randomized trials have not consistently demonstrated any differences in reflux or health related quality of life scores, so routine use of these stents cannot be recommended as yet.[21]

Endoscopic dilation

Mechanical dilation of esophageal tumors improves dysphagia in 80–90% of patients. In experienced hands, the procedure carries a perforation risk less than 1%.[22] Unfortunately, the tumor invariably re-occludes the lumen and so the palliative effect of dilation alone lasts only 3–4 weeks. The role of mechanical dilation in the palliation of dysphagia due to esophageal cancer is primarily as an adjunctive measure to aid in placement of esophageal stents.[22]

Tumor ablation

Laser therapy

Nd:YAG laser therapy delivers an intense beam of light that heats and vaporizes tumor tissue, thereby restoring patency to the esophageal lumen. Dysphagia relief is often immediate. Laser therapy offers similar dysphagia relief when compared to esophageal stents. An early study suggested that laser therapy was associated with fewer complications than esophageal stenting.[23] A limitation of this retrospective study was that many of the patients in the stenting group received a plastic endoprosthesis rather than SEMS. A prospective randomized study subsequently concluded that laser therapy carried a higher risk of fistula formation, bleeding, and need for repeat intervention when compared to esophageal stents.[24] Therefore, this therapy is not widely utilized.

Photodynamic therapy (PDT)

Photodynamic therapy involves intravenous injection of a photosensitizing agent that is preferentially taken up by neoplastic cells, followed by endoscopic application of laser therapy to the malignant stricture. PDT appears to be effective at palliating dysphagia, but its widespread acceptance is limited by the high cost of the photosensitizing agent and the requirement for patients to avoid sunlight for several weeks to avoid skin phototoxicity.[25] Furthermore, patients require repeat intervention within a mean interval of two months.[26]

Cryoablation

During cryoablation, liquid nitrogen or carbon dioxide at super cold temperatures (−76 to −158°C) is sprayed directly on the tumor for 20–40 s. The tissue is then allowed to thaw before spraying again for 20–40 s. Typically, 2–4 freeze-thaw cycles of liquid nitrogen or 4–8 freeze-thaw cycles of carbon dioxide are administered. These freeze-thaw cycles cause intracellular disruption and ischemia, which leads to ablation of tumor tissue (thermal ablation). High quality data has demonstrated the safety and effectiveness of this technology in Barretts esophagus and early esophageal cancer.[27] The published literature on the efficacy of this modality for esophageal cancer palliation is primarily from smaller case series.[27] Further research is necessary to clarify the role of cryoablation in esophageal cancer palliation.

Brachytherapy

Esophageal brachytherapy is intraluminal delivery of radiation therapy. The radioactive source is advanced down to the tumor through a nasogastric or orogastric tube, and radiation therapy is delivered for a short duration (less than 5 min). Because brachytherapy precisely delivers the radiation dose to the tumor in an internal fashion, it can better spare normal surrounding tissues such as the lungs, heart, and liver compared with external beam radiation therapy.[28] A multicenter randomized trial comparing SEMS to a single dose of brachytherapy at 12 Gray found that dysphagia improved more rapidly with esophageal stents, but long-term relief was better after brachytherapy.[19] Additionally, there were fewer complications and higher quality of life scores with brachytherapy than SEMS. Despite the evidence in favor of brachytherapy for patients with high performance status, the ease of SEMS insertion as first-line therapy and the need for SEMS rescue in a significant number of patients initially treated with radiation have limited the application of brachytherapy in the United States. In addition, this method of local radiotherapy is unavailable in the majority of hospitals in the United States.[5]

Nutrition support in esophageal cancer

In addition to the catabolic effects of the tumor, esophageal cancer causes luminal narrowing and dysphagia. As a result, malnutrition occurs in 80% of patients with esophageal cancer.[29] The decision to proceed with enteral or parenteral nutrition support in patients with advanced incurable disease requires careful consideration of the goals of such support.[30] Enteral nutrition preserved gut integrity and reduces bacterial translocation. Enteral nutrition is also less expensive than parenteral nutrition. Enteral nutrition is therefore preferred to parenteral nutrition, particularly since patients with esophageal cancer typically have a functional gut below the tumor. Naso-enteric feeding is the least invasive form of enteral nutrition support. However, naso-enteric tubes are less frequently used for long-term nutritional palliation because they cause sinusitis and are typically not well accepted by patients being managed with a palliative intent. The complication rate for gastrostomy tube placement in esophageal cancer patients compares favorably to complication rates for gastrostomy tubes placed for non-malignant purposes.[31] A percutaneous gastrostomy can be considered as standard definitive nutritional palliation, particularly in patients unsuitable for esophageal stenting. If endoscopic placement of a gastrostomy is not feasible due to obstructing esophageal tumor, then radiologic or surgical approaches provide an alternative means of placement. Jejunostomy tube feeding is an option for patients with esophageal cancer and significant gastroparesis.

Palliation of Malignant Biliary Obstruction

Introduction

Etiologies of malignant biliary obstruction include pancreatic adenocarcinoma, cholangiocarcinoma, gallbladder cancer, liver metastases (most frequently from gastrointestinal cancers, breast cancer, and lung cancer), ampullary carcinoma, hepatocellular carcinoma, neuroendocrine tumors, cystic pancreatic neoplasms, and malignant hilar adenopathy.[32] Pancreatic adenocarcinoma is the most common malignancy associated with biliary obstruction, and is the fourth leading cause of cancer related death in both men and women. Approximately 75–80% of patients with pancreatic adenocarcinoma have unresectable disease at diagnosis.[33] Palliative mechanical decompression to relieve jaundice is a mainstay of therapy in these patients with biliary obstruction due to advanced unresectable neoplasia.

Until the 1960s, surgical bypass (hepaticojejunostomy) was the primary method of palliating jaundice in patients with malignant biliary obstruction. Percutaneous biliary drainage was first reported in 1969, and began to be used with increased frequency in the 1970s.[34] In 1979, the first series of 10 patients with endoscopically placed plastic stents was reported.[35]

A Cochrane review of 21 trials comparing surgical bypass to endoscopically placed plastic stents in patients with malignant biliary obstruction reported similar technical success in the two groups.[36] Patients who received plastic stents had significantly fewer complications and consequently, a trend towards decreased mortality.[36,37]

Randomized and observational studies suggest that technical success rates and overall mortality is similar using either an endoscopic or a percutaneous approach; complications may be lower in patients receiving an endoscopic stent.[38,39] Furthermore, studies assessing quality of life using standardized surveys such as the Short Form 36 (SF-36) have documented improved scores after endoscopic stenting.[40]

Endoscopic decompression has therefore become the preferred approach for palliation of jaundice in patients with malignant biliary obstruction. Percutaneous biliary drainage remains an important salvage therapy if endoscopic stenting is unsuccessful (e.g. duodenal obstruction that does not permit passage of the duodenoscope) or obstruction is primarily within the intrahepatic bile ducts. Endoscopic ultrasound (EUS) guided transpapillary or transluminal biliary drainage is another safe and feasible alternative when ERCP is unsuccessful.[41] However, EUS guided drainage is a technically complex procedure and is therefore not widely available.[42]

Plastic stents

Plastic biliary stents are composed of Polyurethane, Polyethylene, or Teflon. These stents range in diameter from 7 French to 11.5 French and 5–15 cm in length.[43] In patients with malignant biliary obstruction, straight plastic stents are typically preferred to single and double pigtail stents because of their larger caliber. These straight stents typically have flaps at each end to anchor the stents and prevent migration, and the majority of straight plastic biliary stents have side holes to facilitate the free flow of bile. These stents are relatively inexpensive and generally easy to remove if necessary. The major limitation of plastic stents is that they tend to occlude within a median of 4–5 months, even with larger diameter 10 French stents.[44] The currently accepted rationale is that insertion of a stent across the sphincter of Oddi eliminates the barrier that prevents microbial colonization. Once microbes colonize the stent and reduce its diameter, other materials like cholesterol crystals and dietary plant fiber accumulate within the stent and cause occlusion.[45] A number of strategies have been evaluated to reduce plastic stent occlusion including antibiotics (to reduce microbial colonization), ursodiol (to reduce cholesterol crystal accumulation), polymer coating, and double layer stents (to reduce coefficient of friction).[46–49] Unfortunately, none of these strategies reliably reduce plastic stent occlusion.

Metal stents

In 1991, uncovered metal stents were first introduced (Figs. 1c, 1d, 1g, 1h). Because of their larger 10 mm (30 French) caliber, metal stents remain patent much longer than plastic stents.[50] However, metal stents can be 15–40 times more expensive than plastic stents. The reduced number of endoscopic retrograde cholangiography (ERCP) procedures a patient would require due to stent occlusion typically offsets the increased cost of a metal stent. In patients with biliary obstruction due to unresectable disease, metal stents are cost-effective when compared to plastic stents if a patient's anticipated survival is greater than three months or the cost of an endoscopic ERCP exceeds $1820.[51]

Metal stent occlusion can occur after a median of 10–12 months, in large measure due to tumor ingrowth between the stent scaffolding. In an attempt to minimize tumor ingrowth, partially and fully covered metal stents were designed but prospective and randomized studies have not demonstrated any difference in stent patency between covered and uncovered metal stents.[50,52,53] An initial concern with covered metal stents was that they increase risk of pancreatitis or cholecystitis by blocking the pancreatic or cystic ducts respectively. However, in the randomized and prospective trials, there was no increase in either of these complications with covered metal stents when compared to uncovered metal stents.[53,54] Covered metal stents do tend to migrate more frequently than uncovered metal stents. Nevertheless, fully covered metal stents are utilized with increasing frequency in part due to the off label ability to remove these stents.

When metal stent occlusion does occur in patients with malignant biliary obstruction, endoscopic options include mechanical cleaning, plastic stent reinsertion, and metal stent re-insertion. Published data on management of stent occlusion are all retrospective observational studies. A meta-analysis of the published literature on management of stent occlusion did not find an increase in stent patency with metal stents when compared to plastic stents, likely because a patient's life expectancy at that stage is often less than three to six months.[55]

Unilateral versus bilateral drainage

A single stent is generally sufficient in patients with jaundice due to common bile duct obstruction, as is typical in patients with pancreatic adenocarcinoma and Bismuth I cholangiocarcinoma. Consensus is lacking regarding unilateral versus bilateral stenting in patients with malignant hilar obstruction (e.g. due to Bismuth II, III, and IV cholangiocarcinoma). Only 25–30% of the liver needs to be drained to achieve adequate palliation of obstructive jaundice.[56] Therefore, a single stent into one lobe of the liver should provide adequate palliation of jaundice, provided the drained lobe is free of disease. Several studies have attempted to address whether unilateral or bilateral drainage is preferred for palliation of obstructive jaundice in patients with hilar cholangiocarcinoma. Early studies reported a higher incidence of cholangitis and shorter survival with unilateral drainage. Since then, however, technical modifications such as avoiding contrast injection into the undrained segments and peri-procedural antibiotics have enhanced the safety of the unilateral drainage. A randomized controlled trial performed in patients with cholangiocarcinoma reported a higher technical success rate and lower rate of early complications in patients randomized to unilateral drainage when compared to patients randomized to bilateral drainage. The incidence of late complications and overall survival was similar in the two groups.[57] Nevertheless, some authors have suggested bilateral drainage for selected patients with Bismuth II cholangiocarcinoma because of their expected prolonged survival.[58]

Newer modalities

A number of newer endoscopic therapies have been proposed to palliate malignant obstructive jaundice. These include drug eluting stents, photodynamic therapy, intraluminal brachytherapy, high intensity intraductal ultrasound, and radiofrequency ablation. The published human data on all of these techniques are limited, and so the exact role for any of these modalities in the palliation of malignant obstructive jaundice has yet to be defined.

Drug eluting stents

Although a smaller study suggested improved stent patency with paclitaxel eluting covered metal stents, a larger prospective study did not demonstrate any increase in patency or survival with drug eluting stents when compared to non-drug eluting covered metal stents.[59] Newer stents that elute gemcitabine have been designed but have not as yet been formally studied.[59]

Photodynamic therapy

Photodynamic therapy involves the administration of a photosensitizer that preferentially accumulates in neoplastic tissue. The photosensitizer is activated by endoscopically applying laser light to the malignant stricture.[60] Smaller studies in patients with unresectable cholangiocarcinoma, those who received a stent plus photodynamic therapy had a longer survival and improved quality of life compared to biliary stenting alone.[60,61] Larger studies are required to clarify the role of photodynamic therapy in malignant biliary obstruction. Even if larger studies demonstrate that photodynamic therapy is efficacious, this modality is limited by the high cost of the photosensitizing agent. Also, patients need to avoid any sunlight exposure for several weeks after therapy in order to avoid the phototoxic side effect of dermatitis.

Intraluminal brachytherapy

The rationale for intraluminal brachytherapy is the ability to achieve higher doses of radiation (10.4 to 20 Grays) than external beam radiation without damaging surrounding organs. Iridium-192 seeds are mounted on a catheter and the seeds are placed directly across the malignant stricture. Studies assessing this modality for palliation have yielded mixed results. In some studies, intraluminal brachytherapy demonstrated a survival benefit.[62] However, when used in combination with external beam radiation therapy, the risk of cholangitis approached 50%.[63]

High intensity intraductal ultrasound (HIDUS)

Localized ablation of tumor cells using high intensity ultrasound appears effective in patients with prostate cancer. High intensity ultrasound is performed in the bile duct by mounting an ultrasound probe over a guidewire and positioning the probe directly within the stricture. In a pilot study of 10 patients with malignant biliary obstruction, there was a reduction in stricture length and tumor size as determined by ERCP and endoscopic ultrasound.[63]

Intraductal radiofrequency ablation (RFA)

Case reports and case series have demonstrated the feasibility of introducing an 8 French radiofrequency ablation catheter over a 0.035 inch guidewire and delivering energy of 10W for 90s at 400kz with a 1 min cool down period.[64] The largest case series from the United Kingdom reported improvement in stricture diameter following RFA. All patients had metal stents placed after RFA was performed. Cases of RFA to treat metal stent occlusion have also been reported.[64] Bile duct injury is a potential concern with this technique, since the depth of coagulative necrosis is deeper than in other organs like the esophagus.

Palliation of Malignant Gastroduodenal Obstruction

Introduction

Pancreatic adenocarcinoma is the most common cause of malignant gastroduodenal obstruction in the United States.[65] Other frequent causes of duodenal obstruction include cholangiocarcinoma and metastatic disease.[65] Gastric outlet obstruction due to gastric cancer occurs more frequently in Asia. Primary duodenal adenocarcinoma and ampullary carcinoma are less frequent causes of duodenal obstruction. Palliative interventional therapies for malignant gastroduodenal obstruction include surgery, gastroduodenal stenting, and gastrostomy tube placement for venting. Pharmacologic adjuncts for management of pain, nausea, and vomiting include analgesics (opioids and non-opioids), anti-secretory drugs (octreotide, scopolamine, and glocopyrrolate), and anti-emetics.[66]

Surgical gastrojejunostomy

The traditional operation for malignant pylorus or duodenal obstruction is an open gastrojejunostomy. Over the last two decades, there has been a trend towards minimally invasive laparascopic gastrojejunostomy. In experienced hands, the minimally invasive approach appears to offer similar operating times, shorter hospitalization, and fewer complications than the open approach.[67–69]

Gastroduodenal stents

Self-expandable metallic stents (SEMS) designed specifically to palliate gastric outlet and duodenal obstruction have been available since the 1990s. In prospective trials, technical placement is successful in 90% of patients, and 80% of patients experience clinical improvement.[70–72] Uncovered and covered enteral stents have been designed, but only uncovered metal stents are available in the United States. Duodenal stents are 20–27 mm in diameter, 6–12 cm in length, and have proximal and distal flanges with a 27 mm diameter. These stents can be deployed through the working channel of a therapeutic gastroscope or a colonoscope.[73] Complete stent expansion usually occurs in 24 to 48 hours. Following successful stent placement, patients are generally advised to avoid meat and fiber to prevent stent occlusion with food. After a duodenal stent has been placed, obtaining biliary access can be challenging. Therefore, patients with known or impending biliary obstruction should have a biliary SEMS placed before enteral stenting is performed.[74,75]

Stents versus surgical gastrojejunostomy

A systematic review that included two randomized trials, six comparative studies, and 36 observational studies found no differences between enteral stenting and surgical gastrojejunostomy with regards to technical success, or early complications, or late complications.[76] Initial clinical success was higher and duration of hospitalization was shorter in the stent group. On the other hand, recurrent obstructive symptoms were less common in the surgical bypass group (i.e. more durable palliation with surgery).[76] Although formal cost-effectiveness analyses have not been performed, median cost in a Medicare database was $12,000 lower in patients who received an enteral stent when compared to gastrojejunostomy.[77]

Based on these data, enteral stents are the first-line intervention for relieving malignant gastroduodenal obstruction in patients with anticipated survival less than six months. Surgical gastrojejunostomy should be considered in patients expected to live longer than six months who are reasonable surgical candidates.

Venting gastrostomy tube

Endoscopic, radiologic, or surgical placement of a gastrostomy tube is an option in patients who are expected to survive less than one month or who have rapidly progressive disease, overt ascites, carcinomatosis, or multiple sites of obstruction.[78] The gastrostomy allows the patient to drain gastric secretions. Patients are also able to ingest a clear liquid diet for pleasure, since they can subsequently drain the clear liquids through the gastrostomy. In this setting, the gastrostomy tube is not intended for nutritional support. In some instances, extending a small bore jejunostomy tube through the gastrostomy and past the site of obstruction is feasible. In these patients, the jejunal extension can be used to provide enteral nutrition.

Palliation of Obstruction due to Malignant Colorectal Cancer

Introduction

Intra-luminal obstruction occurs in 7–29% of patients with colorectal cancer.[79] Ovarian cancer is the most common extra-luminal cause of malignant colorectal obstruction. Peritoneal carcinomatosis from other pelvic or gastrointestinal malignancies can also cause colorectal obstruction. Patients with malignant large bowel obstruction due to colorectal cancer or extra-luminal malignant obstruction tend to have advanced disease and are often poor operative candidates. Malignant large bowel obstruction can be managed surgically or with placement of a colorectal stent.

Surgery

Right-sided malignant obstruction is typically managed with a one-stage surgical resection and primary anastomosis. Surgical options for managing malignant left-sided colorectal obstruction include the following techniques: loop colostomy or loop ileostomy and subsequent resection (2-or 3-staged procedure), Hartman's procedure (primary resection with end colostomy), and primary resection and anastomosis.

Studies comparing loop colostomy or ileostomy to Harman's procedure have found a longer hospitalization with the staged procedure without any statistically significant differences in morbidity or mortality.[80,81] Hartman's procedure also exposes the patient to fewer operations than a staged resection. Therefore, Hartman's procedure is generally preferable to a staged resection.

Hartman's procedure is technically easier than primary resection and anastomosis, and eliminates the risk of anastamotic dehiscence. However, with Hartman's procedure a second operation would be necessary to reverse the ostomy, and 80% of colon cancer patients are unable to have the stoma reversed.[82] Primary resection and anastomosis allows for a single definitive surgery, and may be associated with better long-term outcomes than Hartman's procedure.[83]

A randomized trial comparing total colectomy to subtotal colectomy found no differences in mortality or complications with either approach.[84] Diarrhea was more frequent in the total colectomy group, so the investigators recommended subtotal colectomy over total colectomy. In the 1980s, segmental resection was proposed as an alternative to subtotal colectomy. In the absence of right colon perforation or cecal ischemia, segmental resection is generally preferred over subtotal colectomy because this technique better preserves normal bowel function.[85] Mechanical bowel preparation prior to surgery is simpler and reduces the duration of surgery when compared to intra-colonic irrigation, but both methods of bowel cleansing are associated with similar morbidity and mortality.[86]

In summary, segmental primary resection with anastamosis is a safe option in malignant left-sided colorectal obstruction and appears to be associated with best outcomes. Hartman's procedure could be considered in patients at high surgical risk, particularly if the surgeon is not a colorectal subspecialist or is relatively inexperienced at performing primary resection and anastomosis. Total or subtotal colectomy should be reserved for impending or actual perforation of the right colon.[86] Loop colostomy without plan for further operations can be considered for palliation in extremely poor operative candidates in whom a Hartman's procedure or primary resection and anastomosis would carry a prohibitive operative risk.

Colonic stents

The use of a colonic self-expandable metallic stent (SEMS) was first reported in 1990. Since that time, several retrospective, prospective and randomized trials have been published describing the efficacy of colonic SEMS. Colonic stents can be utilized as both a bridge to surgery and an alternative to surgery in the palliative setting.[87] Colonic stents are primarily utilized for left-sided lesions (distal to splenic flexure) at least 5 cm from the anal verge (Figs. 1e, 1f). While there are case series of successful right-sided colonic stenting, colonic SEMS are infrequently placed in right-sided malignant colorectal obstruction because of the technical difficulty of navigating a stent or a colonoscope to the right side in an unprepped, obstructed colon.[88,89]

Covered and uncovered metal colonic stents have been designed, but only uncovered metal stents are currently available in the United States. Most colonic SEMS are deployed through the scope (TTS), although an over the wire (OTW) stent that cannot fit through the scope is also available.[90] Colonic SEMS range in length from 4–12 cm, and have a diameter of 20–25 mm at the body and 20–35 mm at the proximal flanges. These stents are ideally deployed with at least 2 cm exposed distal and proximal to the obstructing lesion. Dilation prior to stent placement is not recommended because this maneuver greatly increases the risk of perforation. Following successful stent placement, patients should avoid foods that are high in fiber and take mineral oil supplements or laxatives in order to minimize the risk of stent occlusion by feces.[90]

In a systematic review of 88 non-randomized studies, stent placement was technically successful in 96% of patients, and clinical success was achieved in a median of 92% of patients.[91] The median duration of stent patency was 106 days. The most common complications were reocclusion (12%), stent migration (11%), and perforation (5%).[91]

The angiogenesis inhibitor bevacizumab may be associated with an increased risk of colonic perforation after colonic SEMS placement.[92,93]

Bevacizumab is frequently included in first-line chemotherapy for metastatic colorectal cancer. Although the exact etiology of increased perforation risk with bevacizumab is unclear, investigators have proposed a number of potential explanations. One possibility is that bevacizumab causes thrombosis of smaller splanchnic or mesenteric vessels, leading to bowel ischemia.[94] Another possible mechanism is decreased bowel mucosa healing due to vascular endothelial growth factor (VEGF) inhibition.[94] Finally, the tumor may provide some degree of stability to the bowel wall and the stent. Regression of tumor with chemotherapy can create an area of disruption susceptible to perforation.[94]

Colonic stents versus surgery

A randomized controlled trial comparing colonic stents to palliative surgery in patients with metastatic colorectal cancer was terminated prematurely because of excessive complications in patients assigned to colorectal stenting.[95] In this study, colonic perforation occurred in 6 of 11 patients who received a colonic stent and only 1 of 10 patients managed surgically. A number of randomized trials comparing emergent colonic stenting to emergency surgery in patients with acute malignant colonic obstruction have also been performed. A Cochrane review of five randomized trials did not find any differences in mortality or complication rates, although average time for clinical relief was significantly longer in the colonic stent group (3.7 days in the stent group versus 0.7 days in the surgery group).[96] A more recent meta-analysis of eight randomized trials comparing colonic stents as a bridge to surgery versus emergency surgery found that the stent group had a lower incidence of complications, higher rate of primary anastomosis, lower stoma creation rate, and decreased incidence of intensive care admission compared to the emergency surgery group.[97]

Taken together, these results suggest that colonic stenting is a reasonable option for palliation in patients who are not surgical candidates. Colonic stenting can also be considered in patients with acute malignant colonic obstruction who are at higher risk of complications from emergency surgery. Their role in patients who are reasonably fit and willing to undergo a palliative operation is less clear. Emerging data suggest that colonic stenting should probably be avoided in patients who are receiving or will receive bevacizumab.

Take Home Messages

- **Esophagus**
  - Endoscopic stenting is the most frequently employed strategy for palliation of malignant dysphagia; partially covered self-expandable metal stents are the preferred stent design in this setting.
  - Stent placement across a large bulky tumor in the proximal or mid esophagus can cause tracheal compression. In these patients, placement of a tracheal stent prior to esophageal stenting should be considered.
  - Covered metal stents are the first-line therapy for malignant tracheo-esophageal fistula.
  - Dysphagia improves more rapidly with SEMS compared to brachytherapy. Brachytherapy provides longer-term relief, causes fewer complications, and is associated with higher quality of life scores compared to SEMS.
- **Biliary**
  - Endoscopic stent placement is the preferred approach for palliation of jaundice in patients with malignant biliary obstruction. Percutaneous biliary drainage remains an important salvage therapy if endoscopic stenting is unsuccessful or obstruction is primarily within the intrahepatic bile ducts. EUS guided drainage is a new alternative modality for the traditional percutaneous method.
  - Metal stents have a longer patency but are more expensive than plastic stents. Metal stents are cost-effective compared to plastic stents in patients with anticipated survival longer than three months.
  - Whether to place unilateral versus bilateral stents in patients with malignant hilar obstruction is an area of controversy. A randomized controlled trial reported higher technical success rates and lower rate of early complications with unilateral drainage.

- ♦ A number of newer endoscopic therapies have been proposed to palliate malignant obstructive jaundice such as drug eluting stents, photodynamic therapy, intraluminal brachytherapy, high intensity ultrasound, and radiofrequency ablation. The published human data on all of these techniques are limited.

- **Gastroduodenal**
  - ♦ Enteral stents are the first-line intervention for palliating malignant gastroduodenal obstruction in patients with anticipated survival less than six months.
  - ♦ Surgical gastrojejunostomy should be considered in patients expected to live longer than six months who are reasonable surgical candidates; laprascopic gastrojejunostomy is associated with similar operating times, shorter hospitalization, and fewer complications than the open approach.
  - ♦ Endoscopically placing a biliary stent is technically challenging once an enteral stent is in place; patients with known or impending biliary obstruction should have a biliary SEMS placed before enteral stenting is performed.
  - ♦ Endoscopic, radiologic, or surgical placement of a gastrostomy tube is an option in patients who are expected to survive less than one month or who have rapidly progressive disease, overt ascites, carcinomatosis, or multiple sites of obstruction.

- **Colorectal**
  - ♦ Surgery is the preferred approach for palliation of right-sided colonic approach; in select cases right-sided colonic stent placement may be feasible.
  - ♦ Colonic stenting is a reasonable option for palliation of left-sided colonic obstruction in patients who are not surgical candidates. Colonic stenting can also be considered in patients with acute malignant colonic obstruction who are at higher risk of complications from emergency surgery.
  - ♦ The role of colonic stents in patients who are reasonably fit and willing to undergo a palliative operation is less clear.

References

1. Mougey, A., and Adler, D.G., Esophageal stenting for the palliation of malignant dysphagia. *J Support Oncol*, 2008. **6**(6): 267–73.
2. Sihvo, E.I., Luostarinen, M.E., and Salo, J.A., Fate of patients with adenocarcinoma of the esophagus and the esophagogastric junction: a population-based analysis. *Am J Gastroenterol*, 2004. **99**(3): 419–24.
3. Muller, J.M. *et al.*, Surgical therapy of oesophageal carcinoma. *Br J Surg*, 1990. **77**(8): 845–57.
4. Hirai, T. *et al.*, Bypass operation for advanced esophageal cancer — an analysis of 93 cases. *Jpn J Surg*, 1989. **19**(2): 182–8.
5. Sharma, and Kozarek, R., Role of esophageal stents in benign and malignant diseases. *Am J Gastroenterol*, 2010. **105**(2): 258–73; quiz 274.
6. Parker, C.H., and Peura, D.A., Palliative treatment of esophageal carcinoma using esophageal dilation and prosthesis. *Gastroenterol Clin North Am*, 1991. **20**(4): 717–29.
7. Knyrim, K. *et al.*, A controlled trial of an expansile metal stent for palliation of esophageal obstruction due to inoperable cancer. *N Engl J Med*, 1993. **329**(18): 1302–7.
8. Roseveare, C.D. *et al.*, Metal stents improve dysphagia, nutrition and survival in malignant oesophageal stenosis: a randomized controlled trial comparing modified Gianturco Z-stents with plastic Atkinson tubes. *Eur J Gastroenterol Hepatol*, 1998. **10**(8): 653–7.
9. Vakil, N. *et al.*, A prospective, randomized, controlled trial of covered expandable metal stents in the palliation of malignant esophageal obstruction at the gastroesophageal junction. *Am J Gastroenterol*, 2001. **96**(6): 1791–6.
10. Saranovic, D. *et al.*, Fluoroscopically guided insertion of self-expandable metal esophageal stents for palliative treatment of patients with malignant stenosis of esophagus and cardia: comparison of uncovered and covered stent types. *Dis Esophagus*, 2005. **18**(4): 230–8.
11. Sabharwal, T. *et al.*, A randomised prospective comparison of the Flamingo Wallstent and Ultraflex stent for palliation of dysphagia associated with lower third oesophageal carcinoma. *Gut*, 2003. **52**(7): 922–6.
12. Siersema, P.D. *et al.*, A comparison of 3 types of covered metal stents for the palliation of patients with dysphagia caused by esophagogastric carcinoma: a prospective, randomized study. *Gastrointest Endosc*, 2001. **54**(2): 145–53.

13. Seven, G. *et al.*, Partially versus fully covered self-expanding metal stents for benign and malignant esophageal conditions: a single center experience. *Surg Endosc*, 2013. **27**(6): 2185–92.
14. Conigliaro, R. *et al.*, Polyflex stents for malignant oesophageal and oesophagogastric stricture: a prospective, multicentric study. *Eur J Gastroenterol Hepatol*, 2007. **19**(3): 195–203.
15. Verschuur, E.M. *et al.*, New design esophageal stents for the palliation of dysphagia from esophageal or gastric cardia cancer: a randomized trial. *Am J Gastroenterol*, 2008. **103**(2): 304–12.
16. Chen, Y.H. *et al.*, Comparative study of esophageal stent and feeding gastrostomy/jejunostomy for tracheoesophageal fistula caused by esophageal squamous cell carcinoma. *PLoS One*, 2012. **7**(8): e42766.
17. Shin, J.H. *et al.*, Esophagorespiratory fistula: Long-term results of palliative treatment with covered expandable metallic stents in 61 patients. *Radiology*, 2004. **232**(1): 252–9.
18. Baron, T.H., Expandable metal stents for the treatment of cancerous obstruction of the gastrointestinal tract. *N Engl J Med*, 2001. **344**(22): 1681–7.
19. Homann, N. *et al.*, Delayed complications after placement of self-expanding stents in malignant esophageal obstruction: treatment strategies and survival rate. *Dig Dis Sci*, 2008. **53**(2): 334–40.
20. Dua, K.S. *et al.*, Self-expanding metal esophageal stent with anti-reflux mechanism. *Gastrointest Endosc*, 2001. **53**(6): 603–13.
21. Homs, M.Y. *et al.*, Esophageal stents with antireflux valve for tumors of the distal esophagus and gastric cardia: a randomized trial. *Gastrointest Endosc*, 2004. **60**(5): 695–702.
22. Egan, J.V. *et al.*, Esophageal dilation. *Gastrointest Endosc*, 2006. **63**(6): 755–60.
23. Gevers, A.M. *et al.*, A comparison of laser therapy, plastic stents, and expandable metal stents for palliation of malignant dysphagia in patients without a fistula. *Gastrointest Endosc*, 1998. **48**(4): 383–8.
24. Konigsrainer, A. *et al.*, Expandable metal stents versus laser combined with radiotherapy for palliation of unresectable esophageal cancer: a prospective randomized trial. *Hepatogastroenterology*, 2000. **47**(33): 724–7.
25. Moghissi, K. *et al.*, The role of photodynamic therapy (PDT) in inoperable oesophageal cancer. *Eur J Cardiothorac Surg*, 2000. **17**(2): 95–100.

26. Litle, V.R. *et al.*, Photodynamic therapy as palliation for esophageal cancer: experience in 215 patients. *Ann Thorac Surg*, 2003. **76**(5): 1687–92; discussion 1692–3.
27. Vignesh, S. *et al.*, Endoscopic therapy of neoplasia related to Barrett's esophagus and endoscopic palliation of esophageal cancer. *Cancer Control*, 2013. **20**(2): 117–29.
28. Shridhar, R. *et al.*, Radiation therapy and esophageal cancer. *Cancer Control*, 2013. **20**(2): 97–110.
29. Larrea, J. *et al.*, The nutritional status and immunological situation of cancer patients. *Nutr Hosp*, 1992. **7**(3): 178–84.
30. Mercadante, S., Nutrition in cancer patients. *Support Care Cancer*, 1996. **4**(1): 10–20.
31. Grilo, A., Santos, C.A., and Fonseca, J., Percutaneous endoscopic gastrostomy for nutritional palliation of upper esophageal cancer unsuitable for esophageal stenting. *Arq Gastroenterol*, 2012. **49**(3): 227–31.
32. Weir, H.K. *et al.*, Annual report to the nation on the status of cancer, 1975–2000, featuring the uses of surveillance data for cancer prevention and control. *J Natl Cancer Inst*, 2003. **95**(17): 1276–99.
33. Siegel, R., Naishadham, D., and Jemal, A., Cancer statistics, 2013. *CA Cancer J Clin*, 2013. **63**(1): 11–30.
34. Molnar, W., and Stockum, A.E., Relief of obstructive jaundice through percutaneous transhepatic catheter — a new therapeutic method. *Am J Roentgenol Radium Ther Nucl Med*, 1974. **122**(2): 356–67.
35. Osnes, M. *et al.*, Nonoperative internal drainage of obstructive common bile ducts. *Arch Surg*, 1979. **114**(7): 862–5.
36. Moss, A.C., Morris, E., and Mac Mathuna, P., Palliative biliary stents for obstructing pancreatic carcinoma. *Cochrane Database Syst Rev*, 2006. (1): CD004200.
37. Moss, A.C. *et al.*, Malignant distal biliary obstruction: a systematic review and meta-analysis of endoscopic and surgical bypass results. *Cancer Treat Rev*, 2007. **33**(2): 213–21.
38. Speer, A.G. *et al.*, Randomised trial of endoscopic versus percutaneous stent insertion in malignant obstructive jaundice. *Lancet*, 1987. **2**(8550): 57–62.
39. Pinol, V. *et al.*, Percutaneous self-expanding metal stents versus endoscopic polyethylene endoprostheses for treating malignant biliary obstruction: randomized clinical trial. *Radiology*, 2002. **225**(1): 27–34.

40. Abraham, N.S., Barkun, J.S., and Barkun, A.N., Palliation of malignant biliary obstruction: a prospective trial examining impact on quality of life. *Gastrointest Endosc*, 2002. **56**(6): 835–41.
41. Dhir, V. *et al.*, Multicenter study on endoscopic ultrasound-guided expandable biliary metal stent placement: choice of access route, direction of stent insertion, and drainage route. *Dig Endosc*, 2013.
42. Kedia, P., Gaidhane, M., and Kahaleh, M., Endoscopic guided biliary drainage: how can we achieve efficient biliary drainage? *Clin Endosc*, 2013. **46**(5): 543–551.
43. Pfau, P.R. *et al.*, Pancreatic and biliary stents. *Gastrointest Endosc*, 2013. **77**(3): 319–27.
44. Wagh, M.S. *et al.*, Multicenter Randomized Trial of 10-French versus 11.5-French Plastic Stents for Malignant Biliary Obstruction. *Diagn Ther Endosc*, 2013. **2013**: 891915.
45. Donelli, G. *et al.*, Plastic biliary stent occlusion: factors involved and possible preventive approaches. *Clin Med Res*, 2007. **5**(1): 53–60.
46. Galandi, D. *et al.*, Ursodeoxycholic acid and/or antibiotics for prevention of biliary stent occlusion. *Cochrane Database Syst Rev*, 2002. (3): CD003043.
47. van Berkel, A.M. *et al.*, A prospective randomized trial of Tannenbaum-type Teflon-coated stents versus polyethylene stents for distal malignant biliary obstruction. *Eur J Gastroenterol Hepatol*, 2004. **16**(2): 213–7.
48. van Berkel, A.M. *et al.*, A prospective randomized study of hydrophilic polymer-coated polyurethane versus polyethylene stents in distal malignant biliary obstruction. *Endoscopy*, 2003. **35**(6): 478–82.
49. Katsinelos, P. *et al.*, Prospective randomized study comparing double layer and Tannenbaum stents in distal malignant biliary stenosis. *Acta Gastroenterol Belg*, 2010. **73**(4): 445–50.
50. Jaganmohan, S. and Lee, J.H., Self-expandable metal stents in malignant biliary obstruction. *Expert Rev Gastroenterol Hepatol*, 2012. **6**(1): 105–14.
51. Moss, A.C. *et al.*, Do the benefits of metal stents justify the costs? A systematic review and meta-analysis of trials comparing endoscopic stents for malignant biliary obstruction. *Eur J Gastroenterol Hepatol*, 2007. **19**(12): 1119–24.
52. Isayama, H. *et al.*, A prospective randomised study of "covered" versus "uncovered" diamond stents for the management of distal malignant biliary obstruction. *Gut*, 2004. **53**(5): 729–34.

53. Telford, J.J. *et al.*, A randomized trial comparing uncovered and partially covered self-expandable metal stents in the palliation of distal malignant biliary obstruction. *Gastrointest Endosc*, 2010. **72**(5): 907–14.
54. Park do, H. *et al.*, Covered versus uncovered wallstent for malignant extrahepatic biliary obstruction: a cohort comparative analysis. *Clin Gastroenterol Hepatol*, 2006. **4**(6): 790–6.
55. Shah, T. *et al.*, Management of occluded metal stents in malignant biliary obstruction: similar outcomes with second metal stents compared to plastic stents. *Dig Dis Sci*, 2012. **57**(11): 2765–73.
56. Abu-Hamda, E.M. and Baron, T.H., Endoscopic management of cholangiocarcinoma. *Semin Liver Dis*, 2004. **24**(2): 165–75.
57. De Palma, G.D. *et al.*, Unilateral versus bilateral endoscopic hepatic duct drainage in patients with malignant hilar biliary obstruction: results of a prospective, randomized, and controlled study. *Gastrointest Endosc*, 2001. **53**(6): 547–53.
58. Singhal, D., van Gulik, T.M., and Gouma, D.J., Palliative management of hilar cholangiocarcinoma. *Surg Oncol*, 2005. **14**(2): 59–74.
59. Shah, T., Drug-eluting stents in malignant biliary obstruction: where do we stand? *Dig Dis Sci*, 2013. **58**(3): 610–2.
60. Lee, T.Y., Cheon, Y.K., and Shim, C.S., Current status of photodynamic therapy for bile duct cancer. *Clin Endosc*, 2013. **46**(1): 38–44.
61. Cheon, Y.K. *et al.*, Longterm outcome of photodynamic therapy compared with biliary stenting alone in patients with advanced hilar cholangiocarcinoma. *HPB (Oxford)*, 2012. **14**(3): 185–93.
62. Chen, Y. *et al.*, HDR-192Ir intraluminal brachytherapy in treatment of malignant obstructive jaundice. *World J Gastroenterol*, 2004. **10**(23): 3506–10.
63. Ishii, H. *et al.*, Relief of jaundice by external beam radiotherapy and intraluminal brachytherapy in patients with extrahepatic cholangiocarcinoma: results without stenting. *Hepatogastroenterology*, 2004. **51**(58): 954–7.
64. Wadsworth, C.A., Westaby, D., and Khan, S.A., Endoscopic radiofrequency ablation for cholangiocarcinoma. *Curr Opin Gastroenterol*, 2013. **29**(3): 305–11.
65. Shone, D.N. *et al.*, Malignancy is the most common cause of gastric outlet obstruction in the era of H2 blockers. *Am J Gastroenterol*, 1995. **90**(10): 1769–70.

66. Ripamonti, C. and Mercadante, S., How to use octreotide for malignant bowel obstruction. *J Support Oncol*, 2004. **2**(4): 357–64.
67. Choi, Y.B., Laparoscopic gatrojejunostomy for palliation of gastric outlet obstruction in unresectable gastric cancer. *Surg Endosc*, 2002. **16**(11): 1620–6.
68. Bergamaschi, R. *et al.*, Open versus laparoscopic gastrojejunostomy for palliation in advanced pancreatic cancer. *Surg Laparosc Endosc*, 1998. **8**(2): 92–6.
69. Navarra, G. *et al.*, Palliative antecolic isoperistaltic gastrojejunostomy: a randomized controlled trial comparing open and laparoscopic approaches. *Surg Endosc*, 2006. **20**(12): 1831–4.
70. van Hooft, J.E. *et al.*, Efficacy and safety of the new WallFlex enteral stent in palliative treatment of malignant gastric outlet obstruction (DUOFLEX study): a prospective multicenter study. *Gastrointest Endosc*, 2009. **69**(6): 1059–66.
71. Masci, E. *et al.*, Enteral self-expandable metal stent for malignant luminal obstruction of the upper and lower gastrointestinal tract: a prospective multicentric study. *J Clin Gastroenterol*, 2008. **42**(4): 389–94.
72. Piesman, M. *et al.*, Improved oral intake after palliative duodenal stenting for malignant obstruction: a prospective multicenter clinical trial. *Am J Gastroenterol*, 2009. **104**(10): 2404–11.
73. Varadarajulu, S. *et al.*, Enteral stents. *Gastrointest Endosc*, 2011. **74**(3): 455–64.
74. Aadam, A.A. and Martin, J.A., Enteral stents in malignant bowel obstruction. *Gastrointest Endosc Clin N Am*, 2013. **23**(1): 153–64.
75. Hamada, T. *et al.*, Duodenal metal stent placement is a risk factor for biliary metal stent dysfunction: an analysis using a time-dependent covariate. *Surg Endosc*, 2013. **27**(4): 1243–8.
76. Jeurnink, S.M. *et al.*, Stent versus gastrojejunostomy for the palliation of gastric outlet obstruction: a systematic review. *BMC Gastroenterol*, 2007. **7**: 18.
77. Roy, A. *et al.*, Stenting versus gastrojejunostomy for management of malignant gastric outlet obstruction: comparison of clinical outcomes and costs. *Surg Endosc*, 2012. **26**(11): 3114–9.
78. Soriano, A., and Davis, M.P., Malignant bowel obstruction: individualized treatment near the end of life. *Cleve Clin J Med*, 2011. **78**(3): 197–206.

79. Deans, G.T., Krukowski, Z.H., and Irwin, S.T., Malignant obstruction of the left colon. *Br J Surg*, 1994. **81**(9): 1270–6.
80. De Salvo, G.L. *et al.*, Curative surgery for obstruction from primary left colorectal carcinoma: primary or staged resection? *Cochrane Database Syst Rev,* 2004. (2): CD002101.
81. Kronborg, O., Acute obstruction from tumour in the left colon without spread. A randomized trial of emergency colostomy versus resection. *Int J Colorectal Dis*, 1995. **10**(1): 1–5.
82. Zorcolo, L. *et al.*, Safety of primary anastomosis in emergency colo-rectal surgery. *Colorectal Dis*, 2003. **5**(3): 262–9.
83. Villar, J.M. *et al.*, Surgical options for malignant left-sided colonic obstruction. *Surg Today*, 2005. **35**(4): 275–81.
84. Single-stage treatment for malignant left-sided colonic obstruction: a prospective randomized clinical trial comparing subtotal colectomy with segmental resection following intraoperative irrigation. The SCOTIA Study Group. Subtotal Colectomy versus On-table Irrigation and Anastomosis. *Br J Surg*, 1995. **82**(12): 1622–7.
85. Ansaloni, L. *et al.*, Guidelenines in the management of obstructing cancer of the left colon: consensus conference of the world society of emergency surgery (WSES) and peritoneum and surgery (PnS) society. *World J Emerg Surg*, 2010. **5**: 29.
86. Kam, M.H. *et al.*, Systematic review of intraoperative colonic irrigation vs. manual decompression in obstructed left-sided colorectal emergencies. *Int J Colorectal Dis*, 2009. **24**(9): 1031–7.
87. Cirocchi, R. *et al.*, Safety and efficacy of endoscopic colonic stenting as a bridge to surgery in the management of intestinal obstruction due to left colon and rectal cancer: a systematic review and meta-analysis. *Surg Oncol*, 2013. **22**(1): 14–21.
88. Dronamraju, S.S. *et al.*, Role of self-expanding metallic stents in the management of malignant obstruction of the proximal colon. *Dis Colon Rectum*, 2009. **52**(9): 1657–61.
89. Tal, A.O. *et al.*, Self-expandable metal stent for malignant colonic obstruction: Outcome in proximal vs. left sided tumor localization. *Z Gastroenterol*, 2013. **51**(6): 551–7.
90. Baron, T.H., Wong Kee Song, L.M., and Repici, A., Role of self-expandable stents for patients with colon cancer (with videos). *Gastrointest Endosc*, 2012. **75**(3): 653–62.

91. Watt, A.M. *et al.*, Self-expanding metallic stents for relieving malignant colorectal obstruction: a systematic review. *Ann Surg*, 2007. **246**(1): 24–30.
92. Small, A.J., Coelho-Prabhu, N., and Baron, T.H., Endoscopic placement of self-expandable metal stents for malignant colonic obstruction: long-term outcomes and complication factors. *Gastrointest Endosc*, 2010. **71**(3): 560–72.
93. Manes, G. *et al.*, Endoscopic palliation in patients with incurable malignant colorectal obstruction by means of self-expanding metal stent: analysis of results and predictors of outcomes in a large multicenter series. *Arch Surg*, 2011. **146**(10): 1157–62.
94. Choi, Y.I. *et al.*, Intestinal perforation in colorectal cancers treated with bevacizumab (Avastin). *Cancer Res Treat*, 2008. **40**(1): 33–5.
95. van Hooft, J.E. *et al.*, Early closure of a multicenter randomized clinical trial of endoscopic stenting versus surgery for stage IV left-sided colorectal cancer. *Endoscopy*, 2008. **40**(3): 184–91.
96. Sagar, J., Colorectal stents for the management of malignant colonic obstructions. *Cochrane Database Syst Rev*, 2011(11): CD007378.
97. Zhang, Y. *et al.*, Self-expanding metallic stent as a bridge to surgery versus emergency surgery for obstructive colorectal cancer: a meta-analysis. *Surg Endosc*, 2012. **26**(1): 110–9.

Chapter 7

Endoscopic Diagnosis and Treatment of Esophageal Malignancies

Fan Zhang, Virginia O. Shaffer, Qiang Cai and Hong Xu

What is New

- Esophagus tumors can be endoscopically diagnosed from superficial changes of mucosa to the cellular level, even subcellular level, and beyond the mucosa through the whole wall and adjacent organs.
- Minimally invasive endoscopic therapies can treat earlier stage esophageal cancer less traumatically than surgery.

Introduction

One of the most common gastrointestinal malignancies is esophageal cancer, which is among the leading ten causes of cancer-related death worldwide. It includes squamous carcinoma and adenocarcinoma. The former accounts for the majority of cancer in the esophagus; it has an insidious onset and poor prognosis. The latter is associated with Barrett's esophagus having long and obvious symptoms. Esophageal squamous cell carcinoma (ECC) is more common in older people with highest incidence between ages of 60–70 years. Men usually have greater morbidity than

Table 1. Non-epithelial esophageal masses.

Tumors	Leiomyoma, gastrointestinal stromal tumors (GIST), lipomyoma, hemangioma, fibroma, lymphangioma, lymphoma, carcinoid tumor, metastatic cancer
Non-tumors	Cyst, varices, inflammatory granuloma

women.[1] Other malignant tumors of the esophagus including sarcomas, lymphoma, primary melanoma, and endocrine cell carcinoma are very rare. Endoscopy plays a crucial role in the diagnosis and treatment of esophageal cancer.

Non-epithelial orientated tumors are not common, but not extremely rare. They can be managed without difficulty by an experienced endoscopist. The clinical presentation of patients with tumors varies from mild or no symptoms to death. The most troublesome part of diagnosis is that a malignant lesion can have the appearance of an innocuous lump with seemingly benign features. Non-epithelial esophageal masses are listed in Table 1.

Advancement in Diagnosis

Diagnostic endoscopy

Chromoendoscopy

Early esophageal cancer presents as flatten, patchy inflammatory changes of mucosa, mild erosion, or elevated lesions. Early detection and treatment lead to much better prognosis than that of advanced esophageal cancer. [2–5] In white light endoscopy, those early cancer lesions are very difficult to find. Traditionally, Lugol's iodine and methylene blue have been used as chromoendoscopy to find the early cancer, and then biopsies are performed. More accurate real time diagnosis can be made with the following advance techniques to reduce the numbers of biopsy, the procedural time, and to avoid or decrease the patients' discomfort from the application of staining chemicals. Narrow-band imaging (NBI), Olympus, Fujinon intelligent color enhancement (FICE), and i-Scan system, Pentax are advance techniques that have been used in recent years. FICE and i-Scan system are developed from computed spectral estimation technology, which processes the reflected photons to reconstitute virtual images for a choice of different wavelengths of red, green, and blue (RGB) signaling. The NBI system depends on optical filters within the light source, using a frame sequential lighting method.

Narrow-band imaging (NBI) can be used to differentiate patterns of mucosa capillary loops to diagnose and predict extension in squamous cell carcinoma. Muto *et al.* and Yoshida *et al.* observed morphological patterns in the intrapapillary capillary loops with NBI with/without magnification.[6,7] Takenaka *et al.* found that the sensitivity, specificity and accuracy of NBI in detection of esophageal squamous cell carcinoma and high-grade intraepithelial neoplasia were 90.9%, 95.4% and 95.1%, respectively.[8]

Computed virtual chromoendoscopy with flexible spectral imaging color enhancement (FICE) is a new dyeless imaging technique that the visibilities of enhances mucosal and vascular patterns. However, a method for selecting a suitable wavelength for a particular condition has not been established. Combined acetic acid and FICE is a promising method for screening high-grade dysplasia and early cancer in Barrett's esophagus.[9,10]

I-Scan technology is the newly developed image-enhanced endoscopy technology from PENTAX, Japan. It consists of three types of algorithms: surface enhancement (SE), contrast enhancement (CE), and tone enhancement (TE). SE enhances light-dark contrast by obtaining luminance intensity data for each pixel and applying an algorithm that allows detailed observation of a mucosal surface structure. CE digitally adds blue color in relatively dark areas, by obtaining luminance intensity data for each pixel and applying an algorithm that allows detailed observation of subtle irregularities around the surface. Both enhancement functions work in real time without impairing the original color of the organ, therefore, SE and CE are suitable for screening endoscopy to detect esophageal tumors at an early stage. TE dissects and analyzes the individual RGB components of a normal image. The algorithm then alters the color frequencies of each component and recombines the components to a single, new color image, which is designed to enhance minute mucosal structures and subtle changes in color. TE works in real-time and consists of three modes such as TE-e for esophageal tumors. TE is mainly for detailed examination of the lesions that are detected in a screening endoscopy.[11]

Qumseya *et al.*[12] using meta-analysis and systematic review found that advanced imaging techniques such as chromoendoscopy and virtual chromoendoscopy significantly increase the diagnostic yield for identification of dysplasia or early cancer in patients with BE.

Optic coherence tomography

Optic coherence tomography (OCT) is an endoscopic, optical analogue of high frequency B-mode ultrasonography.[13] However, instead of using sound waves to generate images, OCT uses light waves. OCT is an optical signal acquisition and processing method that can capture high resolution, three-dimensional images within any optical scattering media, such as biological tissue. Cross-sectional images are obtained by measuring the intensity of back-scattered light from various depths of tissue using a technique called low-coherence interferometry. Just as in B-mode ultrasonography, a quantitative measurement of backscattering is performed at each axial depth and these measurements are repeated at different transverse positions. In this manner, a linear or radial two-dimensional map of backscattering strength is acquired and used to produce a high resolution image. OCT has attracted interest in a variety of medical applications, including ophthalmic scanning, diagnosis of epithelial lesions, bronchoscopic examinationand evaluation of atherosclerosis in blood vessels.[14–16]

OCT is usually performed by introducing a linear or radial catheter into the accessory channel of a standard endoscope. As in ultrasound, a water interface or tissue contact is not required to produce an image. Newer OCT systems are capable of producing a 512 × 512 pixel image within one-quarter of a second. Not only are OCT images obtained in real-time, but these images also have a 10-fold greater resolution (approximately 7 to 20 μm) than other modalities such as endoscopic ultrasound which allows for visualization of many microscopic mucosal features such as villi, crypts and glands.[17] However, although these tissue elements can be viewed in OCT, the sampling depth of OCT is limited to 1–2 mm due to scattering of light by tissue. Additionally, the resolution of OCT is not sufficient to visualize abnormalities such as nuclear dysplasia.

Characteristics features with OCT that may be signs of dysplasia or regenerative changes include incomplete surface maturation and irregular glands.[16–19]

OCT has been studied in examination of the esophagus and the gastroesophageal junction. Normal esophageal tissue on OCT imaging shows an easily recognizable horizontal, layered structure. OCT features which predict the presence of intestinal metaplasia are: (1) the absence of the layered structure of normal squamous epithelium and the presence of the vertical crypt-and-pit morphology of normal gastric mucosa; (2) a disorganized architecture with inhomogeneous back-scattering of the signal and an irregular mucosal surface; and (3) the presence of submucosal glands characterized at the OCT imaging as pockets of low reflectance below the epithelial surface.[20–22] Use of these simple criteria is limited, however, as the presence of the crypt-and-pit architecture in normal or inflamed gastric mucosa may make it difficult to discriminate between esophageal metaplasia and normal or inflamed gastric mucosa. Also, it is difficult to identify high-grade dysplasia utilizing OCT; the increased nuclear-to-cytoplasmic ratio occurring in dysplasia can alter the light reflection characteristics, giving a more inhomogeneous back-scattering of the signal. Poneros *et al.*[20] were able to improve diagnosis of high grade dysplasia by using two parameters of tissue reflectivity as an indicator of dysplasia. These criteria retrospectively diagnosed high grade dysplasia with 100% sensitivity and 85% specificity.

Endocytoscopy

Endocytoscopy (EC) is based on the principle of light contact microscopy. This imaging technology enables real-time visualization of the cellular structures of the superficial epithelial layer in a plane parallel to the mucosal surface. In order to visualize cellular and subcellular structures (e.g., nuclei) with EC, it is necessary to pre-stain the mucosa with an absorptive contrast agent, such as 0.5% to 1% methylene blue, cresyl violet or 0.25% toluidine blue. Often, the mucosa is treated with a mucolytic such as N-acetylcysteine prior to staining. After the stain is applied to the mucosal surface, the tip of the endoscope is placed in direct contact with the dye-stained mucosal surface and then the target mucosa is scanned with condensed normal white light. A fixed-focus, high-power objective lens projects highly magnified images from a minute sampling site (<0.5 mm diameter) on to a charge coupled device.[23–25] With this method, cytological details can be directly visualized, making direct observation of living cells feasible.

Endocytoscopic diagnosis is based on the assessment of several cytological and architectural features, such as the density, size and arrangement of cells; the size and shape of nuclei; the nucleus-to-cytoplasm ratio; and the staining pattern. For example, squamous cell carcinoma of the esophagus is distinguished by increased density of cells and marked heterogeneity in staining in nuclear staining and size, as opposed to the orderly cellular arrangement and homogenous staining pattern seen in normal squamous esophageal epithelium.[23,25]

An EC study by Eberl *et al.*[26] showed that the sensitivity and specificity for the evaluation of 25 patients with neoplastic esophageal lesions by blinded pathologists was 81% and 100% respectively. These improved results are likely due to the presence of identified neoplastic lesions, whereas in the Pohl study there were no visible lesions present.[27] It is important to note that image quality remains an issue with EC. However, advances in this technology are combining EC with other endoscopic tools, such as NBI, to screen Barrett's esophagus and to isolate suspicious areas of the mucosa for further evaluation and biopsy.

Confocal laser microendoscopy

Confocal laser endoscopy (CLE) is one of the newest endoscopic technologies. High resolution microendoscopy, endoscopic techniques such as NBI and chromoendoscopy, are used to highlight suspicious areas of mucosa for biopsy and histological analysis, CLE offers the endoscopist the ability to make a real-time, *in vivo* histological assessment of GI mucosa. CLE is based on the excitation of a fluorophore in a specimen using a laser which sequentially scans specific points on the specimen in a raster pattern whereby the focused spot traverses a line rapidly from left to right and the line is swept top to bottom, mapping out a square.[4] The

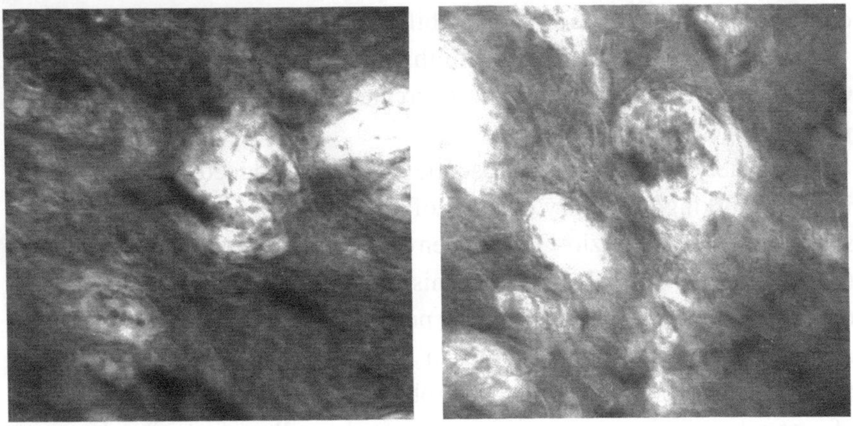

Fig. 1. Photos of an esophageal squamous cell carcinoma in a CLE (Fluorescein sodium contrast).

emission of the fluorophore at the point of illumination is recorded to create the pixels of an image. Emitted light is also channeled through a pinhole such that light which is not focused at a specific depth is unable to reach the detector. Thus, confocal microscopy is able to scan specific optical depths within the specimen and provide a clear, two-dimensional image of the examined tissue.[28]

CLE integrates a confocal laser microscope either in the tip of a video endoscope or as a probe that can be passed through the channel of any endoscope.[2] One widely used CLE system is an endoscopic system with embedded CLE technology manufactured by Pentax (Tokyo, Japan). This system is available both for upper GI endoscopy and colonoscopy.[10] In the embedded CLE technology (eCLE), a confocal laser microscope is integrated directly into the end of a video endoscope. Images are obtained by using a laser which delivers an excitation wavelength of 488 nm. The pixels are collected every 0.7 μm (to give 0.7 μm lateral resolution) for a total field of view of 475 μm and can be collected through various sections of the mucosa in 7 μm increments to a depth of 250 μm. The current equipment is able to achieve this at a rate of 0.8 to 1.6 frames/s. This system is capable of providing both excellent image clarity and the ability of using the confocal endomicroscope similar to a conventional endoscope. Image stabilization achieved by application of suction is used to produce high quality images during eCLE. Consequently, a "suction polyp" is created that targets biopsy of tissue in the imaged area.[29]

Alternately, a confocal microscope can be introduced as a mini-probe into the working/accessory channel of an endoscope; a probe-based CLE system (pCLE), Cellvizio-GI, has been created by Mauna Kea Technologies (Paris, France). The advantage of this system, unlike the eCLE technology, is that the confocal microscopy probe can be used with any commercial endoscope and, subsequently, a variety of wide-field technologies (Narrow Band Imaging, etc.). The probe is placed into the biopsy channel of a standard endoscope and then retracted to allow for tissue biopsy.[29] Depending on the system used, pCLE can scan with 1–3.5 μm lateral resolution for a total field of view of 240–600 μm, which does not compare well with the embedded systems. In addition, pCLE systems are unable to varify the depth at which they collect data and thus lack axial resolution. However, these tradeoffs allow the probe based system to operate with a much faster scanning rate (12 frames/s compared to the 0.8–1.2 frames/s in eCLE).

To obtain images using either confocal endomicroscopic tools, eCLE or pCLE, the patient must be given a fluorescent contrast agent. This can either be given intravenously (IV) or sprayed onto the mucosa directly. The most common contrast agent is 10% fluorescein by IV. Fluorescein aptly highlights the vasculature, lamina propria and intracellular spaces, allowing visualization of vessel pattern and cellular architecture.[30] Fluorescein and its metabolites are excreted by the kidney. Adverse side effects of fluorescein are rare but may include hypotension without shock (0.5%), nausea (0.39%), injection site erythema (0.35%), diffuse self-limited rash (0.04%) or mild epigastric pain (0.09%). Anaphylaxis has been reported but is uncommon. Acriflavine hydrochloride (0.05% in saline) and cresyl violet (0.13% in acetic acid) are two contrast agents that are applied topically to the mucosa during CLE. Acriflavine is used to stain cellular nuclei which fluorescein is unable to. However, since acriflavine accumulates in the nuclei, there is a potential mutagenic risk associated with it. Cresyl violet causes cytoplasmic enrichment which in turn leads to negative visualization of nuclear morphology. It also provides pit pattern characterization of mucosal lesions and so can be used for chromoendoscopy as well.[28,31] Notably, fluorescein does not provide direct nuclear visualization and the appreciation of nucleus-to-cytoplasm ratio cannot be used for the diagnosis and grading of intraepithelial neoplasias.

Kiesslich *et al.*[32] demonstrated that the eCLE diagnosed Barrett's-related neoplasia during endoscopy with a sensitivity of 92.9% and a specificity of 98.4%. Additionally, Dunbar *et al.*[33] conducted a prospective, randomized, double-blinded, crossover study analyzing the diagnostic yield of CLE-targeted biopsies. This study compared four-quadrant random biopsies with CLE-targeted biopsies in 39 patients. They demonstrated that CLE improved the diagnostic yield for detecting neoplasia in BE patients, particularly for endoscopically unapparent neoplastic lesions. CLE detected 33.7% of neoplastic lesions vs 17.2% of lesions detected with random biopsies. Additionally, two-thirds of patients in the routine surveillance group did not need any biopsies when examined with CLE due to absence of neoplasia during *in vivo* imaging. The Kiesslich *et al.*[32] study also reported a potential reduction in number of mucosal biopsies needed; only 30 of 156 (19.2%) CLE sites in 63 patients examined would have required a mucosal biopsy for confirmation of diagnosis of neoplasia. Ongoing work by us and others continue to study the advantages of CLE in diagnosing dysplasia in Barrett's esophagus.

Staging

Endoscopic ultrasonography

The overall accuracy of computed tomogram (CT) for staging esophageal cancer is excellent for advanced disease. Liver metastases and findings consistent with adjacent organ invasion can be reliably noted on CT scan as well as by magnetic resonance imaging (MRI). The sensitivity and specificity for detecting bronchotracheal and pericardial invasion exceed 90–95% in most series. However, CT imaging does not reliably detect local and regional lymph node metastases and "early" (T1–T2) tumors. The emergence of endoscopic ultrasonography (EUS) offers the most significant advancement in the preoperative staging of esophageal cancer. EUS is performed using a modified upper endoscope with an ultrasound transducer housed within the tip. At frequencies ranging from 7.5 to 12 MHz, EUS depicts five layers of the esophageal wall corresponding to its distinct histologic features. Malignant tumors are identified as hypoechoic masses with irregular margins that disrupt the normal esophageal architecture. The depth of tumor invasion is defined by the outermost margin of the hypoechoic mass. Suspicious appearing lymph nodes are identified as hypoechoic rounded structures within the mediastinum and near the esophagus. Fine needle aspiration (FNA) of lymph nodes can be obtained through some EUS scopes for definitive diagnosis of malignant involvement. EUS can accurately diagnose early cancers, that is, those classified as T1–T2. The overall accuracy of EUS for predicting the extent of esophageal cancers approaches 80–90% for T and 70–80% for N classification.[34]

There are several limitations of EUS for staging esophageal cancer. Overstaging of a T2 lesion can sometimes happen when there is significant peritumoral inflammation, whereas understaging sometimes occurs largely due to microscopic invasion beyond the muscularis propria. EUS is also very reliable in diagnosing adjacent organ invasion (i.e., invasion to pleura or aorta); however, limited depth of penetration of EUS results in incomplete assessment for distant metastases. In addition, about 30% of esophageal cancers produce severe esophageal obstruction and cannot be traversed with the regular ultrasound endoscope at the time of presentation. Generally, these tumors can be accurately staged with EUS after dilation of the stricture; and when this occurs, they are almost always advanced tumors, that is, T3 or greater. Recently, the development of through-the-scope miniprobes and wire-guided small-diameter blind ultrasound probes has overcome the problems with tumor strictures in most cases. In addition, as these small caliber ultrasound probes utilize higher scanning frequencies (12–20 MHz), the detection and accuracy of staging for T2 tumors has improved significantly.[34]

A large number of studies[35–37] have looked into the staging accuracy of EUS and CT scan. It has been demonstrated that EUS is more accurate than CT scan for locoregional staging (both T and N classification). EUS appears to be superior in defining abdominal lymph node metastases (especially celiac axis nodes), although CT scan is still the better imaging study to detect distant organ metastases. Nonetheless, CT scan should be considered as complementary to EUS and should be combined with EUS to determine the extent of extraesophageal invasion into the mediastinum and distant metastases. The ideal algorithm for managing these patients should include a CT scan of chest and abdomen, and, if negative for metastasis, an EUS should be done to rule out locally advanced disease.

Takizawa *et al.*[34] showed that EUS is a more accurate technique than contrast-enhanced CT for detecting abnormal lymph nodes. Sensitivity of CT was lower than that of EUS alone or CT + EUS. But some metastatic lymph nodes in the neck and the abdomen are only detectable by CT. Therefore, both EUS and CT should be undertaken for routine examination prior to treatment of esophageal cancer.

Contrast-enhanced EUS

Contrast-enhanced EUS (CE-EUS) is composed of two main categories: CE power-Doppler EUS (CED-EUS) and CE harmonic EUS (CEH-EUS). After injection of contrast materials, increased intensity of week flow signal can be examined with color or power Doppler. Therefore, by using CED-EUS, differentiation of vascular-rich area and hypovascular area is possible with clarity. After development of harmonic imaging method, it is possible to get images of microcirculation and parenchymal perfusion with CEH-EUS. The use of CE-EUS allows a better visualization and differentiation of hypoenhanced masses suggestive of pancreatic adenocarcinoma and hyperenhanced lesions indicative of inflammatory masses.[38–40]

Nomura *et al.*[40] compared enhanced EUS with EUS and found that enhancement of the third and fifth layers was observed in all normal esophageal and gastric walls. Esophageal carcinomas were not enhanced. Enhancement was observed in five gastric carcinomas that had abundant, enlarged, and winding vascular beds. In all esophageal carcinomas and the other 25 gastric carcinomas, the tumors per se were not enhanced, but enhancement of the third and fifth layers around the lesions clearly demarcated the tumor boundaries. As a result, accuracy for detection of the depth of gastric carcinoma improved from 76.7% for EUS to 90% for CE-EUS. All gastric myogenic tumors were enhanced, and irregularly shaped sonolucent areas within these tumors became clear, but they could not distinguish between leiomyoma and leiomyosarcoma.

Although EUS has improved the diagnostic of potential malignancies, gastric lesions with suspicion of gastrointestinal stromal tumors (GIST) or benign lesions like lipoma or leiomyoma can often not be accurately differentiated by EUS, therefore, requiring tissue sampling with the risk of bleeding especially in GIST. As with the newest generation of EUS machines, contrast-enhanced harmonic endoscopic ultrasound (CEH-EUS) has become a new option to determine perfusion characteristics. Kannengiesser *et al.* study showed that CEH-EUS could discriminate GIST from benign lesions with good accuracy.[41] In the future, CEH-EUS-guided discrimination may lead to individualized diagnostic and therapeutic strategies in handling gastrointestinal submucosal lesions.

EUS elastography

Tissue elastic imaging represents a technique that allows calculation and visualization of hardness of tissue. Real-time tissue elastography with ultrasonographic approach is combined to EUS. With this technique, the real-time visualization of the calculated strain value can provide information on tissue hardness at the area of interest and the distribution pattern of tissue hardness as well. In addition to EUS image, the information can guide in the selection of the most probable malignant lymph node for EUS-FNA.[42,43]

Advancement in therapy

En bloc resection remains the definitive surgical cure for esophageal cancer. The operation consists of removal of a tissue block completely surrounded by normal tissue. Locally advanced tumors (T1N1, T2N1, T3N0, and T3N1) are resectable but incurable. These tumors are associated with a high recurrence rate following surgery. The optimal intervention in these patients remains controversial, and practices vary widely depending on the local surgical expertise and the assessment of the patient's preexisting medical condition. Whereas endoscopy has mainly been used to diagnose cancers, new technologies, such as photodynamic therapy and endoscopic mucosal resection, have provided endoscopic treatments with the potential of curing early stage tumors of the esophagus.

Endoscopic mucosal resection (EMR)

The development of EMR was sparked by the need to treat superficial flat and polypoid neoplasm of the gastrointestinal (GI) mucosa with minimally invasive procedures. Long-term studies have demonstrated that EMR outcomes are similar to those of surgery, which has led to acceptance of EMR as a standard treatment, especially in early stage GI cancers. The availability of EUS to determine the depth of tumor invasion and lymph node metastases as well as chromoendoscopic techniques to reveal tumor borders otherwise not visible without staining further facilitate the application of EMR.

Numerous EMR techniques have been described, such as injection and snare cautery, injection with precut, EMR with a cap, or EMR with band ligation. Nevertheless, the general principles are the same. EMR involves expansion of the submucosal layer and lifting of the mucosa to allow for a safe longitudinal resection. Injection of an expansion solution (typically

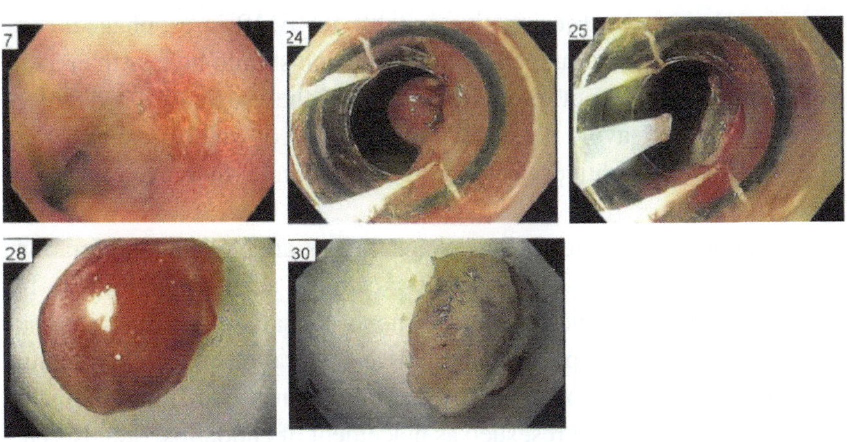

Fig. 2. Endoscopic mucosal resection for T1 esophageal cancer.

normal saline) into the submucosa creates a bleb and increases the distance between the mucosa and muscularis propia. This lifting of the mucosa is essential to prevent transmural burning or perforation. A snare is placed over the base of the "neopolyp" and the mucosa is resected with electrocautery. The cancerous lesion is removed en bloc and allows for a complete detailed histopathologic analysis.

In esophageal cancers, EMR has been applied mainly for squamous cell carcinoma and much less for Barrett's esophagus-related adenocarcinoma. EMR is indicated when the lesion is superficial and without evidence of lymph node metastasis. Although conventional EUS is accurate in determining tumor depth and lymph node metastasis of large or bulky lesions, it is less precise for small, flat, or depressed tumors. Therefore, in these instances, high-frequency ultrasound probes have been recommended. The application of Lugol's solution further assists in visual distinction between a cancerous lesion and normal mucosa (squamous cell carcinoma or dysplasia does not stain). Once the lesion is identified and staged, approximately 20 mL of saline is injected into the submucosa, causing more than half-circumferential mucosal lifting. EMR can then be safely performed. EMR should be avoided if the lesion cannot be lifted by submucosal saline injection (non-lifting sign), which does occur when a tumor has indeed invaded the muscularis propia or when there has been fibrosis due to prior intervention. There is no consensus on the maximal lesion size suitable for EMR in esophageal cancer. However, it is recommended that the lesion should be less than 3 cm in height and should not exceed one-third of the esophageal circumference in width to avoid the late complication of stenosis. For larger lesions, other alternatives, such as photodynamic therapy, should be considered.

The major complications of esophageal EMR are bleeding, perforation, and stenosis. Bleeding during EMR is almost always controllable by injection of a low-concentration epinephrine-saline solution, thermal coagulation, or endoscopic clipping. Large perforations invariably require immediate surgery, although small perforations may be manageable with more conservative measures, such as placement of endoclips. Stenosis can occur when circumferential resection has been attempted.

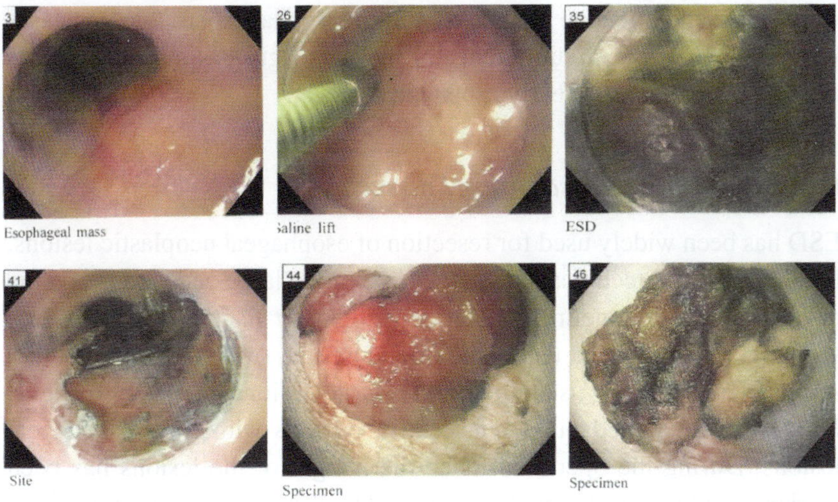

Fig. 3. Endoscopic submucosal dissection for T1 esophageal cancer.

Endoscopic submucosal dissection (ESD)

Early esophageal cancer that could be resected by ESD is the lesion restricted in the M1, M2, M3, or SM1. High grade intraepithelial neoplasia of squamous cell and Barrett's dysplasia, larger than 15 mm, can also be treated by ESD.

ESD in esophagus is more challenging than that in stomach and colon. Narrow space, lack of serosa, pulse of the aorta and heart, and compression of adjacent spine, trachea and aorta require a lot of experience and technique to complete the procedure. Lugol's iodine or NBI both can be used to define the lesion. CO_2 pump could substitute the air pump to decrease the incidence of emphysema or shorten the duration of emphysema occuring. Circumferential ESD of esophagus could lead to post operation stricture. Intra-lesional steroid injection or covered metal stent placement may decrease the stricture's incidence. Lee WJ *et al.*[44] presented a case of a single session of intra-lesional steroid injection performed immediately after near-circumferential ESD to prevent post-ESD stricture. After a follow-up period of six months, the patient had good outcomes without dysphagia. Wen J *et al.*[45] found that esophageal stents were a safe and effective method to prevent esophageal strictures in cases where >75 % of the circumference of the esophagus has mucosal defects after ESD treatment for early esophageal cancer.

Endoscopic submucosal tunnel dissection

ESD has been widely used for resection of esophageal neoplastic lesions, but there are still technical challenges in treating large ones. Based on the development of tunneling technique, Linghu *et al.*[46] reported the first series in which the new technique of endoscopic submucosal tunnel dissection (ESTD) was used to remove large lesions in the esophagus. ESTD was attempted in 11 consecutive patients with early esophageal lesions. During the operation, once the margin of the lesions has been marked, a submucosal tunnel was created by submucosal dissection from the oral incision to the anal incision. Bilateral resection was then performed to remove the lesion completely from the tunnel. The average length of the five lesions was 5.7 cm, and their extent from one third to four fifths of the lumen circumferentially. Operative time ranged from 50 to 120 min (mean, 77 min). En bloc resection with negative lateral and basal margins was achieved in all lesions without complications. Wang L *et al.*[47] also practiced ESTD in the treatment of submucosal lesion of esophagus. Operating time was significantly shorter for ESTD than for ESD, while incision healing was faster for ESTD than for ESD. Hospital stay was also shorter or ESTD than for ESD. The ESTD technique is feasible and promising to be effective and safe in the appropriate tumors in the esophagus.

Cryotherapy

Endoscopic cryotherapy using liquid nitrogen is a novel method of destruction of BE tissue. Initial reports suggest that this therapy is well-tolerated and effective in inducing neosquamous epithelium in subjects with BE. The system uses –196°C liquid nitrogen by using a low-pressure, disposable 7F spray catheter directly to the tissue targeted for treatment at a cooling rate of 25 W. The system enables the physician to control the duration of the cryogen spray to the selected site by depressing a foot pedal. Before

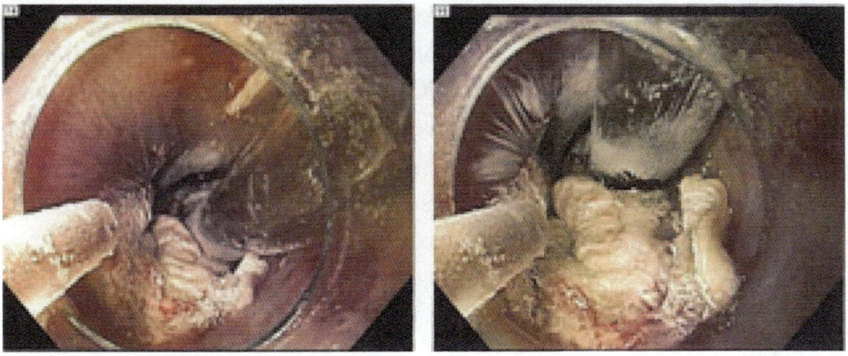

Fig. 4. Cryotherapy for T1 esophageal cancer after endoscopic mucosal resection.

the administration of the liquid nitrogen, a dual lumen decompression tube was placed in the gastric antrum to evacuate nitrogen gas by both passive venting and active suction. To administer the liquid nitrogen, a polyamide catheter was introduced through the working channel of an adult endoscope and positioned 3 to 4 mm beyond the distal tip of the endoscope (or at the distal edge of a clear, friction-fit cap, if used). Gas flow was initiated by depressing a foot pedal. The treatment area was limited to 2 to 3 cm of mucosa in a hemi-circumferential or one third circumferential pattern so that freezing could be maintained without reperfusion during the treatment. In situations when the decompression tube blocks the flow of cryogen onto selected sites, the endoscope tip was used to gently reposition the tube out of the path of the spray. The endoscopist monitored the endoscopic appearance of the tissue, and when white frost was noted in the treatment area, a timer was actuated to track the freeze time. Treatment dosimetry was either 3 cycles of 20 s or 4 cycles of 10 s. During the intervening thaw cycles, the tissue reperfused, with return to its normal salmon color. Monitoring of the abdomen was performed by a nurse or technician for any signs of abdominal distention. Typical initial treatments involve 3 to 5 treatment sites, depending on the length of lesion.[48]

Sonia Gosain *et al.*[49] treated patients with liquid nitrogen spray cryotherapy every 8 weeks until complete eradication of high grade dysphasia (HGD) and intestinal metaplasia (IM). Surveillance endoscopy with biopsies was performed for at least two years. All patients included in the study had complete initial eradication of endoscopic and histologically apparent BE. Complete eradication of HGD and IM were 100% and 84% in two-year follow-up. Recurrent HGD was found in six patients, with completed eradication of HGD in five after repeat treatment. One patient progressed to adenocarcinoma and subsequently downgraded to HGD after repeat cryotherapy. No serious adverse events occurred. Stricture was seen in three patients, all successfully dilated.

Ablation

Tumor ablation treatments available for palliation include radiofrequency ablation (RFA), photodynamic therapy (PDT), chemical sclerosant injection, monopolar and bipolar electrocautery, argon plasma coagulation (APC), and neodymium: yttrium-aluminum-garnet (Nd: YAG) laser. The simplest and least expensive intervention for esophageal cancer ablation is the injection of a chemical sclerosant during endoscopy. Absolute alcohol is the most widely employed chemical agent and created results similar to laser therapy. The major problem with chemical injection is the inability to localize the injected agent as the sclerosant agent tracks along the tissue planes, causing damage to normal tissue and, sometimes, resulting in perforations. Patients may experience temporary worsening of symptoms until adequate tumor necrosis occurs.[50,51]

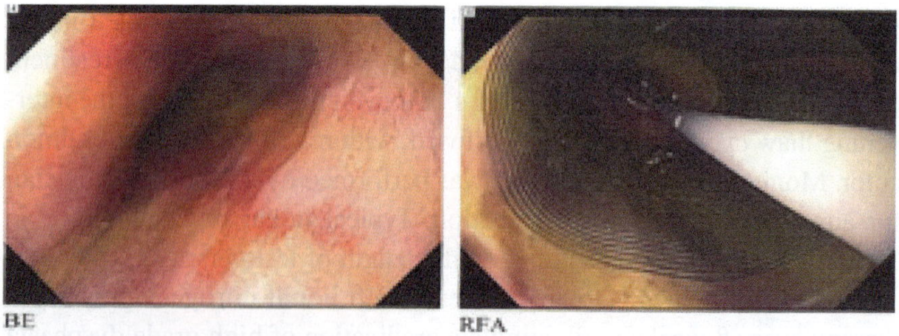

Fig. 5. Radiofrequency ablation for T1 esophageal cancer after endoscopic mucosal resection.

Two RFA techniques are being used depending on the type and location of metaplastic changes: circumferential or focal. The circumferential method based on a balloon system (HALO360) was used for circular, metaplastic lesions on large surfaces, while the focal method based on the HALO90 system mounted on the endoscopic tip was used for smaller focal lesions. Radiofrequency energy was supplied to the tissue via a bipolar electrode; 12 J/cm^2 was applied for dysplastic lesions while 10 J/cm^2 was applied for intestinal metaplasia. The depth of ablative damage involved all mucosa and superficial part of submucosa. Atilla Ertan *et al.*[51] compared efficacy, safety, and cost-comparison of RFA and PDT in the treatment of high grade dysplasia of Barrett's dysplasia (BD). A complete histological resolution response of BD (CR-D) was defined as all biopsies at the last endoscopy session, negative for dysplasia and concluded that RFA had higher rate of CR-D without any serious adverse events and was less costly than PDT for endoscopic treatment of BD.

Photodynamic therapy (PDT) has emerged as an attractive palliative treatment for esophageal cancer and its complications. PDT has been successful in reducing tumor bulk and in opening the esophageal lumen in patients with complete obstruction, a situation in which Nd: YAG laser therapy was considered too risky. PDT has also been utilized as a salvage therapy in patients whose esophageal stents have failed because of tumor ingrowth/overgrowth.

The treatment begins with an intravenous injection of a photosensitive chemical, porfimer sodium (Photofrin). It is administered at a dose of 2 mg/kg of body weight and preferentially concentrates in the tumor tissue. After 40–50 hours following the injection, the area of the esophageal cancer is exposed to a red light at a wavelength of 630 nm, delivered from a continuous-wave dye laser via an optical fiber diffuser for a total cumulative light dose of 300 J/cm. The red light has been chosen for greatest depth of penetration (5 mm). The process initiates a photochemical reaction and the effect takes place over the next hours to days, ultimately resulting in necrosis of the tumor. Improvement in the dysphagia is usually noted within 5–7 days, although some patients may experience worsening of dysphagia initially due to local tissue inflammation and edema. A major issue with PDT is retention of the photosensitive dye in the skin (up to 6 weeks), which requires patients to avoid direct sun exposure or risk severe sunburn. Other complications following PDT include fever, leukocytosis, nausea, and pleural effusion. Severe complications, which fortunately are uncommon, include atrial arrhythmias, stricture formation, hemorrhage, and perforation. The advantage of PDT in early esophageal cancer (T1 or T2 disease) is the overall greater than 80% cure rate. Gray *et al.*[52] concluded the long term efficacy of PDT as an ablative therapy of high grade dysplasia in Barrett's esophagus was good, and found that PDT successfully ablated HGD in 84% of patients and could therefore still be considered an effective salvage treatment for this condition in patients with co-morbidities precluding them for surgical resection.

Monopolar and bipolar electrocautery are falling out of favor and are rarely used at the present time as they are difficult to control the depth of treatment. A newer method,[53] argon plasma coagulation, uses ionized argon gas to convey electrical energy to achieve thermal desiccation of tumor tissue has been used. Unfortunately, the effect is generally superficial, and it is less efficient in relieving dysphagia in advanced esophageal cancer than other tissue ablation methods.

High-power Nd: YAG laser can provide palliation of dysphagia by coagulating and vaporizing malignant tissue under endoscopic control. Tumors amenable to laser therapy are exophytic or polypoid, preferably located in a straight segment of the esophagus such as in the mid-esophagus or lower esophagus, and shorter than 5 cm. Multiple endoscopic laser treatment sessions may be required to reduce the size of the intra-luminal tumor, which improves swallowing. Periodic follow-up is performed to reduce any recurrent intra-luminal tumor growth.

Dilation

Esophageal dilation is most commonly performed with either expandable through-the-scope balloons or wire-guided polyvinyl bougies under fluoroscopy. A small percentage of patients can be successfully dilated to allow for soft diet consumption. However, the benefit from dilation is usually of short duration, and other methods are usually required for more prolonged symptom relief. One of the major complications of esophageal dilation is perforation.

Esophageal prostheses

Placement of esophageal prostheses (stents) is another appealing method for the palliation of malignant strictures and provides effective relief of dysphagia in most cases. The prostheses are usually inserted surgically or endoscopically with fluoroscopic guidance. A wide variety of stents have been developed and modified over the years that provide good mechanical support for maintaining esophageal lumen patency and reduce complications such as stent migration and tumor ingrowth. At present, the expandable metal stents are the most widely applied form of prostheses. The principal merits of such stents are the ease of insertion and the remarkably low risk of esophageal perforation. Covering the stent with a polymer sheet effectively reduces tumor ingrowth and provides for treatment of tracheoesophageal fistulas, while the outer flange diameters have been increased, thereby making a funnel-shaped stent that adheres to the esophageal wall to significantly lower the rate of migration. Early complications of expandable metal stents have included incomplete expansion, perforation, bleeding, and pain. Late complications include tumor overgrowth/ingrowth, ulceration, food impaction, and stent migration. Patients who have received prior radiation and chemotherapy are more prone to develop complications. Stents that cross into the gastric cardia may cause significant gastroesophageal reflux that can usually be controlled with proton-pump inhibitors; however, a new stent has been developed that prevents reflux via a valve mechanism.[54] In cases where patients develop an airway fistula, such as bronchoesophageal or tracheoesophageal fistula, stent placement is the optimum therapy.[55] Furthermore, a second stent may be placed in the airway if there is significant stenosis causing dyspnea or an esophageal stent is placed at the upper esophagus.

Take Home Messages

- Regular surveillance of the esophagus with high definition white light endoscopy and the appropriate associated techniques, such as NBI, may be able to find the cancer at an early stage.
- With EMR, ESD, RFA, and other techniques, early lesions can be treated by endoscopy in a minimally invasive way.

- Endoscopic techniques can also be used in late stage cancers with the application of endoscopic prostheses or dilation for palliation.

References

1. Parkin, D.M., Bray, F., Ferlay, J. *et al.*, Global cancer statistics, 2002. *CA Cancer J Clin*, 2005. **55**: 74–108.
2. Reddymasu, S.C., Sharma, P., Advances in endoscopic imaging of the esophagus. *Gastroenterol Clin North Am*, 2008. **37**: 763–74, vii
3. Waxman, I., Konda, V.J., Endoscopic techniques for recognizing neoplasia in Barrett's esophagus: which should the clinician use? *Curr Opin Gastroenterol*, 2010. **26**: 352–60.
4. Wong Kee Song, L.M., Wilson, B.C., Endoscopic detection of early upper GI cancers. *Best Pract Res Clin Gastroenterol*, 2005. **19**: 833–56.
5. Toyoda, H., Rubio, C., Befrits, R., Hamamoto, N., Adachi, Y., Jaramillo, E., Detection of intestinal metaplasia in distal esophagus and esophagogastric junction by enhanced-magnification endoscopy. *Gastrointest Endosc*, 2004. **59**: 15–21.
6. Muto, M., Nakane, M., Katada, C. *et al.*, Squamous cell carcinoma in situ at oropharyngeal and hypopharyngeal mucosal sites. *Cancer*, 2004. **101**(6): 1375–81.
7. Yoshida, T., Inoue, H., Usui, S. *et al.*, Narrow-band imaging system with magnifying endoscopy for superficial esophageal lesions. *Gastrointestinal Endoscopy*, 2004; **59**(2): 288–95.
8. Takenaka, R., Kawahara, Y., Okada, H. *et al.*, Narrow-band imaging provides reliable screening for esophageal malignancy in patients with head and neck cancers. *Am J Gastroenterol*, 2009. **104**(12): 2942–48.
9. Inoue, M., Miyake, Y., Odaka, T. *et al.*, Objective evaluation of visibility in virtual chromoendoscopy for esophageal squamous carcinoma using a color difference formula. *J Biomed Opt*, 2010. **15**(5): 056019.
10. Camus, M., Coriat, R., Leblanc, S. *et al.*, Helpfulness of the combination of acetic acid and FICE in the detection of Barrett's epithelium and Barrett's associated neoplasias. *World J Gastroenterol,* 2012; **18**(16): 1921–5.
11. Kodashima, S., Fujishiro, M., Novel image-enhanced endoscopy with i-scan technology. *World J Gastroenterol*, 2010; **16**(9): 1043–9.

12. Qumseya, B.J., Wang, H., Badie, N. *et al.*, Advanced imaging technologies increase detection of dysplasia and neoplasia in patients with barrett's esophagus: a meta-analysis and systematic review. *Clin Gastroenterol Hepatol*, 2013. **11**(12): 1562–70.
13. Chen, J., Lee, L., Clinical applications and new developments of optical coherence tomography: an evidence-based review. *Clin Exp Optom*, 2007. **90**: 317–35.
14. Mogensen, M., Thrane, L., Jørgensen, T.M., Andersen, P.E., Jemec, G.B., OCT imaging of skin cancer and other dermatological diseases. *J Biophotonics*, 2009. **2**: 442–51.
15. Williamson, J.P., McLaughlin, R.A., Phillips, M.J., Armstrong, J.J., Becker, S., Walsh, J.H., Sampson, D.D., Hillman, D.R., Eastwood, P.R., Using optical coherence tomography to improve diagnostic and therapeutic bronchoscopy. *Chest*, 2009. **136**: 272–76
16. Farooq, M.U., Khasnis, A., Majid, A., Kassab, M.Y., The role of optical coherence tomography in vascular medicine. *Vasc Med*, 2009. **14**: 63–71
17. Das, A., Sivak, M.V., Chak, A., Wong, R.C., Westphal, V., Rollins, A.M., Willis, J., Isenberg, G, Izatt, J.A., High-resolution endoscopic imaging of the GI tract: a comparative study of optical coherence tomography versus high-frequency catheter probe EUS. *Gastrointest Endosc*, 2001. **54**: 219–24
18. Hsiung, P.L., Pantanowitz, L., Aguirre, A.D., Chen, Y., Phatak, D., Ko, T.H., Bourquin, S., Schnitt, S.J., Raza, S., Connolly, J.L., Mashimo, H., Fujimoto, J.G., Ultrahigh-resolution and 3-dimensional optical coherence tomography *ex vivo* imaging of the large and small intestines. *Gastrointest Endosc*, 2005. **62**: 561–74.
19. Winkler, A.M., Rice, P.F., Weichsel, J., Watson, J.M., Backer, M.V., Backer, J.M., Barton, J.K., *In vivo*, dual-modality OCT/LIF imaging using a novel VEGF receptor-targeted NIR fluorescent probe in the AOM-treated mouse model. *Mol Imaging Biol*, 2010.
20. Poneros, J.M., Diagnosis of Barrett's esophagus using optical coherence tomography. *Gastrointest Endosc Clin N Am*, 2004. **14**: 573–88, x.
21. Testoni, P.A., Mangiavillano, B., Optical coherence tomography in detection of dysplasia and cancer of the gastrointestinal tract and bilio-pancreatic ductal system. *World J Gastroenterol*, 2008. **14**: 6444–52.

22. Zagaynova, E., Gladkova, N., Shakhova, N., Gelikonov G., Gelikonov V., Endoscopic OCT with forward-looking probe: clinical studies in urology and gastroenterology. *J Biophotonics,* 2008. **1**: 114–128
23. Fujishiro, M, Kodashima, S, Takubo, K, Kakushima N, Omata M., Detailed comparison between endocytoscopy and horizontal histology of an esophageal intraepithelial squamous cell carcinoma. *Dis Esophagus,* 2008. **21**: 181–5.
24. Kwon, R.S., Wong Kee Song, L.M., Adler, D.G., Conway, J.D., Diehl, D.L., Farraye, F.A., Kantsevoy, S.V., Kaul, V., Kethu, S.R., Mamula, P., Pedrosa, M.C., Rodriguez, S.A., Tierney, W.M., Endocytoscopy. *Gastrointest Endosc,* 2009. **70**: 610–3.
25. Inoue, H., Kudo, S.E., Shiokawa, A., Technology insight: laser scanning confocal microscopy and endocytoscopy for cellular observation of the gastrointestinal tract. *Nat Clin Pract Gastroenterol Hepatol,* 2005. **2**: 31–7.
26. Eberl, T., Jechart, G., Probst, A., Golczyk, M., Bittinger, M., Scheubel, R., Arnholdt H., Knuechel, R., Messmann, H., Can an endocytoscope system (ECS) predict histology in neoplastic lesions? *Endoscopy*, 2007. **39**: 497–501.
27. Pohl, H., Koch, M., Khalifa, A., Papanikolaou, I.S., Scheiner, K., Wiedenmann, B., Rösch, T., Evaluation of endocytoscopy in the surveillance of patients with Barrett's esophagus. *Endoscopy*, 2007. **39**: 492–6.
28. Neumann, H., Kiesslich, R., Wallace, M.B., Neurath, M.F., Confocal laser endomicroscopy: technical advances and clinical applications. *Gastroenterology*, 2010. **139**: 388–92, 392.e1–2.
29. Dunbar, K., Canto, M., Confocal endomicroscopy. *Curr Opin Gastroenterol*, 2008. **24**: 631–7.
30. Kiesslich, R., Goetz, M., Vieth, M., Galle, P.R., Neurath, M.F., Confocal laser endomicroscopy. *Gastrointest Endosc Clin N Am*, 2005. **15**: 715–31.
31. Wallace, M.B., Meining, A., Canto, M.I., Fockens, P., Miehlke, S., Roesch, T., Lightdale, C.J., Pohl, H., Carr-Locke, D., Löhr, M., Coron, E., Filoche, B., Giovannini, M., Moreau, J., Schmidt, C., Kiesslich, R., The safety of intravenous fluorescein for confocal laser endomicroscopy in the gastrointestinal tract. *Aliment Pharmacol Ther*, 2010. **31**: 548–52.
32. Kiesslich, R., Gossner, L., Goetz, M., Dahlmann, A., Vieth, M., Stolte, M., Hoffman, A., Jung, M., Nafe, B., Galle, P.R., Neurath, M.F., *In vivo* histology of Barrett's esophagus and associated neoplasia by confocal laser endomicroscopy. *Clin Gastroenterol Hepatol*, 2006. **4**: 979–87.

33. Dunbar, K.B., Okolo, P., Montgomery, E., Canto, M.I., Confocal laser endomicroscopy in Barrett's esophagus and endoscopically inapparent Barrett's neoplasia: a prospective, randomized, double-blind, controlled, crossover trial. *Gastrointest Endosc*, 2009. **70**: 645–54.
34. Takizawa, K., Matsuda, T., Kozu, T. *et al.*, Lymph node staging in esophageal squamous cell carcinoma: a comparative study of endoscopic ultrasonography versus computed tomography. *J Gastroenterol Hepatol*, 2009. **24**(10): 1687–91.
35. Feng, X.Y., Wang, W., Luo, G.Y. *et al.*, Comparison of endoscopic ultrasonography and multislice spiral computed tomography for the preoperative staging of gastric cancer results of a single institution study of 610 Chinese patients. *PLoS One*. 2013. **8**(11): e78846.
36. Mehmedović, A., Mesihović, R., Saray, A., Vanis, N., Gastric cancer staging: EUS and CT. *Med Arch*, 2014. **68**(1): 34–6.
37. Yen, T.J., Chung, C.S., Wu, Y.W. *et al.*, Comparative study between endoscopic ultrasonography and positron emission tomography-computed tomography in staging patients with esophageal squamous cell carcinoma. *Dis Esophagus*, 2012. **25**(1): 40–7.
38. Hirooka, Y., Itoh, A., Kawashima, H. *et al.*, Diagnosis of pancreatic disorders using contrast-enhanced endoscopic ultrasonography and endoscopic elastography. *Clin Gastroenterol Hepatol*, 2009. **7**(11 Suppl): S63–7.
39. Ishikawa, T., Itoh, A., Kawashima, H. *et al.*, Usefulness of EUS combined with contrast enhancement in the differential diagnosis of malignant versus benign and preoperative localization of pancreatic endocrine tumors. *Gastrointest Endosc*, 2010. **71**: 951–9.
40. Nomura, N., Goto, H., Niwa, Y. *et al.*, Usefulness of contrast-enhanced EUS in the diagnosis of upper GI tract diseases. *Gastrointest Endosc*, 1999. **50**(4): 555–60.
41. Kannengiesser, K., Mahlke, R., Petersen, F. *et al.*, Contrast-enhanced harmonic endoscopic ultrasound is able to discriminate benign submucosal lesions from gastrointestinal stromal tumors. *Scand J Gastroenterol*, 2012. **47**(12): 1515–20.
42. Xu, W., Shi, J., Zeng, X. *et al.*, EUS elastography for the differentiation of benign and malignant lymph nodes: a meta-analysis. *Gastrointest Endosc,* 2011. **74**: 1001–9.

43. Gheonea, D.I., S ftoiu, A., Beyond conventional endoscopic ultrasound: elastography, contrast enhancement and hybrid techniques. *Curr Opin Gastroenterol*, 2011; **27**: 423–9.
44. Lee, W.J., Jung, H.Y., Kim do, H. *et al.*, Intralesional steroid injection to prevent stricture after near-circumferential endosopic submucosal dissection for superficial esophageal cancer. *Clin Endosc*, 2013. **46**(6): 643–6.
45. Wen, J., Yang, Y., Liu, Q. *et al.*, Preventing Stricture Formation by Covered Esophageal Stent Placement after Endoscopic Submucosal Dissection for Early Esophageal Cancer. *Dig Dis Sci*, 2013 Dec 10.
46. Linghu, E. Feng, X. Wang, X. Meng, J. Du, H. Wang, H., Endoscopic submucosal tunnel dissection for large esophageal neoplastic lesions. *Endoscopy*, 2013. **45**: 60–2.
47. Wang, L., Ren, W., Zhang, Z., Yu, J., Li, Y., Song, Y., Retrospective study of endoscopic submucosal tunnel dissection (ESTD) for surgical resection of esophageal leiomyoma. *Surg Endosc*, 2013. **27**(11): 4259–66.
48. Greenwald, B.D., Dumot, J.A., Cryotherapy for Barrett's esophagus and esophageal cancer. *Curr Opin Gastroenterol*, 2011. **27**(4): 363–7.
49. Gosain, S., Mercer, K., Twaddell, W.S. *et al.*, Liquid nitrogen spray cryotherapy in Barrett's esophagus with high-grade dysplasia: long-term results. *Gastrointest Endosc*, 2013. **78**(2): 260–5.
50. Wolf, D.S., Dunkin, B.J., Ertan, A., Endoscopic radiofrequency ablation of Barrett's esophagus. *Surg Technol Int*, 2012. **22**: 83–9.
51. Atilla, Ertan, Irum, Zaheer *et al.* Photodynamic therapy vs radiofrequency ablation for Barrett's dysplasia: efficacy, safety and cost-comparison. *World J Gastroenterol*, 2013. **19**(41): 7106–13.
52. Gray, J., Fullarton G.M., Long term efficacy of Photodynamic Therapy (PDT) as an ablative therapy of high grade dysplasia in Barrett's oesophagus. *Photodyn Ther*, 2013. **10**(4): 561–5.
53. Bashar, J., Q., Waseem, D. *et al.*, Photodynamic Therapy for Barrett's esophagus and esophageal carcinoma. *Clin Endosc*, 2013. **46**: 30–7.
54. Hourneaux de Moura, E.G., Toma, K., Goh, K.L. *et al.*, Stents for benign and malignant esophageal strictures. *Ann N Y Acad Sci*, 2013. **1300**: 119–43.
55. Dasari, B.V., Neely, D., Kennedy, A. *et al.*, The role of esophageal stents in the management of esophageal anastomotic leaks and benign esophageal perforations. *Ann Surg*, 2014. **259**(5): 852–60.

56. Nagami, Y., Tominaga, K., Machida, H. *et al.*, Usefulness of non-magnifying narrow-band imaging in screening of early esophageal squamous cell carcinoma: a prospective comparative study using propensity score matching. *Am J Gastroenterol*, 2014. **109**(6): 845–54.
57. Yoichi, M., Teruo, K., Atlas of spectral endoscopic images. 2007.
58. Shinya, K., Mitsuhiro, F., Novel image-enhanced endoscopy with i-scan technology. *World J Gastroenterol*, 2010. **16**(9): 1043–9.

Chapter 8

Multimodality Management of Esophageal Malignancies beyond Endoscopy

Liza Stapleford and Nabil F. Saba

What is New

- So far, there is no consensus as to the best agent or regimen for chemotherapy of esophageal cancer. In general, combination chemotherapy regimens provide higher response rates than single agents, but provides only modestly longer durations of disease control and life expectancy (weeks to a few months longer).
- The treatment of advanced esophageal cancers has converged, and the majority of patients with esophageal, or esophagogastric junction (EGJ) cancers are treated similarly, regardless of histology.
- Although the therapeutic approach has been relatively similar for both adenocarcinomas and squamous cell carcinomas, given the increasing interest in individualized therapy and the rising use of multimodality therapy, the multidisciplinary tumor board plays a critical role in treating patients with esophageal cancer.
- Cytotoxic chemotherapy can provide symptom palliation, improve quality of life, and prolong survival in patients with advanced esophageal cancer.

Epidemiology

Across the globe in the year 2012, there were approximately 456,000 newly diagnosed cases of esophageal cancer with an estimated 400,000 deaths (4.9% of total cancer deaths).[1] The incidence rates worldwide are doubled in men compared to women (2.4:1 ratio).[1] Survival is poor with the global ratio of mortality to incidence being 0.88.[1] In the United States, esophageal cancer is the seventh most common cause of cancer death in men and is responsible for 12,220 estimated deaths per year, despite only 14,440 cases per year.[2] The incidence and incidence-based mortality of esophageal adenocarcinoma in the United States continues to rise, although the rate of incline has slowed since the 1990s.[3] For early stage cancer, both incidence and incidence-based mortality have leveled off since the 1990s and survival rates have improved with five-year relative survival rising from 5% in the late 1970s to 19% in the early 2000s.[2,3]

Esophageal cancer incidence varies strongly with geographic region, with about 80% of cases occurring in less developed regions and rates differing by more than 20-fold between regions. This is in contrast to the pattern seen in overall cancer incidence where more than 60% of cases occur in highly developed regions.[4] The highest rates of esophageal cancer are in the "Central Asian esophageal cancer belt," which includes the central Asian republics, Mongolia, north-western China, and the Caspian littoral.[5] Age-standardized rates in those regions are as high as 11 per 100,000, while in contrast to rate less than two per 100,000 in low incidence regions like Polynesia, Central America, and Western Africa.[1]

Risk Factors

Over 90% of esophageal cancers have adenocarcinoma or squamous cell carcinoma histology.[6,7] The epidemiology of each subtype is distinct and varies with differences in the geographic populations they involve, the incidence trends, and risk factors. Worldwide, squamous cell carcinoma is the dominant histology. Up until the last 30–40 years, squamous cell carcinoma was the most prevalent histology in developed western countries. However, that trend has now changed with a rapid increase in adenocarcinomas in countries such as the United States, Canada, South Australia, Scotland, Denmark, Iceland, Finland, Sweden and Norway.[8]

The etiology of esophageal cancer is multifactorial and varies based on the histology and geographic area. In the "esophageal cancer belt," the predominant histology is squamous cell carcinoma contributing up to 85–90% of cases.[9,10] Although tobacco use is a known risk factor for squamous cell carcinoma,[11,12] the strength of this association is lower in parts of the "esophageal cancer belt" where tobacco use is less prevalent.[10,13] A common pathogenesis has not been identified in this region, however, a number of risk factors have been associated with higher incidences of squamous cell carcinoma. Some of the etiologic factors identified include areca nut chewing,[14] opium use,[15] consumption of hot beverages,[16] low intake of fruit and vegetables,[17] lower socioeconomic status,[18,19] poor oral hygiene,[20,21] and genetic background.[22,23]

In contrast, the main risk factors for squamous cell carcinoma in the United States and developed western countries are tobacco and alcohol intake.[12,24] Freedman *et al.,* prospectively examined the relationship between alcohol, tobacco, and esophageal cancer in the United States.[11] When compared to non-smokers, current smokers had a significantly increased risk of squamous cell carcinoma [hazard ratio (HR) = 9.27; 95% confidence interval (CI), 4.04–21.29] and adenocarcinoma (HR = 3.7; 95% CI, 1.32–3.16). They also found a significant association between alcohol consumption and squamous cell carcinoma risk (HR = 4.93; 95% CI, 2.69–9.03) for participants who consumed more than three drinks per day as compared to those whose intake was up to one drink per day.

The rapid escalation of adenocarcinoma in the United States and other western developed countries has led to increased interest in studying the pathogenesis of this disease. From the mid 1970's through the early 1990s, the incidence of adenocarcinoma of the esophagus rose >350% among white males in the United States with annual rates going from 0.7 to 3.2 per 100,000.[25] Cases among black males and white females also increased, but to a lesser extent. Tobacco is a known risk factor for esophageal adenocarcinoma with up to 40% of cases being attributable to cigarette smoking.[26] Alcohol consumption has not been associated with adenocarcinomas, and furthermore, consumption of wine and moderate alcohol intake (<1 drink per day) has been found in some studies to be protective.[26,27]

Besides tobacco, Barrett's esophagus, obesity, and gastroesophageal acid reflux (GERD) are the well-studied risk factors for esophageal adenocarcinoma. GERD affects approximately 10–20% of the population in the Western world and is the strongest risk factor for esophageal adenocarcinoma and Barrett's esophagus.[28,29] Additional risk factors include obesity, diet low in fruits and vegetables, and hereditary factors.

Classification and regression tree analysis have been used to explore the interaction between risk factors in adenocarcinoma of the esophagus. A multi-center population-based control study of 282 cases and 687 controls from the northeastern United States found that frequency of GERD symptoms was the most important risk stratification factor with diet and smoking being further risk modifiers.[29] Another case control study investigated the relationship between known environmental risk factors and functional polymorphisms in five apoptotic pathway genes in a group of 305 patients with esophageal adenocarcinoma and 339 controls.[30] Corroborating prior studies, acid reflux was the most significant risk factor they found for esophageal adenocarcinoma. Additionally, it appears that gene-environment interactions may vary based on the presence or absence of reflux symptoms. Further research into the gene-environment interaction may lead to the development of individualized risk modification strategies.

Staging and Work-up

In the early stages, esophageal cancer is often asymptomatic and may be detected on a surveillance endoscopy for Barrett's or other diseases. Patients with locally advanced cancers can develop progressive dysphagia to solid foods. According to the American College of Surgeons patterns of care study from 1994, the most common reported symptoms at the time of diagnosis are dysphagia (74%), weight loss (57.3%), and heartburn (20.5%).[6]

Work-up begins with a thorough history and physical, including assessment of performance status. Laboratory studies including complete blood count and comprehensive metabolic panel are standard as is a nutritional assessment. Weight loss and dysphagia are frequent problems and should be addressed with nutritional support and enteral feeding if necessary.

Baseline nutritional status has been shown to be a prognostic factor for survival after definitive chemoradiation,[31,32] and poorer pre-operative nutritional status has been linked to higher rates of post-operative complications and lower survival.[33] Using recursive partitioning analysis and data from three cooperative group trials testing definitive chemoradiation, pre-treatment weight loss of >10% body weight over six months was found to be a stratification variable for survival.[34]

In many developed countries, esophagoscopy has replaced barium esophagogram as the initial diagnostic test. In an international survey of 250 physicians predominately from Europe, North American and Japan, greater than 98% of physicians routinely ordered both esophagoscopy with biopsy and CT scans while only 50% routinely ordered barium esophagrams.[35] The survey also revealed that geographic differences influence the selection of further staging studies. For example, endoscopic ultrasound (EUS) was routinely employed by ~70% of North American and European responders while the usage rate dropped to 35% in Asian responders.

Tumor staging

Endoscopy is the staging examination of choice, allowing for visual description of the tumor appearance, extent, as well as relationship to the esophagogastric junction (EGJ). Biopsy is often performed simultaneously to confirm the pathologic diagnosis. The greater the number of biopsies performed, the higher the diagnostic yield. A prospective trial of 202 patients found that with seven biopsies, the specimens yielded a correct diagnosis of gastroesophageal cancer in 98% of cases.[36]

Before initiation of treatment, staging studies must be performed to determine the appropriate treatment path and prognosis. The seventh edition of the American Joint Committee on Cancer and International Union against Cancer (AJCC/UICC) staging manual included significant revisions for esophageal cancer staging in order to more accurately reflect prognostic data.[37] Group staging in prior editions was based solely on a systematic progression of tumor (T), lymph nodes (N), and metastatic (M) classifications. Prior to creation of the seventh edition of the AJCC/UICC staging manual, the Worldwide Esophageal Cancer Collaboration (WECC) was formed to gather information on gastroesophageal cancers and generate data-driven revisions.[37] The WECC analyzed data from 4,627 patients with esophageal or EGJ tumors who underwent surgery. For lymph node negative patients, survival was influenced by histology, grade, and tumor location, while for lymph node positive patients, the number of involved lymph nodes was prognostic. New stage groupings incorporated these findings and were published in the seventh edition of the AJCC staging manual.[38]

In addition to endoscopy, clinical staging is frequently determined using a combination of modalities, such as computed tomography (CT) scans, positron emission tomography (PET) scans, and endoscopic ultrasonography (EUS). Supplemental studies can also include bronchoscopy with ultrasonography (EBUS), mediastinoscopy, thoracoscopy, and laparoscopy. EUS allows a detailed view of the five histologic layers of the esophagus and is the best tool for assessing the depth of penetration and the T stage. Multiple trials using EUS have shown the accuracy to be greater than 80% for early stage tumors and >90% for stage T3 and higher.[39–43] EUS has also been shown to have greater accuracy that CT for predicting pathologic T stage.[44,45] The accuracy of EUS for determining depth of penetration can be limited by malignant stenosis.[46] Strategies to overcome this include dilatation and use of miniprobes, which have a much smaller diameter and higher frequency than standard ultrasound probes and can be introduced through the instrument channel of endoscopes. The decreased imaging depth of these probes limits their accuracy for staging more advanced cancers.[47]

For all cancers beyond T1a, both CT and PET scans are recommended.[48] CT may show esophageal thickening, but it is relatively insensitive for detecting depth of invasion into the esophageal wall. In a prospective study that used surgical pathology as the gold standard, the overall sensitivity of CT for correctly staging the primary tumor was 43%.[49] The capability of CT to detect the presence of an esophageal tumor is higher ~67%.[50] CT can rule out the presence of T4 disease by illustrating a clear fat plane between the tumor and adjacent structures.

Given that most esophageal cancers are FDG avid, PET has a relatively high sensitivity for detecting the presence of a primary esophageal tumor with reported rates ranging from 78–91%.[50–52] However, the accuracy may be as low as 43% for determining the specific T stage.[49] False negatives are more likely in patients with superficial (pT1) tumors.[50,51] Conversely, false positives can occur due to esophagitis from GERD or recent manipulation from endoscopy, stent placement, or biopsy. Although PET is not a robust study for determining the specific depth of tumor invasion, there is evidence of a correlation between mean FDG uptake and the depth of invasion, risk of lymph node metastasis, lymphatic invasion, and tumor size.[51]

Lymph node metastases

EUS is a valuable tool for evaluating nodal status, allowing for detailed analysis of lymph node characteristics as well as affording the opportunity for biopsy. Features indicative of a malignant lymph node include diameter >10 mm, a round shape, distinctive border, and hypo echoic internal echo.[53,54] The subjectivity of the criteria make assessment by EUS alone less accurate than assessment with EUS and fine-needle aspiration (EUS-FNA). A review in 2003 of published studies by Murata *et al.* found that the specificity, sensitivity, and accuracies of EUS alone for diagnosing malignant lymph nodes were 49–99%, 33–99%, and 71–96%, while the respective values for EUS-FNA were 81–97%, 83–100%, and 83–97%.[55] Two more recent meta-analyses looking at the accuracy of EUS for diagnosing malignant lymph nodes, found pooled sensitivities of 85%[42]and 80%[56] and specificities of 85% and 70%, respectively.

CT scans predominately rely on size criteria for detecting potential metastatic spread to regional lymph nodes. The historic criterion for enlarged lymph nodes varies based on location: a short axis measurement greater than 1 cm for intrathoracic and intrabdominal nodes, a short axis greater than 0.5 cm for supraclavicular nodes, and greater than 0.6 cm for retrocrural lymph nodes. However, lymph node size alone can be misleading as normal sized nodes can contain cancer and lymph nodes may be enlarged due to inflammation. A meta-analysis published in 2008 found no significant differences between the pooled sensitivities and specificities on EUS, CT and PET for detecting regional lymph node metastases in esophageal cancer.[56] The authors suggest that the three tests may be complementary because EUS has the highest sensitivity, but CT and PET are more specific. A more recent meta-analysis from Sgourakis *et al.* evaluated 84 studies and also found that the diagnostic performance of EUS, CT, and PET was similar, although EUS had significantly higher sensitivity and lower specificity than CT and PET.[57] Across the 20 studies looking at CT, the pooled sensitivity and specificity for the detection of regional lymph node metastases were 52% and 81%, respectively.

Anatomic location affects the accuracy of diagnostic imaging modalities to detect malignant lymph nodes. False-negatives can occur with CT and PET in cases where lymph nodes lie immediately adjacent to the primary tumor.[58] A study evaluating preoperative assessment of nodal metastases found that EUS was significantly more accurate than CT or MRI for the assessment of upper para-esophageal and infra-aortic lymph nodes, while CT was more accurate for lower paraesophageal and mediastinal lymph nodes.[59] A wide variation in abilities of CT for detecting lymph node metastases was noted based on anatomic nodal group with ranges of accuracy, sensitivity, and specificity of 68–96%, 8–75%, and 60–98%, respectively. For EUS, the variation is often based on the physical distance: accuracy drops as the distance between the node and the esophageal wall increases.

The reported accuracy of PET for detecting regional lymph nodes is variable, and overall PET has little added utility beyond the combination of CT and EUS in staging regional lymph nodes.[60] Studies evaluating the role of PET in nodal staging are limited by small patient numbers due to the fact that many patients receive neoadjuvant therapy between the initial PET and surgery, thus limiting the comparison of radiographic and pathologic findings. The reported accuracy ranges from 48–84%[50,51,58,61] in four studies using histopathology as the gold standard. In two meta-analyses of 13 studies[57] and 10 studies,[56] the pooled sensitivities were 59% and 57% and the pooled specificities were 81% and 85%, respectively.

Distant metastases

The seventh addition of the AJCC staging manual[38] reclassified metastatic disease by removing the M1a and M1b descriptors and including only a M0 or M1 categorization. The change was driven by data showing that patients with positive non-regional lymph nodes (former M1a) have a better prognosis after resection than those with visceral metastases.[62,63] Distant metastases from esophageal cancer are most commonly seen in the liver, lung, and bones.[64] Staging for distant metastatic disease includes CT, PET-CT, EUS, and diagnostic laparoscopy. The percentage of patients diagnosed with metastatic esophageal cancer is ~35% according to SEER data from 2002–2008.[2] The percentage of patients diagnosed pathologically confirmed stage IV disease is lower and the overall incidence will be lower with stage migration in the new staging system. A patterns of care study published by the American College of Surgeons in 2000, reported the incidences of clinical, pathologic, and combined Stage IV disease as 38.7%, 12.3%, and 31.7%, respectively.[6]

PET improves preoperative staging and is a valuable tool for assessing distant metastases. Prospective studies have shown that PET detects distant metastases in up to 15% of patients who were found to be M0 based on CT and endoscopy.[65,66] The ACOSOG Z0060 trial included 262 patients with resectable esophageal cancer with no evidence of distant metastatic disease on CT and randomized them to plus or minus PET.[52] PET found pathologically confirmed distant metastatic disease in 4.8% of patients, but there were an additional 9.5% of patients who had M1b disease on PET without pathologic confirmation. The authors recommend confirmation of PET-detected metastases in potential surgical candidates, given that the false positive rate was 3.7%.

Overall PET is more accurate than CT for detecting distant metastases. In a series of 91 patients referred for surgical resection, PET for detection of distant metastases had a sensitivity of 69%, specificity of 93%, and accuracy of 84%, while the respective values for CT were significantly less at 46%, 74%, and 63% ($p < 0.01$).[67] In a meta-analysis of 10 studies including 588 patients, the pooled sensitivity and specificity of PET and CT were 71% and 93% and 52% and 91%, respectively.[56] Summary receiver operating characteristics analysis revealed that the diagnostic performance of PET for the detection of distant metastases was significantly higher than that of CT [relative diagnostic odds ratio = 2.26(95% CI, 1.09–4.71); $p < 0.03$)]. Most of the published studies have looked only at PET, but limited data suggests that integrated PET/CT units likely improve accuracy over P*ET al*one by combing metabolic and anatomic information.[68,69]

Therapy

While adenocarcinomas and squamous cell carcinomas have varying epidemiology, pathogenesis, and clinical behavior, the therapeutic approach has been relatively similar for both histologies. In recent years, there has been a paradigm shift as there is increasing recognition of the value of tailoring therapy based on histology. The emphasis on individualized therapy extends beyond considerations of tumor histology to include tumor biology, location, response to neo-adjuvant treatment, and patient co-morbidities. Given the increasing interest in individualized therapy and the rising use of multimodality therapy, the multidisciplinary tumor board plays a critical role in treating patients with esophageal cancer.

Early stage (T1-T2N0)

Surgery is a critical component of treatment for early stage esophageal cancers. Surgical morbidity and mortality has decreased over the past few decades likely due to improvements in technology and better patient selection. An analysis of the Nationwide Inpatient Sample from 1998 to 2006 revealed a reduction in the United States in-hospital mortality from 12% to 7%.[70] An inverse relationship between mortality and surgical volume has also been established. Mortality rates following esophagectomy are lower in centers that perform a higher volume of surgeries per year.[71,72] While this is likely due to multiple factors, there is evidence to suggest that operative mortality and survival after surgery are related to the surgeon's experience and volume of cases.[73,74] Mortality rates for open esophagectomy at many high-volume centers are <5%.[75–77]

Esophagectomy is the initial treatment for clinical T1bN0 cancers and may also be considered for T2N0 patients. Endoscopic treatment or esophagectomy can be used for T1a tumors. Endoscopic mucosal resection (EMR) is indicated for T1a lesions that are small (<2 cm), well-differentiated, and involve less than a third of the circumference of the esophagus. A detailed discussion of endoscopic treatments can be found in Chapter 7. When considering endoscopic treatments, it is important to consider that the risk of lymph node metastases increases as the depth of tumor invasion into the esophagus increases. While T1a tumors may be amenable to endoscopic therapy due to a low (0–7%) incidence of lymph node metastases, the risk for T1b tumors ranges from 21% to 50%.[78–81]

The management of T2N0 tumors is controversial.[82,83] Options include initial surgical resection with adjuvant therapy for pathologically upstaged tumors versus neoadjuvant treatment prior to surgery. Accurate staging can be a challenge for patients with early stage tumors. A recent retrospective review from the Cleveland Clinic analyzed outcomes for 61 patients with clinical T2N0 cancer after EUS and CT+/– PET.[84] Of the 53 patients who were treated with surgery up front, only 7 (13%) had pathologic T2N0 disease. Of the remaining 46 patients, 63% were overstaged and 37% were understaged. Based on these findings, the recommendation was to treat these cT2N0 patients with initial surgery and consider adjuvant therapy for those found to have pathologic upstaging.

Four randomized trials (Table 1) published within the past 20 years have evaluated the role of neoadjuvant concurrent chemoradiotherapy for early stage esophageal cancers.[85–88] All four trials randomized patients to surgery alone or neoadjuvant chemoradiotherapy followed by surgery. Bossett *et al.*[85] included only squamous cell cancers and found no difference in survival between the two arms. Cancer and Leukemia group B (CALGB) 9781[86] was designed to randomize 500 patients with stages I–III esophageal cancer, but was closed prematurely due to slow accrual with only 56 patients enrolled. Intent-to-treat analysis showed a median survival benefit for trimodality therapy (4.48 vs. 1.79 years, $p = 0.002$). There was no significant difference in perioperative mortality with trimodality therapy, and the pathologic complete response (pCR) rate with preoperative treatment was 40%. The Federation Francophone De Cancerologie Digestive (FFCD) 9901 trial[88] randomized 195 patient with Stage I-II esophageal cancer to preoperative fluorouracil and cisplatin plus 45Gy radiation versus surgery alone. Results, which are only available in abstract form, showed that neoadjuvant therapy increased perioperative mortality (7.3% vs. 1.1%, $p = 0.054$) and had an inferior median survival (32 vs. 44 months).

The Dutch CROSS trial[87] was published in 2012 and its findings support the role for preoperative chemoradiotherapy in patients with disease greater than T1N0. A total of 366 patients with T1N1 or T2-3N0-1 esophageal or GE junction tumors were randomized to either surgery

Table 1. Role of neoadjuvant concurrent chemoradiotherapy for early stage esophageal cancers.

Trial	n	Patients	Algorithm	Median survival (months)	p	Mortality (%)	Histology	pCR(%)
FFCD 9901	195	T1-T2N0-1, T3N0	S	43.8	0.66	1.1	SSC & AC	—
			CMT→S	31.8		7.3		
CROSS	366	T1N1, T2-3N0-1	S	24	0.003	4	SSC & AC	29
			CMT→S	49.4		4		
CALGB 9781	56	T1-3N0-1	S	1.79 yrs	0.002	4	SSC & AC	33
			CMT→S	4.48		0		
Bossett	282	T1-T2N0-1, T3N0	S	18.6	—	3.6	SSC	26
			CMT→S	18.6		12.3		

alone or surgery following weekly carboplatin(AUC 2 mg/ml/min) and paclitaxel (50 mg/m^2 of body surface area) and concurrent radiotherapy (41.4Gy in 23 fractions). The chemoradiotherapy was fairly well-tolerated with a 7% incidence of grade 3 or higher hematologic toxicity and less than 13% incidence of grade 3 or higher non-hematologic toxicities. Of the 161 patients treated with preoperative chemoradiotherapy, 47 patients (29%) had a pathologic complete response. The rate of complete resection (R0) was also significantly higher in the trimodality arm (92% v 69%, $p <$ 0.001). Post-operative morbidity and mortality were comparable, with a 4% rate of in hospital mortality in both arms. With a median follow-up of 45 months, the median overall survival was significantly higher in the trimodality arm (49.4 vs. 24 months, $p = 0.003$).

In summary, there is limited data on patients with clinical T2N0 esophageal cancer and no randomized trials that address this group of patients exclusively. The existing data indicates that cT2N0 patients are subject to frequent inaccuracies in staging and, therefore, have a relatively high incidence of subclinical lymph node disease and have considerable heterogeneity in outcomes. In the study from Rice *et al.*[84] of the Cleveland Clinic, the 53 patients with cT2N0 who underwent upfront surgery had 5- and 10-year overall survival rates of 50% and 30%, respectively. When the patients were divided into overstaged (28 patients) and understaged (10 patients), the overall survival at five years was >70% and ~10%, respectively. Stiles *et al.*[89] reviewed 102 patients with surgically treated cT2-3N0, 38% of whom had induction therapy. In the 63 patients treated with surgery alone, subclinical lymph node metastases were found in 55% of cT2 and 78% of cT3 cancers. On multivariate analysis, the presence of pathologic nodal disease was the strongest predictor of overall survival (relative risk 2.73, confidence interval: 1.29 to 5.78). With advances in staging and further study of prognostic factors, it may be possible to determine which patients with cT2N0 disease would derive benefit from preoperative or adjuvant treatment.

For patients who are medically inoperable or decline surgery, definitive chemoradiotherapy is a potentially curative alternative. A retrospective study from Japan of patients with clinical T1bN0 squamous cell carcinoma of the esophagus compared outcomes of 102 patients treated with esophagectomy and 71 patients treated with definitive chemoradiotherapy.[90]

There was no statistically significant difference in overall survival, but the surgical patients had a significantly higher progression-free survival at five years (73.8% vs. 60.6%, $p = 0.0117$) with lower rates of local and regional recurrence.

Locally advanced, resectable (T3-4aN0, T1-4aN1-3)

Due to the overall poor outcomes, the majority of patients with locally advanced disease will receive multimodality therapy. While resection alone is an option, there is significant data to support a survival advantage for patients who have pathologic complete responses after neoadjuvant therapy.[91,92] Part of the difficulty in achieving consensus treatment algorithms lays in the heterogeneous nature of the inclusion criteria and treatment protocols for esophageal clinical trials. The majority of trials have included both squamous cell carcinoma and adenocarcinoma of the esophagus as well as the EGJ.

Despite the increased incidence of EGJ tumors, the studies that focused on this disease location are lacking. These tumors have been rather included in both esophageal and gastric trials and accounted for no more than 30% of patients on gastric cancer trials. The classification of EGJ tumors has also varied over time. The AJCC sixth edition grouped EGJ and gastric cardia tumors as primary gastric tumors, providing there was less than 2 cm of esophageal involvement. However, the seventh edition broadens the category of esophageal cancers to include both EGJ tumors and tumors within the proximal 5 cm of the stomach that extend into the EGJ or distal esophagus. The Siewart classification system is favored by surgeons and divides EGJ tumors into three types.[93,94] Siewert Type I tumors are located in the distal esophagus with the tumor epicenter 1 to 5 cm above the anatomic EGJ. Type II tumors arise from the gastric cardia with their epicenter within 1 cm above or 2 cm below the EGJ. Type III is defined as a subcardial tumor with an epicenter 2 to 5 cm below the EGJ.

The specific approach for an esophageal or EGJ carcinoma is influenced by disease stage, histology, location of the primary tumor, and physician or geographic practice patterns. For example, neoadjuvant chemoradiotherapy is frequently used in North America for EGJ tumors while neoadjuvant chemotherapy is preferred in other parts of the world.

While there is little data to support different treatment pathways based on histology, the inclusion of surgery after neoadjuvant treatment is better established for adenocarcinoma than squamous cell carcinoma.[82,95]

Neoadjuvant radiation

There are five older phase III trials that studied the role of preoperative radiation in esophageal cancer.[96–100] Four of the trials did not show significant survival benefit for adding neoadjuvant radiation. A Scandinavian study[99] showed a benefit but the study suffered from weak design and data analysis. A meta-analysis published in 2005 of the 1,147 patients from these five randomized trials found no statistically significant benefit to preoperative radiation.[101]

Neoadjuvant chemotherapy

Multiple trials have examined the benefit of pre- or peri-operative chemotherapy (Table 2). Four trials have demonstrated a survival benefit using a cisplatin based regimen.[102–105] Two of the trials[103,104] included only adenocarcinomas, with at least 85% of the tumors classified as EGJ or gastric. The largest trial from the Medical Research Council (MRC) in Europe consisted of two-thirds adenocarcinoma and one-third squamous carcinoma.[102] The only trial to show a significant survival benefit for neoadjuvant chemotherapy solely in squamous cell carcinoma was the Rotterdam Esophageal Study Group, which randomized 169 patients with operable esophageal cancers to surgery plus or minus neoadjuvant cisplatin and etoposide.[105]

Several meta-analyses have been published to estimate the survival benefit of neoadjuvant chemotherapy for esophageal cancer (Table 2). Gebski *et al.*[106] analyzed eight randomized trials with 1,724 patients and found a hazard ratio for neoadjuvant chemotherapy of 0.90 (95%CI, 0.81–1.00; $p = 0.05$). This translates to a two-year absolute survival benefit of 7%. When analyzed separately by histology, the benefit was limited to adenocarcinoma. Sjoquist *et al.*[107] updated this meta-analysis to include nine trials with 1,981 patients. Again neoadjuvant chemotherapy significantly improved survival (HR 0.87; 95%, 0.79–0.96; $p = 0.005$), but the

Table 2. The benefit of pre- or peri-operative chemotherapy.

Author	Trial	Tumor Location	Algorithm	*n*	Chemotherapy	Survival (5yr)%	*p*	Histology
Allum	MRC: OE02	Esophagus or EGJ (74% lower 1/3 or cardia)	S C→S	402 400	CF	17 23	0.03	SSC (31%) AC (67%)
Kelson	INT: 0113	Esophagus or EGJ	S C→S→C	227 216	CF	21 20	NS	SSC (47%) AC (53%)
Cunningham	MRC: Magic	Lower 1/3 Eso (15%), EGJ (11%), or Gastric (74%)	S C→S→C	253 250	ECF	23 26	0.009	AC
Roth	—	Mid to lower esophagus	S C→S→C	20 19	BVC	MS 9 months	NS	SCC
Ychou	FNCLCC/ FFCD: ACCORD-07	Lower 1/3 Eso (11%), EGJ (64%), or Gastric (25%)	S C→S→C	111 113	CF	24 38	0.02	AC

Boonstra	—	Esophagus	S C→S	84 85	C/VP-16	17 26	0.03	SCC
Schuhmacher	EORTC: 40954	Cardia/EGJ (53%) or Gastric (47%)	S C→S→C	72* 72*	CF	70 (2yr) 73	0.466	AC
Kranzfelder	Meta-analysis (2011)	Esophagus	S C→S→+/–C	950 757	—	HR 0.93 (0.8–2.08)	0.368	SCC
Sjoquist	Meta-analysis (2011)	—	S C→S→+/–C	1981	—	HR 0.87 (0.79–0.96)	0.005 (AC only)	SSC & AC
Gebski	Meta-analysis (2007)	—	S C→S→+/–C	848 876	—	HR 0.90 (0.81–1.00)	0.05 (AC only)	SSC & AC

benefit was limited to adenocarcinoma. Kranzfelder *et al.*[108] evaluated the benefit of neoadjuvant chemotherapy in resectable squamous cell carcinoma of the esophagus in eight randomized trials with 1,707 patients but found no statistically significant benefit.

The most recently published randomized trial supporting preoperative chemotherapy is the Dutch CROSS trial, which randomized 366 patients with resectable gastroesophageal cancer to surgery alone or 5 weeks of radiation (41.4 Gy) with weekly concurrent carboplatin and paclitaxel.[87] The majority of patients had adenocarcinoma (75%) of the distal esophagus or EGJ (> 80%). Preoperative treatment did not increase postoperative morbidity or mortality and had acceptable rates of grade 3 or worse toxicity (7% hematologic, <13% non-hematologic). Patients in the trimodality arm had a 29% rate of pCR and had a significantly higher rate of R0 resection (92% vs. 69%, $p < 0.001$). Overall survival was significantly better in the trimodality arm (three-year survival 58% vs. 44%, $p = 0.0003$).

Neoadjuvant chemoradiotherapy

While neoadjuvant chemotherapy improves the R0 resection rate, it generally produces a pathologic complete response in less than 10% of patients (~0–7%).[104,105,109–111] Pathologic response and R0 resections after induction therapy have been associated with significantly improved survival for esophageal cancer.[91] The combination of chemotherapy and radiation can improve pCR rates but also potentially increases toxicity. A number of randomized trials have evaluated if there is a survival benefit to adding neoadjuvant chemoradiation prior to surgery for potentially resectable gastro-esophageal cancer (Table 3). Only three of these trials have shown a statistically significant survival benefit, and they predominantly consisted of adenocarcinoma histology.[86,87,112] Many of the other trials consisted of solely or predominantly squamous cell histology. Overall, these trials are difficult to compare due to heterogeneity in staging work-up, histology, tumor location, radiation dose/fractionation, and chemotherapy regimen.

Of the three trials that showed a significant survival benefit to neoadjuvant chemoradiotherapy, two have some noted weaknesses. The study by

Table 3. Evaluations of the survival benefit of neoadjuvant chemoradiation for potentially resectable gastro-esophageal cancer

Author	Trial	Algorithm	*n*	Median survival	3-yr OS	*p*	PCR rate (%)	Histology (%)
van Hagen	CROSS	S	188	24	44	0.003	29.00	AC (75%)
		CMT→S	178	49	58			SSC (25%)
Tepper	CALGB 9781	S	26	54	16 (5yr)	0.002	40	AC (75%)
		CMT→S	30	21	39 (5yr)			SSC (25%)
Urba	University of Michigan	S	50	17.6	16	0.15	28	AC (75%)
		CMT→S	50	16.9	30			SSC (25%)
Bossett	EORTC	S	139	18.6	NS	0.78	26	SSC
		CMT→S	143	18.6				
Walsh	—	S	55	11	6	0.01	25	AC
		CMT→S	58	16	32			
Burmeister	TROG	S	128	22.2	NS	0.57	16	AC (62%)
		CMT→S	128	19.3				SSC (37%)
Mariette	FFCD 9901	S	98	43.8	55	0.66	28.60	AC (~30%)
		CMT→S	97	31.8	49			SSC (~70%)
Nygaard	—	S	41	NR	9	0.3	NR	SCC
		CMT→S	47		17			
Le Prise	—	S	45	NR	14	NS	11	SCC
		CMT→S	41		19			
Lee	—	S	50	27.3	57	0.69	43	SCC
		CMT→S	51	28.2	55			

Walsh *et al.*[112] randomized 113 patients with adenocarcinoma to surgery plus or minus neoadjuvant chemoradiotherapy. The chemoradiotherapy consisted of 40Gy given over 15 days with two cycles of chemotherapy using fluorouracil and cisplatin. Over 85% of patients had tumors of the lower third of the esophagus or cardia. A complete pathological response was seen in 13 of the 52 patients (25%) in the neoadjuvant arm who went to surgery. With a median follow-up of 10 months, the multimodal therapy improved overall survival at three years from 6% to 32%. Criticisms of this trial include the short follow-up, the lower than expected survival seen in the surgery arm, the unconventional radiation fractionation, and the limited staging work-up.

The Cancer and Leukemia Group B (CALGB) 9781 was a randomized Intergroup trial designed to test trimodality therapy versus esophagectomy in patients with surgically resectable esophageal or EGJ cancer stages I–III.[86] Patients in the trimodality arm received two cycles of cisplatin and fluorouracil with concurrent radiation to 50.4 Gy, which was followed by surgery unless patients progressed. Planned enrollment was 500 patients, but only 56 patients were enrolled and the trial was closed early for poor accrual. For the 25 patients treated with preoperative chemoradiotherapy, the pCR rate was 40%. With a median follow-up of six years, five-year survival for the trimodality arm was 39% (95% CI, 21–57%) vs. 16% (95% CI, 5–33%) in the surgery arm. The chief criticism of this trial is the limited sample size.

Several recent meta-analyses have examined benefit of adding preoperative chemoradiotherapy to surgery (Table 4). The most recently published and largest meta-analysis from Sjoquist *et al.*[107] pooled 12 randomized trials comparing neoadjuvant chemoradiotherapy versus surgery alone in 1,854 patients with resectable esophageal cancer. The hazard ratio for all-cause mortality with neoadjuvant chemoradiotherapy was 0.78 (95% CI, 0.70–0.88; $p < 0.001$) and the benefit was statistically significant for both adenocarcinomas and squamous cell carcinomas. An indirect comparison analyzed the benefits of neoadjuvant chemotherapy versus neoadjuvant chemoradiotherapy. While the benefit of chemotherapy was not as strong as chemoradiotherapy, the difference was not statistically significant (HR 0.88; 95% CI, 0.76–1.01; $p = 0.07$).

Table 4. Benefits of preoperative chemoradiotherapy.

Author	Trial	Algorithm	n	Median survival	p	Histology
Gebski	Meta-analysis (2007)	S	586	HR 0.81 (0.70-0.93)	0.002	SSC & AC
		CMT→S	623			
Jin	Meta-analysis (2009)	S	649	OR 1.46 (1.07-1.99)	0.02 (AC only)	SSC & AC
		CMT→S	659			
Kranzfelder	Meta-analysis (2011)	S	545	HR 0.81 (0.70-0.95)	0.008	SCC
		CMT→S	554			
Sjoquist	Meta-analysis (2011)	S	952	HR 0.78 (0.70-0.88)	<0.0001	SSC & AC
		CMT→S	980			

Neoadjuvant chemotherapy versus chemoradiotherapy

In addition to the indirect comparison offered in the above meta-analysis, there have been two randomized trials comparing neoadjuvant chemotherapy with neoadjuvant chemoradiotherapy. Both trials were closed prematurely due to slow accrual and, therefore, were underpowered to show a survival difference.

The Australian trial was a randomized phase II trial comparing preoperative cisplatin and 5-fluorouracil versus the same chemotherapy with 35Gy of radiation given over three weeks.[110] Seventy-five patients with adenocarcinoma of the esophagus or EGJ were enrolled. The addition of radiation improved the pCR rate (13% vs. 0%, $p = 0.01$) and the reduced rate of R1 resection (0% vs. 11%, $p = 0.04$), however progression free and median overall survival were similar (32 months vs. 29 months, $p = 0.83$).

The German Preoperative Chemotherapy or Radiochemotherapy in Esophago-gastric Adenocarcinoma Trial (POET) randomized 126 patients with adenocarcinoma of the lower esophagus or EGJ to preoperative treatment consisting of either 15 weeks of chemotherapy or 12 weeks of chemotherapy followed by three weeks or chemoradiotherapy.[109] The addition of preoperative radiation improved the pCR rate (15.6% vs. 2%, $p = 0.03$) and overall survival at three years (47.4% vs. 27.7%, $p = 0.07$).

A meta-analysis of preoperative chemotherapy with and without radiation in patients with gastroesophageal adenocarcinoma combined aggregate and individual patient data from 14 randomized controlled trials.[113] The pooled hazard ratio was 0.81 (95% CI, 0.73–0.89; $p < 0.0001$) for preoperative chemotherapy or chemoradiotherapy compared to surgery alone. The addition of radiation increased the magnitude of effect, but the difference was not statistically significant.

Adjuvant radiation

Five randomized trials have evaluated post-operative radiation following surgery for esophageal cancer. A systematic review pooled the results of the five trials and found no significant difference in mortality with the addition of adjuvant radiation after surgery.[114] Radiation reduced local failures in three of the trials, but was associated with increased morbidity.

Adjuvant chemotherapy

Adjuvant chemotherapy may be considered for patients with pathologically positive lymph nodes who did not receive neoadjuvant treatment. A limited number of trials have studied the benefit of adjuvant chemotherapy after resection of esophageal cancer. A multi-center French trial randomized 120 patients with squamous cell carcinoma of the esophagus to post-operative cisplatin and 5-fluorouracil versus observation.[115] The surgery was considered palliative for all patients based on the presence of any of the following: pathologic nodal disease, positive margins, or distant metastases. There was no survival difference between the two arms (median survival 14 months).

Two randomized trials from Japan evaluated the benefit of post-operative chemotherapy for resected squamous cell carcinoma of the esophagus. The initial trial included 205 patients and found no survival benefit with the addition of adjuvant cisplatin and vindesine.[116] A follow-up trial randomized 242 patients post-resection to observation versus two cycles of cisplatin and 5-fluorouracil.[117] Chemotherapy did not significantly improve overall survival, but it did increase disease free survival at five years (55% vs. 45%, $p = 0.037$). The disease free survival benefit of chemotherapy was more pronounced in the subset of patients with positive lymph nodes.

The Japanese Oncology Group organized a trial (JCOG 9907) to compare pre- versus post-operative chemotherapy.[118] Patients with clinical stage II or III squamous cell esophageal cancer were randomized to preoperative chemotherapy ($n = 164$) or surgery ($n = 166$) with post-operative for node positive patients. At the planned interim analysis, the trial was halted because overall survival was superior in the pre-operative chemotherapy arm. With a median follow-up of 62 months, five-year overall survival was 55% in the neoadjuvant arm versus 43% in the adjuvant arm ($p = 0.04$).

Adjuvant chemoradiotherapy

Adjuvant chemoradiotherapy for node-positive patients with adenocarcinomas of the EGJ is the standard of care in the United States; however the ideal treatment for squamous cell cancers and patients with upper thoracic tumors is not clear. The Intergroup trial 0116 randomized 556 patients with Stage IB-IV (AJCC 3rd edition) adenocarcinoma of the EGJ (~20%) or stomach (~80%) to chemoradiotherapy or observation following resection with negative margins.[119] The adjuvant therapy consisted of one cycle of 5-fluorouracil with leucovorin followed by two additional cycles with concurrent radiation to 45Gy. Three-year survival was 50% in the chemoradiotherapy arm and 41% in the surgery alone arm (HR for death in surgery alone arm 1.35; 95% CI, 1.09–1.66; $p = 0.005$). Of note, only 10% of patients had an extensive (D2) lymph node dissection and 54% had less than the N1 lymph nodes dissected (D0).

Two smaller randomized trials addressed the benefit of post-operative chemoradiotherapy in patients with resected squamous cell carcinoma. A Japanese trial compared post-operative chemotherapy alone versus with concurrent radiation in 45 patients with completely resected squamous cell carcinoma of the thoracic esophagus.[120] The addition of radiation did not yield a survival or local control benefit, although the study was underpowered to analyze survival. A three arm study from China randomized 238 patients with stage II–III thoracic squamous cell esophageal cancer to pre-operative chemoradiotherapy, post-operative chemoradiotherapy, or surgery alone.[121] Progression-free survival and overall survival were both significantly better in patients receiving chemoradiotherapy compared to surgery alone. No significant differences were detected between the pre- and post-operative chemoradiotherapy arms.

Role of surgery

While surgery is a mainstay of therapy for early stage esophageal cancer, the role of resection in locally advanced cancer is uncertain. Two randomized trials have evaluated the benefit of surgery following chemoradiation for squamous cell carcinoma of the esophagus. The German Oesophageal Cancer Study Group gave induction chemotherapy to all and randomized 172 patients to chemoradiotherapy to 40Gy followed by surgery versus chemoradiotherapy to 65Gy.[122] Patients in the surgical arm had better local control (two-year local progression free survival 64% vs. 41%, $p = 0.003$) but similar overall survival at three years (31% vs. 24%)

and increased treatment-related mortality (13% vs. 4%, $p = 0.03$). The French FFCD 9102 trial randomized 259 patients to chemoradiation with or without surgery.[123] All patients received two cycles of cisplatin and 5-fluorouracil and concomitant radiation (46Gy in 4.5 weeks or 15Gy x2 split course). Patients with a response were randomized to surgery or additional chemoradiation. Surgery did not improve survival (median 17.7 months vs. 19.3), but did reduce local failures (33.6% vs. 43%, $p = 0.0014$) at the cost of increased treatment-related mortality (9.3% vs. 0.8%, $p = 0.002$).

Management of locally advanced, unresectable disease

The gold standard treatment for unresectable, non-metastatic esophageal cancer is concurrent chemotherapy and radiation. Chemotherapy can improve the therapeutic ratio by increasing tumor cell kill and potentially treating microscopic disease outside of the radiation field.[124,125] Initial trials utilized a variety of chemotherapeutic agents and had mixed results.[126–129]

The Radiation Therapy Oncology Group (RTOG) conducted a landmark randomized controlled trial (RTOG 85-01) in patients with squamous cell carcinoma of the esophagus staged T1-3N0-1M0.[130] The trial randomized 129 patients to radiation therapy alone to a dose of 64Gy in 32 fractions versus chemoradiotherapy consisting of four cycles of 5-fluorouracil and cisplatin combined with 50Gy delivered in 25 fractions. The randomization portion of the trial was closed early due to an interim analysis that showed a significant survival benefit for chemoradiotherapy; however, an additional 69 patients were enrolled in the chemoradiotherapy arm. Updated results revealed a significant overall survival benefit at five years for the chemoradiotherapy arm (27% vs. 0%, $p < 0.001$).[131] Despite the survival advantage of concurrent chemotherapy, almost half of patients (26/56) had persistent or recurrent local disease.

The high rate of local failure seen with chemoradiotherapy has driven attempts to intensify therapy. Intergroup 0123 attempted to improve on the results of RTOG 85-01 by escalating the dose of radiation.[132] A total of 236 patients with T1-4N0-1M0 esophageal cancer were treated with the same chemotherapy regimen as RTOG 85-01 and randomized to concurrent radiation with a dose of 64.8Gy or 50.4Gy. There was no significant survival or local control advantage seen in the high dose arm. Treatment-related mortality was higher in the 64Gy arm, although it was unclear if this was due to the higher radiation dose. While ongoing trials are researching the benefit of novel chemotherapy and biologic agents in combination with radiation, the current standard of care for unresectable esophageal cancer is 50Gy of radiation with concurrent chemotherapy.

Metastatic

Approximately 35% of patients with esophageal cancer have metastatic disease at presentation.[2,133] Treatment goals include prolonging survival and maintaining or improving quality of life. One of the most common symptoms is dysphagia. The normal esophageal lumen measures ~25 mm in functional diameter and symptoms of dysphagia to solids appears when the diameter is decreased to 13 mm.[134] Palliative local therapy for dysphagia can include radiation, stenting, dilatation, surgery, cryotherapy, argon laser, Nd:YAG laser therapy, and photodynamic therapy. Selection of a local therapy modality involves consideration of tumor location, patient's performance status, prior treatments, and expertise of treating physicians.[135]

In the metastatic setting, the goals of chemotherapy are to improve overall survival and palliate symptoms. A meta-analysis evaluated the effectiveness of chemotherapy versus best supportive care in advanced EGJ and gastric cancer.[136] Combined results from three randomized trials with 184 patients showed a survival benefit for chemotherapy that equated to an improvement in median survival from 4 to 11 months (HR 0.37; 95% CI, 0.24–0.55). Results from these and other trials have been applied to esophageal cancer due to the inclusion of lower esophageal and EGJ carcinomas in these trials and the lack of recent phase III trials for metastatic esophageal cancer. A Cochrane review of the efficacy of chemotherapy versus supportive care in advanced or metastatic esophageal cancer identified only two randomized control trials with 38 patients.[137] The authors concluded that there was a lack of evidence to support chemotherapy for metastatic esophageal cancer and that further phase III trials should incorporate EGJ tumors to increase statistical power.

Selection of chemotherapeutic agents depends on the patient's performance status and co-morbidities. Single agent chemotherapy has response rates of about 15% to 35% and no proven survival benefit.[138] Combination regimens have shown higher response rates than monotherapy, but without significant changes in survival. Patients with good performance status who receive combination chemotherapy have a median survival on the order of 8 to 11 months.[139–141] The most commonly used and studied combination is cisplatin and fluoropyrimidines, which produce response rates of ~20–70% and median survival of ~8–14 months.[141,142] A randomized, multinational phase II/III trial of advanced gastric and EGJ cancer patients randomized 317 patients to cisplatin and fluorouracil with or without docetaxel (DCF).[143] The addition of docetaxel significantly improved response rates, time to progression, and overall survival (9.2 months vs. 8.6 months, $p = 0.02$). High grade toxicity was also increased with three drug regimen, prompting efforts to find a more tolerable regimen.

The REAL-2 trial randomized 1002 patients with gatroesophageal cancer to one of four epirubicin containing regimens: epirubicin, cisplatin, and fluorouracil (ECF); epirubicin, cisplatin, and capecitabine (ECX); epirubicin, oxaliplatin, and capecitabine (EOX); epirubicin, oxaliplatin, and fluorouracil (EOF).[144] Response rates and progression-free survival were similar for all four regimens, but overall survival was prolonged with EOX compared to ECF (median 11.2 months vs. 9.9, $p = 0.02$). These results have prompted some to recommend EOX as the new standard first-line treatment for metastatic esophageal cancer in patients with good performance status.

Overall, there remains a lack of consensus as to the ideal regimen for metastatic esophageal cancer. Standard combination regimens such as DCF and ECF require central venous access and an ambulatory infusion pump. Results from the REAL-2 affirm that infusional fluorouracil can be replaced with capecitabine without compromising outcomes. Similarly, oxaliplatin can replace cisplatin with equivalent outcomes and less renal toxicity. Patients with poor performance status can receive single agent chemotherapy with fluorouracil, irinotecan, or low-dose weekly taxanes.

The human epidermal growth factor receptor 2 (HER2) protein is overexpressed in 7–34% of esophagogastric cancers.[145–149] The ToGA trial was a phase III, open-label, randomized controlled trial that evaluated the addition of trastuzumab to cisplatin and a fluoropyrimidine in patients with locally advanced, recurrent, or metastatic esophagogastric adenocarcinoma.[150] Trastuzumab in combination with chemotherapy significantly improved median survival over chemotherapy alone (13.8 months vs. 11 months, $p = 0.046$). Based on this trial, recommendations for advanced gastroesophageal cancer include testing for HER2 overexpression or gene amplification and treatment with Trastuzumab if patients are Her-2-neu positive.

Future Directions

Ongoing trials are investigating the combination of a number of targeted agents with chemotherapy in both the metastatic and less advanced disease states. Combination therapy for resectable disease has improved outcomes, but the ideal treatment regimen for patients with stages II–III disease in unknown. The likelihood of outcomes improving with existing regimens is low. Therefore, attention is focused on novel chemotherapies and biologic agents. In addition, research is focusing on PET and other novel methods to predict treatment response at early in therapy.

Take Home Messages

- Endoscopic mucosal resection and endoscopic submucosal dissection are indicated for T1a lesions, well-differentiated, and involve less than a third of the circumference of the esophagus. Surgery is a critical component of treatment for more advance stage esophageal cancers.
- Due to the overall poor outcomes, the majority of patients with locally advanced disease will receive multimodality therapy.
- The gold standard treatment for unresectable, non-metastatic esophageal cancer is concurrent chemotherapy and radiation.
- For the patients with the metastatic disease, the goals of chemotherapy are to improve overall survival and palliate symptoms. Palliative local therapy for dysphagia include radiation, stenting, dilatation, surgery, cryotherapy, argon laser, Nd:YAG laser therapy, and photodynamic therapy.

References

1. Ferlay, J., Soerjomataram, I., Ervik, M., Dikshit, R., Eser, S., Mathers, C., Rebelo, M., Parkin, D.M., Forman, D., Bray, F., GLOBOCAN 2012 v1.0, Cancer Incidence and Mortality Worldwide: IARC CancerBase No. 11 [Internet]. Lyon, France: International Agency for Research on Cancer. Available from: http://globocan.iarc.fr; 2013. Accessed on 1/7/2014.
2. Siegel, R., Naishadham, D., Jemal, A., Cancer statistics, 2013. *CA*, 2013. **63**(1): 11–30.
3. Hur, C., Miller, M., Kong, C.Y. *et al.*, Trends in esophageal adenocarcinoma incidence and mortality. *Cancer*, 2013. **119**(6): 1149–58.
4. Bray, F., Ren, J.S., Masuyer, E., Ferlay, J., Global estimates of cancer prevalence for 27 sites in the adult population in 2008. *Internat J Cancer*, 2013. **132**(5): 1133–1145.
5. Melhado, R.E., Alderson, D., Tucker, O., The changing face of esophageal cancer. *Cancers*, 2010. **2**(3): 1379–404.
6. Daly, J.M., Fry, W.A., Little, A.G. *et al.*, Esophageal cancer: results of an American College of Surgeons Patient Care Evaluation Study. *J Am College Surgeons*, 2000. **190**(5): 562–72; discussion 572–63.
7. Lu, C.L., Lang H.C., Luo, J.C. *et al.*, Increasing trend of the incidence of esophageal squamous cell carcinoma, but not adenocarcinoma, in Taiwan. *Cancer Causes Control*, 2010. **21**(2): 269–74.
8. Vizcaino, A.P., Moreno, V., Lambert, R., Parkin, D.M., Time trends incidence of both major histologic types of esophageal carcinomas in selected countries, 1973–1995. *Internat J Cancer*. 2002. **99**(6): 860–8.
9. Gholipour, C., Shalchi, R.A., Abbasi, M., A histopathological study of esophageal cancer on the western side of the Caspian littoral from 1994 to 2003. *Dis Esophagus*, 2008. **21**(4): 322–7.
10. Islami, F., Kamangar, F., Nasrollahzadeh, D., Moller, H., Boffetta, P., Malekzadeh, R., Oesophageal cancer in Golestan Province, a high-incidence area in northern Iran — a review. *Eur J Cancer*, 2009. **45**(18): 3156–65.
11. Freedman, N.D., Abnet, C.C., Leitzmann, M.F. *et al.*, A prospective study of tobacco, alcohol, and the risk of esophageal and gastric cancer subtypes. *Am J Epidemiol*, 2007. **165**(12): 1424–33.
12. Castellsague, X., Munoz, N., De Stefani, E. *et al.*, Independent and joint effects of tobacco smoking and alcohol drinking on the risk of esophageal cancer in men and women. *Internat J Cancer*, 1999. **82**(5): 657–64.

13. Lin, Y., Totsuka, Y., He, Y. *et al.*, Epidemiology of esophageal cancer in Japan and China. *J Epidemiol*, 2013. **23**(4): 233–42.
14. Akhtar, S. Areca nut chewing and esophageal squamous-cell carcinoma risk in Asians: A meta-analysis of case-control studies. *Cancer Causes Control*, 2013. **24**(2): 257–65.
15. Nasrollahzadeh, D., Kamangar, F., Aghcheli, K. *et al.*, Opium, tobacco, and alcohol use in relation to oesophageal squamous cell carcinoma in a high-risk area of Iran. *Brit J Cancer*, 2008. **98**(11): 1857–63.
16. Islami, F., Boffetta, P., Ren, J.S., Pedoeim, L., Khatib, D., Kamangar, F., High-temperature beverages and foods and esophageal cancer risk a systematic review. *Internat J Cancer*, 2009. **125**(3): 491–524.
17. World Cancer research Fund/American Institute for Cancer Research. *Food, Nutrition, Physical Activity, and the Prevention of Cancer: A Global Perspective*, Washington DC: AICR, 2007.
18. Tran, G.D., Sun, X.D., Abnet, C.C. *et al.*, Prospective study of risk factors for esophageal and gastric cancers in the Linxian general population trial cohort in China. *Internat J Cancer*, 2005. **113**(3): 456–63.
19. Islami, F., Kamangar, F., Nasrollahzadeh, D. *et al.*, Socio-economic status and oesophageal cancer: results from a population-based case-control study in a high-risk area. *Internat J Epidemiol*, 2009. **38**(4): 978–88.
20. Abnet, C.C., Kamangar, F., Islami, F. *et al.*, Tooth loss and lack of regular oral hygiene are associated with higher risk of esophageal squamous cell carcinoma. *Cancer Epidemiol, Biomarkers Prevention*, 2008. **17**(11): 3062–8.
21. Guha, N., Boffetta, P., Wunsch, Filho V. *et al.*, Oral health and risk of squamous cell carcinoma of the head and neck and esophagus: results of two multicentric case-control studies. *Am J Epidemiol*, 2007. **166**(10): 1159–73.
22. Chang, J., Huang, Y., Wei, L. *et al.*, Risk prediction of esophageal squamous-cell carcinoma with common genetic variants and lifestyle factors in Chinese population. *Carcinogenesis*, 2013. **34**(8): 1782–6.
23. Akbari, M.R., Malekzadeh, R., Shakeri, R. *et al.*, Candidate gene association study of esophageal squamous cell carcinoma in a high-risk region in Iran. *Cancer Res*, 2009. **69**(20): 7994–8000.
24. Brown, L.M., Hoover, R., Silverman, D. *et al.*, Excess incidence of squamous cell esophageal cancer among US Black men: role of social class and other risk factors. *Am J Epidemiol*, 2001. **153**(2): 114–22.

25. Devesa, S.S., Blot, W.J., Fraumeni, J.F. Jr., Changing patterns in the incidence of esophageal and gastric carcinoma in the United States. *Cancer*, 1998. **83**(10): 2049–53.
26. Gammon, M.D., Schoenberg, J.B., Ahsan, H. *et al.*, Tobacco, alcohol, and socioeconomic status and adenocarcinomas of the esophagus and gastric cardia. *J Nat Cancer Institute*, 1997. **89**(17): 1277–84.
27. Freedman, N.D., Murray, L.J., Kamangar, F. *et al.*, Alcohol intake and risk of oesophageal adenocarcinoma: a pooled analysis from the BEACON Consortium. *Gut*, 2011. **60**(8): 1029–37.
28. Wheeler, J.B., Reed, C.E., Epidemiology of esophageal cancer. *Surg Clin North Am*, 2012. **92**(5): 1077–87.
29. Navarro, Silvera, S.A., Mayne, S.T., Gammon, M.D. *et al.*, Diet and lifestyle factors and risk of subtypes of esophageal and gastric cancers: classification tree analysis. *Ann Epidemiol*, 2014. **24**(1): 50–7.
30. Zhai, R., Chen, F., Liu, G. *et al.*, Interactions among genetic variants in apoptosis pathway genes, reflux symptoms, body mass index, and smoking indicate two distinct etiologic patterns of esophageal adenocarcinoma. *J Clin Oncol*, 2010. **28**(14): 2445–51.
31. Clavier, J.B., Antoni, D., Atlani, D. *et al.*, Baseline nutritional status is prognostic factor after definitive radiochemotherapy for esophageal cancer. *Dis Esophagus*, 2012.
32. Di Fiore, F., Lecleire, S., Pop, D. *et al.*, Baseline nutritional status is predictive of response to treatment and survival in patients treated by definitive chemoradiotherapy for a locally advanced esophageal cancer. *Am J Gastroenterol*, 2007. **102**(11): 2557–63.
33. Nozoe, T., Kimura, Y., Ishida, M., Saeki, H., Korenaga, D., Sugimachi, K., Correlation of pre-operative nutritional condition with post-operative complications in surgical treatment for oesophageal carcinoma. *Eur J Surgical Oncol*, 2002. **28**(4): 396–400.
34. Thomas, C.R., Jr., Berkey, B.A., Minsky, B.D. *et al.*, Recursive partitioning analysis of pretreatment variables of 416 patients with locoregional esophageal cancer treated with definitive concomitant chemoradiotherapy on Intergroup and Radiation Therapy Oncology Group trials. *Internat J Radiation Oncol, Biol, Physics*, 2004. **58**(5): 1405–10.
35. Boone, J., Livestro, D.P., Elias, S.G., Borel Rinkes, I.H., van Hillegersberg, R., International survey on esophageal cancer: Part II. staging and neoadjuvant therapy. *Dis Esophagus*, 2009. **22**(3): 203–10.

36. Graham, D.Y., Schwartz, J.T., Cain, G.D., Gyorkey, F., Prospective evaluation of biopsy number in the diagnosis of esophageal and gastric carcinoma. *Gastroenterology*, 1982. **82**(2): 228–31.
37. Rice, T.W., Rusch, V.W., Ishwaran H., Blackstone, E.H., Worldwide Esophageal Cancer C. Cancer of the esophagus and esophagogastric junction: data-driven staging for the seventh edition of the American Joint Committee on Cancer/International Union Against Cancer Cancer Staging Manuals. *Cancer*, 2010. **116**(16): 3763–73.
38. Edge, S.B. B.D., Compton C.C., Fritz, A.G., Greene, F.L., Tritti, A. (eds.), *AJCC Cancer Staging Manual. 7th ed.* New York: Springer; 2009.
39. Murata, Y., Suzuki, S., Hashimoto, H., Endoscopic ultrasonography of the upper gastrointestinal tract. *Surgical Endoscopy*, 1988. **2**(3): 180–83.
40. Rosch, T., Lorenz, R., Zenker, K. *et al.*, Local staging and assessment of resectability in carcinoma of the esophagus, stomach, and duodenum by endoscopic ultrasonography. *Gastrointestinal Endoscopy*, 1992. **38**(4): 460–67.
41. Lightdale, C.J., Kulkarni, K.G., Role of endoscopic ultrasonography in the staging and follow-up of esophageal cancer. *J Clin Oncol*, 2005. **23**(20): 4483–89.
42. Puli, S.R., Reddy, J.B., Bechtold, M.L., Antillon, D., Ibdah, J.A., Antillon, M.R., Staging accuracy of esophageal cancer by endoscopic ultrasound: A meta-analysis and systematic review. *World J Gastroenterol*, 2008. **14**(10): 1479–90.
43. Grimm, H., Binmoeller, K.F., Hamper, K., Koch, J., Henne-Bruns, D., Soehendra, N., Endosonography for preoperative locoregional staging of esophageal and gastric cancer. *Endoscopy*, 1993. **25**(3): 224–30.
44. Vilgrain, V., Mompoint, D., Palazzo, L. *et al.*, Staging of esophageal carcinoma: comparison of results with endoscopic sonography and CT. *AJR. Am J Roentgenol*, 1990. **155**(2): 277–81.
45. Botet, J.F., Lightdale, C.J., Zauber, A.G., Gerdes, H., Urmacher, C., Brennan, M.F., Preoperative staging of esophageal cancer: comparison of endoscopic US and dynamic CT. *Radiology*, 1991. **181**(2): 419–25.
46. Hordijk, M.L., Zander, H., van Blankenstein, M., Tilanus, H.W., Influence of tumor stenosis on the accuracy of endosonography in preoperative T staging of esophageal cancer. *Endoscopy*, 1993. **25**(2): 171–75.

47. Hunerbein, M., Ghadimi, B.M., Haensch, W., Schlag, P.M., Transendoscopic ultrasound of esophageal and gastric cancer using miniaturized ultrasound catheter probes. *Gastrointestinal Endoscopy*, 1998. **48**(4): 371–75.
48. Varghese, T.K., Jr., Hofstetter, W.L., Rizk, N.P. *et al.*, The society of thoracic surgeons guidelines on the diagnosis and staging of patients with esophageal cancer. *Ann Thoracic Surgery*, 2013. **96**(1): 346–56.
49. Lowe, V.J., Booya, F., Fletcher, J.G. *et al.*, Comparison of positron emission tomography, computed tomography, and endoscopic ultrasound in the initial staging of patients with esophageal cancer. *Mol Imag Biol*, 2005. **7**(6): 422–30.
50. Rasanen, J.V., Sihvo, E.I., Knuuti, M.J. *et al.*, Prospective analysis of accuracy of positron emission tomography, computed tomography, and endoscopic ultrasonography in staging of adenocarcinoma of the esophagus and the esophagogastric junction. *Ann Surgical Oncol*, 2003. **10**(8): 954–60.
51. Kato, H., Kuwano, H., Nakajima, M. *et al.*, Comparison between positron emission tomography and computed tomography in the use of the assessment of esophageal carcinoma. *Cancer*, 2002. **94**(4): 921–28.
52. Meyers, B.F., Downey, R.J., Decker, P.A. *et al.*, The utility of positron emission tomography in staging of potentially operable carcinoma of the thoracic esophagus: results of the American College of Surgeons Oncology Group Z0060 trial. *J Thoracic Cardiovas Surgery*, 2007. **133**(3): 738–45.
53. Bhutani, M.S., Hawes, R.H., Hoffman, B.J., A comparison of the accuracy of echo features during endoscopic ultrasound (EUS) and EUS-guided fine-needle aspiration for diagnosis of malignant lymph node invasion. *Gastrointestinal Endoscopy*, 1997, **45**(6): 474–9.
54. Murata, Y, Muroi, M, Yoshida, M., Ide, H., Hanyu, F., Endoscopic ultrasonography in the diagnosis of esophageal carcinoma. *Surgical Endoscopy*, 1987. **1**(1): 11–6.
55. Murata, Y., Ohta, M., Hayashi, K., Ide, H., Takasaki, K., Preoperative evaluation of lymph node metastasis in esophageal cancer. *Ann Thoracic Cardiovas Surgery*, 2003. **9**(2): 88–2.
56. Van Vliet, E.P., Heijenbrok-Kal, M.H., Hunink, M.G., Kuipers, E.J., Siersema, P.D., Staging investigations for oesophageal cancer: A meta-analysis. *Brit J Cancer*, 2008. **98**(3): 547–57.

57. Sgourakis, G., Gockel, I., Lyros, O., Hansen, T., Mildenberger, P., Lang, H., Detection of lymph node metastases in esophageal cancer. *Ex Rev Anticancer Ther*, 2011. **11**(4): 601–12.
58. Flanagan, F.L., Dehdashti, F., Siegel, B.A. *et al.*, Staging of esophageal cancer with 18F-fluorodeoxyglucose positron emission tomography. *Am J Roentgenology*, 1997. **168**(2): 417–24.
59. Chandawarkar, R.Y., Kakegawa, T., Fujita, H., Yamana, H., Hayabuthi, N., Comparative analysis of imaging modalities in the preoperative assessment of nodal metastasis in esophageal cancer. *J Surgical Oncol*, 1996. **61**(3): 214–17.
60. Bruzzi, J.F., Munden, R.F., Truong, M.T. *et al.*, PET/CT of esophageal cancer: its role in clinical management. *Radiographics*, 2007. **27**(6): 1635–52.
61. Lerut, T., Flamen, P., Ectors, N. *et al.*, Histopathologic validation of lymph node staging with FDG-PET scan in cancer of the esophagus and gastroesophageal junction: A prospective study based on primary surgery with extensive lymphadenectomy. *Ann Surgery*, 2000. **232**(6): 743–52.
62. Korst, R.J., Rusch, V.W., Venkatraman, E. *et al.*, Proposed revision of the staging classification for esophageal cancer. *J Thoracic Cardiovas Surgery*, 1998. **115**(3): 660–9; discussion 669–70.
63. Tong, D.K., Kwong, D.L., Law, S., Wong, K.H., Wong, J., Cervical nodal metastasis from intrathoracic esophageal squamous cell carcinoma is not necessarily an incurable disease. *J Gastrointestinal Surgery*, 2008. **12**(10): 1638–45; discussion 1645.
64. Quint, L.E., Hepburn, L.M., Francis, I.R., Whyte, R.I., Orringer, M.B., Incidence and distribution of distant metastases from newly diagnosed esophageal carcinoma. *Cancer*, 1995. **76**(7): 1120–5.
65. Downey, R.J., Akhurst, T., Ilson, D. *et al.*, Whole body 18FDG-PET and the response of esophageal cancer to induction therapy: results of a prospective trial, *J Clin*, 2003. **21**(3): 428–32.
66. Flamen, P., Lerut, A., Van Cutsem, E. *et al.*, Utility of positron emission tomography for the staging of patients with potentially operable esophageal carcinoma. *J Clin Oncol*, 2000. **18**(18): 3202–10.
67. Luketich, J.D., Friedman, D.M., Weigel, T.L. *et al.*, Evaluation of distant metastases in esophageal cancer: 100 consecutive positron emission tomography scans. *Ann Thoracic Surgery*, 1999. **68**(4): 1133–6; discussion 1136–7.

68. Krause, B.J., Herrmann, K., Wieder, H., zum Buschenfelde, C.M. 18F-FDG PET and 18F-FDG PET/CT for assessing response to therapy in esophageal cancer, *J Nuclear Med*, 2009; **50**(Suppl 1): 89S–96S.
69. Bar-Shalom R., Guralnik, L., Tsalic, M. *et al.*, The additional value of PET/CT over PET in FDG imaging of oesophageal cancer. *Eur J Nuclear Med Mol Imag*, 2005. **32**(8): 918–24.
70. Kohn, G.P., Galanko, J.A., Meyers, M.O., Feins, R.H., Farrell, T.M. National trends in esophageal surgery — are outcomes as good as we believe? *J Gastrointestinal Surgery*, 2009. **13**(11): 1900–10; discussion 1910–20.
71. Markar, S.R., Karthikesalingam, A., Thrumurthy, S., Low, D.E., Volume-outcome relationship in surgery for esophageal malignancy: systematic review and meta-analysis 2000–2011. *J Gastrointestinal Surgery*, 2012, **16**(5): 1055–63.
72. Birkmeyer, J.D., Siewers, A.E., Finlayson, E.V. *et al.*, Hospital volume and surgical mortality in the United States. *New Eng J Med*, 2002. **346**(15): 1128–37.
73. Birkmeyer, J.D., Stukel, T.A., Siewers, A.E., Goodney, P.P., Wennberg, D.E., Lucas, F.L., Surgeon volume and operative mortality in the United States. *N Eng J Med*, 2003. **349**(22): 2117–27.
74. Derogar, M., Sadr-Azodi, O., Johar, A., Lagergren, P., Lagergren, J., Hospital and surgeon volume in relation to survival after esophageal cancer surgery in a population-based study. *J Clin Oncol*, 2013. **31**(5): 551–7.
75. Ruol, A., Castoro, C., Portale, G. *et al.*, Trends in management and prognosis for esophageal cancer surgery: twenty-five years of experience at a single institution. *Arch Surgery*, 2009. **144**(3): 247–54; discussion 254.
76. Orringer, M.B., Marshall, B., Chang, A.C., Lee, J., Pickens, A., Lau, C.L.. Two thousand transhiatal esophagectomies: changing trends, lessons learned. *Ann Surgery*, 2007. **246**(3): 363–72; discussion 372–64.
77. van Heijl, M., van Lanschot, J.J., Blom, R.L. *et al.*, Outcomes of 16 years of oesophageal surgery: Low postoperative mortality and improved long-term survival. *Nederlands tijdschrift voor geneeskunde*, 2010. **154**: A1156.
78. Ancona, E., Rampado, S., Cassaro, M. *et al.*, Prediction of lymph node status in superficial esophageal carcinoma. *Ann Surg Oncol*, 2008. **15**(11): 3278–88.

79. Pennathur, A., Farkas, A., Krasinskas, A.M. *et al.*, Esophagectomy for T1 esophageal cancer: outcomes in 100 patients and implications for endoscopic therapy. *Ann Thoracic Surgery*, 2009. **87**(4): 1048–1054; discussion 1054–45.
80. Sepesi, B., Watson, T.J., Zhou, D. *et al.*, Are endoscopic therapies appropriate for superficial submucosal esophageal adenocarcinoma? An analysis of esophagectomy specimens. *J Am College Surgeons*, 2010. **210**(4): 418–27.
81. Leers, J.M., DeMeester, S.R., Oezcelik, A. *et al.*, The prevalence of lymph node metastases in patients with T1 esophageal adenocarcinoma a retrospective review of esophagectomy specimens. *Ann Surgery*, 2011. **253**(2): 271–8.
82. Lutz, M.P., Zalcberg, J.R., Ducreux, M. *et al.*, Highlights of the EORTC St. Gallen International Expert Consensus on the primary therapy of gastric, gastroesophageal and oesophageal cancer — differential treatment strategies for subtypes of early gastroesophageal cancer. *Euro J Cancer*, 2012. **48**(16): 2941–53.
83. Ajani, J.A., Barthel, J.S., Bentrem, D.J. *et al.*, Esophageal and esophagogastric junction cancers. *J Nat Comprehensive Cancer Network*, 2011. **9**(8): 830–87.
84. Rice, T.W., Mason, D.P., Murthy, S.C. *et al.*, T2N0M0 esophageal cancer. *J Thoracic Ccardiovas Surgery*, 2007. **133**(2): 317–24.
85. Bosset, J.F., Gignoux, M., Triboulet, J.P. *et al.*, Chemoradiotherapy followed by surgery compared with surgery alone in squamous-cell cancer of the esophagus. *N Eng J Med.*, 1997. **337**(3): 161–7.
86. Tepper, J., Krasna, M.J., Niedzwiecki, D. *et al.*, Phase III trial of trimodality therapy with cisplatin, fluorouracil, radiotherapy, and surgery compared with surgery alone for esophageal cancer: CALGB 9781. *J Clin Oncol*, 2008. **26**(7): 1086–92.
87. van Hagen, P., Hulshof, M.C., van Lanschot, J.J. *et al.*, Preoperative chemoradiotherapy for esophageal or junctional cancer. *N Eng J Med*, 2012. **366**(22): 2074–84.
88. Robb, W.B. M.C., Dahan, L. *et al.*, Surgery alone vs chemoradiotherapy followed by surgery for stage I and I.I. oesophageal cancer: final analysis of a randomised controlled phase III trial — FFCD 9901 (OC-086). *Gut*, 2012. **61**; A37–8.

89. Stiles, B.M., Mirza, F., Coppolino, A. *et al.*, Clinical T2-T3N0M0 esophageal cancer: the risk of node positive disease. *Ann Thoracic Surgery*, 2011. **92**(2): 491–6; discussion 496–8.
90. Motoori, M., Yano, M., Ishihara, R. *et al.*, Comparison between radical esophagectomy and definitive chemoradiotherapy in patients with clinical T1bN0M0 esophageal cancer. *Ann Thoracic Surgical Oncol*, 2012, **19**(7): 2135–41.
91. Berger, A.C., Farma, J., Scott, W.J. *et al.*, Complete response to neoadjuvant chemoradiotherapy in esophageal carcinoma is associated with significantly improved survival. *J Clin Oncol*, 2005. **23**(19): 4330–7.
92. Donahue, J.M., Nichols, F.C., Li, Z. *et al.*, Complete pathologic response after neoadjuvant chemoradiotherapy for esophageal cancer is associated with enhanced survival. *Ann Thoracic Surgery*, 2009. **87**(2): 392–8; discussion 398–9.
93. Siewert, J.R., Stein, H.J., Classification of adenocarcinoma of the oesophagogastric junction. *Brit J Surgery*, 1998. **85**(11): 1457–9.
94. Siewert, J.R., Feith, M, Stein, H.J., Biologic and clinical variations of adenocarcinoma at the esophago-gastric junction: relevance of a topographic-anatomic subclassification. *J Surgical Oncol.*, 2005. **90**(3): 139–46; discussion 146.
95. Allum, W.H., Blazeby, J.M., Griffin, S.M. *et al.*, Guidelines for the management of oesophageal and gastric cancer. *Gut*, 2011. **60**(11): 1449–72.
96. Arnott, S.J., Duncan, W, Kerr, G.R. *et al.*, Low dose preoperative radiotherapy for carcinoma of the oesophagus: results of a randomized clinical trial. *Radiotherapy Oncol*, 1992. **24**(2): 108–13.
97. Gignoux, M., Roussel, A., Paillot, B. *et al.*, The value of preoperative radiotherapy in esophageal cancer: results of a study of the EORTC. *World J Surgery*, 1987. **11**(4): 426–32.
98. Launois, B., Delarue, D., Campion, J.P., Kerbaol, M., Preoperative radiotherapy for carcinoma of the esophagus. *Surgery Gynecology Obstetrics*, 1981. **153**(5): 690–2.
99. Nygaard, K., Hagen, S., Hansen, H.S. *et al.*, Pre-operative radiotherapy prolongs survival in operable esophageal carcinoma: a randomized, multicenter study of pre-operative radiotherapy and chemotherapy. The second Scandinavian trial in esophageal cancer. *World J Surgery*, 1992. **16**(6): 1104–19; discussion 1110.

100. Wang, M., Gu, X.Z., Yin, W.B., Huang, G.J., Wang, L.J., Zhang, D.W., Randomized clinical trial on the combination of preoperative irradiation and surgery in the treatment of esophageal carcinoma: report on 206 patients. *Inter J Radiation Oncol, Biol, Physics.*, 1989. **16**(2): 325–7.
101. Arnott, S.J., Duncan, W., Gignoux, M. *et al.*, Preoperative radiotherapy for esophageal carcinoma. *Cochrane Database Systematic Rev*, **2005**(4): CD001799.
102. Allum, W.H., Stenning, S.P., Bancewicz, J., Clark, P.I., Langley, R.E., Long-term results of a randomized trial of surgery with or without preoperative chemotherapy in esophageal cancer. *J Clin Oncol*, 2009. **27**(30): 5062–7.
103. Cunningham, D., Allum, W.H., Stenning, S.P. *et al.*, Perioperative chemotherapy versus surgery alone for resectable gastroesophageal cancer. *N Eng J Med*, 2006. **355**(1): 11–20.
104. Ychou, M, Boige V, Pignon, J.P. *et al.*, Perioperative chemotherapy compared with surgery alone for resectable gastroesophageal adenocarcinoma: an FNCLCC and FFCD multicenter phase III trial. *J Clin Oncol*, 2011, **29**(13): 1715–21.
105. Boonstra, J.J., Kok, T.C., Wijnhoven, B.P. *et al.*, Chemotherapy followed by surgery versus surgery alone in patients with resectable oesophageal squamous cell carcinoma: Long-term results of a randomized controlled trial. *BMC Cancer*, 2011. **11**: 181.
106. Gebski, V., Burmeister, B., Smithers, B.M. *et al.*, Survival benefits from neoadjuvant chemoradiotherapy or chemotherapy in oesophageal carcinoma: a meta-analysis. *Lancet Oncol*, 2007. **8**(3): 226–34.
107. Sjoquist, K.M., Burmeister, B.H., Smithers, B.M. *et al.*, Survival after neoadjuvant chemotherapy or chemoradiotherapy for resectable oesophageal carcinoma: an updated meta-analysis. *Lancet Oncol.* 2011. **12**(7): 681–92.
108. Kranzfelder, M., Schuster, T., Geinitz, H., Friess, H., Buchler, P., Meta-analysis of neoadjuvant treatment modalities and definitive non-surgical therapy for oesophageal squamous cell cancer. *Brit J Surgery*, 2011. **98**(6): 768–83.
109. Stahl, M., Walz, M.K., Stuschke, M. *et al.*, Phase III comparison of preoperative chemotherapy compared with chemoradiotherapy in patients with locally advanced adenocarcinoma of the esophagogastric junction. *J Clin Oncol*, 2009. **27**(6): 851–6.

110. Burmeister, B.H., Thomas, J.M., Burmeister, E.A. *et al.*, Is concurrent radiation therapy required in patients receiving preoperative chemotherapy for adenocarcinoma of the oesophagus? A randomised phase II trial. *Eur J Cancer*, 2011. **47**(3): 354–60.
111. Schuhmacher, C., Gretschel, S., Lordick, F. *et al.*, Neoadjuvant chemotherapy compared with surgery alone for locally advanced cancer of the stomach and cardia: European Organisation for Research and Treatment of Cancer randomized trial 40954. *J Clin Oncol*, 2010. **28**(35): 5210–18.
112. Walsh, T.N., Noonan, N., Hollywood, D., Kelly, A., Keeling, N., Hennessy, T.P. ,A comparison of multimodal therapy and surgery for esophageal adenocarcinoma. *N Eng J Med*, 1996. **335**(7): 462–67.
113. Ronellenfitsch, U., Schwarzbach, M., Hofheinz,s R. *et al.*, Preoperative chemo(radio)therapy versus primary surgery for gastroesophageal adenocarcinoma: systematic review with meta-analysis combining individual patient and aggregate data. *Euro J Cancer*, 2013. **49**(15): 3149–58.
114. Malthaner, R.A., Wong, R.K., Rumble, R.B., Zuraw, L., Members of the Gastrointestinal Cancer Disease Site Group of Cancer Care Ontario's Program in Evidence-based C. Neoadjuvant or adjuvant therapy for resectable esophageal cancer: a systematic review and meta-analysis. *BMC Med*, 2004. **2**: 35.
115. Pouliquen, X., Levard, H., Hay, J.M., McGee, K., Fingerhut, A., Langlois-Zantin O., 5-Fluorouracil and cisplatin therapy after palliative surgical resection of squamous cell carcinoma of the esophagus. A multicenter randomized trial. French Associations for Surgical Research. *Ann Surgery*, 1996. **223**(2): 127–33.
116. Ando, N., Iizuka, T., Kakegawa, T. *et al.*, A randomized trial of surgery with and without chemotherapy for localized squamous carcinoma of the thoracic esophagus: the Japan Clinical Oncology Group Study. *J Thoracic Cardiovas Surgery*, 1997. **114**(2): 205–09.
117. Ando, N., Iizuka, T., Ide, H. *et al.*, Surgery plus chemotherapy compared with surgery alone for localized squamous cell carcinoma of the thoracic esophagus: a Japan Clinical Oncology Group Study — JCOG9204. *J Clin Oncol*, 2003. **21**(24): 4592–96.
118. Ando, N., Kato, H., Igaki, H. *et al.*, A randomized trial comparing postoperative adjuvant chemotherapy with cisplatin and 5-fluorouracil versus preoperative chemotherapy for localized advanced squamous cell carcinoma

of the thoracic esophagus (JCOG9907). *Annals of Surgical Oncol*, 2012. **19**(1): 68–74.

119. Macdonald, J.S., Smalley, S.R., Benedetti, J. *et al.*, Chemoradiotherapy after surgery compared with surgery alone for adenocarcinoma of the stomach or gastroesophageal junction. *N Eng J Med*, 2001. **345**(10): 725–30.
120. Tachibana, M., Yoshimura, H., Kinugasa, S. *et al.*, Postoperative chemotherapy vs chemoradiotherapy for thoracic esophageal cancer: a prospective randomized clinical trial. *Eur J Surgical Oncol*, 2003. **29**(7): 580–87.
121. Lv, J., Cao, X.F., Zhu, B., Ji L., Tao, L., Wang D.D., Long-term efficacy of perioperative chemoradiotherapy on esophageal squamous cell carcinoma. *World J Gastroenteroly*, 2010. **16**(13): 1649–54.
122. Stahl, M., Stuschke, M., Lehmann, N. *et al.*, Chemoradiation with and without surgery in patients with locally advanced squamous cell carcinoma of the esophagus. *J Clin Oncol*, 2005. **23**(10): 2310–17.
123. Bedenne, L., Michel, P., Bouche, O. *et al.*, Chemoradiation followed by surgery compared with chemoradiation alone in squamous cancer of the esophagus: FFCD 9102. *J Clin Oncol*, 2007. **25**(10): 1160–68.
124. Steel, G.G., Peckham, M.J., Exploitable mechanisms in combined radiotherapy-chemotherapy: the concept of additivity. *Internat J Radiation Oncol Biol Physics*, 1979. **5**(1): 85–91.
125. Wilson, G.D., Bentzen, S.M., Harari, P.M., Biologic basis for combining drugs with radiation. *Sem Radiation Oncol*, 2006. **16**(1): 2–9.
126. Wobbes, T., Baron, B., Paillot, B. *et al.*, Prospective randomised study of split-course radiotherapy versus cisplatin plus split-course radiotherapy in inoperable squamous cell carcinoma of the oesophagus. *Euro J Cancer*, 2001. **37**(4): 470–77.
127. Araujo, C.M., Souhami, L., Gil, R.A. *et al.*, A randomized trial comparing radiation therapy versus concomitant radiation therapy and chemotherapy in carcinoma of the thoracic esophagus. *Cancer*, 1991. **67**(9): 2258–61.
128. Slabber, C.F., Nel, J.S., Schoeman, L., Burger, W., Falkson, G., Falkson, C.I., A randomized study of radiotherapy alone versus radiotherapy plus 5-fluorouracil and platinum in patients with inoperable, locally advanced squamous cancer of the esophagus. *Am J Clin Oncol*, 1998. **21**(5): 462–65.
129. Smith, T.J., Ryan, L.M., Douglass, H.O., Jr. *et al.*, Combined chemoradiotherapy vs. radiotherapy alone for early stage squamous cell carcinoma of

the esophagus: a study of the Eastern Cooperative Oncology Group. *Internat J Radiation Oncol Biol Physics*, 1998. **42**(2): 269–76.

130. Herskovic, A., Martz, K., al-Sarraf, M. *et al.*, Combined chemotherapy and radiotherapy compared with radiotherapy alone in patients with cancer of the esophagus. *N Eng J Med*, 1992. **326**(24): 1593–98.
131. Cooper, J.S., Guo, M.D., Herskovic, A. *et al.*, Chemoradiotherapy of locally advanced esophageal cancer: long-term follow-up of a prospective randomized trial (RTOG 85–01). Radiation Therapy Oncology Group. *JAMA*, 1999. **281**(17): 1623–27.
132. Minsky, B.D., Pajak, T.F., Ginsberg, R.J. *et al.*, INT 0123 (Radiation Therapy Oncology Group 94–05) phase III trial of combined-modality therapy for esophageal cancer: high-dose versus standard-dose radiation therapy. *J Clin Oncol*, 2002. **20**(5): 1167–74.
133. Zhang, Y., Epidemiology of esophageal cancer. *World J Gastroenterology*, 2013. **19**(34): 5598–06.
134. Boyce, H.W., Jr., Palliation of dysphagia of esophageal cancer by endoscopic lumen restoration techniques. *Cancer Control*, 1999. **6**(1): 73–83.
135. Javle, M., Ailawadhi, S., Yang, G.Y., Nwogu, C.E., Schiff, M.D., Nava, H.R., Palliation of malignant dysphagia in esophageal cancer: a literature-based review. *J Supportive Oncol*, 2006, **4**(8): 365–73, 379.
136. Wagner, A.D., Unverzagt, S., Grothe, W. *et al.*, Chemotherapy for advanced gastric cancer. *Cochrane Database Systematic Rev*, 2010. (3): CD004064.
137. Homs, M.Y., v d Gaas, A., Siersema, P.D., Steyerberg, E.W., Kuipers, E.J., Chemotherapy for metastatic carcinoma of the esophagus and gastro-esophageal junction. *Cochrane Database Systematic Rev.*, 2006; (4): CD004063.
138. Grunberger, B., Raderer, M., Schmidinger, M., Hejna, M., Palliative chemotherapy for recurrent and metastatic esophageal cancer. *Anticancer Res*, 2007. **27**(4C): 2705–14.
139. Waddell, T., Chau, I., Cunningham, D. *et al.*, Epirubicin, oxaliplatin, and capecitabine with or without panitumumab for patients with previously untreated advanced oesophagogastric cancer (REAL3): a randomised, open-label phase 3 trial. *Lancet Oncol*, 2013. **14**(6): 481–89.
140. Ilson, D.H., Ajani, J., Bhalla, K. *et al.*, Phase II trial of paclitaxel, fluorouracil, and cisplatin in patients with advanced carcinoma of the esophagus. *J Clin Oncol*, 1998. **16**(5): 1826–34.

141. Bleiberg, H., Conroy, T., Paillot, B. *et al.*, Randomised phase II study of cisplatin and 5-fluorouracil (5-FU) versus cisplatin alone in advanced squamous cell oesophageal cancer. *Euro J Cancer*, 1997. **33**(8): 1216–20.
142. Lee, J., Im, Y.H., Cho, E.Y. *et al.*, A phase II study of capecitabine and cisplatin (XP) as first-line chemotherapy in patients with advanced esophageal squamous cell carcinoma. *Cancer Chemotherapy Pharmacology*, 2008. **62**(1): 77–84.
143. Van Cutsem, E., Moiseyenko, V.M., Tjulandin, S. *et al.*, Phase III study of docetaxel and cisplatin plus fluorouracil compared with cisplatin and fluorouracil as first-line therapy for advanced gastric cancer: a report of the V325 Study Group. *J Clin Oncol*, 2006. **24**(31): 4991–97.
144. Cunningham, D., Starling, N., Rao, S. *et al.*, Capecitabine and oxaliplatin for advanced esophagogastric cancer. *N Eng J Med*, 2008. **358**(1): 36–46.
145. Hu, Y., Bandla, S., Godfrey, T.E. *et al.*, HER2 amplification, overexpression and score criteria in esophageal adenocarcinoma. *Modern Pathol*, 2011, **24**(7): 899–07.
146. Prins, M.J., Ruurda, J.P., van Diest, P.J., van Hillegersberg, R., Ten Kate, F.J., The significance of the HER-2 status in esophageal adenocarcinoma for survival: an immunohistochemical and an in situ hybridization study. *Ann Oncol*, 2013. 24(5): 1290–97.
147. Gravalos, C., Jimeno, A., HER2 in gastric cancer: a new prognostic factor and a novel therapeutic target. *Ann Oncol*, 2008. **19**(9): 1523–29.
148. Hofmann, M., Stoss, O., Shi, D. *et al.*, Assessment of a H.E.R2 scoring system for gastric cancer: results from a validation study. *Histopathology*. 2008, **52**(7): 797–05.
149. Tanner, M., Hollmen, M., Junttila, T.T. *et al.*, Amplification of HER-2 in gastric carcinoma: association with Topoisomerase II alpha gene amplification, intestinal type, poor prognosis and sensitivity to trastuzumab. *Ann Oncol*, 2005. **16**(2): 273–8.
150. Bang, Y.J., Van Cutsem, E., Feyereislova, A. *et al.*, Trastuzumab in combination with chemotherapy versus chemotherapy alone for treatment of HER2-positive advanced gastric or gastro-oesophageal junction cancer (ToGA): a phase 3, open-label, randomised controlled trial. *Lancet*, 2010, **376**(9742): 687–97.

Chapter 9

Endoscopic Diagnosis and Treatment of Gastric Malignancies

Ke Tao, Virginia O. Shaffer, Qiang Cai and Hong Xu

What is New

- Confocal endoscopy offer histological evaluation *in vivo*.
- Endoscopic ultrasonography (EUS) locoregional staging plays an important role in staging and treatment strategy.
- Endoscopic resection of flat lesions leads to five-year survival rates up to 90%.
- Comparing endoscopic mucosal resection (EMR), endoscopic submucosal dissection (ESD) has higher en bloc resection rate and higher complication rate.

Introduction

Despite decreases in incidence and mortality, gastric cancer remains the second leading cause of cancer-related deaths worldwide.[1] According to the WHO, 736,000 deaths were caused by gastric cancer in 2008. Gastric cancer deaths occurred more in low- and middle-income countries. High-risk areas, with age-standardized incidence ranging from 30 to 85 cases per 100,000 in men and 15 to 40 cases per 100,000 in women, include

Japan, China, Portugal, Peru, Italy, Costa Rica, Ecuador, Colombia, Estonia, and Latvia.[2] Low-risk areas, with age-standardized incidence ranging from 4 to 8 per 100,000 in men and 2 to 4 cases per 100,000 in women, include Kuwait, Israel, and United States.[2] As with most other cancers, there are many risk factors associated with gastric cancer, including age, sex, race, *Helicobacter pylori* infection, cigarette smoking, alcohol consumption, etc.

Most epidemiology studies subclassify tumor by sites of the stomach, separating cases into cardia and uncardia (including the fundus, body, and pyloric antrum) gastric cancer. Gastric cardia cancer is thought to have a different etiology from non-cardia cancer.[3] Gastric cardia cancer has dramatically increased in incidence in United States and Europe since 1970s.[4,5] In United States, about 50% of gastric cancer in men are cardia cancer . There is a difference between eastern (Japan) and western cancers by histological classification. Lauren developed a histological classification of gastric cancer — intestinal and diffused. The diffused type accounts for approximately 30% of gastric cancer.[3] It is also thought that these two histological types of tumors have different etiologies.[6] According to Japanese research society committee, gastric cancer is divided into papillary, tubular carcinomas (these two are considered as well-differentiated), poorly differentiated and signet ring carcinoma (these two are considered poorly differentiated). Intestinal type (differentiated type) gastric cancer is more prevalent among patients with early-stage gastric cancer but not common among patients with advanced gastric cancer who require chemotherapy.[7]

The prognosis is strongly related to the tumor stage, and particularly to lymph node involvement.[8] The majority of gastric cancer patients present with an advanced tumor stage because symptoms and clinical signs develop very late and are nonspecific.[9] Warning symptoms, such as gastrointestinal bleeding, rapid weight loss, or epigastric pain are known to occur very late and indicate an advanced stage of the disease.[10]

Gastric Cancer Diagnosis by Endoscopy

Upper gastrointestinal endoscopy provides a sensitive and specific method for diagnosis of gastric tumors. The size and location of any lesions in the stomach should be carefully documented during endoscopy. All mucosal lesions such as ulcers, polyps, strictures, and thickened gastric folds should be biopsied. One study has shown that accurate histological diagnosis of gastric adenocarcinoma is possible in 95% of cases when four biopsies are taken from a specific lesion. Diagnostic accuracy increases to 98% when seven biopsies are taken, and if seven or eight biopsies and cytologic brushings or aspirates are taken diagnostic accuracy approaches 100%. Because visual endoscopic assessment of malignancy only is inaccurate, it is recommended that cytology and at least four to seven biopsies be obtained from all gastric mucosal lesions.

Several endoscopic features of gastric ulcers are more commonly associated with malignancies. However, differentiation of benign and malignant gastric ulcers by endoscopic appearance alone is not reliable. The size of an ulcer is an important risk factor for malignancy, as up to 20% of ulcers over 3 cm in diameter have been shown to be malignant. Other endoscopic features more frequently associated with malignancy include an irregular base, an irregular ulcer margin (which can be interrupted by tumor nodules), and disruption or abrupt cut-off folds adjacent to the ulcer. All gastric ulcers (with the possible exception of superficial ulceration associated with aspirin and other non-steroidal anti-inflammatory drugs) should be followed with repeat endoscopy and biopsy until healed.

Gastric adenocarcinomas have also been classified according to their gross appearance. The original classification system was proposed by Borrmann in 1926 and consisted of protruding, flat or depressed types of cancers, with the protruding type considered to have a better prognosis. This classification was modified by the Japanese Research Society for Gastric Cancer in 1981. The relationship of tumor contour and prognosis has not been consistent.

The majority of gastric polyps are benign, and again there are no reliable endoscopic features to differentiate benign from malignant. Polyp size >1 cm is a risk factor for the presence of neoplasia (adenoma) or malignancy. Biopsy of small polyps (<1 cm) is sufficient for diagnosis. Larger polyps should be biopsied to determine if neoplastic; however this may miss neoplastic foci within the polyp. Before removal of large polyps by endoscopic polypectomy or surgery, the physician must consider the histology obtained on biopsy, clinical symptoms attributable to the polyp, and the patient's age and medical status, in order to determine if polyp removal warrants the risk of the procedure. Endoscopic removal of large gastric polyps may be associated with a 4% risk of post-polypectomy bleeding, which may require surgery.

Gastric cancer may be missed by upper gastrointestinal endoscopy. Characteristics of the gastric cancers missed by upper gastrointestinal endoscopy are early cancer, small size, and Borrmann type III or IV advanced cancers.[11] Treatment of early gastric cancer is more cost-effective than advanced gastric cancer. Patients will have a better life after treatment if cancer is diagnosed at an early stage.

Therefore, it is important to find the precancerous lesion and the early gastric cancer in the stomach. Chromoscopy improves the detection of flat lesions which contain dysplasia in screeming examination of patients with inflammatory bowel diseases.[12] This is true in patients with gastric cancer. Ohkawa *et al.* investigated 109 gastric lesions using autofluorescence imaging (AFI), where all 56 neoplastic lesions and 87.5% of adenomas were recognized as having abnormal AFI.[13] Autofluorescence endoscopy has a high specificity, but lower sensitivity. By now, endoscopists still mainly use white light endoscope (WLE) to examine the suspicious leisions.

Biopsies are essential in the histological diagnosis. Histopathology examination is still the "Gold Standard" for gastric cancer diagnosis. In general, judging the nature of suspicious gastric mucosal lesions and whether a biopsy is needed on endoscopy depends on the endoscopist's skill and experience. Endomicroscopy enables the endoscopist to obtain real-time *in vivo* histology during ongoing endoscopy, thereby creating "optical biopsies." Impersonal diagnostic criteria could be established by using confocal laser endomicroscopy (CLE), which would contribute to the diagnosis and management of suspicious lesions. CLE could enable targeted biopsy, thereby avoiding unnecessary biopsies and mistaken diagnosis. Yan-qing Li directed a study demonstrating that CLE was able to visualize precisely the structure of the pit, and discriminate between normal mucosa, gastritis and gastric cancer.[14] CLE is a useful tool for *in vivo* diagnosis of precancerous conditions and gastric cancer.[15] CLE provides histopathological information during the procedure to help determine whether lesions should be resected.

CLE images need fluorescence agent. CLE with fluorescein only provides anatomical images. Recently, several researchers have applied CLE in the field of molecular imaging with fluorescently labeled antibodies or peptides.[16–18] Targeted imaging using a fluorescent labeled biomarker is the newest direction of CLE examination.

CLE may get high concordance with histopathology, but it is costly. There are other endoscopic methods with lower concordance with pathology. Magnification endoscopy and chromoendoscopy with optical image enhancement help endoscopists exam the gastric mucosa in detail.[19–21] Magnification endoscopy and optical image enhancement highlight the mucosal microvasculature. Normal gastric mucosa, gastritis and gastric cancercorrespond to different types of microvasculature. The combination of both magnification endoscopy and optical image enhancement has made it possible to detect and differentiate non-neoplastic and neoplastic lesions with a much greater degree of accuracy than standard WLE.

Since its introduction in 2004, CLE has emerged as a valuable tool for gastrointestinal endoscopic imaging. Currently, two CLE-based systems are available including an integrated endoscopy system (Pentax Endomicroscopy System, city and country) and a probe-based system (Cellvizio Endomicroscopy System, Mauna Kea Technologies, Paris, France).

Staging

For the diagnosis of gastric malignant lesion, it is important to determine the tumor stage, T stage. As the endoscopic treatment develops, earlier stage cancer within gastrointestinal epithelial layer could be resected by endoscopy.

EUS is able to increase the accuracy of preoperative staging by determining the mucosal depth of invasion and possibly the involvement of regional lymph nodes. Several studies have compared EUS, computed tomogram, and subsequent operative staging. EUS demonstrated 83–88% accuracy for determining depth of invasion compared with 35% accuracy for CT. For determining nodal involvement, EUS is 66–72% accurate compared with 45% accuracy for CT. One meta-analysis demonstrates the sensitivity, specificity, positive likelihood ratio, negative likelihood ratio, and diagnostic odds ratio of EUS on T staging were 0.86 (95% CI, 0.81–0.90), 0.91 (95% CI, 0.89–0.93), 9.8 (95% CI, 7.5–12.8), 0.15 (95% CI, 0.11–0.21), and 65 (95% CI, 41–105), respectively.[22]

Gastric Carcinoma Endoscopic Treatment

There are two kinds of treatment methods: endoscopic lesion resection including polypectomy, EMR and ESD, and lesion destroying techniques which include argon plasma coagulation, radiofrequency ablation, laser treatment etc. For the treatment of early gastric cancer, endoscopic resection is a better choice. After resection, histopathologic results allow for detailed evaluation of the lesion. If the lesion was completed resected, follow-up only is necessary, otherwise, further surgical intervention may be needed.

Endoscopic mucosal resection (EMR)

The technique of EMR, which was called "strip biopsy," was first reported in 1984,[23] paving the way for endoscopic treatment for EGC. EMR is widely accepted because of its minimal invasion, low cost, well patient tolerance, and improved patient quality of life after the procedure.

According to current guidelines,[24] absolute indications for endoscopic resection include differentiated EGCs less than 20 mm in diameter and small (≤10 mm), depressed EGCs without ulceration or scarring. Moreover, these lesions must be confined to the mucosa, with no lymphatic or vascular involvement.

The standard procedure includes lesion stain, submucosal injection, snare resection and hemostasis with endo-clips. For lesion that larger than 20 mm, piecemeal EMR is an alternative. Other types of mucosal resection include ligation EMR which ligate the suspicious mucosa first then resects.

A meta-analysis of 25 studies and 5,221 cases revealed that *en-bloc* resection was achieved in 62.85% of removed lesions and tumor-free vertical and lateral margins were achieved in 58.6%.[25] *En-bloc* resection rates by conventional polypectomy snare have been reported to be between 7% and 34% for large sessile polyps,[26,27] EMR is a better modality for sessile and flat lesions.

Endoscopic submucocal dissection (ESD)

ESD was introduced in 2003. Currently, ESD is becoming the main procedure for the resection of early gastric cancer (EGC) in east Asia. In the beginning, ESD was performed in the stomach and esophagus. Since there are more flat colonic lesions in east Asia, now endoscopists are resecting flat or serrated lesions in the colon in addition to the lesions in the upper gastrointestinal tract.

Indications for ESD are differentiated cancer with no lymphatic or vascular involvement, including: (1) mucosal cancers without ulcerative findings, regardless of tumor size; (2) mucosal cancers with ulcerative findings ≤30 mm; and (3) minute (≤500 μm from the muscularis mucosae), and submucosal invasive cancers ≤30 mm.

The steps in ESD procedure are: (1) mark the border of the lesion; (2) inject and lift the lesion submucosally shown in Fig. 1; (3) dissect circumferentialy; (4) dissect submucosally; (5) obtain wound surface hemostasis. Either APC or the electric knife could be used to mark the lesion. Normal saline with addition of methylene blue and norepinephine are used for the submucosal injection. Adding sodium hyaluronate could keep the mucosa elevated for a longer time, which will make the submucosal layer easier to dissect. During ESD, different kinds of electric knives are used — different knives have their own special function and are used under different circumstances.

A meta-analysis showed a superior histologically complete resection rate in the ESD group than in the EMR group, even for the lesions <20 mm.[28] ESD is technically difficult to perform, and the procedural time is longer than EMR. The recurrence rate and the complication rate are almost the same with EMR. In Japan, endoscopic resection of EGC leads to five-year survival rates up to 90%.[29]

The standard indication of ESD as mentioned above is a lesion without lymphatic or vascular involvement. However, most (approximately 91%) of the patients with potential risk of lymph-nodal metastasis (LNM)

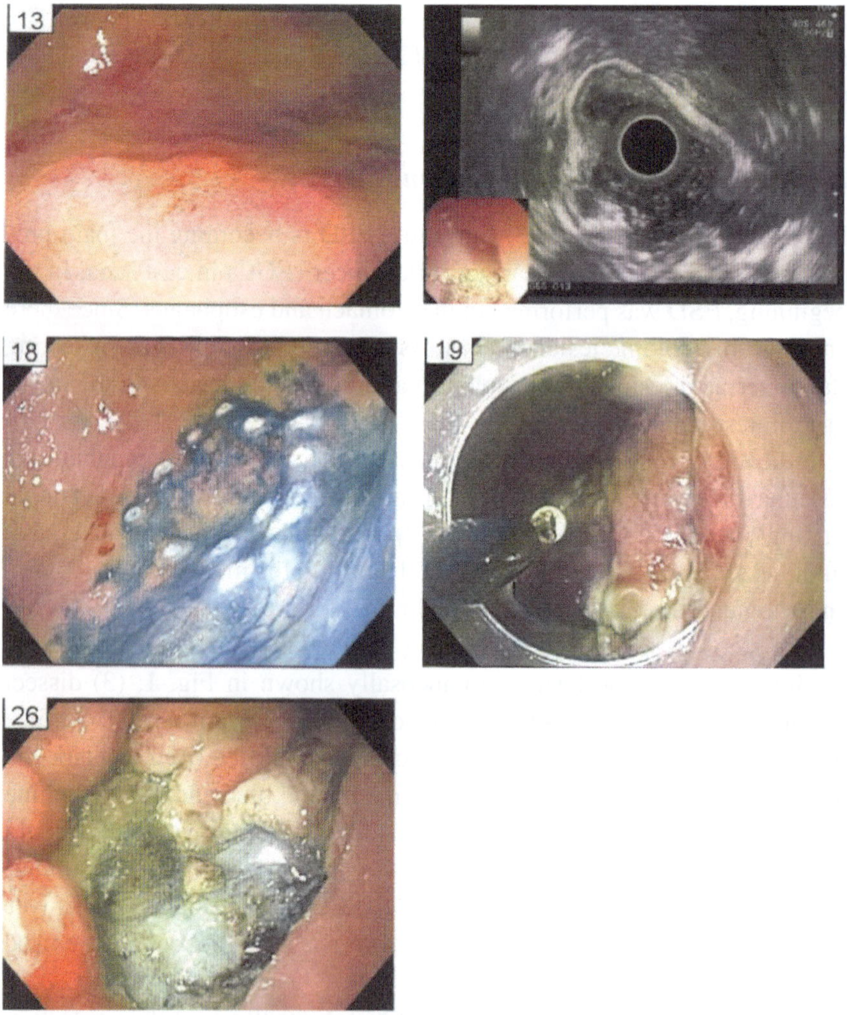

Fig. 1. Endoscopic submucosal resection for a T1 gastric adenocarcinoma.

assessed before surgery are eventually found to have no nodal metastases after "unnecessary" gastrectomy.[30] So, the combination of ESD and laparoscopic lymph node dissection (LLND) could eliminate unnecessary gastrectomy. ESD allows for complete removal of the primary tumor, and LLND confirms the absence of LNM in these patients. ESD and LLND may be the new direction in treating these lesions, especially after emerging of the mini laparoscope.

Palliative treatment

Palliation of obstructive or bleeding complications due to disseminated or recurrent gastric cancer represents a difficult management problem. For obstruction of the distal esophagus, endoscopic laser therapy or prosthetic wire mesh stents have been used successfully, or percutaneous endoscopic gastrostomy (PEG) tubes can be placed to maintain nutrition when stent cannot be placed. For obstruction of the distal stomach, a gastrojejunostomy or partial gastrectomy can be performed. Palliative resection may provide superior results compared with palliative bypass, however, at the expense of increased morbidity. Palliation of obstructing cancer at the gastric outlet may also be managed by wire mesh stents placed by endoscopy. Laser or thermal cautery therapy may be used for persistently bleeding lesions.

Take Home Messages

- Early diagnosis of gastric cancer is more cost-effective.
- New endoscopic methods help detect early stage gastric cancer.
- Magnifying techniques offer better evaluation of gastric lesions.
- EUS is of great value for tumor staging.
- Compared with EMR for early gastric cancer, ESD showed considerable advantages regarding en bloc resection rate, histologically complete resection rate, and local recurrence, even for small lesions.

References

1. Ferlay, J., Bray, F., Pisani, P., Parkin, D.M., *Globacan 2000: Cancer Incidence, Mortality and Prevalence Worldwide*. Version 1.0. IARC Cancer Base No. 5.Lyon: IARC Press; 2001.
2. Parkin, D., Muir, C., *Cancer Incidence in Five Continents*. Schottenfeld, D., Frqumeni, J. (eds.). Lyon, France, IARC Scientific Pulications, 1992. 707–24.

3. Lam, S., Ninth Seah Cheng Siang Memorial Lecture: Gastric cancer Where are we now? *Ann Acad Med Singapore*, 1999. **28**: 881–9.
4. Tredaniel, J., Boffetta, P., Buiatti, E. *et al.*, Tobacco smoking and gastric cancer: Review and meta-analysis. *Int J Cancer*, 1997. **72**(4): 565–73.
5. Devesa, S., Blot, W., Fraumeni, J., Changing patterns in the incidence of esophageal and gastric carcinoma in the United States. *Cancer*, 1998. **83**(10): 2049–53.
6. Lauren, P., The two histological main types of gastric carcinoma: Diffuse and so-called intestinal-type carcinoma: An attempt at a histoclinical classification. *Acta Pathol Microbiol Scand*, 1965. **64**: 31–49.
7. Nishida, T., Treatment of gastric cancer in Asia: The missing link. *Lancet Oncol*, 2009. **10**(11): 1027–8.
8. Coburn, N.G., Lymph nodes and gastric cancer. *J Surg Oncol*, 2009. **99**(4): 199–206.
9. Shah, M.A., Kelsen, D.P., Gastric cancer: a primer on the epidemiology and biology of the disease and an overview of the medical management of advanced disease. *J Natl Compr Cancer Netw*, 2010. **8**(4): 437–447.
10. Fung, W.P., Khoo, O.T., Tye, C.Y., The clinical presentation of gastric cancer: A review of 110 cases (1963–1970). *Singapore Med J*, 1972. **13**(3): 141–5.
11. Hsu, Y.-C., Hsu, C.-Y., Hsu, Lin, H.-J., Clinical and Endoscopic Characteristics of Gastric Cancer Missed By Upper Gastrointestinal Endoscopy. *Gastrointest Endosc*, 2009. **69**(5): Page AB112.
12. Bruno, M.J., Magnification endoscopy, high resolution endoscopy, and chromoscopy; towards a better optical diagnosis. *Gut*, 2003. **52**(Suppl IV): iv7–11.
13. Ohkawa, A., Miwa, H., Namihisa, A., Kobayashi, O., Nakaniwa, N., Ohkusa, T., Ogihara, T., Sato, N., Diagnostic performance of light-induced fluorescence endoscopy for gastric neoplasms. *Endoscopy*, 2004. **36**(6): 515–21.
14. Zhang, J.N., Li, Y.Q., Zhao, Y.A., Yu, T., Zhang, J.P., Guo, Y.T., Liu, H., Classification of gastric pit patterns by confocal endomicroscopy. *Gastrointestinal Endoscopy*, 2008. **67**(6): 843–53.
15. Kiesslich, R., Goetz, M., Burg, J. *et al.*, Diagnosing Helicobacter pylori *in vivo* by confocal laser endoscopy. *Gastroenterology*, 2005. **128**(7): 2119–23.
16. Goetz, M., Ziebart, A., Foersch, S. *et al.*, *In vivo* molecular imaging of colorectal cancer with confocal endomicroscopy by targeting epidermal growth factor receptor. *Gastroenterology*, 2010. **138**(2): 435–46.

17. Foersch, S., Kiesslich, R., Waldner, M.J. *et al.*, Molecular imaging of VEGF ingastrointestinal cancer *in vivo* using confocal laser endomicroscopy. *Gut*, 2010. **59**(8): 1046–55.
18. Hsiung, P.L., Hardy, J., Friedland, S. *et al.*, Detection of colonic dysplasia *in vivo* using a targeted heptapeptide and confocal microendoscopy. *Nat Med*, 2008. **14**(4): 454–8.
19. Nonaka, K., Arai, S., Ban, S. *et al.*, Prospective study of the evaluation of the usefulness of tumor typing by narrow band imaging for the differential diagnosis of gastric adenoma and well-differentiated adenocarcinoma. *Dig Endosc*, 2011. **23**(2): 146–52.
20. Nakayoshi, T., Tajiri, H., Matsuda, K. *et al.*, Magnifying endoscopy combined with narrow band imaging system for early gastric cancer: Correlation of vascular pattern with histopathology (including video). *Endoscopy*, 2004. **36**(12): 1080–4.
21. Yokoyama, A., Inoue, H., Minami, H. *et al.*, Novel narrow-band imaging magnifying endoscopic classification for early gastric cancer. *Dig Liver Dis*, 2010. **42**(10): 704–8.
22. Mocellin, S., Marchet, A., Nitti, D., EUS for the staging of gastric cancer: A meta-analysis. *Gastrointestinal Endoscopy*, 2011. **73**(6): 1122–34.
23. Tada, M., Murakami, A., Karita, M. *et al.*, Endoscopic resection of early gastric cancer. *Endoscopy*, 1993. **25**(7): 445–50.
24. Shimada, Y., JGCA (The Japan Gastric Cancer Association). Gastric cancer treatment guidelines. *Jpn J Clin Oncol*, 2004. **34**(1): 58.
25. Srinivas, R.P., Yasuo, K., Takuji, G., Daphne, A., Yutaka, S., and Mainor R A., Meta-analysis and systematic review of colorectal endoscopic mucosal resection. *World J Gastroenterol*, 2009. **15**(34): 4273–7.
26. Church, J.M., Avoiding surgery in patients with colorectal polyps. *Dis Colon Rectum*, 2003. **46**(11): 1513–6.
27. Stergiou, N., Riphaus, A., Lange, P., Menke, D., Köckerling, F., Wehrmann, T., Endoscopic snare resection of large colonic polyps: How far can we go? *Int J Colorectal Dis*, 2003. **18**(2): 131–5.
28. Lian, J., Chen, S., Zhang, Y., Qiu, F., A meta-analysis of endoscopic submucosal dissection and EMR for early gastric cancer. *Gastrointestinal Endoscopy*, 2012. **76**(4): 763–70.
29. Miyahara, R., Niwa, Y., Matsuura, T. *et al.*, Prevalence and prognosis of gastric cancer detected by screening in a large Japanese population: Data

from a single institute over 30 years. *J Gastroenterol Hepatol*, 2007. **22**(9): 1435–42.

30. Gotoda, T., Yanagisawa, A., Sasako, M., Ono, H., Nakanishi, Y., Shimoda, T., Kato, Y., Incidence of lymph node metastasis from early gastric cancer. The estimation using a large number of cases in two large centers. *Gastric Cancer*, 2000. **3**(4): 219–25.

Chapter 10

Management of Gastric and Gastroesophageal Junction Adenocarcinoma beyond Endoscopy

Gopi K. Prithviraj, Amit Mahipal and Richard Kim

What is New

- The current standard of care in the first-line treatment of advanced or metastatic gastroesophageal junction or gastric cancer is dependent on geographic location, but continues to include a platinum plus fluoropyrimidine backbone.
- HER2-neu status should be assessed in all patients with metastatic gastric cancer. Trastuzumab is recommended in combination with chemotherapy in HER-2 overexpressed patients with metastatic gastric cancer.
- Ramucirumab, a fully human IgG-1 monoclonal antibody against VEGFR-2 has recently shown an overall survival benefit as a single agent or in combination with paclitaxel in refractory gastric cancer.
- Other targeted therapies, including epidermal growth factor receptor (EGFR) inhibitors, c-Met tyrosine kinase inhibitors, and PI3 kinase inhibitors are currently being examined in the preclinical and clinical settings.

Introduction

Gastric cancer, including cancer of the gastroesophageal junction (GEJ), is a global health problem with approximately 1 million people diagnosed every year worldwide.[1] In the United States, an estimated 22,220 new cases will be diagnosed and 10,990 patients will die secondary to gastric cancer in 2014.[2] There are approximately 72,269 people currently living with gastric cancer in the United States.[3] The median age at diagnosis is 69 years of age, with the percentage of new cases highest in persons 75–84 years old.[3] At the time of diagnosis, 25% of the cases are localized (confined to primary site), 20% are regional (spread to regional lymph nodes), 34% are metastatic.[3] The relative five-year survival of patients of all stages diagnosed with gastric cancer is 27.7%.[3] The only potentially curative treatment involves surgical resection of gross and microscopic disease. However, even in surgically resected patients, relapse is common at both distant and regional sites. Despite advances in diagnosis and treatment, the clinical outcome for advanced gastric and GEJ cancer remains poor, with a five-year relative survival of only 3.9%.[3]

Chemotherapy remains the primary treatment modality for the treatment of metastatic or unresectable gastric and GEJ adenocarcinoma. Chemotherapy is administered in this setting for palliation purposes with the hope of improving patients' symptomatology and life expectancy. Chemotherapy compared to best supportive care has been demonstrated to significantly improve overall survival in patients with metastatic gastric cancer.[4] Chemotherapy regimens in advanced gastric and gastroesophageal junction adenocarcinoma are selected dependent on the patient's performance status, medical comorbidities, and HER2-neu status. Various chemotherapy regimens consisting of one to three-drug combinations are approved; however, two-drug cytotoxic regimens are preferred in the treatment of advanced gastric cancer due to lower toxicity and are recommended by National Comprehensive Cancer Network (NCCN). Three-drug cytotoxic regimens are reserved for patients with excellent performance status.[5] The chemotherapy backbone in the management of first-line advanced gastric/GEJ cancers remains cisplatin and fluoropyrimidine-based regimens; however, alternative therapies can be used dependent on patient-specific factors. In this chapter, we will review the current recommendations for first- and second-line chemotherapy regimens for advanced gastric and GE junction adenocarcinomas, as well as the role of newer targeted therapies.

First Line Chemotherapy (Table 1)

Taxane based regimens

DCF: Docetaxel, cisplatin, and 5-fluorouracil

The role of this triple chemotherapy regimen consisting of docetaxel, cisplatin and 5-fluorouracil (5-FU) was elucidated in a multinational randomized phase III study of 457 patients. DCF significantly improved time to progression (5.6 vs. 3.7 months), response rate (37% vs. 25%), and median overall survival (9.2 vs. 8.6 months) when compared to cisplatin and fluorouracil combination in patients with previously untreated advanced gastric cancer. However, there was a noted increase in toxicity, particularly hematologic toxicity, diarrhea, neuropathy and fatigue.[6] Febrile neutropenia was reported in 29% of the patients. Growth factors were not utilized in this study. Due to concern for toxicities, in clinical practice, the DCF regimen is sometimes modified with the substitution of carboplatin or oxaliplatin in place of cisplatin or with the addition of growth factor support.[7] A modified DCF regimen was examined in a multicenter phase II study of previously untreated patients with metastatic gastroesophageal carcinoma and compared to standard DCF with growth factor support. This trial demonstrated similar efficacy and less toxicity with modified DCF regimen. There was reduced incidence of neutropenia, nausea, vomiting, and diarrhea, as well as fewer toxicity-related hospitalizations.[8]

Carboplatin and paclitaxel

Carboplatin and paclitaxel combination has demonstrated activity in phase I/II trials as first- and second-line therapy in advanced gastric and esophageal cancers.[9–13] Gadgeel *et al.* reported a 33% objective response rate in a phase II trial of 27 patients with advanced gastric cancer treated with carboplatin and paclitaxel, with a median response duration of

Table 1. Selected trials for first-line therapy for advanced or metastatic gastric or gastroesophageal cancer.

Author (year)	Trial	N	Regimen	RR (%)	OS (months)	PFS/TTP (months)
Webb (1997)[14]	III	274	ECF	45*	8.9*	7.4*
			FAMTX	21	5.7	3.4
Gadgeel (2003)[9]	II	27	Carboplatin and paclitaxel	33	7.5	4.9
Van Cutsem (2006)[6]	III	445	DCF	37*	9.2*	5.6*
			CF	25	8.6	3.7
Cunningham (2008)[16]	III	1002	ECF	40.7	9.9	6.2
			ECX	46.4	9.9	6.7
			EOF	42.4	9.3	6.5
			EOX	47.9	11.2	7.0
Louvet (2010)[19]	III	416	FOLFIRI	N/A	9.7	5.8
			ECX	N/A	9.5	5.3
Ajani (2010)[23]	III	1053	Cisplatin and S-1	29.1	8.6	4.8
			Cisplatin and infusional 5-FU	31.9	7.9	5.5
Bang (2010)[33]	III	594	Trastuzumab + chemotherapy	47.3*	13.8*	6.7*
			Chemotherapy alone	34.5	11.1	5.5

N/A = Not available, RR = response rate, OS = overall survival, PFS = progression free survival, TTP = time to progression, ECF = epirubicin, cisplatin, fluorouracil; FAMTX = fluorouracil, doxorubicin, methotrexate; DCF = docetaxel, cisplatin, fluorouracil; CF = cisplatin, fluorouracil; ECX = epirubicin, cisplatin, capecitabine; EOF = epirubicin, oxaliplatin, fluorouracil; EOX = epirubicin, oxaliplatin, capecitabine; FOLFIRI = Bolus 5-FU, Infusional 5-FU, leucovorin, irinotecan.
* indicates statistically significant *p* value in favor of the regimen.

4.9 months and median survival of 7.5 months.[9] In advanced esophageal cancer, this combination resulted in a 43% objective response rate in a study of 35 patients with a median response duration of 2.8 months and median survival of 9 months.[10] Overall, carboplatin and paclitaxel combination is well-tolerated, with neutropenia as the major grade 3 toxicity.[10]

Anthracycline-based regimens

ECF: Epirubicin, cisplatin, and 5-fluorouracil

ECF has been an established regimen in the treatment of advanced gastric cancer since 1997.[14] When compared to the standard of care at that time (FAMTX- 5-FU, doxorubicin, and methotrexate), ECF showed a survival advantage (8.9 vs 5.7 months), response advantage (45% vs. 21%), and improved quality of life. Common toxicities included alopecia, nausea and emesis, and hematologic adverse events.[14]

Modifications of ECF regimens: Epirubicin, oxaliplatin and 5-FU (EOF); or epirubicin, cisplatin, and capecitabine (ECX); or Epirubicin, oxaliplatin and capecitabine (EOX)

The ECF regimen can be modified with the substitution of oxaliplatin in place of cisplatin, and/or the substitution of capecitabine for 5-FU.[15,16] The Randomized ECF for Advanced and Locally Advanced Esophagogastric Cancer 2 (REAL-2) trial was a phase III randomized noninferiority trial designed to determine if 5-FU could be replaced by capecitabine, and cisplatin replaced by oxaliplatin, in the ECF regimen for untreated advanced esophagogastric cancer.[16] The REAL-2 study concluded that capecitabine and oxaliplatin were as effective as 5-FU and cisplatin in this patient population, with noninferiority in overall survival. Capecitabine and 5-FU had similar toxicities except for neutropenia and hand-foot syndrome. Use of oxaliplatin instead of cisplatin was associated with a lower incidence of neutropenia, renal insufficiency, and thromboembolic disease and slightly higher rates of neuropathy and diarrhea.[16]

Irinotecan-based regimens

5-Fluorouracil and irinotecan

A modified FOLFIRI regimen with leucovorin plus 5-FU and irinotecan given every two weeks can be used in the treatment of recurrent or metastatic gastric cancer in the first-line setting. In a phase II study of modified FOLFIRI (irinotecan with biweekly, low dose leucovorin and bolus and continuous infusion 5-FU) in the first-line treatment of metastatic gastric cancer, the median OS was 10.3 months with an overall response rate of 38.6%. Major toxicities included anemia and neutropenia.[17,18]

In the phase III intergroup FFCD-GERCOR-FNCLCC 03-07 study, FOLFIRI has been shown to have a prolonged time to treatment failure with equivalent progression-free survival and overall survival to ECX (epirubicin, cisplatin, capecitabine) in a randomized controlled trial of 416 patients with locally advanced or metastatic gastric adenocarcinoma. Grade 3 and 4 toxicities occurred more frequently with ECX (85% vs. 70%), resulting in higher rate of discontinuation then FOLFIRI (16.7% vs. 3.5%).[19]

S-1-based regimens

S-1 is an oral dihydropyrimidine dehydrogenase (DPD) inhibitory oral fluoropyrimidine which is effectively used as monotherapy and in combination therapy in Asian countries in the treatment of advanced gastric cancer. In the SPIRITS (S-1 plus cisplatin versus S-1 alone for first-line treatment of advanced gastric cancer) study, which is a randomized phase III trial conducted in Japan, the study showed that the combination of cisplatin and S-1 was superior over S-1 as a single agent.[20] However, results have not been replicable in Europe and the United States.[21] The safety analysis of the FLAGS Multicenter phase III comparison of cisplatin/S-1 (CS) with cisplatin/5-FU (CF) as first-line therapy in patients with advanced gastric cancer study showed that S-1 combination was associated with decreased rates of neutropenia, stomatitis, diarrhea, and renal adverse events.[22] Some of the toxicity difference can be explained by the fact that the dose of cisplatin was only 75 mg/m^2 in the S-1 arm compared to 100 mg/m^2 in the 5-FU arm. However, cisplatin and S-1 did not show superiority in overall survival when compared to cisplatin and infusional 5-FU in the treatment of advanced gastroesophageal adenocarcinoma in this study.[23]

The rationale for the differences in response to S-1 containing regimens between Asian and European/American countries is not yet known; however, this may be due to the difference in the histology (intestinal vs diffuse) of the tumor. The phase III, multicenter randomized DIGEST trial (Diffuse gastric and esophagogastric junction cancer S-1 trial) is currently recruiting participants to evaluate the safety and efficacy of S-1 and cisplatin compared to 5-FU and cisplatin in patients with metastatic diffuse gastric and GE junction cancers in the first-line setting in Europe and the United States.[24]

Alternative first-line regimens

When compared to 5-FU, leucovorin, and cisplatin, the regimen of 5-FU, leucovorin, and oxaliplatin has similar median overall survival in patients with metastatic gastroesophageal carcinoma. The combination of fluorouracil, leucovorin, and oxaliplatin was found to have reduced toxicity when compared to 5-FU, leucovorin, and cisplatin with decreased rates of anemia, vomiting, nausea, fatigue, and renal failure.[25] Capecitabine and cisplatin is noninferior for progression-free survival when compared to 5-FU and cisplatin in the first-line treatment of advanced gastric cancers.[26]

Other regimens in the first-line treatment of unresectable gastric cancer include the doublet regimens of paclitaxel and cisplatin, docetaxel and cisplatin, docetaxel and irinotecan, or the single-agent regimens of docetaxel or paclitaxel.[5]

Second Line Chemotherapy (Table 2)

The choice of a second-line chemotherapeutic regimen is dependent on what agent(s) were used in the first-line setting, as well as performance status of the patient and the side effect profile of the chemotherapy regimen. Typically, single-agent regimens are initially used. Now there are randomized trials demonstrating OS benefit compared to best supportive care (BSC) in refractory setting.

Docetaxel

Docetaxel monotherapy (75 mg/m^2, every three weeks) has been used as second-line chemotherapy for metastatic gastric adenocarcinoma after progression on fluoropyrimidine and platinum combination chemotherapy in the phase II setting. Overall, the regimen has been well-tolerated.[27]

Table 2. Selected trials for second-line therapy for advanced of metastatic gastric or gastroesophageal cancer.

Author (year)	Trial	N	Regimen	RR (%)	OS (months)	PFS/TTP (months)
Jo (2007)[27]	II	154	Docetaxel	14	7.2	2.6
Kang (2012)[32]	III	202	Irinotecan	N/A	3.8	N/A
			BSC	N/A	5.3*	N/A
Roy (2012)[66]	II	85	DI	37.5	8.6	3.8
			DF	33.3	9.4	4.4
Hironaka (2013)[29]	III	219	Paclitaxel	20.9	9.5	3.6
			Irinotecan	13.6	8.4	2.3
Fuchs (2013)[38]	III	355	Ramucirumab	48.7†	5.2*	2.1
			BSC	23.1†	3.8	1.3
Higuchi (2014)[67]	III	130	Irinotecan and cisplatin	22	10.7	3.8*
			Irinotecan	16	10.1	2.8
Wilke (2014)[39]	III	665	Ramucirumab and paclitaxel	28*	9.6*	4.4*
			Paclitaxel	16	7.4	2.9

N/A = Not available, RR = response rate, OS = overall survival, PFS = progression free survival, TTP = time to progression, BSC = best supportive care, DI = Docetaxel and Irinotecan, DF = Docetaxel and 5-FU.

† = disease control rate.

* = statistically significant *p* value in favor of regimen.

The median overall survival with docetaxel is approximately 7–8 months.[27,28] Side effects include neutropenia, fatigue, diarrhea, and peripheral neuropathy.[28]

Paclitaxel

Weekly paclitaxel can be used as second-line treatment of advanced gastric cancer after progression on a fluoropyrimidine plus platinum.[29] The randomized, open-label, phase III WJOG 4007 trial compared second-line weekly paclitaxel with biweekly irinotecan in 219 patients with advanced gastric cancer without severe peritoneal metastasis. This study did not show a statistically significant difference in overall survival between single-agent paclitaxel and single-agent irinotecan in the second-line setting.[29,30]

Irinotecan

When compared to best supportive care, single-agent irinotecan significantly prolonged overall survival in patients with metastatic or locally advanced gastroesophageal junction or gastric adenocarcinoma in a phase III multicenter randomized trial. However, this study was closed prematurely due to poor accrual.[31] In another phase III trial randomly assigning patients to salvage chemotherapy with either docetaxel or irinotecan versus best supportive care alone, the study demonstrated that salvage chemotherapy improved overall survival in patients with advanced gastric cancer who had received one or two prior chemotherapy regimens. There was no difference in median overall survival between docetaxel and irinotecan.[32]

Alternative second-line regimens

Other available regimens in the second-line treatment of unresectable gastric cancer include irinotecan and cisplatin, irinotecan and a flouropyrimidine, docetaxel and irinotecan, mitomycin and irinotecan, mitomycin and fluorouracil, or single-agent etoposide.[5]

Targeted Therapy

Targeted therapy will likely play a large role in the future treatment of gastric cancer. Agents targeting human epidermal growth factor-2 (HER-2), VEGF (vascular endothelial growth factor) receptor antagonists, EGFR (epidermal growth factor receptors), IGF-R (insulin-like growth factor receptors), the P13k/Akt/mTor pathway, the c-met pathway, and fibroblast growth factor receptors are in various stages of development at this time.

Human epidermal growth factor-2 (HER-2) inhibitors

Trastuzumab

Trastuzumab, a human monoclonal antibody against HER-2 (or ERBB2), is recommended in combination with chemotherapy in patients with advanced gastric cancer with known HER2-neu overexpression.[5] Trastuzumab interferes with the HER2 receptor's cancer-promoting effects. The ToGA (A Study of Herceptin (Trastuzumab) in Combination With Chemotherapy Compared With Chemotherapy Alone in Patients With HER2-Positive Advanced Gastric Cancer) trial was a phase III, open-label, randomized controlled trial which compared trastuzumab in combination with chemotherapy to chemotherapy alone in 594 patients with known HER2 overexpression by immunohistochemistry (IHC) or fluorescence *in-situ* hybridization (FISH). The findings from this trial showed improved median overall survival (OS) with trastuzumab in combination with chemotherapy (OS 13.8 months) versus chemotherapy alone (OS 11.1 months) in HER2-positive advanced gastric cancer.[33] Side effects were comparable in both groups, including nausea, vomiting, and neutropenia. There was no significant difference in cardiac adverse effects between groups.[33] As a result of the ToGA trial, trastuzumab is currently recommended to be used in combination with chemotherapy in HER-2 overexpressed patients with metastatic gastric cancer. At this time, the management of trastuzumab-refractory HER-2 positive gastric cancer is unknown. Currently, there is an ongoing clinical trial evaluating afatinib, an EGFR/HER2 tyrosine kinase inhibitor, in patients with trastuzumab refractory HER-2 positive metastatic or recurrent esophagogastric adenocarcinoma.[34]

Lapatinib

Lapatinib is a dual tyrosine kinase inhibitor which inhibits EGFR as well as HER-2. The LOGIC [Lapatinib Optimization Study in ErbB2 (HER2) Positive Gastric Cancer] trial was a phase III randomized, double-blind study which evaluated CapeOx (capecitabine and oxaliplatin) plus lapatinib versus CapeOx alone in the first-line setting in 545 patients with advanced upper gastrointestinal tract adenocarcinomas with HER2 amplification by FISH or IHC.

While this trial did not reach the primary endpoint for overall survival, it did show improvements in overall survival in Asian patients and patients under 60 years of age in subgroup analysis.[35] Preliminary results of the TyTAN [Lapatinib (Tykerb) with paclitaxel (Taxol) in Asian ErbB2+ (HER2+) Gastric Cancer Study] trial, a phase III randomized trial of second-line treatment of Asian patients with HER-2 positive advanced gastric cancer with lapatinib and weekly paclitaxel, showed improved objective response rate and progression-free survival when compared to paclitaxel alone. Overall survival was 11.0 months in the lapatinib plus paclitaxel arm versus 8.9 months in the paclitaxel alone group, however, this was not statistically significant.[36] Despite the fact that HER-2 amplification was required, it did not correlate with HER-2 positivity by IHC; with 35% of patients having tumors which were scored 0 or 1+ by IHC. In the preplanned subgroup analysis among patients with HER-2 or 3+ expressions, patients in the combination group had significantly improved median OS of 14 months compared to 7.6 months in single agent paclitaxel group.

VEGF (vascular endothelial growth factor) receptor antagonists

Ramucirumab

Ramucirumab is a human IgG1 monoclonal antibody and VEGF receptor 2 antagonist which targets the angiogenesis pathway, and functions by preventing ligand binding and pathway activation in endothelial cells.[37] The phase III, international, randomized double-blind placebo controlled REGARD (Ramucirumab Monotherapy for Previously Treated Advanced Gastric or Gastro-oesophageal Junction Adenocarcinoma) trial examined the role of ramucirumab in patients with advanced gastric or gastroesophageal junction adenocarcinomas with evidence of progressive disease on first-line therapy with fluoropyrimidine-containing or platinum-containing regimens. Patients in the ramucirumab plus supportive care group showed an improved median overall survival of 5.2 when compared to 3.8 months in the supportive care plus placebo group. With the exception of a higher rate of hypertension in the ramucirumab group, adverse effects were similar between groups. Ramucirumab is the first single-agent biologic therapy with a survival benefit in patients with unresectable gastric adenocarcinomas who have progressed on first-line treatment.[38]

In the combination setting, the RAINBOW (A Study of Paclitaxel With or Without Ramucirumab in Metastatic Gastric Adenocarcinoma) trial was a global, phase III, randomized, double-blind study which examined ramucirumab plus paclitaxel compared to placebo plus paclitaxel in 665 patients with metastatic gastric or GE junction adenocarcinomas in the second-line setting. In these patients, who had previously progressed on first-line platinum and fluoropyrimidine-containing regimens, there was an overall survival benefit of over two months in the ramucirumab plus paclitaxel group when compared to the paclitaxel plus placebo group (median survival: 9.6 vs. 7.4 months). Statistically significant improvement in time to progression and response rate was also seen. Common adverse events in the ramucirumab plus paclitaxel arm included neutropenia, hypertension, anemia, fatigue, abdominal pain, and asthenia.[39] To date, the RAINBOW trial is the largest trial of second-line therapy in this patient population.

Bevacizumab

The addition of bevacizumab, a recombinant humanized IgG1monoclonal antibody against VEGF, to platinum-based chemotherapy in the first-line treatment of advanced cancer has been studied in multiple phase II trials and one phase III trial, the AVAGAST (A Study of Bevacizumab in Combination With Capecitabine and Cisplatin as First-line Therapy in Patients With Advanced Gastric Cancer) study. In phase II trials, bevacizumab was fairly well-tolerated with promising response rates, progression-free survival, and overall survival trends.[40] Observed toxicities included thromboembolic events, fatigue, and neutropenia.[40,41] The randomized, double-blind, placebo-controlled AVAGAST trial evaluated the efficacy of the addition of bevacizumab to first-line chemotherapy in 774 patients with advanced gastric cancer. While median progression-free survival and overall response rate were significantly improved with bevacizumab versus placebo, the trial did not reach its primary objective for overall survival.[42] There was no significant difference in median overall survival, with OS of 12.1 months in the bevacizumab plus chemotherapy group versus 10.1 months in the placebo plus chemotherapy group (hazard ratio 0.87; 95% CI, 0.73 to 1.03; $p = 0.1002$). While initially promising, at this time there is no improvement in overall survival with the addition of bevacizumab in advanced gastric or gastroesophageal adenocarcinomas.

Sunitinib

Sunitinib is an oral, multitargeted tyrosine kinase inhibitor (TKI) of VEGF-R, platelet-derived growth factor receptors (PDGFRs), c-kit, RET, and Flt3. In the second-line setting, sunitinib has been evaluated in a phase II, open-label, multicenter study of 78 patients with advanced gastric or gastroesophageal junction adenocarcinoma. The median progression free survival with sunitinib was 2.3 months with a median OS of 6.8 months. Adverse events included thrombocytopenia, neutropenia, fatigue, anorexia, nausea, diarrhea, and stomatitis.[43] Another phase II study in 52 pretreated patients with advanced GC reported that sunitinib (50 mg/day for 4 weeks on, 2 weeks off) was well-tolerated in terms of toxicities. However, tumor response was limited, with an overall response rate of 3.9%, median PFS 1.28 months, and median OS 5.81 months.[44]

Sorafenib

Sorafenib, also a multitargeted oral tyrosine kinase inhibitor, targets VEGF-R, RET, PDGFR, Flt3, c-KIT, and colony-stimulating factor receptor 1. Sorafenib has been evaluated for the treatment of advanced gastric cancer in several studies. In the first-line setting, sorafenib was evaluated in a phase I trial in combination with capecitabine and cisplatin in a phase I trial.[45] In this study, the objective response rate was 62.5%, with median PFS of 10 months and overall survival of 14.7 months.[45] In a phase II study of 44 patients with metastatic or advanced gastric or gastroesophageal junction adenocarcinoma, sorafenib was evaluated in combination with docetaxel and cisplatin as first-line therapy. Patients had a median PFS of 5.8 months and median OS of 13.6 months.[46]

As second-line treatment of advanced gastric adenocarcinoma, the GEMCAD study was a multicenter, phase II study of sorafenib in combination with oxaliplatin in 40 patients with advanced gastric cancer who had progressed on cisplatin and fluoropyrimidine therapy. While the regimen was tolerated fairly well, the median progression-free survival was only 3 months and overall survival was 6.5 months. Given these findings, phase III trials of sorafenib in advanced gastric cancer are not being pursued at this time.[47]

Other tyrosine kinase inhibitors, such as vandetanib and telatinib, are currently being investigated in phase I/II trials.

Epidermal growth factor receptor (EGFR) inhibitors

Cetuximab

Cetuximab is a recombinant IgG1 type chimeric monoclonal antibody that binds to the extracellular domain of human EGFR and competitively inhibits the binding of EGF, and other ligands and ligand-induced tyrosine kinase autophosphorylation. The antibody–receptor interaction prevents receptor dimerization, which blocks EGFR tyrosine kinase activation.[48]

Cetuximab in combination with regimens such as FOLFOX (5-FU, leucovorin, oxaliplatin), FOLFIRI (5-FU, leucovorin, irinotecan), and with oxaliplatin and irinotecan showed promise in early phase II studies in advanced gastric adenocarcinomas.[49–51] However, recent phase II and III trials have not shown significant survival benefit with the addition of cetuximab. In a randomized phase II trial of docetaxel plus oxaliplatin (DOCOX) with or without cetuximab in patients with metastatic gastric or GE junction adenocarcinoma, there was no improvement in PFS or OS with the addition of cetuximab.[52] Finally, the phase III, randomized, open label EXPAND trial found that the addition of cetuximab to capecitabine and cisplatin in the first-line treatment of advanced gastric or gastroesophageal junction cancer provided no benefit in progression-free survival when compared to chemotherapy alone.[53]

Panitumumab

Panitumumab is a human immunoglobulin G_2 monoclonal antibody targeting EGFR. In advanced gastric cancer, the phase III REAL3 trial assessed the addition of panitumumab to EOX (epirubicin, oxaliplatin, and capecitabine) chemotherapy in previously untreated patients. Unfortunately, overall survival was higher in patients who did not receive panitumumab (EOX: 11.3 months, EOX + panitumumab: 8.8 months), and patients who received panitumumab had higher rates of grade 3–4 diarrhea, mucositis, and rash.[54] As a result, the addition of panitumumab to this standard regimen is not recommended in patients with advanced esophagogastric cancer at this time.

Other EGFR inhibitors: Matuzumab, gefitinib, erlotonib

Other EGFR inhibitors examined in gastric cancer include matuzumab, gefitinib, and erlotinib. Matuzumab has been studied in a phase I trial in combination with 5-FU, leucovorin, and cisplatin with acceptable safety profiles in EGFR positive patients with advanced gastric and gastroesophageal adenocarcinomas.[55] In a randomized, multicenter phase II trial of matuzumab in addition to ECX (epirubicin, cisplatin, and capecitabine), this combination did not show an increased response in median OS and PFS, therefore phase III trials are not being pursued at this time.[56] Gefitinib and erlotonib, both oral EGFR inhibitors, have been evaluated in small studies in addition to standard therapies, and may be more effective in cancer of the GE junction. Efficacy at this time does not appear to be related the presence of an EGFR mutation.[57]

PI3 kinase pathway inhibitors

Everolimus

Everolimus is an oral mTOR (mammalian target of rapamycin serine-threonine kinase) inhibitor which inhibits the P13K/Akt/mTOR pathway. Everolimus has previously been shown to have activity against gastric cancer in preclinical studies and in phase I trials.[58,59] In a multicenter phase II study of 53 patients with metastatic gastric cancer, everolimus had a disease control rate of 56%, PFS of 2.7 months, and median OS of 10.1 months in patients who had previously progressed on chemotherapy.[60]

Following these studies, the phase III, randomized, double-blind GRANITE-1 [Safety and Efficacy of RAD001 (Everolimus) Monotherapy Plus Best Supportive Care in Patients With Advanced Gastric Cancer] study examined everolimus versus best supportive care in 656 patients with advanced gastric cancer who had previously progressed on at least two lines of systemic chemotherapy. Everolimus did not significantly improve overall survival, with median OS of 5.4 months when compared to 4.3 months in the placebo group. Median PFS was also not significantly changed, with PFS 1.7 months with everolimus and 1.4 months in the placebo group.[61]

The combination of capecitabine and everolimus was studied in a phase II trial of patients with advanced gastric cancer who had progressed on at least two prior cytotoxic regimens. These heavily pretreated patients treated with capecitabine and everolimus had an overall response rate of 10.6% and disease control rate of 48.9%.[62] But since the single-agent everolimus has not shown improvement in PFS or OS, it dampens the enthusiasm of using everolimus in combination with other chemotherapeutic agents in future phase III trials.

C-Met tyrosine kinase inhibitors

C-Met is a cell surface receptor for hepatocyte growth factor (HGF) that is expressed in epithelial and endothelial cells, and is overexpressed in gastric cancer. HGF possesses tyrosine kinase activity, and expression of both c-Met and HER2 proteins in patients with gastric cancer has been associated with poorer survival.[63]

Foretonib

Foretonib (GSK1363089) is an oral tyrosine kinase inhibitor of c-Met and VEGFR-2 which was examined in a phase II trial in patients with advanced, previously treated gastric cancer. Unfortunately, while foretonib was well-tolerated as a single agent, no clinical benefit was seen in these patients with previously treated gastric cancer.[64] Other clinical trials of various c-MET inhibitors, such as tivantinib, are ongoing.

Tivantinib

Tivantinib is a selective small-molecule inhibitor of c-Met which has recently been studied in a phase II trial as monotherapy in second- or third-line therapy in 30 patients with metastatic gastric cancer. With tivantinib, the disease control rate was 36.7%, with median PFS of 43 days. Grade 3 or 4 toxicities included neutropenia and anemia. While tivantinib showed modest efficacy in this patient population, there was no relationship between efficacy and biomarkers such as amplification or expression of c-Met.[65]

Other targeted therapies

Research is currently ongoing in the preclinical and phase I settings for other classes of targeted agents, including fibroblast growth factor receptor (FGFR) inhibitors, Aurora tyrosine kinase inhibitors, polo-like kinase (Plk1) inhibitors, cyclin-dependent kinase inhibitors, heat shock protein 90 inhibitors, and histone deacetylase inhibitors.

Conclusions

Despite advances in research, the prognosis for metastatic gastric or gastroesophageal junction adenocarcinomas remains poor. However, the advent of recent targeted therapies is leading to a changing landscape in the treatment of advanced or metastatic gastric or GE junction cancers. At this time, the current standard of care in the first-line treatment of advanced or metastatic GE junction or gastric cancer is dependent on geographic location, but includes a platinum plus fluoropyrimidine backbone. Trastuzumab, a monoclonal antibody against HER-2, is recommended in combination with chemotherapy in patients with advanced gastric cancer and known HER2-neu overexpression.[5] However, the use of trastuzumab is limited to the 20% of patients with gastric cancer whose tumors overexpress HER2-neu. In the second-line setting, single-agent regimens such as docetaxel, paclitaxel, or irinotecan can be used, depending on patient-specific factors. New found results of the REGARD and RAINBOW trials in the second-line treatment of advanced gastric cancer have provided promising data for ramucirumab and likely will be incorporated into clinical practice.[39]

With the promising recent results of targeted agents such as trastuzumab and ramucirumab, targeted therapy is likely to play a prominent role in the treatment of advanced gastroesophageal junction and gastric cancer in the future. Clinical trials investigating new targeted agents, such as ziv-afibercept and vorinostat, are currently ongoing. More research is needed to determine other possible active agents and the most effective uses of targeted therapies, as prior studies have shown that the use of these agents in unselected patients has not been successful in improving overall survival. Further biomarker-driven trials will likely play an important role in this area. While the current prognosis of metastatic gastric or gastroesophageal junction cancer remains poor, new advances in treatment may lead to significant improvements in patient outcomes and survival.

Take Home Messages

- The absence of a widely accepted standard schedule makes it difficult to establish which is the reference regimen in first-line advanced gastric cancer but continues to include a platinum plus fluoropyrimidine backbone.
- HER2-neu status should be assessed in all patients with metastatic gastric cancer. Trastuzumab is recommended in combination with chemotherapy in HER-2 overexpressed patients with metastatic gastric cancer.
- Accumulating evidence from randomized phase III trials support using salvage chemotherapy in patients with advanced GE or gastric cancer.
- Ramucirumab has recently shown an overall survival benefit in refractory gastric cancer patients either as single agent or in combination with paclitaxel.

References

1. Jemal, A. *et al.*, Global cancer statistics. *CA Cancer J Clin*, 2011. **61**(2): 69–90.
2. Siegel, R. *et al.*, Cancer statistics, 2014. *CA*, 2014. **64**(1): 9–29.

3. SEER Cancer Statistics Factsheets: Stomach Cancer. *National Cancer Institute*. Bethesda, MD, 2013.
4. Wagner, A.D. *et al.*, Chemotherapy for advanced gastric cancer. *Cochrane Database Syst Rev*, 2010. (3): CD004064.
5. NCCN Clinical Practice Guidelines in Oncology, Version 2.2013, *Gastric Cancer*, 2013.
6. Van Cutsem, E. *et al.*, Phase III study of docetaxel and cisplatin plus fluorouracil compared with cisplatin and fluorouracil as first-line therapy for advanced gastric cancer: a report of the V325 Study Group. *J Clin Oncol*, 2006. **24**(31): 4991–7.
7. Van Cutsem, E., Boni, C. *et al.*, Randomized phase II study (GATE study) of docetaxel plus oxaliplatin with or without flourouracil or capecitabine in metastatic or locally recurrent gastric cancer (abstract). *J Clin Oncol*, 2011. **29**(Suppl 15): Abstract 4018.
8. M.A. Shah, S.S., Stoller, R.G., Kemeny, M., Ritch, P.S., Krishnamurthi, S.S., Su, Y.B., Janjigian, Y.Y., Capanu, M., Kelsen, D.P., and MSKCC Gastric Cancer Consortium, Random assignment multicenter phase II study of modified docetaxel, cisplatin, fluorouracil (mDCF) versus DCF with growth factor support (GCSF) in metastatic gastroesophageal adenocarcinoma (GE). *J Clin Oncol*, 2010. ASCO Annual Meeting Abstracts., 2010. **28**(15) (May 20 Supplement).
9. Gadgeel, S.M. *et al.*, Phase II study of paclitaxel and carboplatin in patients with advanced gastric cancer. *Am J Clin Oncol*, 2003. **26**(1): 37–41.
10. El-Rayes, B.F. *et al.*, A phase II study of carboplatin and paclitaxel in esophageal cancer. *Ann Oncol*, 2004. **15**(6): 960–5.
11. Polee, M.B. *et al.*, A phase I and pharmacokinetic study of weekly paclitaxel and carboplatin in patients with metastatic esophageal cancer. *Clin Cancer Res*, 2004. **10**(6): 1928–34.
12. Philip, P.A. *et al.*, A phase II study of carboplatin and paclitaxel in the treatment of patients with advanced esophageal and gastric cancer. *Semin Oncol*, 1997. **24**(6 Suppl 19): S19-86–8.
13. Stathopoulos, G.P. *et al.*, Paclitaxel and carboplatin in pretreated advanced gastric cancer: a phase II study. *Oncol Rep*, 2002. **9**(1): 89–92.
14. Webb, A. *et al.*, Randomized trial comparing epirubicin, cisplatin, and fluorouracil versus fluorouracil, doxorubicin, and methotrexate in advanced esophagogastric cancer. *J Clin Oncol*, 1997. **15**(1): 261–7.

15. Pluschnig, U. *et al.*, Modified EOX (Epirubicin, Oxaliplatin and Capecitabine) as palliative first-line chemotherapy for gastroesophageal adenocarcinoma. *Anticancer Res*, 2013. **33**(3): 1035–9.
16. Cunningham, D. *et al.*, Capecitabine and oxaliplatin for advanced esophago-gastric cancer. *N Engl J Med*, 2008. **358**(1): 36–46.
17. Kim, B.G. *et al.*, A phase II study of irinotecan with biweekly, low dose leucovorin and bolus and continuous infusion 5-fluorouracil (modified FOLFIRI) as first line therapy for patients with recurrent or metastatic gastric cancer. *Am J Clin Oncol*, 2010. **33**(3): 246–50.
18. Rosati, G. *et al.*, Phase II trial of a biweekly regimen of fluorouracil and leucovorin plus irinotecan in patients with previously untreated advanced gastric cancer. *J Chemother*, 2007. **19**(5): 570–6.
19. Louvet, C., G.R., Bonnetain, F. *et al.*, Final results of the intergroup FFCD-GERCOR-FNCLCC 03-07 phase III study comparing two sequences of chemotherapy in advanced gastric cancers. *ESMO* 2010, 2010. **Abstract 4585**.
20. Koizumi, W. *et al.*, S-1 plus cisplatin versus S-1 alone for first-line treatment of advanced gastric cancer (SPIRITS trial): A phase III trial. *Lancet Oncol*, 2008. **9**(3): 215–21.
21. Liu, G.F. *et al.*, S-1-based combination therapy S-1 monotherapy in advanced gastric cancer: A meta-analysis. *World J Gastroenterol*, 2014. **20**(1): 310–8.
22. Ajani, J.A. *et al.*, Combination of cisplatin/S-1 in the treatment of patients with advanced gastric or gastroesophageal adenocarcinoma: Results of non-inferiority and safety analyses compared with cisplatin/5-fluorouracil in the First-Line Advanced Gastric Cancer Study. *Eur J Cancer*, 2013. **49**(17): 3616–24.
23. Ajani, J.A. *et al.*, Multicenter phase III comparison of cisplatin/S-1 with cisplatin/infusional fluorouracil in advanced gastric or gastroesophageal adenocarcinoma study: the FLAGS trial. *J Clin Oncol*, 2010. **28**(9): 1547–53.
24. Shah, M.A. *et al.*, Phase II study of modified docetaxel, cisplatin, and fluorouracil with bevacizumab in patients with metastatic gastroesophageal adenocarcinoma. *J Clin Oncol*, 2011. **29**(7): 868–74.
25. Al-Batran, S.E. *et al.*, Phase III trial in metastatic gastroesophageal adenocarcinoma with fluorouracil, leucovorin plus either oxaliplatin or cisplatin: A

study of the Arbeitsgemeinschaft Internistische Onkologie. *J Clin Oncol*, 2008. **26**(9): 1435–42.

26. Kang, Y.K. *et al.*, Capecitabine/cisplatin versus 5-fluorouracil/cisplatin as first-line therapy in patients with advanced gastric cancer: A randomised phase III noninferiority trial. *Ann Oncol*, 2009. **20**(4): 666–73.
27. Jo, J.C. *et al.*, Docetaxel monotherapy as a second-line treatment after failure of fluoropyrimidine and platinum in advanced gastric cancer: Experience of 154 patients with prognostic factor analysis. *Jpn J Clin Oncol*, 2007. **37**(12): 936–41.
28. Lee, J.L. *et al.*, A phase II study of docetaxel as salvage chemotherapy in advanced gastric cancer after failure of fluoropyrimidine and platinum combination chemotherapy. *Cancer Chemother Pharmacol*, 2008. **61**(4): 631–7.
29. Hironaka, S. *et al.*, Randomized, open-label, phase III study comparing irinotecan with paclitaxel in patients with advanced gastric cancer without severe peritoneal metastasis after failure of prior combination chemotherapy using fluoropyrimidine plus platinum: WJOG 4007 Trial. *J Clin Oncol*, 2013.
30. Kadokura, M. *et al.*, Weekly paclitaxel as second-line chemotherapy in Japanese patients with advanced gastric cancer. *Anticancer Res*, 2013. **33**(10): 4547–52.
31. Thuss-Patience, P.C. *et al.*, Survival advantage for irinotecan versus best supportive care as second-line chemotherapy in gastric cancer — a randomised phase III study of the Arbeitsgemeinschaft Internistische Onkologie (AIO). *Eur J Cancer*, 2011. **47**(15): 2306–14.
32. Kang, J.H. *et al.*, Salvage chemotherapy for pretreated gastric cancer: A randomized phase III trial comparing chemotherapy plus best supportive care with best supportive care alone. *J Clin Oncol*, 2012. **30**(13): 1513–8.
33. Bang, Y.J. *et al.*, Trastuzumab in combination with chemotherapy versus chemotherapy alone for treatment of HER2-positive advanced gastric or gastro-oesophageal junction cancer (ToGA): A phase 3, open-label, randomised controlled trial. *Lancet*, 2010. **376**(9742): 687–97.
34. Janjigian, Y. Afatinib (BIBW 2992) in Patients With Advanced HER2-Positive Trastuzumab-Refractory Advanced Esophagogastric Cancer. February 28, 2014; Available from: www.clinicaltrials.gov.
35. Hecht, J.B., Y. *et al.*, Lapatinib in combination with capecitabine plus oxaliplatin (CapeOx) in HER2-positive advanced or metastatic gastric, esophageal,

or gastroesophageal adenocarcinoma (AC): The TRIO-013/LOGiC Trial. *ASCO Annual Meeting*. 2013. Chicago, IL.

36. Bang, Y.J., A randomized, open-label, phase III study of lapatinib in combination with weekly paclitaxel versus weekly paclitaxel alone in the second-line treatment of HER2 amplified advanced gastric cancer (AGC) in Asian population: Tytan study in 2013. *Gastrointestinal Cancers Symposium* 2013.
37. Jung, Y.D. *et al.*, Effects of combination anti-vascular endothelial growth factor receptor and anti-epidermal growth factor receptor therapies on the growth of gastric cancer in a nude mouse model. *Eur J Cancer*, 2002. **38**(8): 1133–40.
38. Fuchs, C.S. *et al.*, Ramucirumab monotherapy for previously treated advanced gastric or gastro-oesophageal junction adenocarcinoma (REGARD): An international, randomised, multicentre, placebo-controlled, phase 3 trial. *Lancet*, 2013.
39. Wilke H, V.C.E. *et al.*, RAINBOW: A global, phase III, randomized, double-blind study of ramucirumab plus paclitaxel versus placebo plus paclitaxel in the treatment of metastatic gastroesophageal junction (GEJ) and gastric adenocarcinoma following disease progression on first-line platinum- and fluoropyrimidine-containing combination therapy. *J Clin Oncol*, 2014. **32**(suppl 3; abstr LBA7).
40. Shah, M.A. *et al.*, Phase II study of modified docetaxel, cisplatin, and fluorouracil with bevacizumab in patients with metastatic gastroesophageal adenocarcinoma. *J Clin Oncol*, 2011. **29**(7): 868–74.
41. El-Rayes, B.F. *et al.*, A phase II study of bevacizumab, oxaliplatin, and docetaxel in locally advanced and metastatic gastric and gastroesophageal junction cancers. *Ann Oncol*, 2010. **21**(10):1999–2004.
42. Ohtsu, A. *et al.*, Bevacizumab in combination with chemotherapy as first-line therapy in advanced gastric cancer: A randomized, double-blind, placebo-controlled phase III study. *J Clin Oncol*, 2011. **29**(30): 3968–76.
43. Bang, Y.J. *et al.*, Phase II study of sunitinib as second-line treatment for advanced gastric cancer. *Invest New Drugs*, 2011. **29**(6): 1449–58.
44. Moehler, M. *et al.*, An open-label, multicentre biomarker-oriented AIO phase II trial of sunitinib for patients with chemo-refractory advanced gastric cancer. *Eur J Cancer*, 2011. **47**(10): 1511–20.

45. Kim, C. *et al.*, Phase I dose-finding study of sorafenib in combination with capecitabine and cisplatin as a first-line treatment in patients with advanced gastric cancer. *Invest New Drugs*, 2012. **30**(1): 306–15.
46. Sun, W. *et al.*, Phase II study of sorafenib in combination with docetaxel and cisplatin in the treatment of metastatic or advanced gastric and gastroesophageal junction adenocarcinoma: ECOG 5203. *J Clin Oncol*, 2010. **28**(18): 2947–51.
47. Martin-Richard, M. *et al.*, Multicenter phase II study of oxaliplatin and sorafenib in advanced gastric adenocarcinoma after failure of cisplatin and fluoropyrimidine treatment. A GEMCAD study. *Invest New Drugs*, 2013. **31**(6): 1573–9.
48. Martinelli, E. *et al.*, Anti-epidermal growth factor receptor monoclonal antibodies in cancer therapy. *Clin Exp Immunol*, 2009. **158**(1): 1–9.
49. Pinto, C. *et al.*, Phase II study of cetuximab in combination with FOLFIRI in patients with untreated advanced gastric or gastroesophageal junction adenocarcinoma (FOLCETUX study). *Ann Oncol*, 2007. **18**(3): 510–7.
50. Lordick, F. *et al.*, Cetuximab plus oxaliplatin/leucovorin/5-fluorouracil in first-line metastatic gastric cancer: A phase II study of the Arbeitsgemeinschaft Internistische Onkologie (AIO). *Br J Cancer*, 2010. **102**(3): 500–5.
51. Woll, E. *et al.*, Oxaliplatin, irinotecan and cetuximab in advanced gastric cancer. A multicenter phase II trial (Gastric-2) of the Arbeitsgemeinschaft Medikamentose Tumortherapie (AGMT). *Anticancer Res*, 2011. **31**(12): 4439–43.
52. Richards, D. *et al.*, Results of docetaxel plus oxaliplatin (DOCOX) +/– cetuximab in patients with metastatic gastric and/or gastroesophageal junction adenocarcinoma: results of a randomised Phase 2 study. *Eur J Cancer*, 2013. **49**(13): 2823–31.
53. Lordick, F. *et al.*, Capecitabine and cisplatin with or without cetuximab for patients with previously untreated advanced gastric cancer (EXPAND): A randomised, open-label phase 3 trial. *Lancet Oncol*, 2013. **14**(6): 490–9.
54. Waddell, T. *et al.*, Epirubicin, oxaliplatin, and capecitabine with or without panitumumab for patients with previously untreated advanced oesophago-gastric cancer (REAL3): A randomised, open-label phase 3 trial. *Lancet Oncol*, 2013. **14**(6): 481–9.

55. Trarbach, T. *et al.*, Phase I study of matuzumab in combination with 5-fluorouracil, leucovorin and cisplatin (PLF) in patients with advanced gastric and esophagogastric adenocarcinomas. *Invest New Drugs*, 2013. **31**(3): 642–52.
56. Rao, S. *et al.*, Matuzumab plus epirubicin, cisplatin and capecitabine (ECX) compared with epirubicin, cisplatin and capecitabine alone as first-line treatment in patients with advanced oesophago-gastric cancer: a randomised, multicentre open-label phase II study. *Ann Oncol*, 2010. **21**(11): 2213–9.
57. Wainberg, Z.A. *et al.*, Phase II trial of modified FOLFOX6 and erlotinib in patients with metastatic or advanced adenocarcinoma of the oesophagus and gastro-oesophageal junction. *Br J Cancer*, 2011. **105**(6): 760–5.
58. Cejka, D. *et al.*, Everolimus (RAD001) and anti-angiogenic cyclophosphamide show long-term control of gastric cancer growth in vivo. *Cancer Biol Ther*, 2008. **7**(9): 1377–85.
59. Okamoto, I. *et al.*, Phase I clinical and pharmacokinetic study of RAD001 (everolimus) administered daily to Japanese patients with advanced solid tumors. *Jpn J Clin Oncol*, 2010. **40**(1): 17–23.
60. Doi, T. *et al.*, Multicenter phase II study of everolimus in patients with previously treated metastatic gastric cancer. *J Clin Oncol*, 2010. **28**(11): 1904–10.
61. Ohtsu, A. *et al.*, Everolimus for Previously Treated Advanced Gastric Cancer: Results of the Randomized, Double-Blind, Phase III GRANITE-1 Study. *J Clin Oncol*, 2013. **31**(31): 3935–43.
62. Lee, S.J. *et al.*, Phase II trial of capecitabine and everolimus (RAD001) combination in refractory gastric cancer patients. *Invest New Drugs*, 2013. **31**(6): 1580–6.
63. Nakajima, M. *et al.*, The prognostic significance of amplification and overexpression of c-met and c-erb B-2 in human gastric carcinomas. *Cancer*, 1999. **85**(9): 1894–902.
64. Shah, M.A. *et al.*, Phase II study evaluating 2 dosing schedules of oral foretinib (GSK1363089), cMET/VEGFR2 inhibitor, in patients with metastatic gastric cancer. *PLoS One*, 2013. **8**(3): e54014.
65. Kang, Y.K. *et al.*, A phase II trial of a selective c-Met inhibitor tivantinib (ARQ 197) monotherapy as a second- or third-line therapy in the patients with metastatic gastric cancer. *Invest New Drugs*, 2014. **32**(2): 355–61.

66. Roy, A. *et al.*, Docetaxel combined with irinotecan or 5-fluorouracil in patients with advanced oesophago-gastric cancer: A randomised phase II study. *Br J Cancer*, 2012. **107**(3): 435–41.
67. Higuchi, K. *et al.*, Biweekly irinotecan plus cisplatin versus irinotecan alone as second-line treatment for advanced gastric cancer: A randomised phase III trial (TCOG GI-0801/BIRIP trial). *Eur J Cancer*, 2014.

Chapter 11

Endoscopic Diagnosis and Treatment of Colorectal Malignancies

Shuang Wu, Virginia O. Shaffer, Qiang Cai and Hong Xu

What is New

- New endoscopic imaging modalities, such as confocal laser endomicroscopy, and instruments, such as wide-angle and retroflexion colonoscopies, have been developed to detect early colorectal neoplasms.
- Endoscopic submucosal dissection (ESD) is a novel technique that enables en bloc resection of colorectal neoplasm. Many experts believe that it will someday largely replace colectomy for node-negative colorectal epithelial neoplasia.

New Endoscopic Imaging Modalities

Since the majority of colorectal carcinomas arise from premalignant adenomas, improved detection of colonic adenomas could reduce the mobidity of colorectal malignancy. Therefore, many novel imaging modalities have been applied in practice.

Narrow band imaging (NBI), fujinon intelligent chromoendoscopy (FICE), i-scan

Traditionally, chromoendoscopy with methylene blue or indigo carmine has been used for the detection and characterization of colonic polyps. However, its utility is limited by the disadvantage of cumbersome and messy dyes. Several new imaging technologies, especially narrow band imaging (NBI), have been developed to improve detection rate of adenomas, as well as differentiation from nonneoplastic lesions. i-Scan and FICE, developed by Pentax and Fujinon respectively, have similar functions as NBI. Here we introduce NBI as an illustration.

NBI is an optical filter technology that uses narrowed band widths of blue (390–445 nm) and green (530–550 nm) light waves to optimize the absorbance and scattering characteristics of light for improved visibility of capillaries, veins and other tissue structures. Four shorter wavelengths allow less light to penetrate, and thus blue light enhances surface mucosal characteristics. The enhanced contrast provided by NBI can potentially improve the detection and differentiation of colonic lesions.

A study has been conducted to determine the relative effectiveness of NBI and high-resolution white-light endoscopy (HRE) for detecting polyps. NBI had a significantly lower miss rate than HRE though most polyps detected by NBI were hyperplastic. In addition, significant higher numbers of flat and/or serrated sessile adenomas were detected by NBI compared with HRE.[1]

NBI magnifying endoscopic findings are able to reveal pit pattern, which is predictive for the histological features of colorectal neoplasm. Of note, Type VI is an index for adenoma with severe atypia or SM carcinoma. Type-VN is an index for carcinoma with deep SM invasion.

Autofluorescence imaging

Although NBI and other chromoscopic systems are considered to be effective modalities for colorectal lesions detection, they are based on the endoscopist's subject recognition, and thus, accuracy is operator dependent. A new modality — autofluorescence imaging (AFI) system — has been developed.

AFI is a technology which is capable of capturing fluorescence (500–630 nm) emitted from tissues. This device produces an excitation light source of 442 nm and delivers it to tissue surface. The reflection and fluorescence are captured by two high-sensitivity CCDs. Captured signals are transformed into red or blue, which can be displayed on the monitor as a color image in real-time. Studies have shown that the AFI system is able to facilitate differentiation of non-neoplastic lesions from neoplastic lesions. A novel autofluorescence imaging system with computer-assisted color analysis has potential in predicting the depth of invasion of colorectal neoplasia.[2]

Other novel detection modalities include optical coherence tomography (OCT), but its role is still under evaluation and several challenges must be overcome before it can be applied on a large scale.[3]

Confocal laser endomicroscopy (CLE) and endocytoscopy

Confocal laser endomicroscopy (CLE) is a high-resolution technique that allows for analysis at the cellular level. It is capable of providing a 1,000-fold magnification for *in vivo* analysis of the cell morphology and vascular pattern.

Endocytoscopy is another *in vivo* modality that enables cellular level analysis, providing 1,400-fold magnification. In contrast to CLE, which reaches up to 250 μm, endocytoscopy uses contact light microscopy and permits the study of the superficial layer, approximately 50 μm of depth. Some studies have shown high sensitivity and specificity for colon polyps as 91% and 100%, respectively.[4]

These modalities can increase the positive rate of biopsy during endoscopy; however, adequate bowel preparation is essential as presence of stool may limit imaging. Due to the limitation of flexibility, these endoscopes are mainly applied in rectal lesions and their utility is still controversial.

New Endoscopic Devices and Techniques

Colon capsule endoscopy

Conventional colonoscopy is considered to be the ideal technique for colorectal cancer (CRC) screening programs. However, participation is limited by the drawbacks of conventional colonoscopy, such as complication rate, pain, patient's embarrassment or the need of sedation. Non-invasive techniques may be an alternative to conventional colonoscopy.

Capsule endoscopy is one of the latest evolutions in gastrointestinal endoscopy which allows complete investigation of the small bowel. However, it is no longer limited in the detection of lesions in the small intestine. The colonic capsule (Pill Cam Colon) was recently developed with two lenses and cameras taking more frames from both sides. The indications for the colonic capsule examination are colorectal cancer screening and for incomplete colonoscopy.

In spite of some limitations, such as the inability to insufflate and take biopsies, colon capsule endoscopy may be complementary to conventional colonoscopy and could be an appropriate exam for those patients who have received incomplete colonoscopy, or are contraindicated or are unwilling to undergo conventional colonoscopy. Continuous studies are needed to investigate its indications, diagnostic yield, procedure-specific outcome assessment, and cost-effectiveness.

Advanced colonoscopes

Conventional colonoscopes have been widely used for colorectal lesions screening. However, cecal intubation rate vary by endoscopist and region. Furthermore, pain, complications and patient embarrassment can have negative impact on compliance of traditional colonoscopy. New colonoscopes have been developed to improve screening effectiveness, reduce pain and complications, improve *in vivo* lesion classification and increase ease of insertion.

Wide-angle and retroflexion colonoscope

There are a series of wide-angle colonoscopes, including 140°, 170° and 210° as well as a retroscope, also known as the third-eye (TER) that flexes

180° to point backward at the colonoscope to illuminate and visualize the areas behind folds and flexures.[5]

Special colonoscopic devices

Several colonoscopic instruments or accessories, including the aeroscope, the Invendo, Sightline ColonoSight system, NeoGuide Endoscopy System, Quo vadis, and the endotics system (ES), have been developed to decrease examination time, and increase tolerability for patients. These are listed below, but their role remains controversial.

Cap-fitted colonoscopy

Cecal intubation rate and time have great impact on the screening of colorectal neoplasms. A study has showed that caps can improve cecal intubation time and reduce patients' discomfort. An endoscopic cuff, a new endoscopic accessory placed around the tip of colonoscope, has been reported to improve scar assessment by flattening or depressing colon folds close to the lesion/scar.[6]

Endoscopic ultrasonography (EUS)

As developed by the International Union against Cancer (UICC) and American Joint Committee on Cancer(AJCC), the TNM staging system is commonly used in colorectal malignancies. Accurate preoperative staging of colorectal carcinoma is crucial for therapeutic strategy. Endoscopic ultrasonography (EUS) can aid in preoperative staging of lesions.

EUS has the capability to detect the gastrointestinal wall as several concentric layers and allows it to be appropriate for T stage. Identification of T1 malignancies is especially critical with the increasing application of local endoscopic therapies such as EMR, ESD, and photodynamic therapy. The role of EUS in staging is still being evaluated. A recent study has shown that EUS had higher sensitivity in T1 and specificity in T2 than MRI. MRI had higher sensitivity in N staging and was more accurate in pT1~4 N1~2 than EUS. Reference values for surgery of MRI and EUS were 79.7% vs. 76. 7%, respectively. It may be that EUS is good for early-stage cases while MRI is better for locally advanced ones.[7]

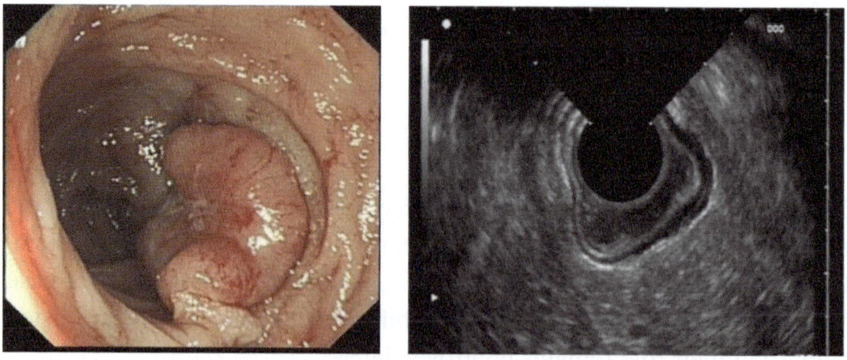

Fig 1. T1 stage rectal carcinoma.

Nevertheless, imaging examinations such MRI or CT scan are not the gold standard. EUS has an overwhelming advantage in that EUS guided fine needle aspiration (EUS-FNA) can be performed to obtain histological or cytological specimens for conclusive preoperative evaluation especially for N stage.

However, EUS for staging of colon tumors is limited by many factors. Owing to the stiffness and limitation of flexibility, cecal intubation usually cannot be achieved by standard echoendoscopes. Therefore, EUS is mainly used to stage rectal carcinomas. In addition, there are cases of rectal stenosis in which echoendoscopes cannot pass the stricture resulting in the failure of completing EUS staging. Ultrasound mini-probes may be used in these situations as alternatives in spite of their penetration limitation. It has been reported that the sensitivity and specificity for colonic carcinoma staging with ultrasound mini-probe were 0.91 and 0.98 for T1 tumors, 0.78 and 0.94 for T2 tumors, 0.97 and 0.90 for T3/T4 tumors; and 0.63 and 0.82 for nodal staging.[8]

Endoscopic Resection of Early Colorectal Neoplasm

Endoscopic resection of colorectal neoplasm includes endoscopic mucosal resection (EMR), a conventional endoscopic therapy of gastrointestinal lesions. However, accurate histopathologic evaluation of the resected specimens is essential to ensure curative potential. Therefore, en bloc resection is more desirable than piecemeal resection.

Endoscopic submucosal dissection (ESD) is a novel endoscopic approach which is increasingly accepted as standard treatment of superficial gastrointestinal neoplasms especially in Asia.

ESD is characterized by three steps: injecting fluid into the submucosa to elevate the lesion from the muscle layer, circumferential cutting of the surrounding mucosa of the lesion, and subsequent dissection of the connective tissue of the submucosa beneath the lesion.

ESD was first used in the resection of early gastric neoplasms, but in recent years ESD has been increasingly applied to the treatment of colon neoplasms. The advantage of ESD over conventional EMR is that it has the potential for a higher rate of en bloc resection regardless of tumor size, facilitating precise histopathological evaluation of the specimen margins. More and more patients will benefit from the endoscopic approach. Nevertheless, indications for ESD should be well defined. Selecting appropriate cases for ESD involves identifying invasion depth of colorectal neoplasms and risk of lymph node metastasis.

The invasion depth of colorectal neoplasms can be predicted by previously referred endoscopic observation such as NBI , magnifying endoscopy and EUS. The risk of submucosal invasion and subsequent lymph node metastasis is critical in determining whether a colorectal neoplastic lesion is appropriate for endoscopic resection.

Classification of submucosal invasion is based on the division of the submucosa (sm) into three layers of equivalent thickness, from sm1 to sm3, superficial to deep. A number of studies have shown that the rate of lymph node metastasis was extremely low (almost nil) if the submucosal depth was less than 1000 μm which corresponds to the sm1 layer.[9] Therefore, even EMR might complete curative potential in such cases since there may be almost no risk of lymph node metastasis.

The specific indications for colorectal ESD are as follows: (1) Large-sized (>20 mm in diameter) lesion in which en bloc resection with snare EMR is difficult, although it is indicative for endoscopic treatment. Nongranular-type LST (LST-NG), particularly those of the pseudodepressed type. Lesion with Vi-type pit pattern. Cancer with submucosal infiltration. Large lesion of the elevated type, suspected to be cancer.

(2) Mucosal lesions with fibrosis caused by biopsy or peristalsis of the lesions. (3) Local residual early cancer after endoscopic resection. (4) Sporadic localized tumors in chronic inflammation, e.g., ulcerative colitis.

The role of ESD for colorectal neoplasms is not as highly accepted as that for gastric neoplasms due to some factors such as operative difficulties. Further studies are needed to clarify the feasibility of ESD for colorectal lesions.

Treatment of Advanced Colorectal Malignancies

Stricture dilation

Malignant strictures are dilated primarily to aid in the successful completion of other endoscopic procedures such as palliative stent placement or endoscopic ultrasonographic tumor staging. Colorectal strictures are most common at surgical anastomoses. Although this complication can be treated effectively by surgery, this is associated with significant technical difficulties, surgical risks and the possibility of repetitive stricture. For this reason, endoscopic dilation has become increasingly widespread, and its good results have led it to become the first choice for the treatment of this condition. This treatment is effective, safe and does not involve further surgery.

Colorectal stenting

Seventy percent of all large bowel obstructions occur in left-sided lesions. Traditionally, 10–30% of these cases presenting with acute obstructive symptoms require urgent surgical decompression. However, emergency colorectal surgery is associated with certain mortality and usually includes a multistage procedure with resection and stoma formation followed by later reversion.

Colonic stenting has been applied as an alternative to surgery for malignant large bowel obstruction. Self-expandable metal stents (SEMSs) are widely used to decompress malignant colorectal obstruction and enable one-stage elective surgery. Complications after stent placement such as

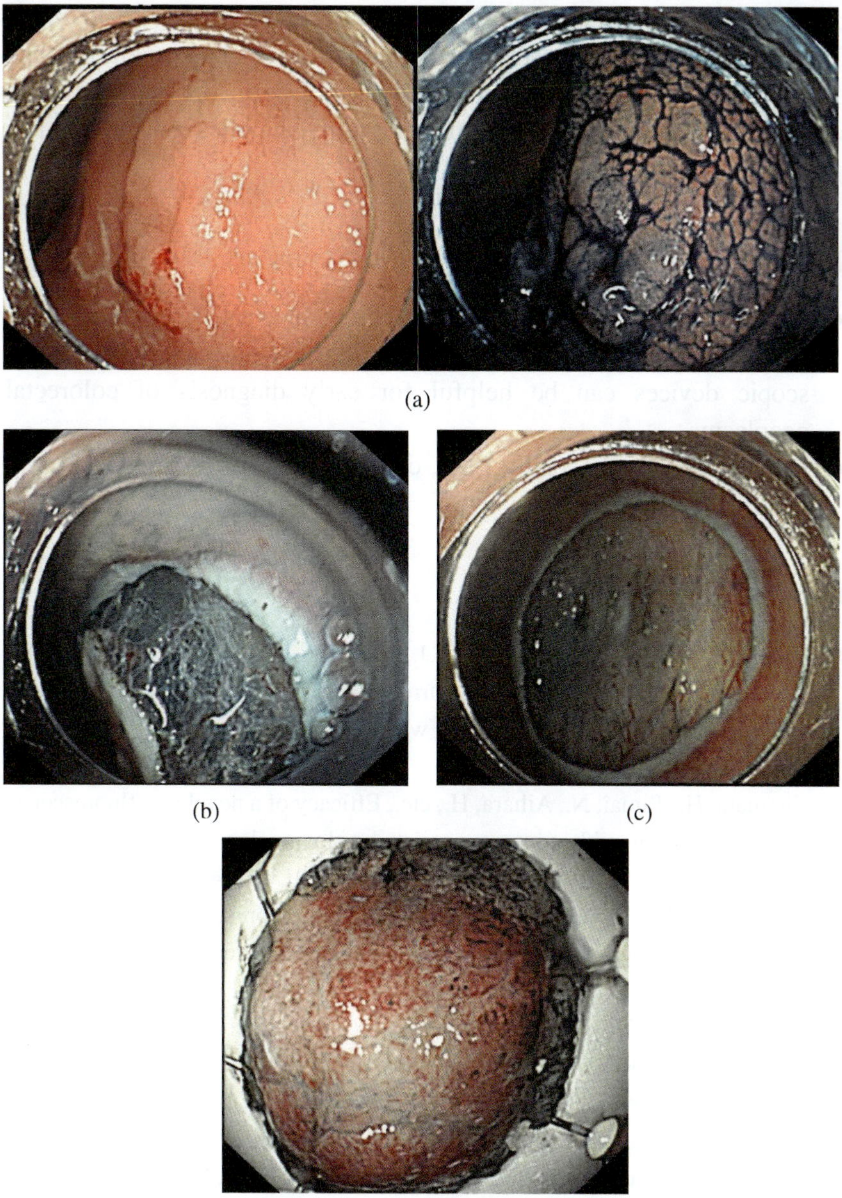

(a)

(b) (c)

(d)

Fig. 2. (a) A flat colon neoplasm. (b) Circumferential cutting of the surrounding mucosa of the neoplasm. (c) Removal of the neoplasm. (d) En bloc resected neoplasm.

bleeding, malposition and perforation can occur early after deployment. Late complications after stent placement include stent migration and occlusion. Given the limited life expectancy of the patient population in whom stents are typically placed, long-term complications or failures have been difficult to assess.

Take Home Messages

- New endoscopic imaging modalities, such as NBI, confocal laser endomicroscopy (CLE), endocytoscopy, EUS and some new endoscopic devices can be helpful for early diagnosis of colorectal neoplasms.
- EMR and ESD, especially ESD, can be useful for treatment of early carcinoma.

References

1. Boparai, K.S., van den Broek, F.J., van, E.S., Fockens, P., Dekker, E., Increased polyp detection using narrow band imaging compared with high resolution endoscopy in patients with hyperplastic polyposis syndrome. *Endoscopy*, 2011. **43**(8): 676–82.
2. Inomata, H., Tamai, N., Aihara, H., etc., Efficacy of a novel autofluorescence imaging system with computer-assisted color analysis for assessment of colorectal lesions. *World J Gastroenterology*, 2013. **19**(41): 7146–53.
3. Iftimia, N., Lyer, A.K., Hammer, D.X., etc., Fluorescence-guided optical coherence tomography imaging for colon cancer screening: a preliminary mouse study. *Biomed Opt Express*, 2012. **3**(1): 178–91.
4. Neumann, H., Fuchs, F.S., Vieth, M., Atreya, R., Siebler, J., Kiesslich, R., Neurath, M.F., Review article: *In vivo* imaging by endocytoscopy. *Aliment Pharmacol Ther*, 2011. **33**(11): 1183–93.
5. Waye, J.D., Heigh, R.I., Fleischer, D.E., Leighton, J.A., Gurudu, S., Aldrich, L.B., Li, J., Ramrakhiani, S., Edmundowicz, S.A., Early, D.S., Jonnalagadda, S., Bresalier, R.S., Kessler, W.R., Rex, D.K., A retrograde-viewing device improves detection of adenomas in the colon: A prospective efficacy evaluation. *Gastrointest Endosc*, 2010. **71**(3): 551–6.

6. Tsiamoulos, Z.P.1, Saunders, B.P., A new accessory, endoscopic cuff, improves colonoscopic access for complex polyp resection and scar assessment in the sigmoid colon. *Gastrointest Endosc*, 2012.**76**(6): 1242–5.
7. Yimei, J., Ren, Z., Lu, X., Huan, Z., A comparison between the reference values of MRI and EUS and their usefulness to surgeons in rectal cancer. *European Review for Medical and Pharmacologicalnces*, 2012. **16**(15): 2069–77.
8. Gall, T.M., Markar, S.R., Jackson, D., Haji, A., Faiz, O., Mini-probe ultrasonography for the staging of colon cancer. A systematic review and meta-analysis. *Colorectal disease*, 2014. **16**(1): 1–8.
9. Kitajimi, K., Fujimori, T., *et al.*, Correlations between lymph node metastasis and depth of submucosal invasion in submucosal invasive colorectal carcinoma: a Japanese collaborative study. *J Gastroenterol*, 2004. **39**(6): 534–43.

Chapter 12

Multimodality Management of Colorectal Malignancies Beyond Endoscopy

John D. Lyons and Virginia O. Shaffer

What is New

- Besides colonoscopy, CT colonography has been explored as an alternative for screening of colorectal cancer.
- Laparoscopy may achieve the same oncologic resection as standard open resection, with a shorter length of stay and quick return of bowel function.
- Preoperative chemoradiation therapy can significantly improve the outcome.

Introduction

The lifetime risk of developing colorectal cancer is approximately 5%. It is projected that there will be 96,830 new colon cancer cases and 40,000 new rectal cancer cases this year. Colorectal cancer is the second leading cause of death in men and women. Survival is based on stage; the earlier the stage of diagnosis, the higher the five-year observed survival rate.

CT Colonography

Screening becomes an important tool for decreasing colorectal cancer deaths. In addition to colonoscopy, other technologies such as CT colonography (CTC) are being explored as methods for colorectal cancer screening.

CTC, or "virtual colonoscopy," provides 3D reconstructions of the large bowel lumen in addition to traditional 2D images to detect polyps and advanced disease. Initial investigations into the practice suggested poor performance, with sensitivities of only 50–60%,[1,2] though improved technology and several modern studies find that CTC may be as good or better than colonoscopy for detection of even small (5–6 mm) polyps.[3–6] While it appears clear that the technology exists to accurately identify early disease with CTC, using such technology for widespread screening remains somewhat controversial. CTC is endorsed by the American Cancer Society and the American College of Radiology,[7] but is not yet recommended by current NCCN screening guidelines.[8] While detection of polyps may be excellent with CTC, how best to subsequently treat them remains in question. Large polyps (>10 mm) and more advanced lesions may be confidently identified and referred for further treatment, but smaller lesions present a greater challenge. Although the majority of small and diminutive polyps will not contain cancer, up to 10% of small polyps will have high-risk pathologic features or carcinoma,[9] and though guidelines for management of patients with multiple small polyps have been proposed,[10] consensus on surveillance or referral for biopsy has not yet been reached. Patients, however, prefer CTC to more invasive traditional colonoscopy,[6,11] and it seems likely that as technology advances and more data accumulates, CTC will find greater utilization as a first-line screening examination.

Treatments for Colorectal Cancer

The main treatments for colorectal cancer are surgery, chemotherapy, and radiation based on location and stage. Each therapy has nuances; some are beyond the scope of this chapter.

Surgery

Resection has traditionally been done in an open fashion; however, with the advances in laparoscopy, a growing number of surgeons resect colorectal malignancies laparoscopically. With the adoption of minimally invasive techniques, a number of specific oncologic questions arose. Could laparoscopy achieve the same oncologic resection as standard open resection with the same lymph node harvest? Would there be higher rates of wound or trocar site recurrence? These questions were answered by the COST trial,[12] which showed the same rates of recurrence and rates of wound recurrence at three years. Overall survival and time to recurrence at all stages were similar in both the laparoscopic and open resection groups. The laparoscopy group had a shorter length of stay, briefer use of parenteral narcotics and oral analgesics.[12] The CLASICC trial randomized patients into a laparoscopy or open resection group. They reported similar rates of in-hospital mortality, transfusion requirements, quality of life, and positive resection margin, except in the low anterior resection group.[13] A phase 3 trial randomized 1,103 patients with rectal cancer to either laparoscopic or open resection. The laparoscopic group had less intraoperative blood loss, 200 vs 400 mL ($p<0.0001$), but took longer 240 vs 188 min ($p<0.0001$). The laparoscopic group had quick return of bowel function, 2 vs 3 days ($p<0.0001$) and hospital stay was shorter, 8 vs 9 days ($p=0.036$). Completeness of resection was similar in both groups, and the median tumor distance to distal resection was also similar. Positive circumferential margin rates were also similar in both groups. In selected patients with rectal cancer treated by skilled surgeons, there is similar resection margins, completeness of resection, and safety profiles for laparoscopy and open resection.[14]

New technologies such as robotic surgery, natural orifice surgery, and single incision surgery raise similar oncologic questions that laparoscopy once did. The answer to some of these questions remains to be determined.

Chemotherapy

Approximately one-third of colon and rectal cancer patients undergoing curative resection will recur. Chemotherapy is adjuvant treatment to hopefully treat unknown microscopic disease or advanced disease not amenable to resection. Several agents have been found to have antineoplastic activity. Among these, 5-fluorouracil (5-FU) has been found to be the most effective single agent.

One of the earliest trials of adjuvant therapy was by the Veterans Administration Surgical Oncology Group randomizing 645 patients who had received surgical resection with curative intent and had no evidence of residual disease.[15] Patients were assigned to either no adjuvant treatment or to receive 5-FU and methyl-CCNU. Overall survival after the fourth year was similar in both groups. However, patients with 1 to 4 positive lymph nodes received benefit from the adjuvant therapy with 51% survival at five years vs 31% for controls.[15] Survival advantage was not seen in patient without positive lymph nodes or with more than five positive lymph nodes.

The National Surgical Adjuvant Breast and Bowel Project (NSABP) Protocol C-01 randomized 1,166 patients with Dukes B and C colon cancer to: no further treatment after curative resection or postoperative chemotherapy consisting of 5-FU, semustine, and vincristine or postoperative BCG.[16] The postoperative chemotherapy arm had overall improvement in disease-free survival and overall survival. At five years, the control group had 1.29 times the risk of treatment failure and 1.3 times the likelihood of dying than the chemotherapy group. When non-cancer related deaths were eliminated, there was no survival difference between the control group and the BCG-treated group.[16]

The North Central Cancer Treatment group randomized 401 resected stage B and C colorectal cancer patients into three groups: no adjuvant treatment or levamisole or levamisole with 5-FU.[17] This trial demonstrated reduced recurrence rates in the 5-FU + levamisole group as compared to control group, but improved survival was only seen in the stage C subset ($p=0.02$).[17] An update of this data showed the number of cancer-related deaths was reduced by 32% ($p<0.004$) for stage C colon cancer.[18] 5-fluorouracil/levamisole became generally accepted as the reference treatment for future trials.

Haller *et al.* randomized patients to low dose leucovorin (LV) + 5-FU, or high dose LV/5FU, or low dose LV, 5FU, levamisole (Lev).[19] The control arm was 5FU/Lev for 12 months. They found no difference in overall survival in the different treatment arms, but did find higher toxicity with the addition of levamisole. Additionally, they found that 6 to 8 months of treatment yielded similar results than a full 12 months of chemotherapy. Arkenau *et al.* compared a regimen of 5FU/LV *vs* 5FU/Lev in stage III curatively resected patients and found the 5FU/LV arm to have improved disease free survival 79.8 *vs* 69.3 months ($p=0.012$). The 5FU/LV arm also had increased median overall survival 88.9 *vs* 78.6 months ($p=0.003$).[20] NSABP protocol C-04 randomized stage 2 and stage 3 patients to 5FU/LV or 5FU/Lev or 5FU/LV/Lev.[21] At five years, patients in the 5FU/LV arm had improved disease survival when compared to the 5FU/Lev arm, 65% *vs* 60% ($p=0.04$). The addition of levamisole to 5FU/LV did not provide additional benefit.[21]

Oxaliplatin, a third generation platinum derivative, became a mainstay of therapy in stage 3 colon cancer with the results of the MOSAIC trial. Andre *et al.* randomized 2,246 patients who had undergone curative resection for stage 2 and stage 3 colon cancer to either 6 months of 5FU/LV or 5FU/LV + oxaliplatin.[22] The addition of oxaliplatin lead to a 23% reduction (p=0.002) in the risk of relapse and increase probability of disease free survival 78.2% *vs* 72.9% (p=0.002). The majority of the benefit was seen in the stage 3 patients.[22] Although some efficacy has been seen with the use of adjuvant therapy in stage 2 disease, it is not routinely used. High-risk features, age, genetic and tumor markers may help differentiate which stage 2 patients would benefit most from additional therapy. Trials are still ongoing.

Saltz *et al.* studied whether irinotecan (CPT-11), a topoisomerase inhibiter, had efficacy in stage 3 disease. This trial randomized 1,264 patients with stage 3 resected colon cancer to 5FU/LV or 5FU/LV + irinotecan. There was no difference in overall survival (OS) or disease free survival (DFS).[23] Colucci *et al.* examined the efficacy of the addition of irinotecan as compared to oxaliplatin in stage 4 disease (FOLFOX4 vs FOLFIRI).[24] They found no difference in overall risk of relapse, time to progression and overall survival.[24]

Antibody therapies such as bevacizumab and cetuximab, have also been tested in the treatment of colon cancer. Bevacizumab is a human monoclonal antibody that blocks vascular endothelial growth factor A and serves as an angiogenesis inhibitor. In one clinical trial, 1,401 patients with stage 4 disease were randomized to FOLFOX (5FU/LV/oxaliplatin) or XELOX (xeloda/LV/oxaliplatin) with or without the addition of bevacizumab.[25] The addition of bevacizumab improved progression-free survival (PFS) 8.0 vs 9.4 months, but there was no difference in overall survival.[25] Another trial randomized 813 patients to a regimen of irinotecan, 5-FU, leucovorin with or without bevacizumab.[26] The addition of bevacizumab improved progression-free survival 10.6 vs 6.2 months ($p<0.001$) and overall survival 20.3 *vs* 15.6 months ($p<0.001$). Cetuximab is a chimeric (mouse/human) monoclonal antibody that is an epidermal growth factor inhibitor. Jonker *et al.* examined 572 stage 4 colorectal cancer patients with EGFR expression to determine if cetuximab improved overall survival.[27] With the addition of cetuximab, overall survival was improved 6.1 *vs* 4.6 months ($p=0.005$). The study of K-ras mutations and the effect they have on response to cetuximab lead to a landmark study in gene directed cancer therapy. Karapetis *et al.* analyzed tumor samples from 394 patients who had been randomly assigned to receive cetuximab plus best supportive care or best supportive care alone.[28] In patients with wild type K-ras tumors, treatment with cetuximab led to improved overall survival 9.5 vs 4.8 months ($p<0.001$), and improved progression-free survival 3.7 *vs* 1.9 months ($p<0.001$). In patients with mutated K-ras tumors, there was no difference in overall survival or progression-free survival with the addition of cetuximab.[28] Other therapeutic agents such as regorafenib, a multikinase inhibitor, are being studied and currently used as third-line agents for treatment refractory malignancy.

Treatment for Rectal Cancer

Despite advances in adjuvant therapies, the mainstay of colorectal cancer treatment is surgery. While segmental resection for colonic and sigmoid malignancies continues today largely unchanged from practice in previous decades (with the exception of a laparoscopic approach), the surgical management of rectal cancers has changed much since the initial description of the abdomino-perineal resection in 1908.[29]

Total mesorectal excision (TME) was first introduced and publicized by Heald in 1982, in a paper titled, "The mesorectum in rectal cancer surgery — the clue to pelvic recurrence?".[30] In it, Heald describes the detailed and complete surgical excision of the entire mesorectum, a structure comprised of fatty lymphovascular surrounding the rectum itself, which in previous iterations of surgical technique had been divided and removed incompletely. By dissecting along the areolar plane between the visceral fascia of the rectum and parietal fascia of the pelvic sidewalls, mesorectum is removed undisturbed. This technique was spurned on by author's own admitted interest in surgical planes,[31] and by prior histologic examinations of mesorectal tissue which had demonstrated microscopic spread of tumor.[30] Remarkably, dissection along this "Holy Plane" and removal of the intact mesorectum allowed the authors to demonstrate a local recurrence rate of 0% at two years, with subsequent follow-up suggesting a five-year local recurrence rate of only 4%.[32] This low rate of local recurrence was in stark contrast to the established behavior of rectal cancer, when treated by surgery alone without complete mesorectal excision has been estimated to recur at a rate as high as 40–50%.[33] Notably, the patients initially treated with TME received no additional therapy in the form of radiation or chemotherapy, but were treated only with careful surgical dissection.

Worldwide use of TME gradually increased, and adoption of the technique allowed other authors and institutions to report similar decreases in rates of local recurrence and improvements in survival,[34–36] eventually solidifying TME as the gold-standard technique for the resection of rectal cancer. Although no randomized trails have been performed comparing TME to prior surgical approaches, and while many of the investigations or trials of TME are retrospective or poorly controlled statistically,[37] the consistency with which adoption of TME has resulted in improving outcomes is overwhelming.[36,38–40] Moreover, lymphoscintigraphy confirms potential mesorectal spread of tumor cells, and the radial margin of resected specimens predicts risk of local recurrence, offering further intuitive support for the basis of mesorectal excision in the treatment of rectal cancers.[41,42]

In addition to TME, radiotherapy offers further benefit to the patient with rectal cancer. Colonic malignancies are not typically amenable to radiation, given the mobile nature of the colon within the peritoneum. The rectum, however, is fixed within the pelvis, allowing radiotherapy to be accurately targeted to rectal malignancies. In recent years, the role of radiation therapy, and combined chemoradiotherapy, has been increasingly clarified. Several large clinical trials have demonstrated that treating rectal cancers with preoperative radiation or chemoradiation can decrease the rate of local disease recurrence, though long-term survival may not be improved.[43–47] The Dutch TME trial, which compared those treated with preoperative radiation and TME to TME alone, showed a two-year recurrence rate of 2.4% in the radiation group, as opposed to 8.2% in the group treated only with surgery.[45] Data from this and other trials has led the NCCN, the American Society of Colon and Rectal Surgeons (ASCRS) and European S3 guidelines to recommend the use of neoadjuvant therapy for the treatment of locally advanced rectal cancer.[48–51]

There remains, however, a substantial amount of debate and ambiguity about which rectal tumors should undergo preoperative treatment. While the data from numerous trials demonstrate improved outcomes with neo-adjuvant radiation and chemoradiation for middle- and low-rectal malignancies, the question of what to do about upper rectal tumors is without a definitive answer.

The basis of the problem is anatomical. The rectum is a pelvic organ, usually 12–15 cm long and lying along the posterior pelvic wall, extending from the sigmoid colon downward toward the anal canal.[52] In contrast to the sigmoid colon more proximally, the rectum is not intraperitoneal. As the fully-peritonealized colon descends toward the pelvis and passes over the sacral promontory, its peritoneal lining reflects back along the walls of the abdominal cavity, leaving the rectum only partially covered, and only on the more proximal portions. The proximal or upper third of the rectum is covered by peritoneum on its anterior and lateral surfaces, while the middle third maintains only an anterior peritoneal lining. The remainder of the rectum (the distal third, the majority of the middle rectum, and the entirely of its posterior length) is completely extraperitoneal, and continues caudally until merging with the anal canal.

Reaching a consensus definition of the rectum, and more specifically its boundaries, in regular and reproducible terms has proven surprisingly difficult. The American Society of Colon and Rectal Surgeons sets forth practice parameters that mention both the splaying of the taeniae coli and passage of the rectosigmoid colon over the sacral promontory as "anatomic" proximal boundaries of the rectum, and further mention that any lesion less than 15 cm from the anal verge on rigid proctoscopy should be classified as "rectal."[49] The aforementioned trials that established the role of neoadjuvant therapy did not include strict definitions of the proximal rectal boundary, but rather defined "upper rectal" tumors as either >10 cm or 10.1–15 or 16 cm from the anal verge. The National Cancer Institute 2000 Guidelines for Colon and Rectal Surgery stated that anything above 12 cm should be treated as colon,[53] implying a more restrictive upper border. This lack of consistency is not only seen in the scientific literature, but is also commonplace in practice. A revealing telephone investigation noted that when surgeons were asked to define the proximal boundary of the rectum, a fairly even distribution of responses was found between the peritoneal reflection, the coalescence of the teniae, the "rectosigmoid junction" and a given distance from the anal verge.[54] While many may invoke the peritoneal reflection as reliable landmark, this "fixture" itself is quite variable, as has been demonstrated in both post-mortem and *in vivo* investigations.[55,56]

This question of rectal and peritoneal anatomy is not trivial. The location of a tumor along the rectosigmoid axis, and variations in peritoneal coverage at that given location, can directly affect tumor staging and treatment. Simply applying a "cutoff" value of 15 cm can easily result in the overstaging and subsequent overtreatment of what is in actuality a completely peritonealized distal colon tumor, and likewise could result in undertreatment of a partially peritonealized rectal tumor.

Moreover, close inspection of the trials establishing benefit of preoperative radiation and chemotherapy reveals conflicting information regarding what should be done with lesions that fall just under 15 cm, or within the upper rectum. The benefit to preoperative radiotherapy shown in the Dutch TME trial was lost when only tumors of the upper third (10.1–15 cm) were considered.[45] The Swedish trial similarly showed a benefit of neoadjuvant XRT over surgery alone, but noted no significant decrease in local recurrence rate for tumors >10 cm from the anal verge.[44] These data would seem to argue that upper rectal lesions, or lesions 10–15 cm from the anal verge at proctoscopy, would potentially best be managed by surgical resection alone, sparing patients the risk of toxicity associated with radiation and chemotherapy. Indeed, data prior to these trials had already suggested that tumors of the upper rectum, when treated without radiation, recur locally and cause cancer-related death significantly less frequently than lower rectal cancers, and at rates similar to surgically excised sigmoid lesions.[57]

There is, however, data to argue the counterpoint. The German trial, in which T3, T4 or node-positive disease was randomized to receive either pre- or post-operative chemoradiotherapy, noted on long-term follow-up that pre- or post-operatively treated upper rectal lesions (10–16 cm), had 10-year local recurrence rates of 2.5% and 2.7%, as opposed to 10.4% when treated with excision alone.[58] This would seem to argue that upper rectal malignancies do benefit from neoadjuvant treatment, and that perhaps they are better treated in the same manner as mid- and low-rectal tumors. Another trial published in 2009 comparing preoperative to selective postoperative chemoradiotherapy demonstrated that, in terms of local recurrence, upper rectal lesions benefited significantly from preoperative treatment, again arguing that they be treated as rectal cancers and not as sigmoid cancers.[46] Further study has suggested that in terms of cancer-specific survival, upper rectal cancers behave significantly more like middle rectal cancers, and that perhaps strategic scoring systems to identify high-risk upper lesions may be useful in determining which patients with upper rectal cancer may benefit from neoadjuvent treatment.[59]

Overall, there is insufficient data to make a clear, evidence-based recommendation on the treatment of upper rectal cancer. The transition of what is a "sigmoid" cancer vs. a "rectal" cancer is unclear and inconsistently defined. Even if a clear distinction were to be made, there is confusing data on the behavior of "upper rectal" cancers. While U.S. guidelines may suggest treating upper rectal cancers effectively as sigmoid lesions,[53] and while there is some amount of evidence to support this approach, the data is hardly overwhelming, and it is likely that some patients with tumors that would benefit from radiation or chemotherapy preoperatively are undergoing simple surgical resection, while others are being subjected to the risks of neoadjuvant chemoradiotherapy unnecessarily. Though factors such as quadrant location of a tumor or histopathological characteristics may be able to offer at least some guidance as to which patients with locally advanced malignancies in this region would benefit from preoperative treatment,[59,60] these lesions are best managed by careful consideration on a patient-to-patient basis.

Similar ambiguity exists with regard to practice of local excision for rectal lesions. Along with adjuvant therapies, endoscopic and transanal surgical techniques have advanced. LAR and APR are significant surgical procedures with defined morbidity and mortality, and the impetus for less invasive surgery is easily understood. The risk of local excision, however, is clear: while en bloc resection allows for removal of regional lymph nodes, local excision does not and residual disease may be left behind.

Local resection vs chemoradiation therapy

Determining preoperatively which patients have tumor confined to bowel wall and which patients have lymph node disease is difficult. Endoscopic ultrasonography (EUS) and MRI may reliably assess depth of tumor penetration, though report accuracies vary from 70% to upwards of 90%,[61,62] or perhaps even higher with newer MRI technology.[63] Similar variability for both modalities is seen in accuracy for nodal spread, with reported values ranging from 60–90%.[61,64] Though newer studies suggest that MRI is becoming more accurate, detecting nodal spread at accuracies above 90%,[65,66] a small series published by Park in 2014 found that MRI missed 35% of nodes harvested at time of resection, and that 15% of these contained metastases.[64] Such shortcomings are magnified by data that finds nodal involvement in 10% of T1 lesions, and in 17% of T2 lesions.[67] Furthermore, though certain histopathological characteristics confer increased risk for nodal involvement, they cannot predict nodal spread with useful clinical accuracy.[68] Given the limitations in preoperative staging, proceeding with local excision, even for early lesions, entails significant risk.

Perhaps not surprisingly, initial long-term follow-up of local resection showed poorer results as compared to radical resection. A review from Chang in 2008 examined results from five comparative investigations and found that local excision consistently demonstrated a higher rate of local recurrence, as well as decreased five-year survival.[69] Similar data suggests local recurrence rates of 12–25% for local excision of T1 lesions versus less than 7% with radical resection. Even poorer results were seen for locally excised T2 lesions, with local recurrence rates nearing 50%.[70–72]

It should be noted, however, that these trials did not include the use of preoperative chemoradiation.

When neoadjuvant treatment is included, outcomes are significantly improved. Studies of preoperative therapy have demonstrated results nearly equivocal to traditional management. One Italian study found no difference in five-year local recurrence or survival when T2N0 tumors were randomized to transanal excision or laparoscopic resection, and another demonstrated three-year disease-free survival of 91% when patients with complete clinical response to neoadjuvant chemoradiation were treated with local excision.[73,74] The distinction of complete clinical response to treatment is an important one. It is prognostic of improved disease-free survival, and investigations have suggested that when complete responders are treated with local excision, outcomes are not significantly different from traditional resection.[75–78] Studies that included incomplete response treated with local excision are less encouraging; though Callender noted no difference in 10-year actuarial local recurrence between local and radical resection (10.6% vs 7.6%, p=0.52), Yu found three-year disease-free survival to be only 85% when T2-3N0 patients underwent neoadjuvant chemoradiation and local resection.[79,80] Similar data indicates a potential recurrence rate of 33% if incomplete responders with T2N0 lesions were to be treated with local surgery.[81] Several investigators have demonstrated that a complete response may be anticipated in roughly 30% of patients treated preoperatively, and is perhaps in these patients that local excision is best utilized.[82–85] Some authors have even suggested that when small tumors respond completely to therapy, non-operative management and observation may be pursued.[76,83] Although NCCN guidelines do not currently include preoperative chemoradiation followed by local excision or observation for small rectal tumors, it seems likely that as larger trials are completed more conservative surgical management will find a place in the treatment of colorectal cancer.[48]

Take Home Messages

- The modern treatment of colorectal cancer includes surgery, chemotherapy, and radiation based on location and stage.

- Laparoscopic operations have proven safe and effective, offering equivalent oncologic outcomes with decreased morbidity. Conclusive results for robotic surgery are still to be obtained. Colon cancers can be treated with segmental resection, and rectal cancers should be removed with total mesorectal excision, a technique that decreases recurrence and improves survival.
- Newer techniques of local or trans-anal excision of early rectal lesions may offer decreased surgical morbidity, but also increase risk of disease recurrence, some of which may be mitigated by neoadjuvant chemoradiation.
- Postoperative chemotherapy should be given to patients with advanced cancers of both the colon and rectum, while rectal cancers will benefit additionally from pre- and post-operative radiation therapy.
- Metastatic colorectal lesions should be tested for genetic mutations, as certain gene profiles have been shown to guide therapy, and newer treatments such as monoclonal antibodies directed at tumor growth factors may also offer some benefit to patients with stage IV disease.

References

1. Cotton, P.B. *et al.*, Computed tomographic colonography (virtual colonoscopy): A multicenter comparison with standard colonoscopy for detection of colorectal neoplasia. *JAMA*, 2004. **291**(14): 1713–9.
2. Rockey, D.C. *et al.*, Analysis of air contrast barium enema, computed tomographic colonography, and colonoscopy: Prospective comparison. *Lancet*, 2005. **365**(9456): 305–11.
3. Pickhardt, P.J. *et al.*, Computed tomographic virtual colonoscopy to screen for colorectal neoplasia in asymptomatic adults. *N Engl J Med*, 2003. **349**(23): 2191–200.
4. Kim, D.H. *et al.*, CT colonography versus colonoscopy for the detection of advanced neoplasia. *N Engl J Med,* 2007. **357**(14): 1403–12.
5. Atkin, W. *et al.*, Computed tomographic colonography versus colonoscopy for investigation of patients with symptoms suggestive of colorectal cancer (SIGGAR): A multicentre randomised trial. *Lancet*, 2013. **381**(9873): 1194–202.

6. Graser, A. *et al.*, Comparison of CT colonography, colonoscopy, sigmoidoscopy and faecal occult blood tests for the detection of advanced adenoma in an average risk population. *Gut*, 2009. **58**(2): 241–8.
7. Levin, B. *et al.*, Screening and surveillance for the early detection of colorectal cancer and adenomatous polyps, 2008: A joint guideline from the American Cancer Society, the US Multi-Society Task Force on Colorectal Cancer, and the American College of Radiology. *Gastroenterology*, 2008. **134**(5): 1570–95.
8. NCCN Clinical Practice Guidelines in Oncology: Colorectal Cancer Screening. Version 2, 2013.
9. Butterly, L.F. *et al.*, Prevalence of clinically important histology in small adenomas. *Clin Gastroenterol Hepatol*, 2006. **4**(3): 343–8.
10. Zalis, M.E. *et al.*, CT colonography reporting and data system: A consensus proposal. *Radiology*, 2005. **236**(1): 3–9.
11. Pickhardt, P.J. *et al.*, Colorectal cancer: CT colonography and colonoscopy for detection — systematic review and meta-analysis. *Radiology*, 2011. **259**(2): 393–405.
12. Clinical Outcomes of Surgical Therapy Study Group, A comparison of laparoscopically assisted and open colectomy for colon cancer. *N Engl J Med*, 2004. **350**(20): 2050–9.
13. Guillou, P.J. *et al.*, Short-term endpoints of conventional versus laparoscopic-assisted surgery in patients with colorectal cancer (MRC CLASICC trial): Multicentre, randomised controlled trial. *Lancet*, 2005. **365**(9472): 1718–26.
14. van der Pas, M.H. *et al.*, Laparoscopic versus open surgery for rectal cancer (COLOR II): Short-term outcomes of a randomised, phase 3 trial. *Lancet Oncol*, 2013. **14**(3): 210–8.
15. Higgins, Jr., G.A. *et al.*, Efficacy of prolonged intermittent therapy with combined 5-fluorouracil and methyl-CCNU following resection for carcinoma of the large bowel. A Veterans Administration Surgical Oncology Group report. *Cancer*, 1984. **53**(1): 1–8.
16. Wolmark, N. *et al.*, Postoperative adjuvant chemotherapy or BCG for colon cancer: Results from NSABP protocol C-01. *J Natl Cancer Inst*, 1988. **80**(1): 30–6.
17. Laurie, J.A. *et al.*, Surgical adjuvant therapy of large-bowel carcinoma: An evaluation of levamisole and the combination of levamisole and fluorouracil. The North Central Cancer Treatment Group and the Mayo Clinic. *J Clin Oncol*, 1989. **7**(10): 1447–56.

18. Moertel, C.G. *et al.*, Levamisole and fluorouracil for adjuvant therapy of resected colon carcinoma. *N Engl J Med*, 1990. **322**(6): 352–8.
19. Haller, D.G. *et al.*, Phase III study of fluorouracil, leucovorin, and levamisole in high-risk stage II and III colon cancer: Final report of Intergroup 0089. *J Clin Oncol*, 2005. **23**(34): 8671–8.
20. Arkenau, H.T. *et al.*, 5-Fluorouracil plus leucovorin is an effective adjuvant chemotherapy in curatively resected stage III colon cancer: Long-term follow-up results of the adjCCA-01 trial. *Ann Oncol*, 2003. **14**(3): 395–9.
21. Wolmark, N. *et al.*, Clinical trial to assess the relative efficacy of fluorouracil and leucovorin, fluorouracil and levamisole, and fluorouracil, leucovorin, and levamisole in patients with Dukes' B and C carcinoma of the colon: Results from National Surgical Adjuvant Breast and Bowel Project C-04. *J Clin Oncol*, 1999. **17**(11): 3553–9.
22. Andre, T. *et al.*, Oxaliplatin, fluorouracil, and leucovorin as adjuvant treatment for colon cancer. *N Engl J Med*, 2004. **350**(23): 2343–51.
23. Saltz, L.B. *et al.*, Irinotecan fluorouracil plus leucovorin is not superior to fluorouracil plus leucovorin alone as adjuvant treatment for stage III colon cancer: Results of CALGB 89803. *J Clin Oncol*, 2007. **25**(23): 3456–61.
24. Colucci, G. *et al.*, Phase III randomized trial of FOLFIRI versus FOLFOX4 in the treatment of advanced colorectal cancer: A multicenter study of the Gruppo Oncologico Dell'Italia Meridionale. *J Clin Oncol*, 2005. **23**(22): 4866–75.
25. Saltz, L.B. *et al.*, Bevacizumab in combination with oxaliplatin-based chemotherapy as first-line therapy in metastatic colorectal cancer: A randomized phase III study. *J Clin Oncol*, 2008. **26**(12): 2013–9.
26. Hurwitz, H. *et al.*, Bevacizumab plus irinotecan, fluorouracil and leucovorin for metastatic colorectal cancer. *N Engl J Med*, 2004. **350**(23): 2335–42.
27. Jonker, D.J. *et al.*, Cetuximab for the treatment of colorectal cancer. *N Engl J Med*, 2007. **357**(20): 2040–8.
28. Karapetis, C.S. *et al.*, K-ras mutations and benefit from cetuximab in advanced colorectal cancer. *N Engl J Med*, 2008. **359**(17): 1757–65.
29. Miles, W.E., A method of performing abdomino-perineal excision for carcinoma of the rectum and of the terminal portion of the pelvic colon. *Lancet*, 1908. **2**:1812–3.
30. Heald, R.J., Husband, E.M., and Ryall, R.D., The mesorectum in rectal cancer surgery — the clue to pelvic recurrence? *Br J Surg*, 1982. **69**(10): 613–6.

31. Heald, R.J., The 'Holy Plane' of rectal surgery. *J R Soc Med*, 1988. **81**(9): 503–8.
32. MacFarlane, J.K., Ryall, R.D., and Heald, R.J., Mesorectal excision for rectal cancer. *Lancet*, 1993. **341**(8843): 457–60.
33. McCall, J.L., Cox, M.R., and Wattchow, D.A., Analysis of local recurrence rates after surgery alone for rectal cancer. *Int J Colorectal Dis*, 1995. **10**(3): 126–32.
34. Bulow, S. *et al.*, Recurrence and survival after mesorectal excision for rectal cancer. *Br J Surg*, 2003. **90**(8): 974–80.
35. Havenga, K. *et al.*, Improved survival and local control after total mesorectal excision or D3 lymphadenectomy in the treatment of primary rectal cancer: An international analysis of 1411 patients. *Eur J Surg Oncol*, 1999. **25**(4): 368–74.
36. Enker, W.E., Total mesorectal excision — the new golden standard of surgery for rectal cancer. *Ann Med*, 1997. **29**(2): 127–33.
37. Dent, O.F. *et al.*, Methodology and reporting in studies of local recurrence after curative excision of the rectum for cancer. *Br J Surg*, 2001. **88**(11): 1476–80.
38. Enker, W.E. *et al.*, Total mesorectal excision in the operative treatment of carcinoma of the rectum. *J Am Coll Surg*, 1995. **181**(4): 335–46.
39. Soreide, O. and Norstein, J., Local recurrence after operative treatment of rectal carcinoma: A strategy for change. *J Am Coll Surg*, 1997. **184**(1): 84–92.
40. Arbman, G. *et al.*, Local recurrence following total mesorectal excision for rectal cancer. *Br J Surg*, 1996. **83**(3): 375–9.
41. Sterk, P. *et al.*, Lymphoscintigraphy in patients with primary rectal cancer: The role of total mesorectal excision for primary rectal cancer — a lymphoscintigraphic study. *Int J Colorectal Dis*, 2002. **17**(3): 137–42; discussion 143.
42. Quirke, P. *et al.*, Local recurrence of rectal adenocarcinoma due to inadequate surgical resection. Histopathological study of lateral tumour spread and surgical excision. *Lancet*, 1986. **2**(8514): 996–9.
43. Sauer, R. *et al.*, Preoperative versus postoperative chemoradiotherapy for rectal cancer. *N Engl J Med*, 2004. **351**(17): 1731–40.
44. Folkesson, J. *et al.*, Swedish Rectal Cancer Trial: long lasting benefits from radiotherapy on survival and local recurrence rate. *J Clin Oncol*, 2005. **23**(24): 5644–50.

45. Kapiteijn, E. *et al.*, Preoperative radiotherapy combined with total mesorectal excision for resectable rectal cancer. *N Engl J Med*, 2001. **345**(9): 638–46.
46. Sebag-Montefiore, D. *et al.*, Preoperative radiotherapy versus selective postoperative chemoradiotherapy in patients with rectal cancer (MRC CR07 and NCIC-CTG C016): A multicentre, randomised trial. *Lancet*, 2009. **373**(9666): 811–20.
47. Peeters, K.C. *et al.*, The TME trial after a median follow-up of 6 years: Increased local control but no survival benefit in irradiated patients with resectable rectal carcinoma. *Ann Surg*, 2007. **246**(5): 693–701.
48. NCCN Clinical Practice Guidelines in Oncology: Rectal Cancer. Version 3. 2014.
49. Monson, J.R. *et al.*, Practice parameters for the management of rectal cancer (revised). *Dis Colon Rectum*, 2013. **56**(5): 535–50.
50. Schmiegel, W. *et al.*, S3-Guidelines Conference "Colorectal Carcinoma" 2004. *Z Gastroenterol*, 2004. **42**(10):1129–77.
51. Valentini, V. *et al.*, Multidisciplinary Rectal Cancer Management: 2nd European Rectal Cancer Consensus Conference (EURECA-CC2). *Radiother Oncol*, 2009. **92**(2): 148–63.
52. *Greenfield's Surgery*. 2011, Philadelphia: Lippincott Williams and Wilkins.
53. Nelson, H. *et al.*, Guidelines 2000 for colon and rectal cancer surgery. *J Natl Cancer Inst*, 2001. **93**(8): 583–96.
54. McMullen, T.P. *et al.*, The investigation of primary rectal cancer by surgeons: Current pattern of practice. *Can J Surg*, 2005. **48**(1): 19–26.
55. Kinugasa, Y. *et al.*, Histological identification of fascial structures posterolateral to the rectum. *Br J Surg*, 2007. **94**(5): 620–6.
56. Najarian, M.M. *et al.*, Determination of the peritoneal reflection using intraoperative proctoscopy. *Dis Colon Rectum*, 2004. **47**(12): 2080–5.
57. Lopez-Kostner, F. *et al.*, Total mesorectal excision is not necessary for cancers of the upper rectum. *Surgery*, 1998. **124**(4): 612–617; discussion 617–8.
58. Sauer, R. *et al.*, Preoperative versus postoperative chemoradiotherapy for locally advanced rectal cancer: Results of the German CAO/ARO/AIO-94 randomized phase III trial after a median follow-up of 11 years. *J Clin Oncol*, 2012. **30**(16): 1926–33.
59. Rosenberg, R. *et al.*, Does a rectal cancer of the upper third behave more like a colon or a rectal cancer? *Dis Colon Rectum*, 2010. **53**(5): 761–70.

60. Popek, S. *et al.*, Preoperative radiation therapy for upper rectal cancer T3,T4/Nx: selectivity essential. *Clin Colorectal Cancer*, 2012. **11**(2): 88–92.
61. Schaffzin, D.M. and Wong, W.D., Endorectal ultrasound in the preoperative evaluation of rectal cancer. *Clin Colorectal Cancer*, 2004. **4**(2): 124–32.
62. Garcia-Aguilar, J. and Holt, A., Optimal management of small rectal cancers: TAE, TEM, or TME? *Surg Oncol Clin N Am*, 2010. **19**(4): 743–60.
63. Group, M.S., Diagnostic accuracy of preoperative magnetic resonance imaging in predicting curative resection of rectal cancer: Prospective observational study. *BMJ*, 2006. **333**(7572): 779.
64. Park, J.S. *et al.*, Accuracy of preoperative MRI in predicting pathology stage in rectal cancers: Node-for-node matched histopathology validation of MRI features. *Dis Colon Rectum*, 2014. **57**(1): 32–8.
65. Hunerbein, M. *et al.*, Prospective comparison of endorectal ultrasound, three-dimensional endorectal ultrasound, and endorectal MRI in the preoperative evaluation of rectal tumors. Preliminary results. *Surg Endosc*, 2000. **14**(11): 1005–9.
66. Matsuoka, H. *et al.*, Comparison between endorectal coil and pelvic phased-array coil magnetic resonance imaging in patients with anorectal tumor. *Am J Surg*, 2003. **185**(4): 328–32.
67. Blumberg, D. *et al.*, All patients with small intramural rectal cancers are at risk for lymph node metastasis. *Dis Colon Rectum*, 1999. **42**(7): 881–5.
68. Chang, H.C. *et al.*, Risk factors for lymph node metastasis in pT1 and pT2 rectal cancer: A single-institute experience in 943 patients and literature review. *Ann Surg Oncol*, 2012. **19**(8): 2477–84.
69. Chang, A.J. *et al.*, Early rectal cancer: Local excision or radical surgery? *J Surg Educ*, 2008. **65**(1): 67–72.
70. Mellgren, A. *et al.*, Is local excision adequate therapy for early rectal cancer? *Dis Colon Rectum*, 2000. **43**(8): 1064–1071; discussion 1071–4.
71. You, Y.N. *et al.*, Is the increasing rate of local excision for stage I rectal cancer in the United States justified? A nationwide cohort study from the National Cancer Database. *Ann Surg*, 2007. **245**(5): 726–33.
72. De Graaf, E.J. *et al.*, Transanal endoscopic microsurgery versus total mesorectal excision of T1 rectal adenocarcinomas with curative intention. *Eur J Surg Oncol*, 2009. **35**(12): 1280–5.
73. Lezoche, G. *et al.*, A prospective randomized study with a 5-year minimum follow-up evaluation of transanal endoscopic microsurgery versus laparoscopic

total mesorectal excision after neoadjuvant therapy. *Surg Endosc*, 2008. **22**(2): 352–8.

74. Pucciarelli, S. *et al.*, Local excision after preoperative chemoradiotherapy for rectal cancer: results of a multicenter phase II clinical trial. *Dis Colon Rectum*, 2013. **56**(12): 1349–56.
75. Maas, M. *et al.*, Long-term outcome in patients with a pathological complete response after chemoradiation for rectal cancer: A pooled analysis of individual patient data. *Lancet Oncol*, 2010. **11**(9): 835–44.
76. Habr-Gama, A. *et al.*, Operative versus nonoperative treatment for stage 0 distal rectal cancer following chemoradiation therapy: Long-term results. *Ann Surg*, 2004. **240**(4): 711–717; discussion 717–8.
77. Kundel, Y. *et al.*, Is local excision after complete pathological response to neoadjuvant chemoradiation for rectal cancer an acceptable treatment option? *Dis Colon Rectum*, 2010. **53**(12): 1624–31.
78. de Campos-Lobato, L.F. *et al.*, Pathologic complete response after neoadjuvant treatment for rectal cancer decreases distant recurrence and could eradicate local recurrence. *Ann Surg Oncol*, 2011. **18**(6): 1590–8.
79. Yu, C.S. *et al.*, Local excision after neoadjuvant chemoradiation therapy in advanced rectal cancer: A national multicenter analysis. *Am J Surg*, 2013. **206**(4): 482–7.
80. Callender, G.G. *et al.*, Local excision after preoperative chemoradiation results in an equivalent outcome to total mesorectal excision in selected patients with T3 rectal cancer. *Ann Surg Oncol,* 2010. **17**(2): 441–7.
81. Perez, R.O. *et al.*, Local excision for ypT2 rectal cancer--much ado about something. *J Gastrointest Surg*, 2007. **11**(11): 1431–1438; discussion 1438–40.
82. Garcia-Aguilar, J. *et al.*, A phase II trial of neoadjuvant chemoradiation and local excision for T2N0 rectal cancer: Preliminary results of the ACOSOG Z6041 trial. *Ann Surg Oncol*, 2012. **19**(2): 384–91.
83. O'Neill, B.D. *et al.*, Non-operative treatment after neoadjuvant chemoradiotherapy for rectal cancer. *Lancet Oncol*, 2007. **8**(7): 625–33.
84. Chau, I. *et al.*, Neoadjuvant capecitabine and oxaliplatin followed by synchronous chemoradiation and total mesorectal excision in magnetic resonance imaging-defined poor-risk rectal cancer. *J Clin Oncol,* 2006. **24**(4): 668–74.
85. Mohiuddin, M. *et al.*, Randomized phase II study of neoadjuvant combined-modality chemoradiation for distal rectal cancer: Radiation Therapy Oncology Group Trial 0012. *J Clin Oncol*, 2006. **24**(4): 650–5.

Chapter 13

Multimodality Management of Oligometastatic Colorectal Cancer

Teviah E. Sachs and Timothy M. Pawlik

What is New

- The role of multimodality treatment for oligometastatic disease is expanding.
- The past decade has seen significant advancements in the therapy of colorectal liver metastasis (CRLM). Improvements in surgical devices, surgical techniques, as well as systemic therapies have broadened the pool of patients with CRLM who are potentially resectable.
- Enhanced ablation and embolization techniques have advanced treatment for difficult lesions.

Background

Colorectal cancer is the second leading cause of cancer in the United States, with approximately 140,000 new cases per year.[1] Nearly twenty percent of patients will present with metastases at the time of diagnosis.[2] The primary site of distant metastases is the liver, followed by lungs and bone, in decreasing frequency. Distant metastases spread most often via hematogenous or lymphatic routes, while trans-peritoneal spread is less common.[3–5] If metastases are widespread, there is little hope for cure and systemic therapy is the treatment of choice. However, when oligometastatic disease — often defined as fewer than five metastases — is encountered, local therapies can be employed to achieve a durable response and a chance at long-term survival.

Traditionally, surgical resection was limited to patients with only liver disease, less than four lesions, and unilobar metastases.[6] However, the past decade has seen significant advancements in the therapy of colorectal liver metastasis (CRLM). Improvements in surgical devices, surgical techniques, as well as systemic therapies have broadened the pool of patients with CRLM who are potentially resectable. Enhanced ablation and embolization techniques have advanced treatment for difficult lesions. Liver first and staged approaches, portal vein embolization or ligation and novel techniques such as associated liver partitioning (ALPPS),[7] have similarly expanded the cohort of patients who potentially can be taken to the operating room with curative intent.

The majority of colorectal metastases — upwards of 70% or more — are found in the liver.[8] While it is not uncommon to have metastases in multiple organ systems at once, direct metastases to other organs without liver involvement are rare. One exception is low-lying rectal lesions where the inferior and middle rectal veins drain directly into the inferior vena cava and metastases can bypass the liver, leading to isolated lung metastases. For patients with CRLM, surgical resection remains the best chance of cure for oligometastatic disease. Five-year survival ranges between 40–70% depending on the burden of disease.[9–12] However, in the case of multiple lesions confined to one organ system, there are a number of questions that arise. Should the primary or the metastasis be approached first? Should a synchronous or a staged resection of the metastases be performed? Should a neoadjuvant or adjuvant therapy be instituted, and if so, which agents should be employed? These, and other questions, have yet to be conclusively defined in the literature. We herein review the management of patients with oligometastatic CRLM.

Operative Considerations

Complete resection of the tumor remains the only chance of cure for patients with metastatic colorectal cancer. In assessing a patient for potential surgery, preoperative planning is important. Laboratory evaluation of liver function, hemoglobin, electrolytes, coagulation factors and nutrition are all recommended. Good quality cross-sectional imaging is necessary in order to identify potentially resectable patients.[13] Both computed tomography (CT) and magnetic resonance imaging (MRI) can be used to assess the extent, as well as distribution, of CRLM in the liver. In patients who are obese, have a fatty liver, or have been heavily pre-treated with systemic chemotherapy, MRI may be a more sensitive imaging modality and is generally preferred.[14] Furthermore, it is imperative to assess for the presence of extra-hepatic disease — as in many cases this is a contraindication to metastasectomy. Local resectability of the liver disease is determined by a thorough assessment of the location and extent of the disease relative to the vascular inflow and outflow, biliary drainage, as well as the future liver remnant (FLR).[15,16] While uncommon, if the metastatic disease compromises both the left and the right sided inflow, then resection is typically not feasible. Similarly, at least one hepatic vein emptying into the inferior vena cava (IVC) is needed for outflow of the remaining liver. While *ex-vivo* resection and re-implantation of complex liver metastases involving the hepatic veins and IVC have been performed successfully,[17,18] it is rarely done. Borderline resectable disease, in which metastases about or involve inflow or outflow structures, can sometimes be converted to resectable disease with neo-adjuvant therapy (Fig. 1).

Another criteria in preoperative assessment of metastatic colorectal liver metastasis is the future liver remnant (FLR). It is estimated that a remnant liver volume of 20–25% is sufficient to preclude liver failure in a healthy patient.[19,20] In patients who have baseline liver dysfunction, such as fibrosis, chemotherapy associated steatosis or steatohepatitis (CASH), the ideal FLR should probably be in the range of 30 to 40%.[21,22] Patients with a small FLR have increased risk of post-operative liver insufficiency or failure.[23] As such, imaging techniques to assess future liver volume should be employed whenever the FLR is suspected to be low (Fig. 2).

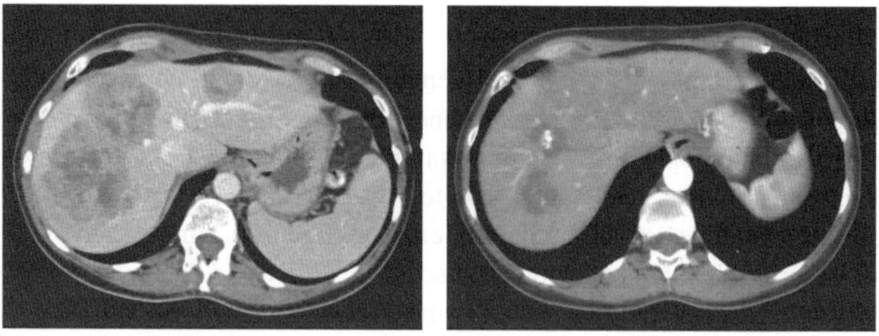

(a) (b)

Fig. 1. Computed Tomography showing extensive colorectal liver metastases to the liver. A lesion abuts the left hepatic vein (a), as well as involving the right hepatic vein. After neo-adjuvant chemotherapy (b) the lesions had all regressed enough to allow resection.

If the FLR is deemed inadequate, portal vein embolization (PVE) should be considered.

Resection

While no randomized trials exist, it is generally accepted that resection of CRLM improves survival and can lead to cure in select patients.[24] Recent series have reported five-year survival up to 40–45% in resectable patients.[25,26] Hepatic resection for CRLM can either be anatomic or non-anatomic. Anatomic resections are based on the segmental inflow and outflow as described by Couinaud.[27,28] Isolated caudate lobe (segment 1) resections for CRLM are occasionally indicated and can be technically more challenging depending on the variable anatomy.[29] Segmentectomy, sectionectomy, hemi-hepatectomy and extended hemihepatectomy are all anatomic resections (Table 1). Non-anatomic resections, or wedge resections, are based on the boundaries of the tumor and are employed in order to retain as much liver parenchyma as possible. Classically, a one centimeter margin was recommended for all resections, and lesser margins were thought to lead to worse recurrence free and overall survival.[30,31] More recently, it has been shown that overall survival is similar for

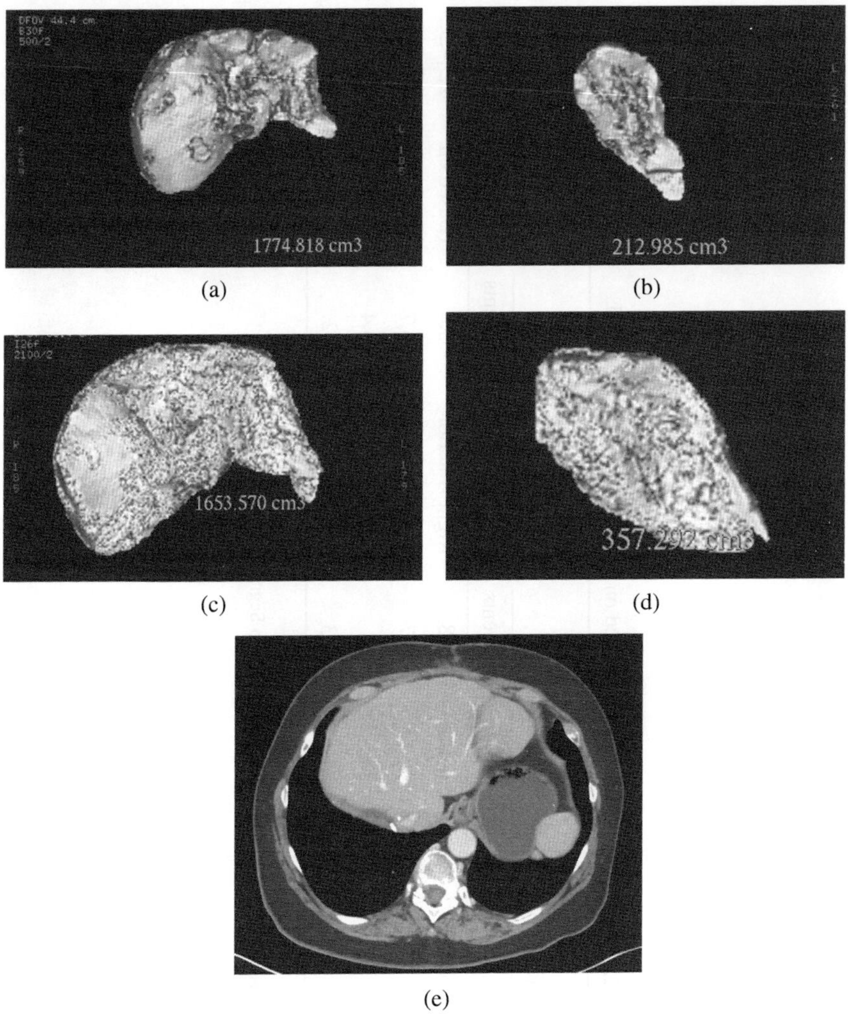

Fig. 2. Computed Tomography 3D volumetric images showing the (a) right and (b) left hemi-livers prior to portal vein embolization (PVE). The left hemi-liver was the future liver remnant in this case. The (c) right and (d) left hemi-livers 8 weeks post PVE. Notice the increase in volume of the future liver remnant. The patient underwent and extended right hepatectomy. A 3-month post-operative image (e) shows the dramatic regenerative capacity of the liver post-resection.

Table 1. Names for liver partitioning based on couinaud segments involved.

Extended hemi-hepatectomy		Hemi-hepatectomy		Sectionectomy		Sectorectomy		Segmentectomy	
Term	Segments	Term	Segments	Term	Segments	Term	Segments	Term	Segments
Right	4,5,6,7,8	Right	5,6,7,8	Right Anterior	5,8	Right Anterior	5,8	(Based on Number)	2,3,4,5, 6,7 or 8
				Left Posterior	6,7	Right Posterior	6,7		
Left	2,3,4,5,8	Left	2,3,4	Left Medial	4	Left Medial	3,4	Caudate*	1
				Left Lateral	2,3	Left Lateral	2		

* also referred to as caudate lobectomy

If including Segment 1 should be stated as such (ie: Left Hepotectomy extended to Segment 1)

R0 resections irrespective of the width of the margin.[32] Other data have suggested that even an R1 margin may not affect overall survival; however, an R1 margin does lead to an increased incidence of intra-hepatic recurrence. As such, a microscopically and macroscopically complete negative margin should be achieved at the time of surgery in order to ensure the best chance at a good long-term outcome.[33,34]

A subset of patients will present with synchronous CRLM, with the primary tumor still in place. Recent literature has demonstrated the safety and efficacy of simultaneous resection of colorectal primary and synchronous liver metastases.[35–40] Moreover, minimally invasive techniques may be employed without detriment to the resection or outcomes.[41–43] In general, simultaneous resections are associated with similar morbidity and mortality compared with staged resections.[38,39] Simultaneous resection does require, however, careful patient selection and particular consideration should be given to the age of the patient, left sided or rectal lesions and the extent of hepatic resection; all of which may lead to increased morbidity and mortality post operatively.[37,38] In addition, data would strongly suggest that long-term oncologic outcomes are comparable between the two approaches.[44–46] It also seems as though the order of resection in a staged approach is not important.[47,48] For example, Brouquet and colleagues demonstrated similar outcomes to traditional combined and staged approaches for the so called "reverse strategy," in which the liver metastases were resected prior to the primary colorectal lesion in a staged approach with neoadjuvant therapy.[48]

Perhaps one of the most novel surgical techniques to be described in the past decade is the associating liver partition and portal vein ligation for staged hepatectomy (ALPPS) procedure. First described by Torres *et al.* in 2012,[2] ALPPS is essentially a two-staged hepatectomy performed during a single hospitalization. The liver and the hilar structures are dissected free of their attachments and the associated right portal vein ligated, along with parenchymal transection and ligation of the segment IV portal, arterial and venous branches. The right and left hepatic veins remain intact. The extended right hemi-liver is sometimes placed in a plastic bag to prevent adhesions and the abdomen is closed. With the right arterial and biliary systems intact, the liver is able to hypertrophy with some reserve in place. Imaging is then performed usually between 6 to 12 days and the

FLR volume is re-assessed. If appropriate, the patient is re-explored, the remaining pedicles are transected and the resection completed. While initially reported for a right-sided resection, it can similarly be performed with a left trisegmentectomy, or even central hepatectomy. [49] While the applicability of the ALPPS procedure has yet to be determined, surgeons should be aware of this technique as it may be applicable to a subset of patients with CRLM.[50,51]

There are no randomized control trials comparing continued systemic therapy versus resection for recurrent disease isolated to the liver. However, there is some data to suggest that in select patients with low burden disease and adequate FLR, recurrent metastasectomy can be done with limited mortality and may lead to improved survival.[52–54]

Portal Vein Embolization (PVE)

Since first described by Makuuchi *et al.* in 1990,[55] PVE has become an adjunct to liver resection in patients whose predicted FLR is small. The liver receives two-thirds of its blood supply via the portal system. PVE redirects the portal flow to the FLR, which can induce subsequent hypertrophy of the non-embolized liver, as was first described by Cantlie over a hundred years ago.[56] In general, PVE is most applicable to patients being considered for an extended right hepatectomy, since the left lateral section and caudate may not represent an adequate FLR.[19–21,57,58] In contrast, while PVE may be indicated in a smaller subset of patients undergoing a planned right hepatectomy, it is rarely needed for a left or extended left hepatectomy due to the typical large volume of the right posterior section.[59] When PVE is indicated, several investigators have shown that it can result in fewer post-operative complications and shorter ICU stay in patients who otherwise would have had a small FLR.[60,61]

Prior to PVE, volumetric assessment (Fig. 2) should be performed in order to calculate the FLR volume.[19,20,57] Volumetric assessments can be accomplished using either computed tomography (CT) or magnetic resonance imaging (MRI), with the choice typically being an institutional preference. The percentage of total liver volume that equals the FLR can be calculated and typically is adjusted for body surface area (Table 2).[59]

Table 2. Percentage of predicted total liver volume required based on extent of hepatic disease.

% TLV	Extent of liver disease
> 20%	Healthy Liver
> 30%	Steatosis/Fibrosis
> 40%	Mild (Childs A) Cirrhosis
Resection Not Recommended	Moderate to Severe (Childs B or C) Cirrhosis

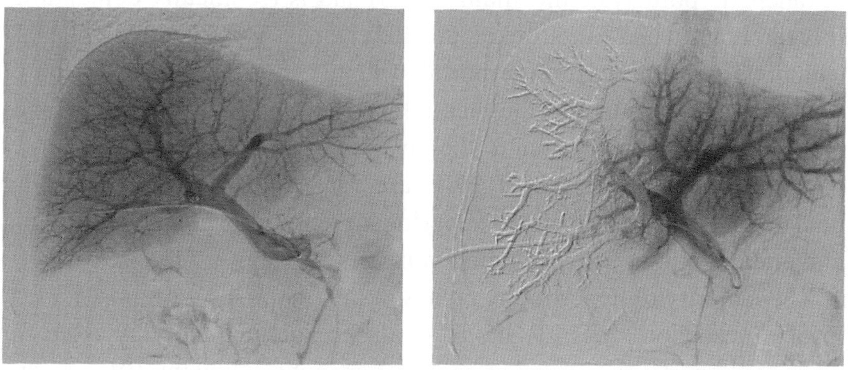

(a) (b)

Fig. 3. Portal Venogram showing the (a) pre-embolization and (b) post-embolization images of a percutaneous ipsilateral trans-hepatic portal venous embolization.

When indicated, PVE is typically performed via a transhepatic, percutaneous approach. In this technique the catheter is inserted through the abdominal wall directly into the hepatic parenchyma and guided into the portal system where embolic material is injected (Fig. 3). A variety of agents have been employed with success and preferences are often institution and operator dependent. These include, but are not limited to, fibrin glue, cyanoacrylate, gelatin sponges, thrombin, metallic coils and microparticles.[62] The transhepatic technique can be performed through the ipsilateral or contralateral hemi-liver. While commonly employed due to the ease of access, the latter approach is less favorable in that it runs the risk of causing permanent injury to the future liver remnant.[62,63] The ipsilateral approach,[61] while more technically demanding as one must traverse the right portal vein branches at sharper angles, is preferred whenever possible as any potentially injured parenchyma will eventually be resected. Moreover, it allows more definitive embolization of the segment IV branches, which improves hypertrophy of the future liver remnant. A second, less common approach is via the internal jugular vein. This transjugular approach, in which a catheter traverses into the vena cava, into the hepatic veins and accesses the portal system trans-sinusoidally, is similar to a transjugular intrahepatic portosystemic shunt (TIPS) and is technically demanding. It is rarely used and literature on its effectiveness is limited.[64,65] The last technique gains access to the portal system via open catheterization of the colic vessels, and was the method utilized by Makuuchi in his landmark paper.[65] However, due to the invasive nature of access, it is rarely employed. Complications of PVE are rare and include subcapsular hematoma, thrombosis of the superior mesenteric or main portal vein, and embolization of non-targeted veins.

The majority of hypertrophy comes in the first 3–4 weeks post-PVE.[58] Prior to resection, the FLR should again be volumetrically assessed for adequate hypertrophy. The degree of hypertrophy following PVE is variable, but most studies have shown an average of approximately 10% increase in liver volume.[58,61] If unsuccessful, as occurs in up to 20% of patients with baseline liver disease,[62,66] repeat PVE can be attempted prior to resection.

Portal vein ligation (PVL) is similar in concept to PVE, but requires an invasive operation and dissection of the hilar structures. It has been proven effective and may produce similar post-operative hypertrophy as does PVE, especially if combined with sclerosis of the portal vein.[67–69] PVL can be done at the time of primary colorectal resection or first stage of a planned two-stage hepatectomy, where the patient is already undergoing an operation. PVL has also been shown to be safe when done laparoscopically.[70] In general, however, due to its invasive nature and increased chance of missed portal vein branches — thereby reducing its efficacy — PVL is less often employed than PVE.

Finally, there are some emerging data describing hepatic vein embolization as an adjunct to portal vein embolization in order to maximize FLR.[71] While technically feasible, it often requires the use of IVC filter or vascular plugs to prevent pulmonary embolism. In addition to the increased technical demands, the efficacy of hepatic vein embolization in inducing hepatic hypertrophy is less well-established and so its application is less common.

Ablation Techniques

Surgical resection of CRLM can be performed in conjunction with ablation of other lesions or, in select cases, ablation alone may be warranted. There are several methods to ablate CRLM. The most common involve hyperthermic ablation techniques: radiofrequency or microwave. While intra-tumoral injections (alcohol, acetic acid) have been described for the treatment of hepatocellular carcinoma, this therapy is less effective for CRLM.[72,73] Cryoablation involves the delivery liquid nitrogen or argon to the lesion causing rapid cooling to a temperature below −40°C, leading to crystallization and destruction of both the tumor and the surrounding vasculature.[74] However, it is subject to substantial heat sync effects, often requires multiple ablations, and has limited efficacy when compared to other ablative techniques.[75,76] While utilized in the past, cryoablation is not currently recommended in the treatment of CRLM.[76]

Radiofrequency ablation (RFA) passes an electrical current through the tumor to create a coagulative necrosis (Fig. 4). RFA has been shown to be most effective for tumors < 3 cm with higher recurrence rates as the lesion size increases (e.g. up to 30–70% local recurrence for lesion > 5 cm).[77–79] Microwave ablation is another type of thermal ablation. With this approach, the generator transmits microwave energy from the electrode causing coagulative necrosis of the tumor. One potential benefit of microwave ablation over RFA is the lower risk of heat-sink effect when applied near large vessels because microwave does not require the transmission of electrical current between electrodes.[80] Both techniques require ultrasound localization of the tumor, and both can injure surrounding tissues, such as visceral structures or the diaphragm when treating dome lesions.[81] There are no studies showing a benefit of one technique over the other,

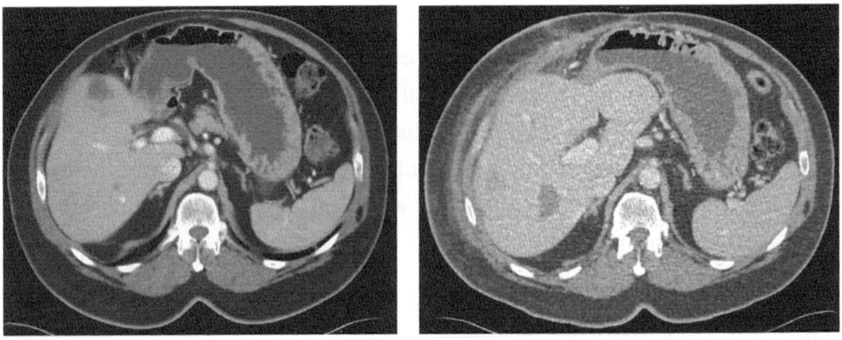

(a) (b)

Fig. 4. Computed Tomography images showing a lesion in segment 6 of the liver (a) prior to and (b) post radio frequency ablation of 3 cm diameter. Note the well-circumscribed area of necrosis post-ablation.

however many centers now favor microwave ablation due to slightly shorter ablation times and the ability to forego patient grounding. Due to the destructive nature of these ablations, follow-up imaging can sometimes be difficult to interpret, and CEA levels are sometimes more informative in suggesting a recurrence.

Despite improvements in ablation techniques, R0 resection remains the best chance of achieving long term recurrence-free and overall survival.[82–86] Overall and recurrence-free survival are 10 to 35% higher with complete resection compared with ablation alone in retrospective analyses[83–85] — even for small, solitary lesions.[82] A true randomized control trial is unlikely due to concerns for both accrual and equipoise. In some cases, ablation may be combined with surgical resection if the total number of lesions cannot be resected or if there are lesions that are surgically inaccessible.[86,87] In these cases, while intra-hepatic recurrence rates are higher, some patients do demonstrate prolonged, durable benefits with regards to both overall and recurrence-free survival.[87] Whether due to selection bias or tumor biology, patients who undergo combined resection and ablation tend to do worse than patients undergoing resection alone.[86]

Systemic Chemotherapy

Systemic chemotherapy plays an important role in the management of patients with CRLM. For patients with advanced unresectable disease, systemic therapy is the backbone of therapy. Systemic chemotherapy, however, is also an important component of the multi-disciplinary care of patients with resectable or potentially resectable disease. Some patients who have advanced disease may benefit from preoperative systemic chemotherapy to down-size / convert their disease to being resectable. In addition, other patients who are surgical candidates with initially resectable disease may sometimes be treated with neoadjuvant systemic therapy. Furthermore, systemic chemotherapy has an important role in the adjuvant post-operative setting for many patients with CRLM.[88]

The major chemotherapeutic options for metastatic colorectal cancer are 5-flourouracil (5-FU) based, alone or in combination with oxaliplatin or irinotecan.[89–101] Alternatively, 5-FU can be substituted with oral formulation flouropyrimidines such as capecitabine and S1.[102–104] Capecitabine is an oral flouropyrimidine that is metabolized into the active form 5-FU. It demonstrates increased activity in tumor cells as opposed to normal cells, leading to a lower toxicity profile,[105] with similar response and overall survival to infusional 5-FU.[106] S-1 is a three drug combination (ftorafur, gimeracil, oteracil) that has shown similar, if not better, response rates compared with capecitabine.[104] However, it has yet to be approved for the use by the FDA, and thus S1 is not available for use in the United States.

The most common first-line treatments for metastatic colorectal cancer are FOLFOX (5-FU, leucovorin, oxaliplatin), FOLFIRI (5-FU, leucovorin, irinotecan) and FOLFOXIRI (5-FU, leucovorin, oxaliplatin and irinotecan).[89,90,107] With the arrival of oxaliplatin in the late 1990's,[108,109] combination chemotherapy for CRLM has become the standard. As a platinum derivative, oxaliplatin acts to crosslink DNA, preventing replication and leading to apoptosis.[110] Its toxicity is mostly related to neuropathy and the severity of symptoms is dose dependent.[111] Although the mechanism is poorly understood, oxaliplatin can lead to sinusoidal obstruction syndrome (SOS) in a subset of patients, which is often termed "blue liver."[112] Initial phase III trials by the French cooperative showed improved progression free survival (PFS) and response rates with a similar overall survival.[97,113] Oxaliplatin is also used in combination with capecitabine (CAPOX) with similar efficacy to FOLFOX,[114,115] albeit with differing toxicity profiles.

Irinotecan is a topoisomerase inhibitor, preventing cancer cell division and leading to cell death.[116] While efficacious as a single agent,[117] it is more effective in combination with flouropyrimidines and leucovorin (FOLFIRI, IFL).[91,118,119] The most common toxicity associated with irinotecan is diarrhea,which can lead to severe dehydration. Patients with Gilbert's syndrome have more severe gastrointestinal and neutropenic complications.[120,121] Unlike oxaliplatin, irinotecan is more associated with steatosis and steatohepatitis.[122] Combination therapy with capecitabine (CAPIRI) is efficacious but is rarely employed as first-line therapy due to severe gastrointestinal complications.[123] It is commonly used as second-line therapy for those patients who progress on oxaliplatin-based therapy, and was shown to have beneficial effects in a small subset of patients in the OPTIMOX-1 study.[124] Whether first-line therapy should be a oxaliplatin- or irinotecan-based regimen remains up for debate,[90,125] and toxicity profiles should be considered prior to initiating either therapy.

Targeted therapies have also demonstrated a significant role in the treatment of metastatic colorectal cancer.[94,98,126–131] Colorectal cancers are most commonly sporadic and up to 60% of these cancers display mutations of the *K-ras* or *B-raf* oncogenes.[132] Among patients who do not demonstrate a *K-ras* mutation (i.e. wild-type *K-ras*), the epidermal growth factor receptors (EGFR) can act as a target for therapies such as cetuximab and panitumumab — monoclonal antibodies that block EGFR and inhibit cell proliferation. Patients who are wild type for *K-ras* have improved progression-free and overall survival with the addition of targeted anti-EGFR therapy to standard chemotherapy.[126–131] Bevacizumab belongs to a separate class of drugs that target the vascular endothelial growth factors (VEGF inhibitors) and also has efficacy in combination with cytotoxic chemotherapy agents for CRLM.[133–135] Side effects of bevacizumab include delayed wound healing, which makes patient selection and timing of surgical therapy critical.[136] Other targeted therapies, such as aflibercept and regorafenib, have similarly demonstrated efficacy, although not as first-line treatment.[137] Recent studies have tried to compare EGFR and VEGF inhibitors, but have not demonstrated clear evidence of superiority for either class of drugs as part of combination first-line therapy. [138,139]

Timing of chemotherapy in relation to resection is not well-defined. Most patients who have a low burden of disease and who are deemed initially resectable are offered surgery "up front." [49] While some patients with initially resectable disease are treated with preoperative systemic chemotherapy, there are no consensus statements or guidelines to delineate who should receive neoadjuvant therapy.[140–142] Patients who have a high risk with surgery or who have borderline resectable — often termed convertible — disease, are often offered chemotherapy as a means to assess tumor biology and aggressiveness, in addition to achieving response. By selecting patients who progress despite systemic therapy, the morbidity of a major operation may possibly be avoided. Patients who do respond — and even those who do not progress — are more likely to benefit from surgery.[57]

Patients with borderline unresectable disease due to close approximation to hepatic venous or portal structures or extent of disease in the liver (Fig. 1) may benefit from chemotherapy in an attempt to "convert" the disease to being resectable. By giving chemotherapy to downsize the extent of disease, between 5 and 30% of patients will have sufficient response such that surgical resection becomes feasible.[143–146] Response is most often classified by factors related to changes on imaging.[147,148] However, even with the best of techniques, imaging response rates do not necessarily correlate to pathologic response rates in as many as 80% of patients.[149,150] Evaluation of patients after initial therapy is recommended at 2-month intervals,[151] and chemotherapy should be stopped once resectability is achieved. The choice of what chemotherapy to use is debatable, but traditional therapies of FOLFOX, FOLFIRI and FOLFOXIRI with or without additional targeted agents, such as cetuximab, are most commonly used.

On occasion, the use of preoperative chemotherapy may result in "disappearing" liver metastases, which can represent a management challenge.[150,152,153] Chemotherapy-induced steatosis or steatohepatitis can darken the background liver on imaging, making it more difficult to follow metastatic lesions.[154] There are a number of studies looking at hepatic recurrence in patients with disappearing liver metastases, with varying results regarding the incidence of a durable complete response after disappearance of the CRLM.[150,155,156] It is generally agreed that if all sites of disease can be resected, intrahepatic recurrence free survival is improved, but the effect on overall survival is less clear,[152] and further study is necessary before a consensus can be achieved.

Intra-Arterial (HIA) Infusion of Chemotherapy

Similar to primary tumors of the liver, CRLM can be targeted for isolated, high dose chemotherapy through the arterial circulation. Floxuridine (FUDR) is the most common agent used either alone or in combination with systemic pyrimidine-based therapy. FUDR is metabolized by the liver, which minimizes — but does not eradicate — risk of high dose chemotherapy affecting other organ systems.[157,158] Hepatic artery infusion (HAI) therapy is typically delivered directly into hepatic circulation via a catheter placed into the gastroduodenal that administers the chemotherapy from a subcutaneous pump.[159] Early reports of thrombosis, hepatic toxicity and gastroduodenal ischemic complications have been minimized with improved selection and application.[160] While HAI has some efficacy as a stand-alone therapy in patients post-metastasectomy, its greatest benefit is found in combination with systemic chemotherapy.[160–163] At high volume, experienced centers where HAI is performed, there is evidence of improved locoregional control and recurrence free survival,[164–166] and even some data to suggest improved overall survival in select patient groups.[167] However, the lack of generalizability in these studies combined with the complexity of care associated with HAI has so far limited its widespread adoption.

While the role of trans-arterial catheter-based therapy for hepatocellular carcinoma is well-accepted, the use of catheter-based trans-arterial therapy (Fig. 5) for colorectal liver metastases is less well-defined. There have been a few randomized control trials, many which lacked adequate controls, that have shown limited benefit over systemic therapies.[168,169] While many different chemotherapeutic regimens have been implemented, the best evidence of significant improvement over systemic

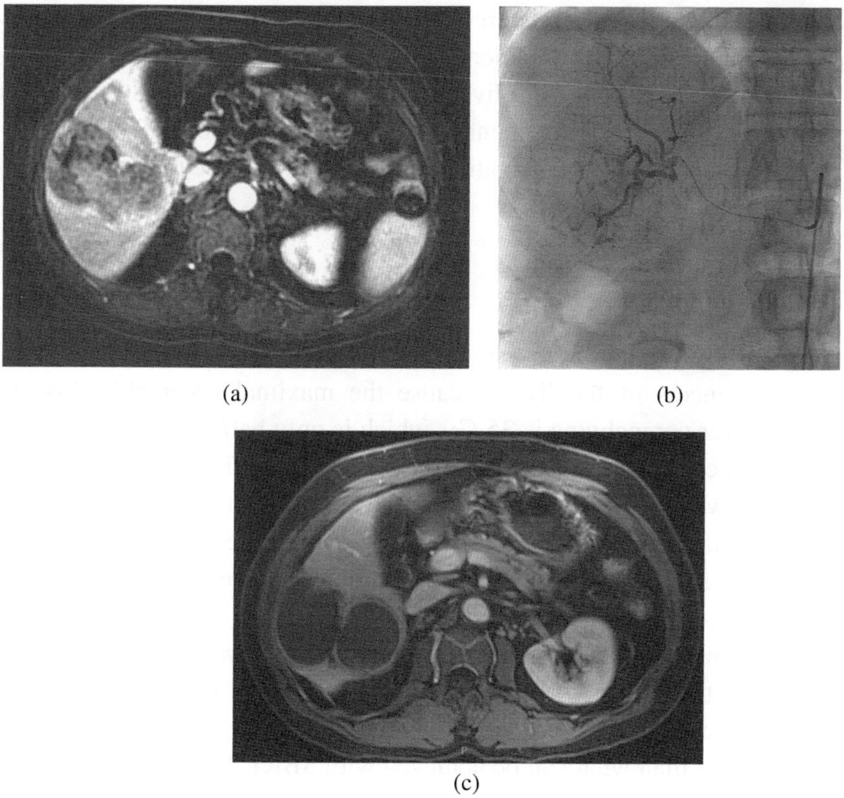

Fig. 5. Magnetic resonance images of (a) two large masses in the right hemi-liver. This patient was treated with trans-arterial chemoembolization (TACE) via selective catheterization of the right hepatic artery (b). Post-procedural images of the lesions (c) several weeks later.

therapy has come with the infusion of drug eluting beads trans-arterial chemoembolization (DEB-TACE).[170–174] In a multi-institutional randomized control trial of 74 patients with CRLM, patients who received treatment with irinotecan loaded beads (DEBIRI) were compared with patients who received systemic irinotecan (FOLFIRI). The DEBIRI group showed significant improvement in progression free survival (7 versus 4 months), overall survival (22 versus 15 months) and duration of improvement in quality of life (8 versus 3 months).[173] In a separate study, Poggi and colleagues administered oxaliplatin loaded microspheres (DEBOX,OEM-TACE) to patients with unresectable intrahepatic cholangiocarcinoma and colorectal liver metastases, with two-third of patients showing stable or improvement in disease burdened by RECIST criteria.[171] However, more investigations are needed to define the role of intra-arterial therapy for CRLM.

Radiation Therapy

External beam radiation therapy (EBRT) has traditionally not been used to treat cancers of the liver because the maximal acceptable dose to healthy liver parenchyma is 35 Gy, which is only half of the dose needed to adequately sterilize CRLM.[175] Using conformational imaging techniques, however, SBRT can maximize the dose to the tumor without added toxicity to the surrounding healthy liver.[176] Recent literature, while sparse, does show some benefit in patients with unresectable disease, especially for metastases to the central nervous system.[177]

Radioembolization involves delivery of radioactive isotopes of iodine (^{131}I) or yttrium-90 (^{90}Y) directly to the tumor via the hepatic arterial system, and can achieve doses of between 50 and 150 Gy, which are much higher than what can be achieved with SBRT.[178] In the case of ^{131}I, lipiodol — a type of contrast medium used to identify hepatic tumors — is labeled with the radioactive iodine, and then the mixture is injected into the feeding vessels of the tumor. For ^{90}Y, glass or resin coated beads are used for delivery. With precise identification of feeding vessels via arteriogram, selective intrahepatic arterial radioembolization can be achieved, thereby sparing non-diseased liver. Both types of intra-arterial radioembolization are effective due to the nature of hepatic tumors, which derive the majority of their blood supply from the arterial system, as compared to normal liver parenchyma that is more heavily supplied by the portal venous system.[179] ^{90}Y based radioembolization can be delivered via glass or resin labeled beads. The glass beads (TheraSphere®) are between 20 and 30 μm, while the resin labeled beads (SIR-Spheres®) range between 20 and 40 μm in size. The one notable difference between the two methods is in the number of beads deployed: between 1 and 8 million for glass coated beads versus between 40 to 80 million for the resin coated beads. While each approach can deliver a similar amount of radiation (measured in Becquerels, Bq), the dose per bead is much smaller in the resin beads (50 Bq) than the glass beads (2500 Bq).[180] In either case, the beads themselves become lodged in the smaller arterioles around the tumor, delivering comparatively high doses of radiation to the diseased parenchyma. There is no comparative data as to which form of ^{90}Y coated bead works more effectively. The EPOCH study, projected for completion by 2016, will compare patients undergoing second-line chemotherapy for unresectable CRLM with or without the addition of TheraSphere®.[181]

^{131}I-lipiodol radioembolization is more commonly used in hepatocellular carcinoma due to the affinity of lipiodol for HCC tumors, and is not utilized much for CRLM.[182] The radiolabeled lipiodol adheres to the tumor cell wall and is transported into the cell. In normal liver parenchyma, the Kupffer cells phagocytose and remove the lipiodol, but tumors are void of Kupffer cells and so the radiolabeled lipiodol remains in the tumor, long after the radiation has decayed. It therefore serves a dual purpose as an effective radioembolic delivery agent as well as acting as a chemoembolic agent, lysing the cells which it has entered and blocking further blood flow to the tumor.[183]

Both ^{90}Y and ^{131}I-lipiodol radioembolization can even be combined with HIA chemotherapy, and have shown some improvement in overall survival as compared to HIA chemotherapy alone, although randomized data are limited.[184–186]

Brachytherapy for colorectal liver metastases is rarely employed, and when performed is most commonly done in conjunction with other treatment modalities.[185,187,188] It requires either intra-operative placement or highly specific CT-guided placement of radioactive seeds into the tumor. Its effectiveness decreases with tumors greater than 4 cm in dimension.[189]

Surveillance

There are limited data to direct surveillance for Stage IV colorectal cancer patients' post-metastasectomy. The majority of expert opinions extrapolate recommendations from the data on Stage II and III colon cancer. Both the National Comprehensive Cancer Network (NCCN)[190] and the American Society of Clinical Oncology (ASCO)[191] recommend intensive follow-up including surveillance imaging, CEA testing and physical exam. The literature, however, is not clear as to the actual benefit of intensive follow-up regimens with regard to long-term survival.[192–194] Detection of recurrent disease can facilitate repeat hepatic resection of CRLM and several series have shown a survival benefit for repeat metastasectomy in select patients with good functional status.[52,195]

Non-Hepatic Oligometastatic Disease

The treatment for non-hepatic oligometastatic colorectal cancer is, first and foremost, systemic therapy. The decision to pursue treatment involving chemotherapy, radiation therapy and locoregional ablative therapy is highly patient dependent. The data on surgical resection for these lesions is limited and consensus on which lesions should undergo resection remains elusive.

Lung

There are no randomized trials to support resection of isolated lung metastases. Even so, there is recent data from several series that have shown benefit in overall survival for select patients.[196–200] The tumor size, number of metastases and time interval between primary resection and appearance of lung metastasis relates to prognosis.[196,199] Survival benefits are also seen in patients who have had synchronous or previous hepatic metastases.[198,201] Still, in patients with metastatic disease, those with lung lesions have a far worse prognosis than those with only liver disease.[202,203] Much like with liver assessment, it is imperative that the post-operative remnant lung function be adequate, or resection should not be planned.

Adrenal

In the rare case of isolated adrenal metastasis, there are a few case reports suggesting improved survival with resection.[204–206] The largest series reports a total of eight patients, with a mean survival of 32 months. However, due to its rarity, the management of oligometastatic colorectal disease to the adrenal gland remains undefined.

Brain

Colorectal metastases to the brain occur infrequently, with an incidence ranging between 0.6 and 4%, and nearly always occur in the setting of metastases to other organs.[207–209] The mainstay of treatment, as with all non-hepatic metastases, is systemic therapy with or without focused radiation.[210] Data regarding resection is limited, but in select cases has shown some benefits in overall survival and symptom improvement.[209,211]

Retroperitoneum

Data regarding resection of oligometastatic disease in the retroperitoneum is limited. A recent review did suggest a benefit in overall (34 to 44 months) and disease-free survival (17 to 21 months) in resected patients.[212] Still, this has likely more to do with tumor biology and is dependent on careful patient selection.[213]

Take Home Messages

- Improvements over the past 20 years in the diagnosis and treatment of colorectal cancer have led to a demonstrable increase in survival.
- The addition of targeted therapies, ablative techniques and staged resections has allowed for the tailoring of treatments to the individual patient.
- Careful preoperative assessment and multidisciplinary involvement is crucial in order to identify the appropriate course for these patients.
- With both recent and future advances in multimodality therapy, patients with oligometastatic colorectal cancer have ever-increasing chances at prolonged survival and even cure of their disease.

References

1. Statistics of the American Cancer Society. http://www.cancer.org/cancer/colonandrectumcancer/detailedguide/colorectal-cancer-key-statistics. Accessed Feb 2014.
2. Siegel, R., Naishadham, D., Jemal, A., Cancer statistics, 2013. *CA*, 2013. **63**(1): 11–30.

3. Weiss, L., Grundmann, E., Torhorst, J. *et al.*, Haematogenous metastatic patterns in colonic carcinoma: an analysis of 1541 necropsies. *J Pathol*, 1986. **150**(3): 195–203.
4. Chambers, A.F., Groom, A.C., MacDonald, I.C., Dissemination and growth of cancer cells in metastatic sites. *Nat Rev. Cancer*, 2002. **2**(8): 563–72.
5. Carmignani, C.P., Sugarbaker, T.A., Bromley, C.M., Sugarbaker, P.H. Intraperitoneal cancer dissemination: mechanisms of the patterns of spread. *Cancer Metastasis Rev*, 2003. **22**(4): 465–72.
6. Hughes, K.S., Simon, R., Songhorabodi, S. *et al.*, Resection of the liver for colorectal carcinoma metastases: a multi-institutional study of patterns of recurrence. *Surgery*, 1986. **100**(2): 278–84.
7. Torres, O.J., Moraes-Junior, J.M., Lima e Lima, N.C., Moraes, A.M., Associating liver partition and portal vein ligation for staged hepatectomy (ALPPS): a new approach in liver resections. *Arquivos brasileiros de cirurgia digestiva : ABCD = Braz Arch Digest Surg*, 2012. **25**(4): 290–2.
8. Patanaphan, V., Salazar, O.M. Colorectal cancer: metastatic patterns and prognosis. *Southern Med J*, 1993. **86**(1): 38–41.
9. Pawlik, T.M., Scoggins, C.R., Zorzi, D. *et al.*, Effect of surgical margin status on survival and site of recurrence after hepatic resection for colorectal metastases. *Ann Surg*, 2005. **241**(5): 715–22, discussion 722–14.
10. Choti, M.A., Sitzmann, J.V., Tiburi, M.F. *et al.*, Trends in long-term survival following liver resection for hepatic colorectal metastases. *Ann Surgery*, 2002. **235**(6): 759–66.
11. Charnsangavej, C., Clary, B., Fong, Y., Grothey, A., Pawlik, T.M., Choti, M.A., Selection of patients for resection of hepatic colorectal metastases: expert consensus statement. *Ann Surg Oncol*, 2006. **13**(10): 1261–8.
12. Bentrem, D.J., Dematteo, R.P., Blumgart, L.H. Surgical therapy for metastatic disease to the liver. *Ann Rev Med*, 2005. **56**: 139–56.
13. Yamada, H., Katoh, H., Kondo, S., Okushiba, S., Morikawa, T., Repeat hepatectomy for recurrent hepatic metastases from colorectal cancer. *Hepatogastroenterology*, 2001; **48**(39): 828–30.
14. Sahani, D.V., Bajwa, M.A., Andrabi, Y., Bajpai, S., Cusack, J.C., Current status of imaging and emerging techniques to evaluate liver metastases from colorectal carcinoma. *Ann Surg*, 2014. **259**(5): 861–72.

15. Scheele, J., Altendorf-Hofmann, A., Stangl, R., Schmidt, K. Surgical resection of colorectal liver metastases: Gold standard for solitary and radically resectable lesions. *Swiss Surg*, 1996. (Suppl 4): 4–17.
16. Wanebo, H.J., Chu, Q.D., Vezeridis, M.P., Soderberg, C. Patient selection for hepatic resection of colorectal metastases. *Arch Surg*, 1996; **131**(3): 322–9.
17. Hemming, A.W., Mekeel, K.L., Zendejas, I., Kim, R.D., Sicklick, J.K., Reed, A.I., Resection of the liver and inferior vena cava for hepatic malignancy. *J Am College Surgeons*, 2013. **217**(1): 115–24; discussion 124–15.
18. Hemming, A.W., Langham, M.R., Reed, A.I., van der Werf, W.J., Howard, R.J., Resection of the inferior vena cava for hepatic malignancy. *Am Surg*, 2001. **67**(11): 1081–7; discussion 1087–8.
19. Vauthey, J.N., Chaoui, A., Do, K.A. *et al.*, Standardized measurement of the future liver remnant prior to extended liver resection: methodology and clinical associations. *Surgery*, 2000. **127**(5): 512–9.
20. Abdalla, E.K., Denys, A., Chevalier, P., Nemr, R.A., Vauthey, J.N., Total and segmental liver volume variations: implications for liver surgery. *Surgery*, 2004. **135**(4): 404–10.
21. Shindoh, J., Tzeng, C.W., Aloia, T.A. *et al.*, Optimal future liver remnant in patients treated with extensive preoperative chemotherapy for colorectal liver metastases. *Ann Surg Oncol*, 2013. **20**(8): 2493–500.
22. Narita, M., Oussoultzoglou, E., Fuchshuber, P. *et al.*, What is a safe future liver remnant size in patients undergoing major hepatectomy for colorectal liver metastases and treated by intensive preoperative chemotherapy? *Ann Surg Oncol*, 2012. **19**(8): 2526–38.
23. van den Broek, M.A., Olde Damink, S.W., Dejong, C.H. *et al.*, Liver failure after partial hepatic resection: definition, pathophysiology, risk factors and treatment. *Liver Internat,* 2008. **28**(6): 767–80.
24. Rougier, P., Milan, C., Lazorthes, F. *et al.*, Prospective study of prognostic factors in patients with unresected hepatic metastases from colorectal cancer. Fondation Francaise de Cancerologie Digestive. *Brit J Surg*, 1995. **82**(10): 1397–400.
25. Cummings, L.C., Payes, J.D., Cooper, G.S., Survival after hepatic resection in metastatic colorectal cancer: a population-based study. *Cancer*, 2007. **109**(4): 718–26.

26. Rees, M., Tekkis, P.P., Welsh, F.K., O'Rourke, T., John, T.G., Evaluation of long-term survival after hepatic resection for metastatic colorectal cancer: a multifactorial model of 929 patients. *Ann Surg*, 2008. **247**(1): 125–35.
27. Couinaud, C., Anatomic principles of left and right regulated hepatectomy: technics. *J Chir (Paris),* 1954. **70**(12): 933–66.
28. Couinaud, C., Plea for exact hepatic segmentation and an anatomic technic of regular resection of the liver. Partial clamping of the hepatic stump. *Presse Med*, 1966. **74**(55): 2849–52.
29. Bartlett, D., Fong, Y., Blumgart, L.H. Complete resection of the caudate lobe of the liver: technique and results. *Brit J Surg*, 1996. **83**(8): 1076–81.
30. Cady, B., Jenkins, R.L., Steele, G.D., Jr. *et al.*, Surgical margin in hepatic resection for colorectal metastasis: a critical and improvable determinant of outcome. *Ann surg*, 1998. **227**(4): 566–71.
31. Ekberg, H., Tranberg, K.G., Andersson, R. *et al.*, Determinants of survival in liver resection for colorectal secondaries. *Brit J Surg*, 1986. **73**(9): 727–31.
32. Reddy, S.K., Zorzi, D., Lum, Y.W. *et al.*, Timing of multimodality therapy for resectable synchronous colorectal liver metastases: a retrospective multi-institutional analysis. *Ann Surg Oncol*, 2009. **16**(7): 1809–19.
33. Wakai, T., Shirai, Y., Sakata, J. *et al.*, Appraisal of 1 cm hepatectomy margins for intrahepatic micrometastases in patients with colorectal carcinoma liver metastasis. *Ann Surg Oncol*, 2008. **15**(9): 2472–81.
34. Nuzzo, G., Giuliante, F., Ardito, F. *et al.*, Influence of surgical margin on type of recurrence after liver resection for colorectal metastases: a single-center experience. *Surgery,* 2008. **143**(3): 384–93.
35. Reddy, S.K., Pawlik, T.M., Zorzi, D. *et al.*, Simultaneous resections of colorectal cancer and synchronous liver metastases: a multi-institutional analysis. *Ann Surg Oncol*, 2007. **14**(12): 3481–91.
36. Martin, R., Paty, P., Fong, Y. *et al.*, Simultaneous liver and colorectal resections are safe for synchronous colorectal liver metastasis. *J Am College Surgeons*, 2003. **197**(2): 233–41; discussion 241–32.
37. Thelen, A., Jonas, S., Benckert, C. *et al.*, Simultaneous versus staged liver resection of synchronous liver metastases from colorectal cancer. *Internat J Colorectal Dis*, 2007. **22**(10): 1269–76.
38. Hopt, U.T., Drognitz, O., Neeff, H., Timing of resection in patients with colorectal carcinoma and synchronous liver metastases. *Zentralblatt fur Chirurgie*, 2009. **134**(5): 425–9.

39. Hillingso, J.G., Wille-Jorgensen, P., Staged or simultaneous resection of synchronous liver metastases from colorectal cancer — a systematic review. *Colorectal Dis*, 2009. **11**(1): 3–10.
40. Brouquet, A., Abdalla, E.K., Kopetz, S. *et al.*, High survival rate after two-stage resection of advanced colorectal liver metastases: response-based selection and complete resection define outcome. *J Clin Oncol*, 2011. **29**(8): 1083–90.
41. Polignano, F.M., Quyn, A.J., Sanjay, P., Henderson, N.A., Tait I.S., Totally laparoscopic strategies for the management of colorectal cancer with synchronous liver metastasis. *Surgical Endoscopy*, 2012. **26**(9): 2571–8.
42. Patriti, A., Ceccarelli, G., Bartoli, A., Spaziani, A., Lapalorcia, L.M., Casciola, L., Laparoscopic and robot-assisted one-stage resection of colorectal cancer with synchronous liver metastases: a pilot study. *J Hepato-biliary-pancreatic Surg*, 2009. **16**(4): 450–7.
43. Kim, S.H., Lim, S.B., Ha, Y.H. *et al.*, Laparoscopic-assisted combined colon and liver resection for primary colorectal cancer with synchronous liver metastases: initial experience. *World J Surg*, 2008. **32**(12): 2701–6.
44. Tanaka, K., Shimada, H., Matsuo, K. *et al.*, Outcome after simultaneous colorectal and hepatic resection for colorectal cancer with synchronous metastases. *Surgery*, 2004. **136**(3): 650–9.
45. Vogt, P., Raab, R., Ringe, B., Pichlmayr, R., Resection of synchronous liver metastases from colorectal cancer. *World J Surg*, 1991. 15(1): 62–7.
46. Fahy, B.N., Fischer, C.P., Synchronous resection of colorectal primary and hepatic metastasis. *J Gastrointestinal Oncol*, 2012. **3**(1): 48–58.
47. de Rosa, A., Gomez, D., Hossaini, S. *et al.*, Stage IV colorectal cancer: outcomes following the liver-first approach. *J Surg Oncol*, 2013. **108**(7): 444–9.
48. Brouquet, A., Mortenson, M.M., Vauthey, J.N. *et al.*, Surgical strategies for synchronous colorectal liver metastases in 156 consecutive patients: classic, combined or reverse strategy? *J Am College Surgeons*, 2010. **210**(6): 934–41.
49. Gauzolino, R., Castagnet, M., Blanleuil, M.L., Richer, J.P., The ALPPS technique for bilateral colorectal metastases: three "variations on a theme". *Updates Surg*, 2013. **65**(2): 141–8.
50. Donati, M., Stavrou, G.A., Oldhafer, K.J., Current position of ALPPS in the surgical landscape of CRLM treatment proposals. *World J Gastroenterol*, 2013. **19**(39): 6548–54.

51. Nadalin, S., Capobianco, I., Li, J., Girotti, P., Konigsrainer, I., Konigsrainer, A., Indications and Limits for Associating Liver Partition and Portal Vein Ligation for Staged Hepatectomy (ALPPS). Lessons Learned from 15 Cases at a Single Centre. *Zeitschrift fur Gastroenterologie*, 2014. **52**(1): 35–42.
52. Wicherts, D.A., de Haas, R.J., Salloum, C. *et al.*, Repeat hepatectomy for recurrent colorectal metastases. *Brit J Surg*, 2013. **100**(6): 808–18.
53. Pessaux, P., Lermite, E., Brehant, O., Tuech, J.J., Lorimier, G., Arnaud, J.P., Repeat hepatectomy for recurrent colorectal liver metastases. *J Surg Oncol*, 2006. **93**(1): 1–7.
54. Yan, T.D., Sim, J., Black, D., Niu, R., Morris, D.L., Systematic review on safety and efficacy of repeat hepatectomy for recurrent liver metastases from colorectal carcinoma. *Ann Surg Oncol*, 2007. **14**(7): 2069–77.
55. Makuuchi, M., Thai, B.L., Takayasu, K. *et al.*, Preoperative portal embolization to increase safety of major hepatectomy for hilar bile duct carcinoma: a preliminary report. *Surgery*, 1990. **107**(5): 521–7.
56. Cantlie, J., On a new arrangement of the right and left lobes of the liver. *Proceedings: The Anatomical Society of Great Britain & Ireland*, 1897. **32**: 4–9
57. Vauthey, J.N., Abdalla, E.K., Doherty, D.A. *et al.*, Body surface area and body weight predict total liver volume in Western adults. *Liver transplant*, 2002. **8**(3): 233–40.
58. Ribero, D., Abdalla, E.K., Madoff, D.C., Donadon, M., Loyer, E.M., Vauthey, J.N., Portal vein embolization before major hepatectomy and its effects on regeneration, resectability and outcome. *Brit J Surg*, 2007. **94**(11): 1386–94.
59. Hemming, A.W., Reed, A.I., Howard, R.J. *et al.*, Preoperative portal vein embolization for extended hepatectomy. *Ann Surg*, 2003. **237**(5): 686–91; discussion 691–83.
60. Farges, O., Belghiti, J., Kianmanesh, R. *et al.*, Portal vein embolization before right hepatectomy: prospective clinical trial. *Ann Surg*, 2003. **237**(2): 208–17.
61. Nagino, M., Nimura, Y., Kamiya, J., Kondo, S., Kanai, M., Selective percutaneous transhepatic embolization of the portal vein in preparation for extensive liver resection: the ipsilateral approach. *Radiology*, 1996. **200**(2): 559–63.
62. Avritscher, R., de Baere, T., Murthy, R., Deschamps, F., Madoff, D.C., Percutaneous transhepatic portal vein embolization: rationale, technique, and outcomes. *Semin Interven Radiol*, 2008. **25**(2): 132–45.

63. Kodama, Y., Shimizu, T., Endo, H., Miyamoto, N., Miyasaka, K., Complications of percutaneous transhepatic portal vein embolization. *J Vascul Interven Radiol*, 2002. **13**(12): 1233–7.
64. Perarnau, J.M., Daradkeh, S., Johann, M., Deneuville, M., Weinling, P., Coniel, C., Transjugular preoperative portal embolization (TJPE) a pilot study. *Hepatogastroenterol*, 2003. **50**(51): 610–3.
65. Smits, M.L., Vanlangenhove, P., Sturm, E.J. *et al.*, Transsinusoidal portal vein embolization with ethylene vinyl alcohol copolymer (Onyx): a feasibility study in pigs. *Cardiovascul Interven Radiol*, 2012. **35**(5): 1172–80.
66. Abulkhir, A., Limongelli, P., Healey, A.J. *et al.*, Preoperative portal vein embolization for major liver resection: a meta-analysis. *Ann Surg*, 2008. **247**(1): 49–57.
67. Broering, D.C., Hillert, C., Krupski, G. *et al.*, Portal vein embolization vs. portal vein ligation for induction of hypertrophy of the future liver remnant. *J Gastrointestinal Surg*, 2002. **6**(6): 905–13; discussion 913.
68. Capussotti, L., Muratore, A., Baracchi, F. *et al.*, Portal vein ligation as an efficient method of increasing the future liver remnant volume in the surgical treatment of colorectal metastases. *Arch Surg*, 2008. **143**(10): 978–82; discussion 982.
69. Aussilhou, B., Lesurtel, M., Sauvanet, A. *et al.*, Right portal vein ligation is as efficient as portal vein embolization to induce hypertrophy of the left liver remnant. *J Gastrointestinal Surg*, 2008. **12**(2): 297–303.
70. Are, C., Iacovitti, S., Prete, F., Crafa, F.M., Feasibility of laparoscopic portal vein ligation prior to major hepatectomy. *HPB*, 2008. **10**(4): 229–33.
71. Hwang, S., Lee, S.G., Ko, G.Y. *et al.*, Sequential preoperative ipsilateral hepatic vein embolization after portal vein embolization to induce further liver regeneration in patients with hepatobiliary malignancy. *Ann Surg*, 2009. **249**(4): 608–16.
72. Giovannini, M., Percutaneous alcohol ablation for liver metastasis. *Semin Oncol.* 2002. **29**(2): 192–5.
73. Riemsma, R.P., Bala, M.M., Wolff, R., Kleijnen, J., Percutaneous ethanol injection for liver metastases. *Cochrane Database Syst Rev*, 2013. **5**: CD008717.
74. Sofocleous, C.T., Sideras, P., Petre, E.N., "How we do it" — a practical approach to hepatic metastases ablation techniques. *Tech Vascul Interven Radiol*, 2013. **16**(4): 219–29.

75. Mala, T., Edwin, B., Tillung, T., Kristian, Hol P., Soreide, O., Gladhaug, I., Percutaneous cryoablation of colorectal liver metastases: potentiated by two consecutive freeze-thaw cycles. *Cryobiology*, 2003. **46**(1): 99–102.
76. Bala, M.M., Riemsma, R.P., Wolff, R., Kleijnen, J., Cryotherapy for liver metastases. *Cochrane Database Syst Rev*, 2013. **6**: CD009058.
77. Feliberti, E.C., Wagman, L.D., Radiofrequency ablation of liver metastases from colorectal carcinoma. *Cancer Control*, 2006. **13**(1): 48–51.
78. Livraghi, T., Solbiati, L., Percutaneous treatment: radiofrequency ablation of hepatic metastases in colorectal cancer. *Tumori*, 2001. **87** (1 Suppl 1): S69.
79. Solbiati, L., Ierace, T., Tonolini, M., Osti, V., Cova, L., Radiofrequency thermal ablation of hepatic metastases. *Eur J Ultrasound*, 2001. **13**(2): 149–58.
80. Wright, A.S., Sampson, L.A., Warner, T.F., Mahvi, D.M., Lee, F.T., Jr., Radiofrequency versus microwave ablation in a hepatic porcine model. *Radiology*, 2005. **236**(1): 132–9.
81. Head, H.W., Dodd, G.D., 3rd, Dalrymple, N.C. *et al.*, Percutaneous radiofrequency ablation of hepatic tumors against the diaphragm: frequency of diaphragmatic injury. *Radiology*, 2007. **243**(3): 877–84.
82. Weng, M., Zhang, Y., Zhou, D. *et al.*, Radiofrequency ablation versus resection for colorectal cancer liver metastases: a meta-analysis. *PloS One*. 2012. **7**(9): e45493.
83. Aloia, T.A., Vauthey, J.N., Loyer, E.M. *et al.*, Solitary colorectal liver metastasis: resection determines outcome. *Arch Surg*, 2006. **141**(5): 460–6; discussion 466–7.
84. Lee, W.S., Yun, S.H., Chun, H.K. *et al.*, Clinical outcomes of hepatic resection and radiofrequency ablation in patients with solitary colorectal liver metastasis. *J Clin Gastroenterol*, 2008. **42**(8): 945–9.
85. Hur, H., Ko, Y.T., Min, B.S. *et al.*, Comparative study of resection and radiofrequency ablation in the treatment of solitary colorectal liver metastases. *Am J Surgery*, 2009. **197**(6): 728–36.
86. Gleisner, A.L., Choti, M.A., Assumpcao, L., Nathan, H., Schulick, R.D., Pawlik, T.M., Colorectal liver metastases: Recurrence and survival following hepatic resection, radiofrequency ablation, and combined resection-radiofrequency ablation. *Arch Surg*, 2008. **143**(12): 1204–12.

87. Kornprat, P., Jarnagin, W.R., DeMatteo, R.P., Fong, Y., Blumgart, L.H., D'Angelica, M., Role of intraoperative thermoablation combined with resection in the treatment of hepatic metastasis from colorectal cancer. *Arch Surg*, 2007. **142**(11): 1087–92.
88. Adam, R., Delvart, V., Pascal, G. *et al.*, Rescue surgery for unresectable colorectal liver metastases downstaged by chemotherapy: a model to predict long-term survival. *Ann surg*, 2004. **240**(4): 644–57; discussion 657–48.
89. Tournigand, C., Cervantes, A., Figer, A. *et al.*, OPTIMOX1: a randomized study of FOLFOX4 or FOLFOX7 with oxaliplatin in a stop-and-Go fashion in advanced colorectal cancer — a GERCOR study. *J Clin Oncol*, 2006. **24**(3): 394–400.
90. Tournigand, C., Andre, T., Achille, E. *et al.*, FOLFIRI followed by FOLFOX6 or the reverse sequence in advanced colorectal cancer: a randomized GERCOR study. *J Clin Oncol,* 2004. **22**(2): 229–37.
91. Douillard, J.Y., Cunningham, D., Roth, A.D. *et al.*, Irinotecan combined with fluorouracil compared with fluorouracil alone as first-line treatment for metastatic colorectal cancer: a multicentre randomised trial. *Lancet*, 2000. **355**(9209): 1041–7.
92. Goldberg, R.M., Sargent, D.J., Morton, R.F. *et al.*, A randomized controlled trial of fluorouracil plus leucovorin, irinotecan, and oxaliplatin combinations in patients with previously untreated metastatic colorectal cancer. *J Clin Oncol*, 2004. **22**(1): 23–30.
93. Goldberg, R.M., Tabah-Fisch, I., Bleiberg, H. *et al.*, Pooled analysis of safety and efficacy of oxaliplatin plus fluorouracil/leucovorin administered bimonthly in elderly patients with colorectal cancer. *J Clin Oncol*, 2006. **24**(25): 4085–91.
94. Goldberg, R.M., Venook, A.P., Schilsky, R.L., Cetuximab in the treatment of colorectal cancer. *Clin Adv Hematol Oncol*, 2004. **2**(11): 1–10; quiz 11–2.
95. Cheeseman, S.L., Joel, S.P., Chester, J.D. *et al.*, A 'modified de Gramont' regimen of fluorouracil, alone and with oxaliplatin, for advanced colorectal cancer. *Brit J Cancer*, 2002. **87**(4): 393–9.
96. Chibaudel, B., Tournigand, C., Artru, P. *et al.*, FOLFOX in patients with metastatic colorectal cancer and high alkaline phosphatase level: an

exploratory cohort of the GERCOR OPTIMOX1 study. *Ann Oncol*, 2009, **20**(8): 1383–6.

97. de Gramont, A., Figer, A., Seymour, M. *et al.*, Leucovorin and fluorouracil with or without oxaliplatin as first-line treatment in advanced colorectal cancer. *J Clin Oncol*, 2000. **18**(16): 2938–47.
98. de Gramont, A., Tournigand, C., Andre, T., Larsen, A.K., Louvet, C., Targeted agents for adjuvant therapy of colon cancer. *Semin Oncol*, 2006. **33**(6 Suppl 11): S42–5.
99. Falcone, A., Ricci, S., Brunetti, I. *et al.*, Phase III trial of infusional fluorouracil, leucovorin, oxaliplatin, and irinotecan (FOLFOXIRI) compared with infusional fluorouracil, leucovorin, and irinotecan (FOLFIRI) as first-line treatment for metastatic colorectal cancer: the Gruppo Oncologico Nord Ovest. *J Clin Oncol*, 2007. **25**(13): 1670–6.
100. Maindrault-Goebel, F., de Gramont, A., Louvet, C. *et al.*, High-dose intensity oxaliplatin added to the simplified bimonthly leucovorin and 5-fluorouracil regimen as second-line therapy for metastatic colorectal cancer (FOLFOX 7). *Eur J Cancer.* 2001. **37**(8): 1000–5.
101. Maindrault-Goebel, F., Tournigand, C., Andre, T. *et al.*, Oxaliplatin reintroduction in patients previously treated with leucovorin, fluorouracil and oxaliplatin for metastatic colorectal cancer. *Ann Oncol*, 2004. **15**(8): 1210–4.
102. Toxicity of fluorouracil in patients with advanced colorectal cancer: effect of administration schedule and prognostic factors. Meta-Analysis Group In Cancer. *J Clin Oncol*, 1998. **16**(11): 3537–41.
103. Hochster, H., Chen, T.T., Lu, J.M. *et al.*, Tolerance and activity of oxaliplatin with protracted topotecan infusion in patients with previously treated ovarian cancer. A phase I study. *Gynecol Oncol*, 2008. **108**(3): 500–4.
104. Hong, Y.S., Park, Y.S., Lim, H.Y. *et al.*, S-1 plus oxaliplatin versus capecitabine plus oxaliplatin for first-line treatment of patients with metastatic colorectal cancer: a randomised, non-inferiority phase 3 trial. *Lancet Oncol*, 2012. **13**(11): 1125–32.
105. Schuller, J., Cassidy, J., Dumont, E. *et al.*, Preferential activation of capecitabine in tumor following oral administration to colorectal cancer patients. *Cancer Chemother Pharmacol,* 2000. **45**(4): 291–7.
106. Hoff, P.M., Ansari, R., Batist, G. *et al.*, Comparison of oral capecitabine versus intravenous fluorouracil plus leucovorin as first-line treatment in 605

patients with metastatic colorectal cancer: results of a randomized phase III study. *J Clin Oncol*, 2001. **19**(8): 2282–92.

107. Adams, R.A., Meade, A.M., Seymour, M.T. *et al.*, Intermittent versus continuous oxaliplatin and fluoropyrimidine combination chemotherapy for first-line treatment of advanced colorectal cancer: results of the randomised phase 3 MRC COIN trial. *Lancet Oncol*, 2011. **12**(7): 642–53.
108. Becouarn, Y., Rougier, P., Clinical efficacy of oxaliplatin monotherapy: phase II trials in advanced colorectal cancer. *Semin Oncol*, 1998. **25**(2 Suppl 5): 23–31.
109. Becouarn, Y., Ychou, M., Ducreux, M. *et al.*, Phase II trial of oxaliplatin as first-line chemotherapy in metastatic colorectal cancer patients. Digestive Group of French Federation of Cancer Centers. *J Clin Oncol*, 1998. **16**(8): 2739–44.
110. Graham, J., Mushin, M., Kirkpatrick, P., Oxaliplatin. *Nat Rev Drug Discov,* 2004. **3**(1): 11–2.
111. Argyriou, A.A., Cavaletti, G., Briani, C. *et al.*, Clinical pattern and associations of oxaliplatin acute neurotoxicity: a prospective study in 170 patients with colorectal cancer. *Cancer*, 2013. **119**(2): 438–44.
112. Vauthey, J.N., Pawlik, T.M., Ribero, D. *et al.*, Chemotherapy regimen predicts steatohepatitis and an increase in 90-day mortality after surgery for hepatic colorectal metastases. *J Clin Oncol*, 2006. **24**(13): 2065–72.
113. Ducreux, M., Malka, D., Mendiboure, J. *et al.*, Sequential versus combination chemotherapy for the treatment of advanced colorectal cancer (FFCD 2000-05): an open-label, randomised, phase 3 trial. *Lancet Oncol*, 2011. **12**(11): 1032–44.
114. Arkenau, H.T., Arnold, D., Cassidy, J. *et al.*, Efficacy of oxaliplatin plus capecitabine or infusional fluorouracil/leucovorin in patients with metastatic colorectal cancer: a pooled analysis of randomized trials. *J Clin Oncol*, 2008. **26**(36): 5910–7.
115. Porschen, R., Arkenau, H.T., Kubicka, S. *et al.*, Phase III study of capecitabine plus oxaliplatin compared with fluorouracil and leucovorin plus oxaliplatin in metastatic colorectal cancer: a final report of the AIO Colorectal Study Group. *J Clin Oncol*, 2007. **25**(27): 4217–23.
116. Pommier, Y., Leo, E., Zhang, H., Marchand, C., DNA topoisomerases and their poisoning by anticancer and antibacterial drugs. *Chem Biol*, 2010. **17**(5): 421–33.

117. Cunningham, D., Pyrhonen, S., James, R.D. *et al.*, Randomised trial of irinotecan plus supportive care versus supportive care alone after fluorouracil failure for patients with metastatic colorectal cancer. *Lancet*, 1998. **352**(9138): 1413–8.
118. Saltz, L., Irinotecan-based combinations for the adjuvant treatment of stage III colon cancer. *Oncology (Williston Park)*, 2000. **14**(12 Suppl 14): 47–50.
119. Saltz, L.B., Cox, J.V., Blanke, C. *et al.*, Irinotecan plus fluorouracil and leucovorin for metastatic colorectal cancer. Irinotecan Study Group. *N Eng J Med*, 2000. **343**(13): 905–14.
120. Carlini, L.E., Meropol, N.J., Bever, J. *et al.*, UGT1A7 and UGT1A9 polymorphisms predict response and toxicity in colorectal cancer patients treated with capecitabine/irinotecan. *Clin Cancer Res*, 2005. **11**(3): 1226–36.
121. Cote, J.F., Kirzin, S., Kramar, A. *et al.*, UGT1A1 polymorphism can predict hematologic toxicity in patients treated with irinotecan. *Clin Cancer Res*, 2007. **13**(11): 3269–75.
122. Fong, Y., Bentrem, D.J., CASH (Chemotherapy-Associated Steatohepatitis) costs. *Ann Surg*, 2006. **243**(1): 8–9.
123. Borner, M.M., Bernhard, J., Dietrich, D. *et al.*, A randomized phase II trial of capecitabine and two different schedules of irinotecan in first-line treatment of metastatic colorectal cancer: efficacy, quality-of-life and toxicity. *Ann Oncol*, 2005. **16**(2): 282–8.
124. Bidard, F.C., Tournigand, C., Andre, T. *et al.*, Efficacy of FOLFIRI-3 (irinotecan D1,D3 combined with LV5-FU) or other irinotecan-based regimens in oxaliplatin-pretreated metastatic colorectal cancer in the GERCOR OPTIMOX1 study. *Ann Oncol*, 2009. **20**(6): 1042–7.
125. Colucci, G., Gebbia, V., Paoletti G *et al.*, Phase III randomized trial of FOLFIRI versus FOLFOX4 in the treatment of advanced colorectal cancer: a multicenter study of the Gruppo Oncologico Dell'Italia Meridionale. *J Clin Oncol*, 2005. **23**(22): 4866–75.
126. Bokemeyer, C., Bondarenko, I., Hartmann, J.T. *et al.*, Efficacy according to biomarker status of cetuximab plus FOLFOX-4 as first-line treatment for metastatic colorectal cancer: the OPUS study. *Ann Oncol*, 2011. **22**(7): 1535–46.
127. Cunningham, D., Humblet, Y., Siena, S. *et al.*, Cetuximab monotherapy and cetuximab plus irinotecan in irinotecan-refractory metastatic colorectal cancer. *N Eng J Med*, 2004. **351**(4): 337–45.

128. Maughan, T.S., Adams, R.A., Smith, C.G. *et al.*, Addition of cetuximab to oxaliplatin-based first-line combination chemotherapy for treatment of advanced colorectal cancer: results of the randomised phase 3 MRC COIN trial. *Lancet*, 2011. **377**(9783): 2103–14.
129. Sobrero, A.F., Maurel, J., Fehrenbacher, L. *et al.*, EPIC: phase III trial of cetuximab plus irinotecan after fluoropyrimidine and oxaliplatin failure in patients with metastatic colorectal cancer. *J Clin Oncol*, 2008. **26**(14): 2311–9.
130. Tveit, K.M., Guren, T., Glimelius, B. *et al.*, Phase III trial of cetuximab with continuous or intermittent fluorouracil, leucovorin, and oxaliplatin (Nordic FLOX) versus FLOX alone in first-line treatment of metastatic colorectal cancer: the NORDIC-VII study. *J Clin Oncol*, 2012. **30**(15): 1755–62.
131. Van Cutsem, E., Kohne, C.H., Lang, I. *et al.*, Cetuximab plus irinotecan, fluorouracil, and leucovorin as first-line treatment for metastatic colorectal cancer: updated analysis of overall survival according to tumor KRAS and BRAF mutation status. *J Clin Oncol*, 2011. **29**(15): 2011–9.
132. Tortola, S., Marcuello, E., Gonzalez, I. *et al.*, p53 and K-ras gene mutations correlate with tumor aggressiveness but are not of routine prognostic value in colorectal cancer. *J Clin Oncol*, 1999. **17**(5): 1375–81.
133. Hurwitz, H., Fehrenbacher, L., Novotny, W. *et al.*, Bevacizumab plus irinotecan, fluorouracil, and leucovorin for metastatic colorectal cancer. *N Eng J Med*, 2004. **350**(23): 2335–42.
134. Hurwitz, H.I., Tebbutt, N.C., Kabbinavar, F. *et al.*, Efficacy and safety of bevacizumab in metastatic colorectal cancer: pooled analysis from seven randomized controlled trials. *Oncologist*, 2013. **18**(9): 1004–12.
135. Giantonio, B.J., Catalano, P.J., Meropol, N.J. *et al.*, Bevacizumab in combination with oxaliplatin, fluorouracil, and leucovorin (FOLFOX4) for previously treated metastatic colorectal cancer: results from the Eastern Cooperative Oncology Group Study E3200. *J Clin Oncol*, 2007. **25**(12): 1539–44.
136. Fuloria, J., Safety profiles of current antiangiogenic therapies for metastatic colorectal cancer. *OncoTargets Therapy*, 2012. **5**: 133–42.
137. Grothey, A., Cutsem, E.V., Sobrero, A. *et al.*, Regorafenib monotherapy for previously treated metastatic colorectal cancer (CORRECT): an international, multicentre, randomised, placebo-controlled, phase 3 trial. *Lancet*, 2013. **381**(9863): 303–12.

138. Randomized comparison of FOLFIRI plus cetuximab versus FOLFIRI plus bevacizumab as first-line treatment of KRAS wild-type metastatic colorectal cancer: German AIO study KRK-0306 (FIRE-3); JCO, 2013 ASCO Annual Meeting Abstracts. **31**(18) (June 20 Supplement).
139. NCT00265850. Cetuximab and/or Bevacizumab Combined With Combination Chemotherapy in Treating Patients With Metastatic Colorectal Cancer. ClinicalTrials.gov.
140. Chua, T.C., Saxena, A., Liauw, W., Kokandi, A., Morris, D.L. Systematic review of randomized and nonrandomized trials of the clinical response and outcomes of neoadjuvant systemic chemotherapy for resectable colorectal liver metastases. *Ann Surg Oncol*, 2010. **17**(2): 492–501.
141. Lam, V.W., Spiro, C., Laurence, J.M. *et al.*, A systematic review of clinical response and survival outcomes of downsizing systemic chemotherapy and rescue liver surgery in patients with initially unresectable colorectal liver metastases. *Ann Surg Oncol,* 2012. **19**(4): 1292–301.
142. Gallagher, D.J., Zheng, J., Capanu, M. *et al.*, Response to neoadjuvant chemotherapy does not predict overall survival for patients with synchronous colorectal hepatic metastases. *Ann Surg Oncol*, 2009. **16**(7): 1844–51.
143. Delaunoit, T., Alberts, S.R., Sargent, D.J. *et al.*, Chemotherapy permits resection of metastatic colorectal cancer: experience from Intergroup N9741. *Ann Oncol*, 2005. **16**(3): 425–9.
144. Adam, R., Aloia, T.A., Is hepatic resection justified after chemotherapy in patients with colorectal liver metastases and lymph node involvement? *J Clin Oncol*, 2009. **27**(8): 1343–5; author reply 1345.
145. Alberts, S.R., Horvath, W.L., Sternfeld, W.C. *et al.*, Oxaliplatin, fluorouracil, and leucovorin for patients with unresectable liver-only metastases from colorectal cancer: a North Central Cancer Treatment Group phase II study. *J Clin Oncol*, 2005. **23**(36): 9243–9.
146. Masi, G., Cupini, S., Marcucci, L. *et al.*, Treatment with 5-fluorouracil/folinic acid, oxaliplatin, and irinotecan enables surgical resection of metastases in patients with initially unresectable metastatic colorectal cancer. *Ann Surg Oncol*, 2006. **13**(1): 58–65.
147. Chung, W.S., Park, M.S., Shin, S.J. *et al.*, Response evaluation in patients with colorectal liver metastases: RECIST version 1.1 versus modified CT criteria. *Am J Roentgenol*, 2012. **199**(4): 809–15.

148. Therasse, P., Arbuck, S.G., Eisenhauer, E.A. *et al.*, New guidelines to evaluate the response to treatment in solid tumors. European Organization for Research and Treatment of Cancer, National Cancer Institute of the United States, National Cancer Institute of Canada. *J Natl Cancer Inst,* 2000. **92**(3): 205–16.
149. Arita, J., Ono, Y., Takahashi, M., Inoue, Y., Takahashi, Y., Saiura, A., Usefulness of contrast-enhanced intraoperative ultrasound in identifying disappearing liver metastases from colorectal carcinoma after chemotherapy. *Ann Surg Oncol*, 2014.
150. Benoist, S., Brouquet, A., Penna, C. *et al.*, Complete response of colorectal liver metastases after chemotherapy: does it mean cure? *J Clin Oncol*, 2006. **24**(24): 3939–45.
151. http://www.nccn.org
152. Bischof, D.A., Clary, B.M., Maithel, S.K., Pawlik, T.M., Surgical management of disappearing colorectal liver metastases. *Brit J Surg*, 2013. **100**(11): 1414–20.
153. Strobel, O., Buchler, M.W., Surgical management of disappearing colorectal liver metastases. *Chirurg*, 2013. **84**(12): 1075.
154. Oliva, M.R., Mortele, K.J., Segatto, E. *et al.*, Computed tomography features of nonalcoholic steatohepatitis with histopathologic correlation. *J Comp Assisted Tomography*, 2006. **30**(1): 37–43.
155. Elias, D., Youssef, O., Sideris, L. *et al.*, Evolution of missing colorectal liver metastases following inductive chemotherapy and hepatectomy. *J Surg Oncol*, 2004. **86**(1): 4–9.
156. Auer, R.C., White, R.R., Kemeny, N.E. *et al.*, Predictors of a true complete response among disappearing liver metastases from colorectal cancer after chemotherapy. *Cancer*, 2010. **116**(6): 1502–9.
157. Ko, Y.J. Karanicolas, P.J. Hepatic arterial infusion pump chemotherapy for colorectal liver metastases: an old technology in a new era. *Curr Oncol*, 2014. **21**(1): e116–21.
158. Karanicolas, P.J., Metrakos, P., Chan, K. *et al.*, Hepatic arterial infusion pump chemotherapy in the management of colorectal liver metastases: expert consensus statement. *Curr Oncol*, 2014. **21**(1): e129–36.
159. Chang, A.E., Schneider, P.D., Sugarbaker, P.H., Simpson, C., Culnane, M., Steinberg, S.M., A prospective randomized trial of regional versus systemic

continuous 5-fluorodeoxyuridine chemotherapy in the treatment of colorectal liver metastases. *Ann Surg*, 1987. **206**(6): 685–93.

160. Goere, D., Benhaim, L., Bonnet S. *et al.*, Adjuvant chemotherapy after resection of colorectal liver metastases in patients at high risk of hepatic recurrence: a comparative study between hepatic arterial infusion of oxaliplatin and modern systemic chemotherapy. *Ann Surg*, 2013. **257**(1): 114–20.
161. Alberts, S.R., Roh, M.S., Mahoney, M.R. *et al.*, Alternating systemic and hepatic artery infusion therapy for resected liver metastases from colorectal cancer: a North Central Cancer Treatment Group (NCCTG)/ National Surgical Adjuvant Breast and Bowel Project (NSABP) phase II intergroup trial, N9945/CI-66. *J Clin Oncol*, 2010. **28**(5): 853–8.
162. Barber, F.D., Mavligit, G., Kurzrock, R., Hepatic arterial infusion chemotherapy for metastatic colorectal cancer: a concise overview. *Cancer Treat Rev,* 2004. **30**(5): 425–36.
163. Bolton, J.S., O'Connell, M.J., Mahoney. M.R. *et al.*, Hepatic arterial infusion and systemic chemotherapy after multiple metastasectomy in patients with colorectal carcinoma metastatic to the liver: a North Central Cancer Treatment Group (NCCTG) phase II study, 92-46-52. *Clin Colorectal Cancer,* 2012. **11**(1): 31–7.
164. Kemeny, M.M., Adak, S., Gray, B. *et al.*, Combined-modality treatment for resectable metastatic colorectal carcinoma to the liver: surgical resection of hepatic metastases in combination with continuous infusion of chemotherapy — an intergroup study. *J Clin Oncol*, 2002. **20**(6): 1499–505.
165. Kemeny, N., Huang, Y., Cohen, A.M *et al.*, Hepatic arterial infusion of chemotherapy after resection of hepatic metastases from colorectal cancer. *N Eng J Med*, 1999. **341**(27): 2039–48.
166. Kemeny, N.E., Ron, I.G., Hepatic arterial chemotherapy in metastatic colorectal patients. *Semin Oncol*, 1999. **26**(5): 524–35.
167. Kemeny, N.E., Gonen, M., Hepatic arterial infusion after liver resection. *N Eng J Med*, 2005. **352**(7): 734–5.
168. Sanz-Altamira, P.M., Spence, L.D., Huberman, M.S. *et al.*, Selective chemoembolization in the management of hepatic metastases in refractory colorectal carcinoma: a phase II trial. *Dis Colon Rectum*, 1997. **40**(7): 770–5.

169. Hunt, T.M., Flowerdew, A.D., Birch, S.J., Williams, J.D., Mullee, M.A., Taylor, I., Prospective randomized controlled trial of hepatic arterial embolization or infusion chemotherapy with 5-fluorouracil and degradable starch microspheres for colorectal liver metastases. *Brit J Surg*, 1990. **77**(7): 779–82.
170. Poggi, G., Amatu, A., Montagna, B. *et al.*, OEM-TACE: a new therapeutic approach in unresectable intrahepatic cholangiocarcinoma. *Cardiovascul Interven Radiol*, 2009. **32**(6): 1187–92.
171. Poggi, G., Quaretti, P., Minoia, C. *et al.*, Transhepatic arterial chemoembolization with oxaliplatin-eluting microspheres (OEM-TACE) for unresectable hepatic tumors. *Anticancer Res*, 2008. **28**(6B): 3835–42.
172. Hong, K., Geschwind, J.F., Locoregional intra-arterial therapies for unresectable intrahepatic cholangiocarcinoma. *Semin Oncol*, 2010. **37**(2): 110–7.
173. Fiorentini, G., Aliberti, C., Tilli, M. *et al.*, Intra-arterial infusion of irinotecan-loaded drug-eluting beads (DEBIRI) versus intravenous therapy (FOLFIRI) for hepatic metastases from colorectal cancer: final results of a phase III study. *Anticancer Res*, 2012. **32**(4): 1387–95.
174. Narayanan, G., Barbery, K., Suthar, R., Guerrero, G., Arora, G., Transarterial chemoembolization using DEBIRI for treatment of hepatic metastases from colorectal cancer. *Anticancer Res*, 2013. **33**(5): 2077–83.
175. Grimm, J., LaCouture, T., Croce, R., Yeo, I., Zhu, Y., Xue, J., Dose tolerance limits and dose volume histogram evaluation for stereotactic body radiotherapy. *J Appl Clin Med Phys*, 2011. **12**(2): 3368.
176. Kirkpatrick, J.P., Kelsey, C.R., Palta, M. *et al.*, Stereotactic body radiotherapy: A critical review for non-radiation oncologists. *Cancer*, 2013.
177. Hiraki, M., Nishimura, J., Ohtsuka, M. *et al.*, Impact of stereotactic body radiotherapy on colorectal cancer with distant metastases. *Oncol Rep*, 2014. **31**(2): 795–9.
178. Dancey, J.E., Shepherd, F.A., Paul, K. *et al.*, Treatment of nonresectable hepatocellular carcinoma with intrahepatic 90Y-microspheres. *J Nuclear Med*, 2000. **41**(10): 1673–81.
179. Breedis, C., Young, G., The blood supply of neoplasms in the liver. *Am J Path*, 1954. **30**(5): 969–77.
180. Lewandowski, R.J., Salem, R., Yttrium-90 radioembolization of hepatocellular carcinoma and metastatic disease to the liver. *Semin Interven Radiol*, 2006. **23**(1): 64–72.

181. Mulcahy, M., A Phase III Clinical Trial Evaluating TheraSphere® in Patients With Metastatic Colorectal Carcinoma of the Liver Who Have Failed First Line Chemotherapy. http://clinicaltrials.gov/show/NCT01483027.
182. Al-Mufti, R.A., Pedley, R.B., Marshall, D. *et al.*, *In vitro* assessment of Lipiodol-targeted radiotherapy for liver and colorectal cancer cell lines. *Brit J Cancer,* 1999. **79**(11–12): 1665–71.
183. Davis, C.R., Interventional radiological treatment of hepatocellular carcinoma. *Cancer Control*, 2010. **17**(2): 87–99.
184. Gray, B., Van Hazel, G., Hope, M. *et al.*, Randomised trial of SIR-Spheres plus chemotherapy vs. chemotherapy alone for treating patients with liver metastases from primary large bowel cancer. *Ann Oncol*, 2001. **12**(12): 1711–20.
185. Sharma, R.A., Van Hazel, G.A., Morgan, B. *et al.*, Radioembolization of liver metastases from colorectal cancer using yttrium-90 microspheres with concomitant systemic oxaliplatin, fluorouracil, and leucovorin chemotherapy. *J Clin Oncol*, 2007. **25**(9): 1099–106.
186. Van Hazel, G., Blackwell, A., Anderson, J. *et al.*, Randomised phase 2 trial of SIR-Spheres plus fluorouracil/leucovorin chemotherapy versus fluorouracil/leucovorin chemotherapy alone in advanced colorectal cancer. *J Surg Oncol*, 2004. **88**(2): 78–85.
187. Collettini, F., Singh, A., Schnapauff, D. *et al.*, Computed-tomography-guided high-dose-rate brachytherapy (CT-HDRBT) ablation of metastases adjacent to the liver hilum. *Eur J Radiol*, 2013. **82**(10): e509–14.
188. Donath, D., Nori, D., Turnbull, A., Kaufman, N., Fortner, J.G., Brachytherapy in the treatment of solitary colorectal metastases to the liver. *J Surg Oncol*, 1990. **44**(1): 55–61.
189. Collettini, F., Lutter, A., Schnapauff, D. *et al.*, Unresectable Colorectal Liver Metastases: Percutaneous Ablation Using CT-Guided High-Dose-Rate Brachytherapy (CT-HDBRT). *Rofo*, 2014.
190. Benson, A.B., 3rd, Bekaii-Saab, T., Chan, E. *et al.*, Metastatic colon cancer, version 3.2013: featured updates to the NCCN Guidelines. *J Natl Compr Canc Netw*, 2013. **11**(2): 141–52; quiz 152.
191. Meyerhardt, J.A., Mangu, P.B., Flynn, P.J. *et al.*, Follow-up care, surveillance protocol, and secondary prevention measures for survivors of

colorectal cancer: American Society of Clinical Oncology clinical practice guideline endorsement. *J Clin Oncol*, 2013. **31**(35): 4465–70.
192. Ohlsson, B., Breland, U., Ekberg, H., Graffner, H., Tranberg, K.G., Follow-up after curative surgery for colorectal carcinoma. Randomized comparison with no follow-up. *Dis Colon Rectum*, 1995. **38**(6): 619–26.
193. Schoemaker, D., Black, R., Giles, L., Toouli, J., Yearly colonoscopy, liver CT, and chest radiography do not influence 5-year survival of colorectal cancer patients. *Gastroenterol*, 1998. **114**(1): 7–14.
194. Primrose, J.N., Perera, R., Gray, A. *et al.*, Effect of 3 to 5 years of scheduled CEA and CT follow-up to detect recurrence of colorectal cancer: the FACS randomized clinical trial. *Jama*, 2014. **311**(3): 263–70.
195. Jones, N.B., McNally, M.E., Malhotra, L. *et al.*, Repeat hepatectomy for metastatic colorectal cancer is safe but marginally effective. *Ann Surg Oncol*, 2012. **19**(7): 2224–9.
196. Blackmon, S.H., Stephens, E.H., Correa, A.M. *et al.*, Predictors of recurrent pulmonary metastases and survival after pulmonary metastasectomy for colorectal cancer. *Ann Thorac Surg*, 2012. **94**(6): 1802–9.
197. Gonzalez, M., Poncet, A., Combescure, C., Robert, J., Ris, H.B., Gervaz, P., Risk factors for survival after lung metastasectomy in colorectal cancer patients: a systematic review and meta-analysis. *Ann Surg Oncol*, 2013. **20**(2): 572–9.
198. Gonzalez, M., Robert, J.H., Halkic, N. *et al.*, Survival after lung metastasectomy in colorectal cancer patients with previously resected liver metastases. *World J Surg*, 2012. **36**(2): 386–91.
199. Lin, B.R., Chang, T.C., Lee, Y.C., Lee, P.H., Chang, K.J., Liang, J.T., Pulmonary resection for colorectal cancer metastases: duration between cancer onset and lung metastasis as an important prognostic factor. *Ann Surg Oncol*, 2009. **16**(4): 1026–32.
200. Rama, N., Monteiro, A., Bernardo, J.E., Eugenio, L., Antunes, M.J., Lung metastases from colorectal cancer: surgical resection and prognostic factors. *Eur J Cardiothorac Surg*, 2009. **35**(3): 444–9.
201. Shah, S.A., Haddad, R., Al-Sukhni, W. *et al.*, Surgical resection of hepatic and pulmonary metastases from colorectal carcinoma. *J Am College Surgeons*, 2006. **202**(3): 468–75.

202. Hopt, U.T., Drognitz, O., Neeff, H., Timing of resection in patients with colorectal carcinoma and synchronous liver metastases. *Zentralbl Chir*, 2009. **134**(5): 425–9.
203. Neeff, H., Horth, W., Makowiec, F. *et al.*, Outcome after resection of hepatic and pulmonary metastases of colorectal cancer. *J Gastrointestinal Surg*, 2009. **13**(10): 1813–20.
204. Mourra, N., Hoeffel, C., Duvillard, P., Guettier, C., Flejou, J.F., Tiret, E., Adrenalectomy for clinically isolated metastasis from colorectal carcinoma: report of eight cases. *Dis Colon Rectum*, 2008. **51**(12): 1846–9.
205. Katayama, A., Mafune, K., Makuuchi, M., Adrenalectomy for solitary adrenal metastasis from colorectal carcinoma. *Jap J Clin Oncol*, 2000. **30**(9): 414–6.
206. Fujita, K., Kameyama, S., Kawamura, M., Surgically removed adrenal metastasis from cancer of the rectum. Report of a case. *Dis Colon Rectum*, 1988. **31**(2): 141–3.
207. Tan, W.S., Ho, K.S., Eu, K.W., Brain metastases in colorectal cancers. *World J Surg*, 2009. **33**(4): 817–21.
208. Hammoud, M.A., McCutcheon, I.E., Elsouki, R., Schoppa, D., Patt, Y.Z., Colorectal carcinoma and brain metastasis: distribution, treatment, and survival. *Ann Surg Oncol*, 1996. **3**(5): 453–63.
209. Byrne, B.E., Geddes, T., Welsh, F.K., John, T.G., Chandrakumaran, K., Rees, M., The incidence and outcome of brain metastases after liver resection for colorectal cancer metastases. *Colorectal Dis*, 2012. **14**(6): 721–6.
210. Esmaeilzadeh. M., Majlesara, A., Faridar, A. *et al.*, Brain metastasis from gastrointestinal cancers: a systematic review. *Internation J Clin Pract*, 2014.
211. Mege, D., Ouaissi, M., Fuks, D. *et al.*, Patients with brain metastases from colorectal cancer are not condemned. *Anticancer Res*, 2013. **33**(12): 5645–8.
212. Ho, T.W., Mack, L.A., Temple, W.J., Operative salvage for retroperitoneal nodal recurrence in colorectal cancer: a systematic review. *Ann Surg Oncol*, 2011. **18**(3): 697–703.
213. Kobayashi, A., Sugito, M., Ito, M., Saito, N., Predictors of successful salvage surgery for local pelvic recurrence of rectosigmoid colon and rectal cancers. *Surg Today*, 2007. **37**(10): 853–9.

Chapter 14

Diagnosis and Staging of Pancreatic Malignancies

Saurabh Chawla, Parit Mekaroonkamol and Field F. Willingham

What is New

- Pancreatic adenocarcinoma is predicted to become the second leading cause of cancer mortality due to increasing incidence and poor survival rates.
- Helical CT, MRI and EUS are all very sensitive modalities for pancreatic tumor detection and are often used in combination for complete staging and optimal management of pancreatic tumors.

Introduction

The pancreas secretes enzymes and hormones which aid in digestion and metabolism. Histologically, the pancreas has a predominant exocrine component composed of acini and ducts compromising most of its substance which is responsible for the secretion of digestive enzymes. A smaller but equally important endocrine component is formed by islet cells responsible for the secretion of peptide hormones such as insulin, glucagon, somatostatin, pancreatic polypeptide and vasoactive intestinal peptide (VIP). In addition, the parenchyma has lymphoid and stromal cells responsible for the integrity of the organ.

Primary neoplastic change can occur in all of the various components of the gland and occasionally, this organ may also be a site of spread of malignancy from other primary sites. Pancreatic ductal adenocarcinoma with its associated variants accounts for 85–90% of all pancreatic neoplasms.[1] Endocrine tumors arising from islet cells are much less frequent (<5%) and, based on the predominant hormone activity, can have myriad presentations. They are now classified as pancreatic neuroendocrine tumors.[2] Finally, there is a subset of less common pancreatic malignant tumors which include rarer subtypes of exocrine, lymphoid and metastatic malignancies. These differ in presentation and prognosis from ductal adenocarcinomas and neuroendocrine tumors. This chapter reviews the recent advances in the clinical presentation, diagnosis and staging of the various malignant pancreatic neoplasms.

Pancreatic Adenocarcinoma

Epidemiology

Pancreatic cancer is the fourth leading cause of cancer related mortality in the United States though it accounts for only 2.8% of new cancer cases.[3,4] This is related to late clinical presentation, aggressive tumor biology and the lack of effective therapies. The median survival is 12 months.[5,6] Consequently, the incidence rate for pancreatic cancer (12.2/100,000 men and women per year) is similar to the number of deaths per year from this malignancy (10.9/100,000 men and women per year) (http://seer.cancer.gov/csr/1975_2010/). While death rates for the four leading cancers in the United States (lung, breast, colorectal and prostate) have continued to decline over the last decade, the incidence and mortality due to pancreatic cancer have shown a slight increase, and it is predicted that pancreatic cancer may become the second leading cause of cancer mortality in the United States by 2020.[7] The key factor in improving this dismal prognosis is early recognition as early tumor stage is associated with significantly better survival with some studies showing up to a 66% survival after surgical resection of small tumors not involving the lymph nodes.[8,9] A detailed review of pancreatic cancer epidemiology is presented in Chapter 1 of this book.

Clinical presentation and its role in diagnosis and staging

In 1865 Dr. Armand Trousseau first reported the association of thromboembolism with visceral malignancy and subsequently, after noticing phlebitis in his left upper arm, diagnosed himself and died shortly thereafter from gastric cancer.[10] Thus, migratory thrombophlebitis became known as Trousseau's syndrome and was one of the earliest described symptoms of pancreatic cancer. To date, most symptoms associated with pancreatic cancer remain vague and non-specific and the clinical presentation is often dependent on tumor location within the pancreas.

In a prospective multicenter series of 185 consecutive patients, pain, asthenia, weight loss and anorexia were the most commonly reported symptoms occurring in over 80% of the patients.[11] Cholestatic symptoms of jaundice and dark colored urine are present in approximately 50% of the patients and are more commonly associated with pancreatic head tumors due to the proclivity of these tumors to compress and obstruct the intra-pancreatic bile duct. These manifestations of obstructive jaundice, along with steatorrhea (25%), may prompt earlier investigation, and therefore pancreatic head tumors may be recognized at an earlier stage as compared to tumors in the body and tail.[11,12] The body/tail tumors often manifest with the insidious onset of abdominal pain which is often unrecognized in the early stages due to its non specific nature. Tumors of the body tend to present with mid epigastric pain, while tumors in the tail may be associated with left sided pain. As the tumor progresses beyond the capsule or infiltrates into the retroperitoneum, the pain may become neural in character and radiate to the back.[13] Pain at presentation may also have a prognostic significance. In a prospective study involving 77 patients, preoperative pain was associated with decreased survival even in patients with otherwise resectable disease as determined by imaging (9.2 months *vs* 21.9 months; $p = 0.045$).[14]

New onset pancreatitis, diabetes mellitus especially in the elderly or paraneoplastic phenomena such as pancreatic panniculitis (erythematous subcutaneous areas of nodular fat necrosis), cicatricial and bullous pemphigoid have also been described as presenting symptoms and should prompt a work-up of pancreatic malignancies in the appropriate clinical context.[15–18]

As with Trousseau's syndrome, some other eponymous physical examination findings are associated with pancreatic cancer and were described after decades of careful observation in the era prior to advent of cross sectional imaging. These signs include left supraclavicular adenopathy (Virchow's node), a palpable periumbilical mass (Sister Mary Joesph's node) and a drop metastasis at Blumer's shelf on digital rectal examination. The presence of these signs suggests metastatic disease and is associated with a poor prognosis.[19] These signs are not specific for pancreatic cancer and have been reported with other intra-abdominal adenocarcinomas. Other non-specific physical findings may include hepatomegaly (39%), palpable abdominal masses (24%) or Courvoisier's sign, the presence of a non-tender palpable distended gall bladder at the right costal margin which may be present in up to 13% of patients.[11]

The diagnosis of pancreatic cancer may be delayed by up to two years after initial presentation. This is because of the non-specific nature of early complaints and the low prevalence of pancreatic cancer amongst patients seen in primary care. This decreases the positive predictive value of most of these symptoms individually to less than 1%. The presence of jaundice is more alarming and prompts an immediate work-up raising its PPV to 22%, and thus may lead to the diagnosis of the malignancy at an earlier stage.[20]

Astute clinical evaluation and advances in imaging and tissue acquisition can now lead to earlier recognition and tissue diagnosis for smaller tumors; however, curative intent surgery is still limited to less than 15% of all tumors.[21] Therefore, there remains an urgent need for earlier diagnosis. Large population-based cohorts have now identified certain modifiable and non-modifiable risk factors which may predict an increased odds of developing pancreatic cancer (Table 1). As with the clinical signs and symptoms, the absolute risk increase in the presence of these factors remains low due to the low prevalence of pancreatic cancer. The recognition of familial pancreatic cancer kindreds and association with genetic syndromes in about 5% of pancreatic cancers has also led to an interest in identifying high-risk individuals (Table 2), who can then be screened to detect premalignant (PanIN, IPMN) or early stage tumors.

Table 1. Risk factors for pancreatic adenocarcinoma.

Risk factor	Odds ratio (95%CI)	Comments	Ref.
Cigarette Smoking		For former smokers, there is a rapid reduction in risk within 2 years of quitting which returns to baseline after 10 years.	(198)
• Current	1.74 (1.61, 1.87)		
• Former	1.2 (1.11,1.29)		
Heavy alcohol use		Conflicting data with heavy alcohol use, no significant correlation with mild to moderate alcohol use	(199, 200)
(> 6 drinks per day)	1.5 (1.2–1.8)		
(> 3 drinks per day)	1.22 (1.12–1.34)		
Body Mass Index		Increased association with central obesity and early adult obesity	(201)
• >30	1.47 (1.23, 1.75)		
Diet	Inconclusive evidence	A "Western" dietary pattern (high intake of saturated fat and/or meat, particularly smoked or processed meats) has been linked to the development of pancreatic cancer in some studies	(202, 203)
Diabetes	1.94 (1.66–2.27)	Relative risk correlated negatively with duration of DM	(100)
Antidiabetic agents	Inconclusive evidence	Recent meta-analysis report no significant association	(204)
• Metformin	Prior studies note protective benefit with Metformin	FDA and European Medicines Agency cite insufficient evidence to confirm increased risk	
• Sulfonylureas			
• Insulin Secreatagogues (GLP 1 Analogues, DPP 4 inhibitors)	Some animal studies and case control studies report increase risk of pancreatic cancer with sulfonylureas and insulin secreatagogues		

(*Continued*)

Table 1. *(Continued)*

Risk factor	Odds ratio (95%CI)	Comments	Ref.
ABO Genotype			(205)
• OO	1.00		
• AO	1.23 (1.10, 1.37)		
• AA	1.49 (1.24, 1.79)		
• BO	1.35 (1.15, 1.59)		
• BB	1.58 (0.97, 2.59)		
• AB	1.44 (1.15, 1.81)		
Occupational factors		Most common reported industries with these exposures include dry cleaning and metal works.	(206)
• Chlorinated HC	MRR 1.4 (1.0, 1.8)		
• PAH	MRR 1.14 (0.89, 1.45)		
• Others-Cadmium, Nitrosamines, Non organochlorine pesticides			
Chronic Pancreatitis	Population attributable fraction 1.34% (95% CI: 0.612–2.07%)	Standardized incidence ratio (the ratio of observed to expected cases) –26.3, with cumulative risk of 4% at 20 years	(207)

Table 2. Hereditary risk factors for pancreatic adenocarcinoma (Adapted from Refs. [13] and [25]).

Risk factor	Gene affected	Comments
Hereditary pancreatitis	Serine Protease 1 (PRSS1) on Chr 7q35	Standardized incidence ratio 87 (42–113) Cumulative risk of developing pancreatic cancer 10% at 50 years 19% at 60 years 54% at 75 years Higher in smokers, and those with DM
Hereditary Breast Cancer (HBOC)	BRCA 2 (13q12q13) BRCA 1, PALB2	BRCA 2 most common mutation in patients with hereditary pancreatic cancer with 3.5-10 fold increase risk of developing cancer
Peutz-Jeghers syndrome	STK11/LKB1 (19p13)	100-fold increased risk, cumulative risk upto 36%
Familial atypical multiple-mole melanoma (FAMMM) syndrome	p16 (9p21)	12–20 fold increased risk, cumulative risk upto 17% by 75 years of age
Ataxia-telangiectasia (AT)	ATM (11q22-23)	Leukemia and lymphoma most commonly associated with AT. Weak association with pancreatic cancer however ATM mutations identified in some familial kindreds
Lynch syndrome	hMSH2, hMLH1	Weak association, noted in some families (<5 fold increased risk)
Family X (pancreatic cancer, pancreatic insufficiency and DM	4q32-34	>80% penentrance, early age of onset
Familial pancreatic cancer	"heterogeneous group of families with at least two first-degree relatives with pancreatic ductal adenocarcinoma in the absence of an accumulation of other cancers or diseases that are known to be familial"	18-fold increased risk with two or more first degree relatives affected 57-fold increased risk with three or more affected family members (two of whom were first-degree relatives) Possible extension of increased risk to even second-degree relatives

Screening for occult pancreatic adenocarcinoma

Population-based screening is not feasible due to the low incidence of pancreatic cancer and lack of a simple reliable non-invasive screening tool.[22] Small cohort studies have therefore focused on high-risk individuals with known genetic syndromes or family history (Table 2) with variable results. One study in 1999 used ERCP, spiral CT, EUS and tumor markers (CEA and CA 19-9) and reported abnormal findings in 7 of the 14 screened individuals who subsequently underwent resection and were found to have widespread dysplasia on histology but no invasive cancers.[23] Other groups have reported a diagnostic yield as low as 1.3% using multiple modalities including MRCP and EUS with FNA.[24] Screening studies to date have included premalignant lesions such as IPMNs and PanINs as these significant; however, it is unclear if early identification and treatment will lead to increased survival as only a fraction of these lesions may progress to invasive cancer.[25] Also, screening protocols utilizing multiple imaging modalities may not be cost-effective and may detect non-pancreatic lesions which will then need to be addressed, raising other financial, medical and ethical considerations.[26]

Recommendations from screening may come from consensus statements from multidisciplinary groups focused on pancreatic cancer research or are individual center based but have yet not been endorsed by gastroenterology and cancer societies. The International Cancer of the Pancreas Screening (CAPS) Consortium, an international multidisciplinary group of 50 experts recommends screening for first-degree relatives (FDRs) of patients with pancreatic cancer from a familial PC kindred with at least two affected FDRs; patients with Peutz–Jeghers syndrome; and p16, BRCA2 and hereditary non-polyposis colorectal cancer (HNPCC) mutation carriers with ≥ 1 affected FDR.[25] EUS and MRI have been shown to be better than CT scan for small lesions and do not involve ionizing radiation. Therefore these modalities are most often used for screening. Other groups have recommended that screening should start at around 40 to 45 years of age or 10–15 years younger than the youngest family member with diagnosed pancreatic cancer and at age 25 in patients with Peutz- Jeghers syndrome.[27] It is also suggested that screening be initiated a decade earlier in smokers due to concern about potentiation of risk with cigarette smoking. Even amongst experts, consensus has not been reached for the age at which to initiate screening or stop surveillance, screening intervals, the need for EUS FNA to evaluate pancreatic cysts or the subsequent management of lesions identified on screening.

Biomarkers for diagnosis and staging

Blood or serum biomarkers are attractive tools in cancer management due to the relatively non-invasive nature and ease of collection. They can be used to diagnose or follow the course of the disease. Several such biomarkers such as CEA, CA 50, 242, CAM 17-1, and DUPAN 2 have been evaluated for early detection, diagnosis and prognosis; however, most have been limited by low specificity and sensitivity.[13,28] It has been shown that the degree of elevation of CA 19-9 can determine prognosis by predicting radiographically occult metastatic disease or recurrence of disease following curative resection.[29] However this marker has limited diagnostic potential due to low sensitivity for detecting early pancreatic cancers. The specificity is also low due to significant elevation in other benign and malignant pancreatico-biliary diseases such as cholestasis, cirrhosis, pancreatitis, and other abdominal malignancies.[30] Furthermore, the utility of CA 19-9 is further diminished because it is not expressed in 5–10% of Caucasian populations with Lewis a-genotype as it requires the presence of Lewis blood group antigen a to be expressed.[31] Better elucidation of the dysplasia carcinoma sequence, identification of gene mutations, proteomic profiling and other molecular events leading to invasive cancer as well as the availability of specific mouse models of pancreatic cancer, have led to increased understanding of early pancreatic cancer and development of an array of tumor markers. These biomarkers are now present at several molecular levels including DNA, RNA, proteins and cells.[28] Most of these are not yet available clinically and are therefore not discussed here. Once identified and validated, these may significantly alter screening and early detection protocols and hopefully improve survival in pancreatic cancer.

Role of imaging in diagnosis and staging

As discussed above, clinical manifestations are often vague and varied and have a poor predictive value for pancreatic cancer. Therefore, imaging has a decisive role in diagnosis, and staging, dictatating further management. An ideal imaging test should be able to detect small lesions, delineate the relationship of surrounding vessels to the lesion and also identify distant metastases, as all of these factors determine resectability and predict survival. While radiologic signs are not pathognomic for pancreatic cancer, histological confirmation by biopsy is not recommended for resectable disease. Tissue acquisition percutaneously, endoscopically or surgically is recommended prior to neoadjuvant therapy or if the diagnosis is in doubt.[32] There is a wide array of radiologic and endoscopic modalities now available for imaging of the pancreas. These include Ultrasonography (US), Computerized Tomography (CT), Magnetic Resonance Imaging (MRI), Positron Emission Tomography (PET), Endoscopic Ultrasound (EUS) and Endoscopic Retrograde Cholangiopancreatography (ERCP). Each of these techniques continues to evolve with technological advancements but availability and expertise vary across centers.

Transabdominal ultrasonography (US)

Traditionally, transabdominal ultrasound has been the initial radiological study performed in patients presenting with jaundice because of its high sensitivity for identifying intra and extrahepatic biliary tract dilation and thus determining the level of obstruction.[33] On ultrasound, adenocarcinoma typically appears as a solid hypoechoic lesion with irregular margins which may be associated with dilated biliary and pancreatic ducts. In a large prospective study involving 900 patients, the sensitivity and specificity of transabdominal US for detecting pancreatic cancer was 90% and 98.8% though there was significant difference in the sensitivity and accuracy of the diagnosis between investigators.[34] Others have reported a lower sensitivity of US for detecting small (<2 cm) lesions and determining vascular involvement or regional metastasis. Besides operator dependence, other factors like obesity, bowel gas and patient discomfort limit the utility of US as an independent modality and therefore it often remains an initial screening test which is complemented by other modalities.[35] Recent advances in US technology including use of contrast agents, tissue harmonic imaging and elastography are thought by some to enhance visualization, differentiation from chronic pancreatitis, and improve staging. These techniques have not yet become mainstream though and further studies are needed to compare them to other existing modalities and define their performance characteristics.[36]

Computerized tomography (CT)

CT scan is the most commonly used imaging technique to evaluate for suspected pancreatic cancer and has supplanted abdominal ultrasound as first-line imaging modality for abdominal complaints in emergency rooms in the United States.[13,37] Abdominal CT scans are widely available and can be rapidly performed. In addition, they are less influenced by factors such as obesity and bowel gas with US examination or respiratory artifacts with MR imaging. They are also less operator dependent than the other two imaging modalities. Multiphasic contrast enhanced examinations are recommended as direct visualization of tumors on CT scan relies on the relative difference in vascular supply between the tumor and the surrounding parenchyma, with solid tumors typically appearing as hypoattenuating or dark lesions. Up to 11% of these lesions may be isoattenuating and may be detected by associated secondary signs such as duct cutoff and upstream ductal dilation.[38] While a standard contrast enhanced CT scan is often initially performed, the pancreatic-protocol technique is the most sensitive for diagnosis of a mass lesion and for the determination of resectability. This technique involves rapid acquisition of images in arterial, portal venous and parenchymal phases of enhancement after administration of intravenous contrast and requires a multidetector row helical CT scanner.[13] The sensitivity of CT scan using these techniques has been reported as high as 100% for tumors larger than 15 mm to 20 mm, but drops to 77% for tumors less than 20 mm.[39,40]

CT also plays an important role in the staging of pancreatic cancer and determining resectability by evaluating for local tumor extension, vascular invasion, and nodal or distant metastasis. The CT criteria for vascular invasion include arterial embedding in tumor, venous obliteration, tumor involvement exceeding half of the circumference of the vessel, vessel wall irregularity, vessel stenosis or a tear drop sign of the superior mesenteric veins.[41,42] Vascular invasion can also be predicted based on the degree of contact between the tumor and the blood vessels.[43] A recent meta-analysis included 18 studies and reported a pooled sensitivity and specificity of CT in diagnosing vascular invasion of 77% and 81%, which increased to 85% and 82% if the analysis was limited to studies conducted after 2003 (2004–2008).[44]

While peripancreatic lymph nodes are well-visualized on CT scan, lymph node shape or size-based criteria are not very sensitive or specific in determining nodal involvement.[45] In one cohort, 9% of lymph nodes less than 5 mm, 36% between 5–10 mm and just 17% of those larger than 10 mm were found to be malignant, suggesting that size of lymph nodes alone should not preclude surgical exploration. Another study found that 72% of resectable tumors had regional nodal involvement compared with only 50% of unresectable tumors.[46]

Hepatic metastatic lesions are best visualized in the portal phase when they appear hypoattenuating, compared to the surrounding parenchyma, and therefore can be missed in the arterial phase which is used to evaluate pancreatic parenchyma, underscoring the importance of a good dual or triple phase exam.[47] CT is very sensitive for liver lesions greater than 1 cm (91%) but both sensitivity and specificity drop in smaller lesions (53.3% and 77.8%), which may represent metastasis in up to 12% of patients.[47,48] This is because smaller masses cannot be reliably differentiated from cysts, hemangiomas or other benign lesions. Peritoneal involvement on CT may be detected by soft tissue infiltration of omentum, nodular bowel wall thickening or peritoneal thickening or more indirectly by the presence of ascites, or with contrast enhancement of peritoneum or mesenteric lymph nodes.[49] As with liver and lymph nodes, a CT scan can identify larger lesions readily but performs less well for smaller lesions where the sensitivity drops to 7–50%.[50] Preoperative imaging using CT scan may miss 20–30% of patients with distant metastases.[51,52]

Role of percutaneous biopsy for diagnosis

Advances in imaging technology and decrease in mortality with pancreaticoduodenectomy has resulted in decreased emphasis being placed on preoperative histopathological confirmation of a pancreatic cancer diagnosis. In some settings, a negative FNA still leads to resection and tumor seeding in potentially resectable tumors can be a concern. Histological confirmation, however, is typically required when neo-adjuvant therapy is planned. While both US and CT allow guided FNA of pancreatic masses, most recent series report sensitivity rates lower than 90%.[53] Further decreased accuracy is reported in lesions less than 3 cm and in pancreatic head and uncinate process masses where FNA may be technically difficult due to intervening vessels.[54] Uncommonly, serious complications such as bile leak, peritonitis, septicemia and pancreatitis have been reported[55,56] and there remains a concern for transperitoneal seeding with malignant cells during needle withdrawal.[57] The advent of EUS guided FNA (see below) circumvents some of these problems as smaller lesions can be better visualized, intervening vessels avoided and the FNA needle does not have to traverse normal peritoneum decreasing the risk of tumor seeding. Image guided percutaneous biopsies remain valuable for sampling metastatic lesions, especially in the liver, which are not always accessible to EUS-FNA.[58]

Magnetic resonance imaging (MRI)

Pancreatic adenocarcinomas are typically hypointense to normal pancreas on precontrast T1-weighted images and early post contrast T1-weighted images and hypointense or isointense on later post contrast T1 weighted images. T2-weighted images are generally less useful as tumors show similar signal intensity to surrounding pancreas;[59] however the T2 sequence can be very helpful in ruling in or out a cystic lesion. While it has been demonstrated that MRI has a superior soft tissue contrast compared to CT scan, a meta-analysis of 68 studies (1990–2003) found MRI to be less sensitive than helical CT (84% vs 91%) for detecting pancreatic adenocarcinoma.[60] More recent single center studies have demonstrated similar accuracy with both modalities for tumor detection and staging.[61–63] MRI remains of value in patients with impaired renal function or iodinated contrast allergy. Also, because of superior soft tissue contrast, MRI is helpful in further defining a small isoattenuating carcinoma, identifying an inflammatory mass, or fatty infiltration of pancreatic head which may be mistaken for a adenocarcinoma on a CT scan.[50,64] For locoregional staging, MRI has increased sensitivity for detection of small (less than 10 mm) hepatic metastasis compared to CT due to its superior ability to characterize small hemangiomas or cysts as definitively benign.[65] Because of the similar performance status between the two modalities, along with other limitations associated with MRI including lack of availability or technical expertise, increased risk of organ motion artifact due to longer scanning time and increased cost, helical CT may be the preferred diagnostic and staging modality in some centers. MRI is critical in certain settings and may be the modality of choice depending on local expertise and preference.

Positron emission tomography (PET)

PET is a nuclear medicine based functional imaging technique that detects emissions of a radionuclide which is attached to a biologically active molecule, most commonly fludeoxyglucose (FDG). Since, this radiotracer is taken up by various tissues in proportion to their metabolic activity, malignant foci which have a higher rate of metabolism show increased activity. PET without CT has poor spatial resolution and low sensitivity for small lesions (<10 mm) and thus does not play a major role in pancreatic tumor diagnosis and staging.[66] PET when combined with CT (co-registration) merges the tumor affinity of PET scanning with spatial recognition of CT and should theoretically enhance the accuracy of CT. On the other hand, high radiotracer uptake in the primary mass may hinder subtle evaluation of surrounding vasculature or lymph nodes. For local diagnosis, studies have reported conflicting data, with sensitivity of PET/CT ranging from 72–85% and specificity from 33–94%. In the typical presentation, PET CT is not recommended for local diagnosis.[63,67] PET-CT has however been shown to be more sensitive for detecting metastatic disease than CT or MRI, especially for occult metastasis to bone, peritoneum and may also detect other synchronous malignancies.[68] With functional imaging, PET-CT has the potential to differentiate between benign and malignant focal lesions, but the study may be falsely negative due to hyperglycemia or diabetes or in small sub-centimeter lesions, while false positive results can occur in intensely inflammatory states such as pancreatitis and psuedocyst infection or with recently placed biliary stents.[50] The usefulness of PET scanning will vary depending upon the pretest probability, the results of the computed tomography and the provider's testing thresholds; therefore further prospective studies and cost-effectiveness analyses are needed to clarify its role.[69] Presently PET-CT is not routinely used as an initial imaging modality with pancreatic tumors, but is a useful adjunct if there remains concern for distant metastatic disease after non functional imaging. Also, given its functional nature it is valuable to follow response to therapy and local recurrence which can be very difficult to judge with non-functional imaging due to fibrotic and necrotic changes after therapy in the tumor bed.[68]

Endoscopic ultrasonography (EUS)

In the late 70s, recognizing the poor sensitivity of transabdominal US, researchers started working on the feasibility of transgastric sonography, which they hoped would give higher frequency US images of the pancreas because of less of air and material artifact. The first prototype endoscopic ultrasound device was reported in 1980.[70] Since then, echoendoscopes have undergone tremendous innovation and improvement and are of two main types — radial and linear. The radial echoendoscope offers 360° views in a plane perpendicular to the transducer while the linear echoendoscope scans in a plane parallel to the axis of the endoscope. Unlike the radial endoscope, the linear echoendoscope has a working channel which can be used for fine needle aspiration or biopsy of a lesion.

Echoendosonography for the pancreas has some unique advantages. The sensitivity of EUS for detecting pancreatic masses ranges from 85% to 100% and is generally considered to be superior to MDCT and MRI.[71,72] EUS outperforms the other modalities for imaging of smaller tumors (<20 mm) where it has reported sensitivity of 90% to 100% compared to 40% to 67% for CT and 33% for MRI.[39,73] Based on these results, EUS should be considered the first-line test for tissue diagnosis for pancreatic mass lesions. EUS may detect lesions missed by cross section scanning and should be considered in patients with clinical suspicion of pancreatic cancer; a non-diagnostic CT or MRIEUS is an accurate modality for loco-regional staging for pancreatic cancer with T stage accuracy ranging from 64–94%.[74,75] and N stage accuracy from 41–86%.[39,46]

The variation in T staging may be due to referral bias because of exclusion of patients with advanced or locally advanced disease in some studies. The N stage accuracy is limited because of poor specificity of EUS criteria for predicting lymph node metastasis, similar to the lack of specificity of the CT criteria.[45,76]

EUS imaging has anatomical limitations precluding evaluation of distant metastasis and therefore CT and MRI remain superior to EUS for assessment of non-nodal metastasis. However, EUS is sensitive for detection and sampling of small liver lesions and ascites which may be missed by other imaging modalities.[77,78]

EUS provides excellent views of the portal and splenic veins and most studies demonstrate sensitivities greater than 80% for tumor invasion of portal vein or portal vein confluence which is superior to CT or MR imaging.[79] EUS sensitivity for superior mesenteric vein (17–83%),[80] superior mesenteric artery (17%)[81] and celiac artery (50%)[82] are however lower compared to CT or MR. Due to anatomic limitations, EUS does not have the ability to follow vessels such as the SMA distally, which may obscure evaluation for some vascular involvement.

The other major advantage of EUS over cross-sectional imaging modalities is the ability to obtain a fine needle aspirate or core biopsy of the suspected pancreatic tumor at the time of the procedure. In a recent meta-analysis of 33 studies, EUS-FNA was found to have a very good sensitivity (85%) and specificity (98%) for pancreatic mass lesions, with no to very few complications (0–2.0%). It is superior to percutaneous tumor sampling due to better accessibility to the tumor mass, the ability to torque and change the needle axis to avoid intervening vessels and lessen risk of tumor seeding (2.2% vs 16.3%).[83,84] When compared to CT or US guided FNA, EUS-FNA has been reported to be more sensitive (84% vs 62%)[85] and accurate[54] for primary pancreatic masses and therefore has become the modality of choice for tumor sampling.

While EUS is an excellent imaging modality with ability for tissue acquisition, it is highly operator dependant and has a steep learning curve.[86] Also the sensitivity of EUS decreases in chronic pancreatitis, with diffusely infiltrating tumor or in patients with a prominent dorsal/ventral split, even in the hands of experienced endosonographers.[79] Like transabdominal ultrasonography, advancements in EUS technology using elastography and contrast enhancement may emerge to improve the diagnostic accuracy of EUS.

EUS Elastography: EUS elastography is based on the premise that compression of tissue produces a smaller strain (displacement) in hard tissue than it does in soft tissue.[87] This difference in strain can then be measured and used to differentiate between different tissue types as in inflammatory psuedotumors, chronic pancreatitis and pancreatic adenocarcinoma. First generation elastography used a qualitative method with a color spectrum from red to blue. However, interpretation was not straightforward because the lesions do not image homogeneously and steadily throughout the procedure affecting inter-observer agreement.[88] The subsequent generation of elastography made this technique more objective by providing numerical measurements of tissue stiffness using artificial neural network analysis.[89] Initial studies, using this technology have been very encouraging with sensitivity and specificity of strain ratio for detecting pancreatic malignancies (100% and 92.9%, respectively, area under the receiver operating curve, 0.983)[90] and malignant lymph nodes.[91] Though, many technical issues remain such as size inequality between the lesion and the reference area, deep position of the target relative to the transducer and degree of transducer compression and angulation, EUS elastography may complement EUS in confirming a diagnosis and determining resectability.[88]

Contrast-Enhanced EUS: Contrast-Enhanced (CE) EUS utilizes microbubbles in an intravenously injected contrast agent to enhance the small, low-velocity vasculature of pancreatic tumors. Harmonic EUS then detects these signals and filters out signals from the tissue to better define pancreatic lesions, which can then be classified based on their enhancement.[92] Ductal adenocarcinomas are typically hypoenhancing while neuroendocrine tumors are hyperenhancing.[93] In a prospective study involving 277 patients, CE-EUS and MDCT did not differ significantly in diagnostic ability with regard to all lesions but CH-EUS was superior to MDCT in diagnosing small (≤2 cm) carcinomas ($p < 0.05$), detecting 12 neoplasms that were missed by MDCT. Also, when CH-EUS was combined with EUS-FNA, the sensitivity of EUS-FNA increased from 92.2% to 100%, suggesting EUS equipped with contrast harmonic imaging may play an important role in the characterization of small tumors and may improve the diagnostic yield of EUS-FNA.[94] Presently contrast agents for this modality have been approved in Europe and Asia but have not yet been FDA approved for use in the United States.

Endoscopic retrograde cholangiopancreatography (ERCP)

The ERCP finding of the double duct sign (strictures in the common bile duct and pancreatic duct with upstream dilation) is common in the setting of pancreatic head mass lesions. Other signs include long irregular pancreatic duct strictures, distal bile duct strictures or pancreatic duct obstruction in the absence of chronic pancreatitis. However, ERCP for diagnostic evaluation has several limitations. Findings on cholangiopancreatography are not very specific to pancreatic cancer.[95] ERCP does not have the ability to evaluate for resectability or staging, has a higher failure rate than other non-invasive imaging modalities, and may result in significant complications or even death.[96] ERCP does have the ability to obtain a tissue diagnosis using brush cytology or forceps biopsy and can provide biliary drainage in patients with obstructive jaundice secondary to pancreatic tumors. The sensitivity of brush cytology is limited by its relatively low and widely variable sensitivity values ranging from 20–60%, inferior to EUS-FNA.[97] Furthermore, most centers now do not prefer preoperative ERCP for biliary drainage in patients with resectable tumors due to increased risk of post-surgical complications.[98] Technological advances such as pancreatoscopy and the introduction of newer methods for cytological evaluation such as immunocytochemistry, flow cytometry, image analysis, fluorescence in situ hybridization (FISH), and mutation analysis may increase the diagnostic yield but are employed in varying degrees depending on operator and center availability. ERCP plays a key role in treatment for patients who require biliary drainage due to cholangitis, pruritus, abdominal pain, or symptomatic biliary obstruction. A normal or low serum bilirubin may be required to receive chemotherapy, and in this setting, many patients can be decompressed with ERCP to enable systemic treatment. Finally, patients with unresectable tumors can receive metal stents for longer term palliation of biliary obstruction. Staging Laparoscopy: 10–40% of patients deemed to have resectable disease on non-invasive imaging are found to be unresectable at the time of laparotomy.[99] This is mainly because of the limited sensitivity of imaging modalities to detect small metastases to the liver or peritoneum.[64] Laparoscopy with or without laparoscopic ultrasound, allows for direct inspection of liver and peritoneal surface and imaging of occult metastasis and vascular involvement and gained popularity as a staging modality when it was shown that it could prevent unnecessary open laparotomy in up to a third of patients.[100,101] However, interpretation of the literature on staging laparoscopy is difficult due to inconsistent use of high quality CT, inclusion of patients with locally advanced disease and lack of co-relation of laparoscopic staging with R_0 resection.[102] While a recent Cochrane review incorporating studies from 1986–2012 reported that staging laparoscopy would decrease the rate of laparotomy for unresectable tumors by 22%, other well-designed single center studies have reported a yield of 2% or less with routine staging laparoscopy.[103–105] While routine staging laparoscopy is not advocated for all resectable tumors, staging laparoscopy is recommended for large primary tumors, lesions in body or tail of pancreas, equivocal radiographic findings suggestive of occult metastatic disease such as low volume ascites, possible carcinomatosis or small hypodense liver lesions not amenable to preoperative biopsy, and subtle clinical or laboratory findings such as hypoalbuminemia, elevated CA 19-9, weight loss or severe pain requiring narcotic analgesia.[102]

Multimodality preoperative staging to determine resectability

As described above, though CT, MR and EUS overall have similar performance characteristics for the diagnosis and staging of pancreatic malignancies, each has unique limitations. Some groups have therefore proposed that optimal preoperative staging may require combination of two or more of these modalities. One prospective study evaluated 62 consecutive patients with helical CT, EUS, MRI and Angiography[106] and reported that helical CT had the highest accuracy for locoregional vascular invasion (83%), distant metastases (88%), tumor TNM stage (46%), and tumor resectability (83%), whereas EUS had the highest accuracy in assessing tumor size ($r = 0.85$) and lymph node involvement (65%). A decision analysis suggested that the best strategy to assess tumor resectability would be based on CT or EUS as the initial test, followed by the alternative technique in potentially resectable cases. A sequential strategy using EUS as a confirmatory technique only after a helical CT has suggested resectability of the tumor was most cost-effective. Similar results have been reported by other authors using both CT[80,107] and MR.[108] Other studies have not found an incremental benefit by combining two modalities in all patients.[39] While no firm consensus exists on the best modalities for preoperative staging, more than one imaging strategy is indicated in patients with equivocal findings prior to referral for surgical resection. If some cases, staging laparoscopy (as described above) is a minimally invasive approach to further evaluate such patients prior to major surgery. A proposed algorithm for diagnostic and staging workup of suspected pancreatic cancer is presented in Fig. 1.

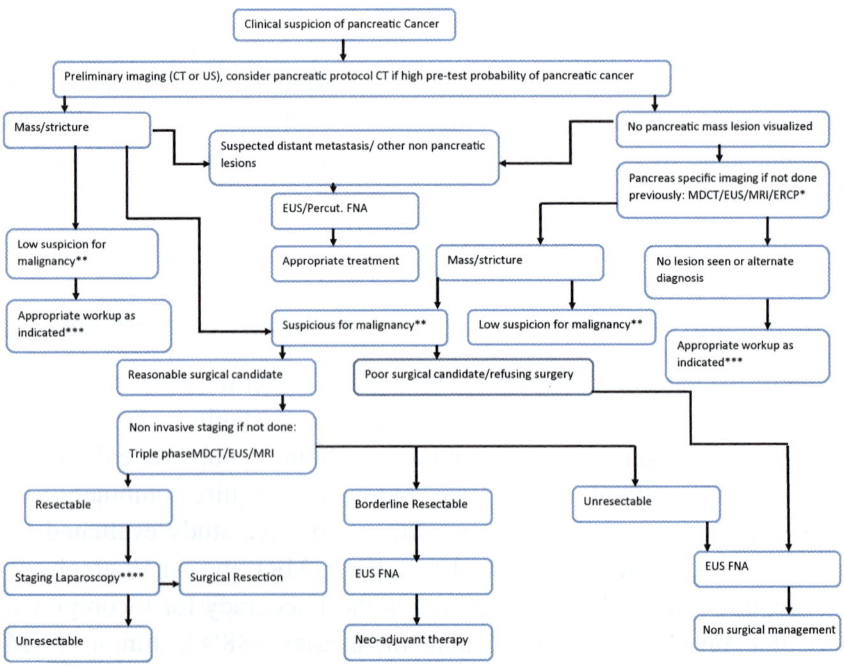

Fig. 1.

Staging systems for pancreatic cancer

Cancer staging systems have been developed to standardize the extent of tumor spread as determined by various modalities. This allows for better communication of disease extent across providers and institutions, aids clinical research by homogenizing treatment groups, and leads to stage based clinical guidelines and prognosis assessment, ultimately resulting in better clinical care. In addition to defining disease extent, staging systems should be able to subgroup varying disease presentations into stages on which treatment recommendations and subsequent prognosis determination can be based.

Globally, the most common staging system used for all cancers, including pancreatic cancer, is the Tumor Node Metastasis (TNM) system of the combined American Joint Committee on Cancer (AJCC)/ International Union Against Cancer (UICC) (Table 3). This system incorporates TNM classification of anatomical spread into a composite stage and has been demonstrated to be an important prognostic tool for pancreatic cancer.[6]

With advances in imaging technology and treatment protocols, the AJCC staging system is periodically revised to more accurately represent prognosis. There was a significant change for pancreatic cancer staging in the 6th edition which standardized the clinical definition of resectability and classified involvement of the superior mesenteric vein, splenic vein and portal vein as T3 from the previously classification of T4, recognizing the potential resectability of these tumors. In the latest (7th) edition of AJCC staging system, while the definitions of TNM and anatomic stage/ prognostic groupings have not been changed, triphasic multislice CT or MR are recommended for staging. Pancreatic neuroendocrine tumors, which were specifically excluded from prior editions, have been included for staging similar to exocrine pancreatic malignancy.[109]

While AJCC staging remains important for prognosis, this system relies on some information which can only be determined through post-surgical pathological evaluation of the resected tumor. Also, it does not completely characterize the relationship of tumor to the adjacent vasculature which is a key component in determining resectability and need for neoadjuvant chemotherapy.[110]

Table 3. TNM classification with AJCC staging and stage based survival of pancreatic adenocarcinoma.

Primary Tumor (T)	
TX	Primary tumor cannot be assessed
T0	No evidence of primary tumor
Tis	Carcinoma *in situ**
T1	Tumor limited to the pancreas, 2 cm or less in greatest dimension
T2	Tumor limited to the pancreas, more than 2 cm in greatest dimension
T3	Tumor extends beyond the pancreas but without involvement of the celiac axis or the superior mesenteric artery
T4	Tumor involves the celiac axis or the superior mesenteric artery (unresectable primary tumor)
Regional Lymph Nodes (N)	
NX	Regional lymph nodes cannot be assessed
N0	No regional lymph node metastasis
N1	Regional lymph node metastasis
Distant Metastasis (M)	
M0	No distant metastasis
M1	Distant metastasis

Anatomic stage/prognostic groups				Median survival** (Months)
Stage 0	Tis	N0	M0	
Stage IA	T1	N0	M0	24.1
Stage IB	T2	N0	M0	20.6
Stage IIA	T3	N0	M0	15.4
Stage IIB	T1	N1	M0	12.7
	T2	N1	M0	
	T3	N1	M0	
Stage III	T4	Any N	M0	10.6
Stage IV	Any T	Any N	M1	4.5

*This also includes the "PanInIII" classification.

**(6)

Therefore, pancreatic cancer is also staged clinically based on tumor resectability as determined by presurgical imaging studies. This staging classifies pancreatic cancer into resectable, borderline resectable, locally advanced and metastatic stages, each of which differ in management and prognosis.

While a broad consensus exists for most categories, societies and institutions may differ on the definition of borderline resectable tumors based on local experience. This is because borderline resectable tumors require neoadjuvant therapy for which high quality phase III trials have not yet been concluded, and advanced surgical techniques like venous and hepatic arterial interposition grafts for tumors encasing veins or abutting arteries are not universally available.[111] These criteria as adopted by the National Comprehensive Cancer Network (NCCN) are listed in Table 4.[32]

AJCC recommends the College of American Pathologists (CAP) checklist for endocrine or exocrine pancreatic tumors as a guideline for pathological evaluation of pancreatic resection specimens to standardize pathological reporting.[109] Besides classifying resection status into R0 (gross complete resection with microscopically negative margins), R1 resection (microscopic residual tumor at margin) and R2 resection (macroscopic residual tumor at margin) which have prognostic implications, it is recommended that pathological staging include SMA margin assessment, perineural and lymphovascular invasion, lymph node status and lymph node ratio (metastatic/total number of nodes examined), and treatment effect for patients who have undergone neoadjuvant therapy, as these components have significant prognostic value.[110]

Pancreatic Neuroendocrine Tumors (PNETs)

Neuroendocrine neoplasms are a group of epithelial neoplasms that are derived from multipotential stem cells of endodermal origin with predominant neuroendocrine differentiation. Neuroendocrine cells are widely distributed throughout the body but those that arise in the pancreas have been traditionally referred to as pancreatic carcinoids, pancreatic neuroendocrine tumors (PNETs), or islet cell tumors. PNETs account for approximately 3% of all pancreatic neoplasms.[112] The term "neuroendocrine tumor" was first proposed by Capella *et al.* in 1995 to be used instead of carcinoid as it conveys the potential malignant nature and

Table 4. NCCN criteria defining resectability status for pancreatic adenocarcinoma.

Resectable:

- No distant metastases
- No radiographic evidence of superior mesenteric vein (SMV) and portal vein abutment, distortion, tumor thrombus, or venous encasement
- Clear fat planes around the celiac axis, hepatic artery, and superior mesenteric artery (SMA)

Borderline Resectable:

- No distant metastases
- Venous involvement of the SMV/portal vein showing tumor abutment with or without impingement and narrowing of the lumen
- Encasement of the SMV/portal vein but without encasement of the nearby arteries, or short segment venous occlusion resulting from either tumor thrombus or encasement but with suitable vessel proximal and distal to the area of vessel involvement allowing for safe resection and reconstruction
- Gastroduodenal artery encasement up to the hepatic artery with either short segment encasement or direct abutment of the hepatic artery, without extension to the celiac axis
- Tumor abutment of the SMA not to exceed 180° of the circumference of the vessel wall

Unresectable:

- Head:
  - Distant metastases
  - 180° SMA encasement, any celiac abutment
  - Unreconstructible SMV/portal occlusion
  - Aortic invasion or encasement
- Body:
  - Distant metastases
  - SMA or celiac encasement >180°
  - Unreconstructible SMV/portal occlusion
  - Aortic invasion
- Tail:
  - Distant metastases
  - SMA or celiac encasement >180°
- Nodal Status:
  - Metastases to lymph nodes beyond the field of resection should be considered unresectable

*Abutment is defined as ≤ 180° and encasement is >180° (32)

histopathology of the tumor more accurately.[113] Even though they share some common histologic appearance, there is a vast heterogeneity among neuroendocrine neoplasms. They differ in biologic behavior, histologic differentiation, and functionality. PNETs can be further categorized into functional and non-functional tumors.[114,115] Functional status is determined by the presence of a specific clinical syndrome, regardless of the level of hormonal secretion.[114,115] Another class of PNETs described in the WHO 2010 classification is mixed adenoneuroendocrine carcinomas, previously described as mixed carcinoid adenocarcinoma or mixed exocrine-endocrine carcinoma. This type of neoplasm comprises both adenocarcinoma and neuroendocrine carcinoma with at least 30% of each component.[116]

Epidemiology

The exact incidence and prevalence of PNETs are unknown and are likely to be underestimated as majority of PNETs are asymptomatic. Tumor detection is frequently incidental and the rapid rise in the incidence of PNETs over the past decade correlates with greater usage of cross-sectional imaging studies.

An overall low incidence of 2.2 cases/10^6 population/year has been reported, while a study of autopsy reports found the incidence to be as high as 10%.[2,117] This variation may also involve evolving classification, improving diagnostic modalities and registry systems that usually include only malignant neoplasms.[13]

PNETs are slightly more common among men (53%) than women (47%) with mean age of diagnosis of 60 years old.[118,119] Up to 75% of PNETs are non-functioning tumors.[120] The incidence of functional PNETs varies by tumor type with insulinoma being the most common (1–4 cases/10^6 population/year), followed by gastrinoma (0.5–2 cases/10^6 population/year), VIPoma (0.05–0.2 cases/10^6 population/year), and glucagonoma (0.01–0.1cases/10^6 population/year).[119] The true incidence of rarer types of PNETs such as somatostatinoma, GRHoma, ACTHoma, PTHrPoma is difficult to estimate given their rarity.

Even though most PNETs are sporadic, some can be hereditary. When there is a family history of PNETs, certain hereditary endocrinopathies should be considered. These includes multiple endocrine neoplasia type I (MEN1), neurofibromatosis type I, tuberous sclerosis, and Von Hippel Lindau syndrome.

Classification

Functional PNETs

Functional PNETs are defined as neuroendocrine tumors that cause clinical hormonal syndromes regardless of peptide/hormonal secreting activity. Non-functional PNETs may secrete numerous substances such as chromogranins, neuron-specific endolase, pancreatic polypeptide (including insulin, gastrin, glucagon, vasoactive intestinal polypeptide), or ghrelin but these substances may not cause (or the level of substances are not high enough to cause) a hormonal syndrome. Each functional PNET has distinct clinical manifestations from hormonal hypersecretion, which will be discussed later on in this chapter.

Non-functional PNETs

Non-functional PNETs can cause clinical symptoms from local tumor compression or metastasis and can present with symptoms such as abdominal pain, jaundice, pruritus, anorexia, nausea, weight loss, watery diarrhea, or peptic ulcer disease. Nearly 50% of non-functional PNETs are diagnosed incidentally on cross sectional imaging for other indications; however, when symptomatic, obstructive symptoms from mass effect may be the most common presentation.[121,122] As non-functional PNETs do not cause hypersecretory syndrome, they tend to be diagnosed later in the course of the disease. The most common presenting symptoms are abdominal pain (up to 78%), and anorexia and nausea (45%).[123,124] Abdominal pain may be caused by the tumor bulk itself, distension of the liver capsule, or direct invasion of the autonomic myenteric plexus or celiac ganglion. Rarely, the tumor can invade the splenic vein causing gastric varices. Tumors arising in pancreatic head may present with obstructive jaundice due to bile duct compression, or gastric outlet obstruction due to compression or infiltration of the duodenum.[123,124]

Functional PNETs

(1) Insulinoma

Pancreatic insulinoma is the most common functioning neuroendocrine tumor of the pancreas.[13] However, it is a rare tumor with an incidence of 1–4 cases/10^6 population/year.[119,125] The median age of patients with insulinoma is 50 years, and it is more prevalent in women (57%) but more aggressive in men.[125,126] Insulinomas typically have an indolent course but metastasis can be found in up to 6% at the initial diagnosis.[125] Insulinomas can occur sporadically or as part of multiple endocrine neoplasia type 1 (MEN-1 syndrome). Six percent of insulinomas are associated with the MEN-1 syndrome.[126] Insulinomas can occur in any part of the pancreas and usually presents as a single pancreatic tumor (87%); however, multiple pancreatic lesions can sometimes be found (7%).[125]

As its name implies, insulinomas are PNETs that secrete proinsulin, which is later cleaved into an active form of insulin. It is believed that the tumor arises from ductular or acinar cells of the pancreas rather than from neoplastic proliferation of islet cells.[127] The hormonal syndrome caused by insulin hypersecretion is known as Whipple's triad, which comprises of low plasma glucose together with hypoglycemic symptoms that are reversible with normalization of the glucose level. Hypoglycemic symptoms include neuroglycopenic symptoms (blurred vision, lightheadedness, dizziness, confusion, amnesia, abnormal behavior, loss of consciousness, seizure) and sympatoadrenal symptoms (palpitation, anxiety, diaphoresis, and tremor), which are results of catecholamine release in response to hypoglycemia. The triad was originally recognized as the clue for diagnosis of insulinoma. Since neuroglycopenic symptoms resolve with food intake, some of the patients with insulinoma also experience weight gain.[128] Hypoglycemic symptoms usually occur in the fasting state (73%); however, 21% of patients reported both fasting and postprandial symptoms and 6% reported only postprandial symptoms.[126]

(2) Gastrinoma

Pancreatic gastrinoma is a type of functional PNET that secretes gastrin as the predominant peptide. Its incidence is 0.5–2 cases/10^6 population/year.

Table 5. Summary of characteristics of functional PNETs.

Functional PNETs	Clinical syndrome	Laboratory diagnostics
Insulinoma	• Whipple's triad • Neuroglycopenic symptoms • Sympatoadrenal symptoms	• Elevate insulin and C-peptide during hypoglycemic episode • Insulin to glucose raio <0.3 • Undetectable sulfonylurea
Gastrinoma	• Zollinger Ellison syndrome • Diarrhea • Hypergastrinemia • Gastric acid hypersecretion • Peptic ulcer diathesis	• Serum gastrin >1000 pg/mL (475 pmol/L) • Gastric pH <2 • Serum gastrin increases >200 pg/mL after secretin stimulation test • Serum gastrin increases >395 pg/mL after calcium stimulation test
VIPoma	• Verner Morrison syndrome/ WDHA syndrome • Watery diarrhea • Hypokalemia • Achlorhydria	• Stool osmolal gap <50 mOsm/kg • VIP >75 ph/mL
Glucagonoma	• Glucagonoma syndrome (4D syndrome) • Dermatitis (Necrolytic migratory erythema) and mucositis • Diabetes mellitus • Deep vein thrombosis • Depression (neuropsychiatric symptoms)	• Glucagon level >1000 pg/mL
Somatostatinoma	• Somatostainoma syndrome • Diabetes mellitus • Gastric hypochlorhydria • Cholelithiasis • Steatorrhea	• Somatostatin level >160 pg/mL
Corticotropinoma	• Cushing syndrome • Diabetes mellitus • Obesity • Hypertension • Hyperpigmentation	• Plasma ACTH >20 pg/mL • Negative high-dose dexamethasone suppression test • Negative CRH stimulation test

(*Continued*)

Table 5. (*Continued*)

Functional PNETs	Clinical syndrome	Laboratory diagnostics
PTHrPoma	• Hyperparathyroidism, Hypercalcemic crisis • Altered mental status, confusion • Abdominal pain • Nausea, vomiting • Ureteric stones • Osteolytic lesion	• Hypercalcemia • Hypophosphatemia • Elevated PTHrP

It is estimated that 0.1–1% of patients with peptic ulcer disease have gastrinoma.[125] Approximately 20% of gastrinomas are associated with the MEN-1 syndrome.[129] Most patients are diagnosed between the ages of 20–50 years old with mean age of symptom onset of 41 years and a slight male preponderance.[130,131] Twenty percent of gastrinomas arise in the pancreas, while the remainders are typically localized in the duodenum. Most of the pancreatic gastrinomas are found in pancreatic head and uncinate process.[132] Even though most of these tumors have an indolent course, up to 33% may have metastatic disease at the initial diagnosis. The most common site of metastasis is the liver, followed by the axial skeletons.[133]

High levels of gastrin stimulate the parietal cells and histamine-releasing enterochromaffin-like cells leading to uncontrolled secretion of gastric acid. Hypersecretion of gastric acid often causes persistent, refractory peptic ulcer disease and gastroesophageal reflux. The hypersecretory state can also cause chronic diarrhea due to inactivation of pancreatic enzymes by the abnormally acidic environment in the duodenum, resulting in malabsorption and maldigestion, leading to steatorrhea. In addition, high level of gastrin interferes with sodium and water absorption in the small intestine, causing secretory diarrhea. Prolonged and untreated hypersecretion of gastrin can lead to complications such as peptic ulcer perforation, gastric outlet obstruction, esophageal strictures, or life-threatening gastrointestinal bleeding. While the most common presenting symptoms are abdominal pain and diarrhea, other symptoms such as anorexia, weight loss, dysphagia, proximal muscle weakness (from hypokalemia), and severe heart burn are also significant symptoms.[131] Endoscopic findings in patients with gastrinomas include prominent gastric fold (94%), multiple duodenal ulcers (75% in proximal duodenum and 14% in distal duodenum), jejunal ulcers (11%), and esophageal and pyloric strictures.[131,134] The clinical syndrome of refractory peptic ulcer disease, high gastrin levels, and a pancreatic tumor was first described by Zollinger and Ellison in 1955. This characteristic presentation of gastrinoma is now known as the Zollinger-Ellison syndrome.[135]

(3) VIPoma

Pancreatic VIPoma is a type of functional PNET that secretes vasoactive intestinal peptide (VIP). It is rarer than insulinoma and gastrinoma with incidence of 0.05–0.2 cases/10^6 population/year.[136] In adults, VIPoma almost exclusively arises within pancreas, while in children, it is not uncommon for the tumor to arise from extrapancreatic locations such as the sympathetic ganglia or adrenal gland, or in the setting of ganglioneuroblastoma.[136] It usually occurs sporadically however, 5% of the tumors are associated with the MEN-1 syndrome. In contrast, only 0.65% of patients with the MEN-1 syndrome have a VIPoma.[137]

Compared to other functional PNETs, VIPomas may have an aggressive presentation. The primary tumor is usually larger than 3 cm and is commonly found in the pancreatic tail (75%). At the time of diagnosis, 60–80% of patients may have metastatic disease.[138,139]

VIP is a 28-amino acid polypeptide that binds to high affinity receptors on intestinal epithelial cells, leading to activation of cellular adenylate cyclase and cAMP production. This results in a cascade of intestinal physiologic responses including secretion of free water along with sodium and chloride, inhibition of reabsorption, and inhibition of gastric secretion. Systemically, VIP also stimulates vasodilation, bone resorption, and hepatic glycogenolysis.[140,141]

The classic features of the VIPoma syndrome include secretory diarrhea (700–4000 of stool output per day with a low stool osmolal gap, not improved with fasting), flushing, lethargy, nausea, vomiting, muscle weakness, muscle cramps, hypokalemia, hypochloridia, and hypercalcemia. The presentation has many names including Verner-Morrison syndrome, watery diarrhea-hypokalemia-achloridia syndrome (WDHA), and pancreatic cholera.[142] Co-secretion with calcitonin has been reported.[143]

(4) Glucagonoma

Glucagonoma is a PNET derived from alpha cells of the pancreas and, similar to insulinoma and VIPoma, arises almost exclusively from pancreas. Tumor cells are abundant with secretory granules of glucagon as evidenced by immunoperoxidase staining and in situ hybridization of glucagon mRNA. The tumor can range in size up to as large as 25 cm. It is commonly found in the pancreatic tail. The mean age of diagnosis is 50 years with slight female preponderance.[144,145] Similar to VIPoma, glucagonomas typically have more aggressive behavior and metastases are commonly found at the initial diagnosis. The common sites of metastases include the liver, bones, and lymph nodes.[146]

Glucagon is an anabolic 29-amino acid polypeptide that stimulates glycogenolysis, gluconeogenesis, ketogenesis, lipolysis, amino acid oxidation and catecholamine secretion. Excessive unregulated secretion of glucagon may therefore lead to hyperglycemia, diabetes mellitus and amino acid depletion. This hypoaminoacidemia is believed to play an important role in the pathophysiology of necrolytic migratory erythema (NME), the hallmark dermatologic manifestation of glucagonoma. NME is a unique dermatologic manifestation that can be seen in up to 70% of patients with glucagonoma.[147] It is described as painful progressive migratory erythematous papules or plaques involving the face, perineum, and extremities. The lesions typically coalesce with central clearing within 1–2 weeks leaving indurated bronze-colored scars. Blistering, crusting, and scaling at the borders are common. Skin biopsy is not necessary but if performed, it should be done at the edge of the lesion. The yield of skin biopsy is low but can reveal the classic superficial necrolysis with separation of the epidermal outer layers and perivascular infiltration with lymphocytes and histiocytes.[148] The pathophysiology of NME is not completely understood but is believed to involve amino acid depletion and excessive anabolism from glucagon hypersecretion. Mucous membranes can be affected by the same process, resulting in glossitis, angular cheilitis, stomatitis, blepharitis, hair thinning, and dystrophic nails. Other features of glucagonoma syndrome include normocytic normochromic anemia (which is believed to be from direct interference of erythropoietin function from glucagon), weight loss, venous thromboembolism, abdominal pain, anorexia, constipation, proximal muscle weakness and neuropsychiatric symptoms such as ataxia, dementia, and optic atrophy.[144,145] When diarrhea is present, concurrent mixed polypeptide hypersecretion such as gastrin, VIP, or serotonin should be suspected. Despite the severe hyperglycemia observed in glucagonoma, diabetic ketoacidosis rarely occurs as the islet beta cells remain intact.[149]

(5) Somatostatinoma

Somatostatinoma is a rare neuroendocrine tumor that is derived from the D-cells of the pancreas. It is typically diagnosed in the fifth decade of life with a roughly equal distribution between men and women. Approximately 45% of somatostatinomas arise in extrapancreatic locations, commonly in the duodenum or periampullary area. Pancreatic somatostatinomas are usually found in the pancreatic head. Only 10% of somatostatinomas are associated with somatostatinoma syndrome.[150,151]

Somatostatin is a 14-amino acid polypeptide with paracrine signaling that inhibits secretion of insulin, glucagon, gastrin, and growth hormone. It also has direct inhibitory effects on cholecystokinin-stimulated pancreatic enzymes, pancreatic bicarbonate, gallbladder contraction, intestinal contractility, intestinal amino acid absorption, and gastric acid secretion.[152] These inhibitory effects lead to the clinical presentation of the somatostatinoma syndrome which includes diabetes mellitus (insulin depletion), cholelithiasis (decreased gall bladder contractility increasing billiary stasis), steatorrhea (decreased active pancreatic enzymes and interference with intestinal absorption), and gastric hypochlorhydria (decreased gastrin secretion). Other symptoms include abdominal pain, anorexia, and obstructive jaundice.[152]

(6) Corticotropinoma (ACTHoma)

Corticotropinoma is a rare neuroendocrine tumor that secretes corticotrophin. The tumor is commonly found in the adrenal gland or pituitary and only 1–16% of corticotropinomas are localized to the pancreas.[153] The tumor has an aggressive behavior and usually metastasizes to the liver. Patients with the tumor may present with florid cushing syndrome, obesity, hypertension, glucose intolerance, osteoporosis, muscular atrophy, and hyperpigmentation. Secretion of multiple hormones from the tumor can also occur.[154]

(7) Parathyroid hormone related peptide producing NET (PTHrPoma)

Pancreatic PTHrPoma is a rare entity with less than 50 cases reported worldwide.[155] Parathyroid hormone related peptide is a single monomeric peptide with multiple isoforms some of which have identical N-terminal domains as parathyroid hormone (PTH) and thus can stimulate PTH receptors.[156] Hypersecretion of PTHrP manifests as hyperparathyroidism and patients can present with malignant hypercalcemia, altered mental status, confusion, constipation, abdominal pain, nausea, vomiting, ureteric stones, osteolytic lesions, and renal failure. It typically presents as a large solitary tumor (median size of 10 cm) and is usually localized to the pancreatic body (32%) or tail (53%).[155]

Diagnostic approaches

PNETs are difficult to diagnose due to vague non-specific clinical symptoms and low incidence. When PNET is suspected, either from clinical symptoms or radiologic findings, a multidisciplinary approach is undertaken to confirm the diagnosis, classify the type of the tumor, determine extent of the disease, and stage the tumor. Diagnostic modalities, including serum biomarkers, radiologic studies, and arterial stimulation venous sampling will be discussed here.

Role of biomarkers

Several circulating biomarkers for neuroendocrine tumors have been evaluated. The most commonly used biomarker for all types of neuroendocrine tumors is chromogranin A (CgA).[157] CgA is elevated in majority of the patients with both functional and non-functional PNETs. The overall diagnostic sensitivity is higher in patients with metastatic disease (60–100%) than in patients with localized disease (29–50%).[158–160] The plasma level of CgA correlates well with tumor burden and therefore is used to monitor response to therapy and progression free survival.[157,161,162]

However, for poorly understood reasons, CgA is not elevated in insulinomas, PNETs associated with MEN-1 syndrome, and poorly differentiated PNETs. CgA can also be falsely elevated in patients with renal failure as it is renally excreted. Moreover, since CgA-containing ECL cells are stimulated by gastrin, any condition that causes gastrin hypersecretion, such as proton-pump inhibitor use, atrophic gastritis, or pernicious anemia can cause elevation of plasma CgA. Due to its high false positive and false negative rates, CgA alone should not be used as a diagnostic marker.[157]

Other biologic markers for PNETs include neuron specific enolase (NSE) and pancreatic polypeptide (PP). NSE is a dimer of the glycolytic enzyme enolase and is present in cytoplasmic neuroendocrine cells. Its level is related to the secretory activity of the tumor. Similar to CgA, it is not specific enough to be a diagnostic marker but it is used for follow-up after treatment. PP is less specific than CgA and NSE but when its level is higher than three times the age-matched normal fasting basal level, its specificity increases and should raise suspicion for a PNET.[157,163,164]

For functional PNETs, specific measurement of laboratory markers is performed to make the diagnosis. For insulinoma, an inappropriately high insulin level during induced or spontaneous hypoglycemia can be demonstrated by an insulin-to-glucose ratio of 0.3 or less. C-peptide and sulfonylurea levels are measured to exclude exogenous insulin use and medication induced hyperinsulinemia (insulin and C-peptide levels should be high while sulfonylurea should be undetectable in hypoglycemia from insulinoma).[144]

The gastrin level is abnormally high in patients with gastrinoma.[130] Since hypergastrinemia is a normal physiologic response to proton-pump inhibitor (PPI) use, atrophic gastritis, pernicious anemia, *H. pylori* infection, food intake, after small bowel resection, and with a high gastric pH, interpretation of high gastrin should be made carefully. It is recommended to measure gastrin levels while fasting and after stopping PPIs for at least 7 days. A gastric pH should be measured as a high gastric pH can cause hypergastrinemia. A serum gastrin level of greater than 1000 pg/mL (475 pmol/L) when the gastric pH is less than 2 is highly suggestive of gastrinoma. In patients with high clinical suspicion who have lower elevations of gastrin (between 100 pg/mL and 1000 pg/mL) and a low gastric pH, a secretin stimulation test can be considered.[130]

The stool osmolal gap should be measured in patients with suspected VIPoma. An osmolal gap less than 50 mOsm/kg in fresh stool sample suggests a secretory diarrhea, together with a high VIP level (>75 pg/mL) and a pancreatic tumor, establishes the diagnosis of VIPoma.[141]

Glucagon is one of the stress hormones therefore, it is elevated in various conditions such as sepsis, burns, trauma, surgery, and fasting. However, these conditions are associated with only moderate elevations of glucagon (less than 500 pg/mL). Patients with NME and/or diabetes mellitus usually have higher concentrations. A glucagon level greater than 1000 pg/mL is highly suggestive of glucagonoma.[147]

For somatostatinomas, somatostatin levels higher than 160 pg/mL with the clinical triad of diabetes, steatorrhea and cholelithiasis as determined by blood glucose, fecal fat and abdominal ultrasound are highly suggestive of the diagnosis.[150]

Radiologic studies

As with pancreatic adenocarcinoma, cross sectional studies such as helical multiphasic contrast-enhanced computed tomography (CT) and magnetic resonance imaging (MRI) are first-line diagnostic modalities of PNETs. Functional PETs are usually small at the time of diagnosis, while non-functional PETs tend to be larger (mean diameter 8.4 cm) and are more likely than functional PETs to demonstrate necrosis, cystic changes and calcifications.[165] Pancreatic duct obstruction and dilation is uncommon with malignant PETs, unlike ductal adenocarcinoma.[165] Intrapancreatic accessory splenic tissue can also present as a hypervascularized mass in pancreatic tail which can sometimes mimick PNETs on CT scan, thus it should be considered in the differential diagnosis. Most NETs are isodense with the pancreas on pre-contrast imaging but show avid contrast enhancement usually in the arterial but occasionally in the portal venous phase, therefore dual or multiphase contrast enhanced CT has a higher sensitivity than conventional CT scanning.[166] As above, the sensitivity of CT increases with tumor size.[39,40] Therefore MDCT has a lower sensitivity (57–63%) for functional tumors which are usually small with a median size of 1.3 cm.[165] CT-negative tumors are small and more likely to be insulinomas, and are better visualized by EUS. EUS has been shown to detect 91% of CT-negative PNETs which typically appear as round, homogenous hypoechoic lesions. Therefore, a sequential approach of CT followed by EUS is recommended and has been reported to have a 100% sensitivity for diagnosing these tumors.[166,167]

On MRI, PNETs have low signal intensity on T1-weighted images and high signal intensity on T2-weighted images. The tumors are most conspicuous on fat suppressed T1 weighted sequences where they appear of low intensity against the bright pancreas.[165] With improvement of MR technology and experience, MRI is comparable to CT for detection of primary PNET and superior for metastatic disease.[168,169] The performance characteristics of various imaging modalities for assessing local spread, resectability and metastasis are similar to those reported earlier for pancreatic adenocarcinomas.

Somatostain-receptor scintigraphy (SRS) or Octreoscan is a nuclear imaging study using radiolabelled octreotide, a somatostatin analog, to detect somatostain receptor-rich neuroendocrine tissue. Application of single proton emission computed tomography (SPECT) or positron emission tomography (PET) CT to SRS has improved its accuracy significantly. However, its sensitivity and specificity are still lower than CT and MRI.[170] Also, certain PNETs such as insulinoma and poorly differentiated PNETs express low levels of somatostatin receptors and are usually undetectable by SRS-SPECT, thus limiting its use as a diagnostic modality.[171,172] Glucagon-like peptide-1 (GLP-1) receptor scintigraphy, a similar nuclear imaging study based on the same principle has promising data in detecting insulinoma but requires further investigation and has not yet been widely accepted. The important advantage of SRS-SPECT is that it can help select patients who have tumor with highly expressed somatostatin receptors who are more likely to respond to somatostain-based therapies such as ^{90}Y-edotreotide or Tyr^{3}-octreotate.

Arterial stimulation venous sampling

Arterial stimulation venous sampling (ASVS) is an invasive test for tumor localization. Its principle is based on a directly selective arterial injection of certain stimulant such as secretin for gastrinoma and calcium gluconate for insulinoma with subsequent measurement of hormonal response of the tumor by venous sampling of the hepatic venous effluent. This invasive technique can be used in an extremely occult functional tumor for tumor localization. Its use has decreased over the past decade as other diagnostic modalities including CT, MRI, and EUS have become more effective.[173] Other adjunct invasive modalities include intraoperative pancreatic ultrasound, which is sometimes required when other modalities fail.[165]

Grading and staging systems

The classification of PNETs has evolved considerably over the past decade. Grading and staging systems proposed by World Health Organization (WHO), European Neuroendocrine Tumor Society (ENETS), and American Joint Committee on Cancer (AJCC) share common schemes with minor differences (Table 6).[109,116,174]

Grading systems reflect the biologic aggressiveness of the tumor as suggested by histologic features (based on proliferative rates) while staging systems reflect the extent of the disease based on vascular invasion, tumor size, and distant metastasis. Both systems are used independently to assess prognosis.

Histologically, PNETs have been traditionally categorized into well-differentiated neuroendocrine tumor and poorly differentiated neuroendocrine carcinoma. Histologic features of well-differentiated neuroendocrine tumors include organized tumor cells in trabecular or gyriform pattern with uniformly round or oval nuclei, coarsely stippled chromatin (salt and pepper chromatin), and finely granular cytoplasm with abundant neurosecretory granules.[175] They tend to have indolent course with much better prognosis and an overall five-year survival rate up to 67%.[176] However, it is not unusual for well-differentiated PNETs to present with metastasized disease.[176]

Table 6. Histologic grading of pancreatic neuroendocrine tumors (109, 116, 174).

Grade	Mitotic count (per 2 mm^2)	Ki-67 labeling index (%)
Low grade (G1)	<2	<3
Intermediate grade (G2)	2–20	3–20
High grade (G3)	>20	>20

Poorly differentiated neuroendocrine carcinomas have a sheet-like or diffuse tumor cell arrangement with non-uniform nuclei, and less cytoplasmic granularity. These tumors have more aggressive behavior with a rapid clinical course that resembles small or large cell neuroendocrine carcinoma of the lung.[175]

Morphology alone cannot predict the tumor behavior as there is a subgroup of well-differentiated PNETs that have a more aggressive clinical course while metastatic tumors may show little or no cellular pleomorphism, hyperchromasia, or increased mitotic activity.[177] For these reasons, the terms "benign" and "malignant" are no longer used for histological grading of PNETs. The WHO has updated their grading system to further subcategorize well-differentiated neuroendocrine tumors into low grade (G1) and intermediated grade (G2) subgroups based on their proliferative rate (mitotic count and Ki-67 index).[116] This grading scheme, together with the staging system is used for prognosis. The parameters used in this grading system are also endorsed by AJCC and ENETS (Table 7).

Poorly differentiated carcinomas are all high-grade neoplasms (G3) and are no longer defined by local vascular invasion or metastasis. The term "neuroendocrine tumor grade 3" can be used but is discouraged as by definition, neuroendocrine tumors are well-differentiated. Similarly neuroendocrine carcinomas should not be classified as grade 1, grade 2, or well-differentiated neuroendocrine carcinoma.[116]

Ki-67 protein is a large nuclear protein that is closely associated with cell cycle regulation and organization of the nucleolus. Ki-67 is expressed in G1, S, G2 and M phases, with a peak level during mitosis, hence its use as a surrogate marker of cellular proliferation.[109,116,174] According to WHO and ENETS guidelines, 2000 cells in the area of the highest proliferative rate (hot spots) should be counted to determine the Ki-67 labeling index.[116,174]

Mitotic count is the most direct marker of proliferative activity of the tumor. It requires no special immunohistochemical staining as compared to Ki-67 labeling index. Performing an average count over 40–50 HPF assuming that 10 HPF equals 2 mm^2 is recommended. However, in limited specimens such as those obtained with fine needle aspiration, this may not be possible as there may be many more Ki67-labeled cells than cells in mitosis. Moreover, there is no standardization among different brands of microscopes and each HPF may not be equal.[178]

Table 7. Comparison between TNM staging systems of AJCC and ENETS (109, 174).

		AJCC	ENETS
Primary tumor (T)	**Tx**	Primary tumor cannot be assessed	Primary tumor cannot be assessed
	T0	No evidence of primary tumor	No evidence of primary tumor
	T1	Tumor limited to pancreas ≤2 cm	Tumor limited to pancreas ≤2 cm
	T2	Tumor limited to pancreas >2 cm	Tumor limited to pancreas 2–4 cm
	T3	Tumor extends beyond the pancreas but without involvement of the celiac axis or the superior mesenteric artery	Tumor limited to the pancreas and is larger than 4 cm or invading duodenum or bile duct
	T4	Tumor involves the celiac axis or the superior mesenteric artery	Tumor invading adjacent organs (stomach, spleen, colon, adrenal gland) or the wall of large vessels (celiac axis or superior mesenteric artery)
Regional lymph node (N)	**Nx**	Regional lymph noe cannot be assessed	Regional lymph noe cannot be assessed
	N0	No regional lymph node metastasis	No regional lymph node metastasis
	N1	Regional lymph node metastasis	Regional lymph node metastasis
Distant metastasis (M)	**Mx**	No Mx categorized	Distant metastasis cannot be assessed
	M0	No distant metastasis	No distant metastasis
	M1	Distant metastasis	Distant metastasis

Staging systems for pancreatic neuroendocrine tumor (109, 174)

AJCC				ENETS			
Stage	T	N	M	Stage	T	N	M
IA	T_1	N_0	M_0	I	T_1	N_0	M_0
IB	T_2	N_0	M_0	IIA	T_2	N_0	M_0
IIA	T_3	N_0	M_0	IIB	T_3	N_0	M_0
IIB	T_1, T_2, T_3	N_1	M_0	IIIA	T_4	N_0	M_0
III	T_4	N_{ANY}	M_0	IIIB	T_{ANY}	N_1	M_0
IV	T_{ANY}	N_{ANY}	M_1	IV	T_{ANY}	N_{ANY}	M_1

If both mitotic count and Ki-67 labeling index are performed and they yield different grades, the neoplasm should be regarded as the higher grade. Other prognostic parameters such as tumor necrosis, lymphovascular and perineural invasion have not been included in grading criteria.[109,174]

There are currently two widely accepted TNM staging systems by AJCC and ENETS with only minor differences in primary tumor (T) staging between the two as shown in Table 7. The prognostic values of both systems have been extensively validated.[179,180] Five-year overall survival rates for stage I, II, III, and IV disease of PNETs are 92%, 84%, 81%, 57%, respectively using AJCC staging and are 100%, 88%, 85%, 57%, respectively using ENETS staging.[180] It is unclear which staging system has better prognostication.

ENETS stages poorly differentiated neuroendocrine carcinoma in the same way as well-differentiated neuroendocrine tumors while AJCC stages poorly differentiated neuroendocrine carcinomas as adenocarcinomas. Also, it is important to note that functionality of the tumor plays no role in staging and grading systems.

Uncommon Pancreatic Tumors

Solid pseudopapillary tumor (SPT)

SPTs are low grade malignant epithelial neoplasms characterized by a solid growth pattern of discohesive polygonal cells which undergo cystic degeneration and psuedopapillae formation.[181] They account for 0.13–2.7% of pancreatic tumors and characteristically affect young females (90% females, mean age 22–28 years) and have a very good prognosis with a five-year survival rate of 95%.[182] These tumors are often diagnosed incidentally when small and become symptomatic only when the tumor has increased in size (mean diameter 6–10 cm) and causes compression of surrounding organs.[183] They have characteristic imaging features though occasionally percutaneous or EUS guided FNA may be required to differentiate them from large necrotic neuroendocrine tumors. On US, they appear as heterogenous, encapsulated mass with solid echogenic and cystic hypoechoic components with peripheral calcifications. CT may show a well-defined, low-attenuation mass with peripheral enhancement and complex cystic components with areas of necrosis and hemorrhage while MRI may show variable signal intensity on T1 weighted images and high signal intensity on T2-weighted images.[184] Local or extended resection, depending on the size of the tumor and involvement of adjacent organs or lymph nodes, is the mainstay of therapy and standard chemotherapeutic regimens are not established.[185]

Acinar cell carcinoma (ACC)

ACC are rare but biologically aggressive malignant tumors arising from the acinar cells in the pancreas. They account for 1–2% of all malignant pancreatic tumors, usually present in the fifth to seventh decades, and are twice as common in men.[186] Tumors tend to be focal, slightly more predominant in the head of the pancreas and are often large (10–15 cm in diameter) at time of diagnosis. Most commonly, they present with nonspecific abdominal symptoms due to the size of the tumor. Because this tumor arises from acinar cells, it is associated with systemic release of pancreatic enzymes including trypsin, chymotrypsin, amylase and lipase although the serum levels of these enzymes may not be elevated.[183] In 10–15% of patients, this tumor can be associated with the lipase hypersecretion syndrome which is a paraneoplastic syndrome characterized by subcutaneous nodules, eosinophilia and arthralgias secondary to lipase hypersecretion.[186] Serum tumor markers such as CA 19-9, AFP and CEA are variably expressed and are not specific to establish a diagnosis, though they may be useful for evaluating recurrence if elevated.[187] These tumors are often hypovascular but well-marginated, exophytic and much larger than adenocarcinoma on imaging, though hypervascular variants which may be confused with NETs have been reported. Therefore, imaging studies are not diagnostic for ACC and FNA or even surgical pathology may be required for establishing a diagnosis.[188] Though metastases to liver and lymph nodes have been reported in up to 50% of patients at presentation, no chemotherapeutic regimen has shown significant benefit.[189] Therefore surgery remains the only treatment of choice and no formal staging system has been used for ACC. Overall, these tumors have a slightly better prognosis than ductal adenocarcinoma with a median survival of 47 months, decreasing to 14 months for unresectable tumors.[186,189]

Primary pancreatic lymphoma (PPL)

PPLs are extremely rare and compromise less than 0.5% of all pancreatic tumors and less than 2% of Extranodal non-Hodgkin's lymphoma (NHL). Histologically, most PPLs are diffuse large cell lymphomas and have been reported more frequently in men, presenting in the fifth or sixth decade.[190] They can be differentiated from secondary involvement of the pancreas by lymphoma which is much more frequent and can occur in up to a third of cases with non-Hodgkin's lymphoma by the following criteria: Absence of superficial or mediastinal lymphadenopathy; normal peripheral leukocyte count; main mass in the pancreas with lymph node involvement confined to the peripancreatic region; and no hepatic or splenic involvement. Unfortunately, it is much more difficult to differentiate them from pancreatic ductal carcinoma because like adenocarcinoma, they usually present with non-specific abdominal symptoms and classic symptoms such as fever, chills and night sweats are uncommon.[190] Also, on imaging they commonly present as solitary masses confined to the head, varying in size from 2–15 cm with mean reported diameter of 8 cm though body or tail tumors and rarely diffuse involvement of the entire gland has also been reported. On CT, the mass is hypodense and homeogenous and can extend into and infiltrate peripancreatic vasculature and surrounding structures. On MRI, they appear as a low signal intensity, homogenous mass on T1 weighted images with subtle post-contrast enhancement, and on T2 weighted images, they show a more heterogenous character with low to intermediate signal amplitude.[191] Certain imaging findings which may help differentiate PPL from pancreatic adenocarcinoma include: a combination of bulky localized tumor in the pancreatic head without significant dilatation of main pancreatic duct; enlargement of lymph nodes below the level of renal veins; invasive tumor growth not respecting anatomic boundaries and infiltrating the retroperitoneum or surrounding organs.[191]

A clinical suspicion of PPL should prompt percutaneous or EUS guided FNA or core biopsy of the lesion with flow cytometry of the specimen, which has been shown to reliably diagnose PPL and differentiate it from other pancreatic tumors. Once diagnosed, PPL is staged as other NHLs using the Ann Arbor Staging system.

Unlikely the pancreatic adenocarcinoma which it can mimic, PPL is usually treated with a combination of chemotherapy and radiation therapy or stem cell transplantation and carries a much better prognosis.[190]

Isolated pancreatic metastasis

Pancreatic metastases occur most commonly from primary tumors in lung, kidney, and breast. Melanomas can also metastasize to the pancreas. Though uncommon, virtually any primary neoplasm can metastasize to the pancreas. The diagnosis is usually evident in the presence of primary tumor, however occasionally isolated metastasis to the pancreas may occur years after resection of the primary tumor and may be mistaken for a primary pancreatic neoplasm. Isolated pancreatic metastases can account for approximately 2% of all pancreatic neoplasms.[192] These lesions may be diagnosed during routine surveillance or by the presence of non-specific symptoms and imaging findings similar to the primary tumor. RCC is the most common primary cancer to metastasize to the pancreas and is characterized by a long disease free interval after nephrectomy before recognition.[183] On CT scan, metastatic RCC appears as a large hypervascular spherical mass with well-defined margins and central low attenuation that can mimic other hypervascular lesions of pancreas such as NET.[193] In patients with a history of resected RCC, this presentation is usually diagnostic and tissue biopsy is not required, though percutaneous or EUS biopsy may be obtained for suspected metastasis from non-RCC malignancies or if diagnostic confusion exists. Resection of isolated pancreatic metastasis from RCC is associated with a good prognosis and with a five-year survival of 68–75%, whereas resection of pancreatic metastasis from other tumor sites carries a worse prognosis with a median survival of two years.[183]

Pancreatoblastoma

Pancreatoblastomas are malignant neoplasms of presumed stem cell origin which most commonly occur in the first decade of life but have been reported in adolescents and rarely adults. Pancreatoblastomas are slow growing tumors usually diagnosed when they are large (mean size 10 cm) with signs and symptoms due to the mass effect from the tumor. Elevation of alpha fetoprotein has been reported in up to 68% of these patients.[194] On imaging, most of these tumors are well-defined and at least partially circumscribed, seen as multilobulated masses with enhancing septa on CT and mixed echotexture on US. On MR, these tumors appear heterogenous with low to intermediate signal intensity on T1 and high signal intensity on T2 weighted images.[195] Distant metastasis is seen in 26% of adults and most commonly involves the liver and lymph nodes.[196] Histologically, pancreatoblastomas are highly cellular neoplasms composed of small uniform epithelial cells arranged in sheets and nests with occasional squamoid nests (corpuscules) which are a useful diagnostic feature of this tumor.[181] Pancreatoblastomas when localized can be excised completely and are associated with good prognosis, especially in children. In adults, despite aggressive treatment, the prognosis is poor with median survival of 18.5 months.[197]

Take Home Messages

- Familial pancreatic cancer kindreds and association with genetic syndromes has been identified in 5% of pancreatic cancer and may be used in early detection of pancreatic tumors in high-risk individuals.
- The 7th edition of the AJCC staging system, recommends triphasic multislice CT or MRI for staging, includes pancreatic neuroendocrine tumors for staging similar to exocrine pancreatic malignancies and has downstaged pancreatic tumor with involvement of superior mesenteric vein, splenic vein and portal vein to T3 recognizing potential resectability of these lesions.
- While most pancreatic neuroendocrine tumors are non functional and are increasingly, incidentally, diagnosed at an earlier stage with greater use of cross sectional abdominal imaging, functional PNETs are neuroendocrine tumors that cause clinical horomonal syndromes and can be recognized clinically by characteristic clinical presentation and serum biomarkers.
- Serum chromogranin A (CgA) correlates well with tumor burden in most patients with both functional and non-functional PNETs (except

insulinomas), and therefore may be used to monitor response to therapy and progression free survival.

- PNETs are prognosticated using staging systems to determine disease extent and grading systems to prognosticate biological aggressiveness.
- Solid psuedopapillary tumors, acinar cell carcinoma, primary pancreatic lymphoma and pancreatoblastomas are much less frequent and more indolent pancreatic tumors which may be differentiated from pancreatic adenocarcinoma by certain clinical and radiological characteristics.
- Isolated pancreatic metastasis may present as solid pancreatic mass and can occur after a long disease free interval after treatment of primary tumor (usually renal cell carcinoma). Resection of isolated pancreatic metastasis from RCC is associated with good prognosis.

References

1. Capella, C., Albarello, L., Capelli, P., Sessa, F., Zamboni, G., Carcinoma of the exocrine pancreas: The histology report. *Digest Liver Dis*, 2011. **43**(Suppl 4): S282–92.
2. Halfdanarson, T.R., Rabe, K.G., Rubin, J., Petersen, G.M., Pancreatic neuroendocrine tumors (PNETs): Incidence, prognosis and recent trend toward improved survival. *Ann Oncol*, 2008. **19**(10): 1727–33.
3. Yeo, T.P., Lowenfels, A.B., Demographics and epidemiology of pancreatic cancer. *Cancer J*, 2012. **18**(6): 477–44.
4. SEER cancer statistics review. Bethesda, Md.: U S Dept of Health and Human Services, Public Health Institute, National Institutes of Health. p. v.
5. Oberstein, P.E., Olive, K.P., Pancreatic cancer: Why is it so hard to treat? *Ther Adv Gastroenterol*, 2013. **6**(4): 321–37.
6. Bilimoria, K.Y., Bentrem, D.J., Ko, C.Y., Ritchey, J., Stewart, A.K., Winchester, D.P. *et al.*, Validation of the 6th edition AJCC Pancreatic Cancer Staging System: Report from the National Cancer Database. *Cancer*, 2007. **110**(4): 738–44.
7. Muniraj, T., Jamidar, P.A., Aslanian, H.R., Pancreatic cancer: A comprehensive review and update. *Disease-a-month*, 2013. **59**(11): 368–402.

8. Nagakawa, T., Konishi, I., Ueno, K., Ohta, T., Akiyama, T., Kayahara, M. *et al.*, Surgical treatment of pancreatic cancer. The Japanese experience. *Internat J Pancreatol*, 1991. **9**: 135–43.
9. Garcea, G., Dennison, A.R., Pattenden, C.J., Neal, C.P., Sutton, C.D., Berry, D.P., Survival following curative resection for pancreatic ductal adenocarcinoma. A systematic review of the literature. *J Pancreas*, 2008. **9**(2): 99–132.
10. Carrier, M., Le Gal, G., Wells, P.S., Fergusson, D., Ramsay, T., Rodger, M.A., Systematic review: The Trousseau syndrome revisited: Should we screen extensively for cancer in patients with venous thromboembolism? *Ann Internal Med*, 2008. **149**(5): 323–33.
11. Porta, M., Fabregat, X., Malats, N., Guarner, L., Carrato, A., de Miguel, A. *et al.*, Exocrine pancreatic cancer: Symptoms at presentation and their relation to tumour site and stage. *Clin Translational Oncol*, 2005. **7**(5): 189–97.
12. Bakkevold, K.E., Arnesjo, B., Kambestad, B., Carcinoma of the pancreas and papilla of Vater: Presenting symptoms, signs, and diagnosis related to stage and tumour site. A prospective multicentre trial in 472 patients. Norwegian Pancreatic Cancer Trial. *Scand J Gastroenterol*, 1992. **27**(4): 317–25.
13. DeVita, V.T., Jr, Lawrence, T.S.R.S.A. DeVita, Hellman, and Rosenberg's *Cancer: Principles & Practice of Oncology*: Wolters Kluwer/Lippincott Williams & Wilkins; 2008. Available from: http://catdir.loc.gov/catdir/enhancements/fy0811/2008006079-d.html Materials specified: Publisher description http://catdir.loc.gov/catdir/enhancements/fy0811/2008006079-d.htmlhttp://www.lww.com/product/DeVita-Hellman-and-Rosenbergs-Cancer/?978-0-7817-7207-5.
14. Kelsen, D.P., Portenoy, R., Thaler, H., Tao, Y., Brennan, M., Pain as a predictor of outcome in patients with operable pancreatic carcinoma. *Surgery*, 1997. **122**(1): 53–9.
15. DiMagno, E.P., Pancreatic cancer: Clinical presentation, pitfalls and early clues. *Annals of Oncology*, 1999. **10**(Suppl 4): 140–2.
16. Mujica, V.R., Barkin, J.S., Go, V.L., Acute pancreatitis secondary to pancreatic carcinoma. Study Group Participants. *Pancreas*, 2000. **21**(4): 329–32.
17. Saruc, M., Pour, P.M., Diabetes and its relationship to pancreatic carcinoma. *Pancreas*, 2003. **26**(4): 381–7.

18. Ostlere, L.S., Branfoot, A.C., Staughton, R.C., Cicatricial pemphigoid and carcinoma of the pancreas. *Clin Exp Dermat*, 1992. **17**(1): 67–8.
19. Yeo, T.P., Hruban, R.H., Leach, S.D., Wilentz, R.E., Sohn, T.A., Kern, S.E. *et al.*, Pancreatic cancer. *Curr Problems Cancer*, 2002. **26**(4): 176–275.
20. Stapley, S., Peters, T.J., Neal, R.D., Rose, P.W., Walter, F.M., Hamilton, W., The risk of pancreatic cancer in symptomatic patients in primary care: A large case-control study using electronic records. *Brit J Cancer*, 2012. **106**(12): 1940–4.
21. Shaib, Y., Davila, J., Naumann, C., El-Serag, H., The impact of curative intent surgery on the survival of pancreatic cancer patients: A US Population-based study. *Am J Gastroenterol*, 2007. **102**(7): 1377–82.
22. Decker, G.A., Batheja, M.J., Collins, J.M., Silva, A.C., Mekeel, K.L., Moss, A.A. *et al.*, Risk factors for pancreatic adenocarcinoma and prospects for screening. *Gastroenterol Hepatol*, 2010. **6**(4): 246–54.
23. Brentnall, T.A., Bronner, M.P., Byrd, D.R., Haggitt, R.C., Kimmey, M.B., Early diagnosis and treatment of pancreatic dysplasia in patients with a family history of pancreatic cancer. *Ann Internal Med*, 1999. **131**(4): 247–55.
24. Langer, P., Kann, P.H., Fendrich, V., Habbe, N., Schneider, M., Sina, M. *et al.*, Five years of prospective screening of high-risk individuals from families with familial pancreatic cancer. *Gut*, 2009. **58**(10): 1410–8.
25. Canto, M.I., Harinck, F., Hruban, R.H., Offerhaus, G.J., Poley, J.W., Kamel, I. *et al.*, International Cancer of the Pancreas Screening (CAPS) Consortium summit on the management of patients with increased risk for familial pancreatic cancer. *Gut*, 2013. **62**(3): 339–47.
26. Verna, E.C., Hwang, C., Stevens, P.D., Rotterdam, H., Stavropoulos, S.N., Sy, C.D. *et al.*, Pancreatic cancer screening in a prospective cohort of high-risk patients: A comprehensive strategy of imaging and genetics. *Clin Cancer Res*, 2010. **16**(20): 5028–37.
27. Greer, J.B., Brand, R.E., Screening for pancreatic cancer: Current evidence and future directions. *Gastroenterol Hepatol*, 2007. **3**(12): 929–38.
28. Kaur, S., Baine, M.J., Jain, M., Sasson, A.R., Batra, S.K., Early diagnosis of pancreatic cancer: Challenges and new developments. *Biomarkers Med*, 2012. **6**(5): 597–612.
29. Locker, G.Y., Hamilton, S., Harris, J., Jessup, J.M., Kemeny, N., Macdonald, J.S. *et al.*, ASCO 2006 update of recommendations for the use of tumor markers in gastrointestinal cancer. *J Clin Oncol*, 2006. **24**(33): 5313–27.

30. Molina, V., Visa, L., Conill, C., Navarro, S., Escudero, J.M., Auge, J.M. *et al.*, CA 19-9 in pancreatic cancer: Retrospective evaluation of patients with suspicion of pancreatic cancer. *Tumour Biol*, 2012. **33**(3): 799–807.
31. Tempero, M.A., Uchida, E., Takasaki, H., Burnett, D.A., Steplewski, Z., Pour, P.M., Relationship of carbohydrate antigen 19-9 and Lewis antigens in pancreatic cancer. *Cancer Res*, 1987. **47**(20): 5501–3.
32. Tempero, M.A., Arnoletti, J.P., Behrman, S., Ben-Josef, E., Benson, A.B., 3rd, Berlin, J.D. *et al.*, Pancreatic adenocarcinoma. *J Nat Comprehensive Cancer Network*, 2010. **8**(9): 972–1017.
33. Brambs, H.J., Claussen, C.D., Pancreatic and ampullary carcinoma. Ultrasound, computed tomography, magnetic resonance imaging and angiography. *Endoscopy*, 1993. **25**(1): 58–68.
34. Karlson, B.M., Ekbom, A., Lindgren, P.G., Kallskog, V., Rastad, J., Abdominal US for diagnosis of pancreatic tumor: Prospective cohort analysis. *Radiology*, 1999. **213**(1): 107–11.
35. Tamm, E.P., Bhosale, P.R., Lee, J.H., Pancreatic ductal adenocarcinoma: Ultrasound, computed tomography, and magnetic resonance imaging features. *Semin Ultrasound CT MR*, 2007. **28**(5): 330–8.
36. Zamboni, G.A., Ambrosetti, M.C., D'Onofrio, M., Pozzi Mucelli, R., Ultrasonography of the pancreas. *Radiologic Clin North Am*, 2012. **50**(3): 395–406.
37. Leschka, S., Alkadhi, H., Wildermuth, S., Marincek, B., Multi-detector computed tomography of acute abdomen. *Eur Radiol*, 2005. **15**(12): 2435–47.
38. Prokesch, R.W., Chow, L.C., Beaulieu, C.F., Bammer, R., Jeffrey, R.B., Jr., Isoattenuating pancreatic adenocarcinoma at multi-detector row CT: Secondary signs. *Radiology*, 2002. **224**(3): 764–8.
39. Legmann, P., Vignaux, O., Dousset, B., Baraza, A.J., Palazzo, L., Dumontier, I. *et al.*, Pancreatic tumors: Comparison of dual-phase helical CT and endoscopic sonography. *Am J Roentgenol*, 1998. **170**(5): 1315–22.
40. Bronstein, Y.L., Loyer, E.M., Kaur, H., Choi, H., David, C., DuBrow, R.A. *et al.*, Detection of small pancreatic tumors with multiphasic helical CT. *Am J Roentgenol*, 2004. **182**(3): 619–23.
41. Hough, T.J., Raptopoulos, V., Siewert, B., Matthews, J.B., Teardrop superior mesenteric vein: CT sign for unresectable carcinoma of the pancreas. *Am J Roentgenol*, 1999. **173**(6): 1509–12.

42. Li, H., Zeng, M.S., Zhou, K.R., Jin, D.Y., Lou, W.H., Pancreatic adenocarcinoma: The different CT criteria for peripancreatic major arterial and venous invasion. *J Comp Assisted Tomography*, 2005. **29**(2): 170–5.
43. Lu, D.S., Reber, H.A., Krasny, R.M., Kadell, B.M., Sayre, J., Local staging of pancreatic cancer: Criteria for unresectability of major vessels as revealed by pancreatic-phase, thin-section helical CT. *Am J Roentgenol*, 1997. **168**(6): 1439–43.
44. Zhao, W.Y., Luo, M., Sun, Y.W., Xu, Q., Chen, W., Zhao, G. *et al.*, Computed tomography in diagnosing vascular invasion in pancreatic and periampullary cancers: A systematic review and meta-analysis. *Hepatobiliary Pancreatic Dis Internat*, 2009. **8**(5): 457–64.
45. Roche, C.J., Hughes, M.L., Garvey, C.J., Campbell, F., White, D.A., Jones, L. *et al.*, CT and pathologic assessment of prospective nodal staging in patients with ductal adenocarcinoma of the head of the pancreas. *Am J Roentgenol*, 2003. **180**(2): 475–80.
46. DeWitt, J., Devereaux, B., Chriswell, M., McGreevy, K., Howard, T., Imperiale, T.F. *et al.*, Comparison of endoscopic ultrasonography and multidetector computed tomography for detecting and staging pancreatic cancer. *Ann Internal Med*, 2004. **141**(10): 753–63.
47. Horton, K.M., Fishman, E.K., Adenocarcinoma of the pancreas: CT imaging. *Radiologic Clin North Am*, 2002. **40**(6): 1263–72.
48. Schwartz, L.H., Gandras, E.J., Colangelo, S.M., Ercolani, M.C., Panicek, D.M., Prevalence and importance of small hepatic lesions found at CT in patients with cancer. *Radiology*, 1999. **210**(1): 71–4.
49. Walkey, M.M., Friedman, A.C., Sohotra, P., Radecki, P.D., CT manifestations of peritoneal carcinomatosis. *Am J Roentgenol*, 1988. **150**(5): 1035–41.
50. Raman, S.P., Horton, K.M., Fishman, E.K., Multimodality imaging of pancreatic cancer-computed tomography, magnetic resonance imaging, and positron emission tomography. *Cancer J*, 2012. **18**(6): 511–22.
51. Liu, R.C., Traverso, L.W., Laparoscopic staging should be used routinely for locally extensive cancer of the pancreatic head. *J Gastrointestinal Surg*, 2004. **8**(8): 923–4.
52. Diehl, S.J., Lehmann, K.J., Sadick, M., Lachmann, R., Georgi, M., Pancreatic cancer: Value of dual-phase helical CT in assessing resectability. *Radiology*, 1998. **206**(2): 373–8.

53. Clarke, D.L., Clarke, B.A., Thomson, S.R., Garden, O.J., Lazarus, N.G., The role of preoperative biopsy in pancreatic cancer. *HPB*, 2004. **6**(3): 144–53.
54. Volmar, K.E., Vollmer, R.T., Jowell, P.S., Nelson, R.C., Xie, H.B., Pancreatic FNA in 1000 cases: A comparison of imaging modalities. *Gastrointest Endosc*, 2005. **61**(7): 854–61.
55. Livraghi, T., Damascelli, B., Lombardi, C., Spagnoli, I., Risk in fine-needle abdominal biopsy. *J Clin Ultrasound*, 1983. **11**(2): 77–81.
56. Livraghi, T., Lombardi, C., Mascia, G., Bile peritonitis: Another complication after fine-needle biopsy. *Diagnost Imag*, 1983. **52**(1): 33–5.
57. Warshaw, A.L., Implications of peritoneal cytology for staging of early pancreatic cancer. *Am J Surg*, 1991. **161**(1): 26–9; discussion 9–30.
58. Crowe, D.R., Eloubeidi, M.A., Chhieng, D.C., Jhala, N.C., Jhala, D., Eltoum, I.A., Fine-needle aspiration biopsy of hepatic lesions: Computerized tomographic-guided versus endoscopic ultrasound-guided FNA. *Cancer*, 2006. **108**(3): 180–5.
59. Miller, F.H., Rini, N.J., Keppke, A.L., MRI of adenocarcinoma of the pancreas. *Am J Roentgenol*, 2006. **187**(4): W365–74.
60. Bipat, S., Phoa, S.S., van Delden, O.M., Bossuyt, P.M., Gouma, D.J., Lameris, J.S. *et al.*, Ultrasonography, computed tomography and magnetic resonance imaging for diagnosis and determining resectability of pancreatic adenocarcinoma: A meta-analysis. *J Comp Assisted Tomography*, 2005. **29**(4): 438–45.
61. Fusari, M., Maurea, S., Imbriaco, M., Mollica, C., Avitabile, G., Soscia, F. *et al.*, Comparison between multislice CT and MR imaging in the diagnostic evaluation of patients with pancreatic masses. *La Radiologia Medica*, 2010. **115**(3): 453–66.
62. Grenacher, L., Klauss, M., Dukic, L., Delorme, S., Knaebel, H.P., Dux, M. *et al.*, Diagnosis and staging of pancreatic carcinoma: MRI versus multislice-CT — a prospective study. *RoFo: Fortschritte auf dem Gebiete der Rontgenstrahlen und der Nuklearmedizin*, 2004. **176**(11): 1624–33.
63. Kauhanen, S.P., Komar, G., Seppanen, M.P., Dean, K.I., Minn, H.R., Kajander, S.A. *et al.*, A prospective diagnostic accuracy study of 18F-fluorodeoxyglucose positron emission tomography/computed tomography, multidetector row computed tomography, and magnetic resonance imaging in primary diagnosis and staging of pancreatic cancer. *Ann Surg*, 2009. **250**(6): 957–63.

64. Wong, J.C., Lu, D.S., Staging of pancreatic adenocarcinoma by imaging studies. *Clin Gastroenterol Hepatol*, 2008. **6**(12): 1301–8.
65. Holalkere, N.S., Sahani, D.V., Blake, M.A., Halpern, E.F., Hahn, P.F., Mueller, P.R., Characterization of small liver lesions: Added role of MR after MDCT. *J Comp Assisted tomography*, 2006. **30**(4): 591–6.
66. Frohlich, A., Diederichs, C.G., Staib, L., Vogel, J., Beger, H.G., Reske, S.N., Detection of liver metastases from pancreatic cancer using FDG PET. *J Nuclear Med*, 1999. **40**(2): 250–5.
67. Buchs, N.C., Buhler, L., Bucher, P., Willi, J.P., Frossard, J.L., Roth, A.D. *et al.*, Value of contrast-enhanced 18F-fluorodeoxyglucose positron emission tomography/computed tomography in detection and presurgical assessment of pancreatic cancer: A prospective study. *J Gastroenterol Hepatol*, 2011. **26**(4): 657–62.
68. Grassetto, G., Rubello, D., Role of FDG-PET/CT in diagnosis, staging, response to treatment, and prognosis of pancreatic cancer. *Am J Clin Oncol*, 2011. **34**(2): 111–4.
69. Orlando, L.A., Kulasingam, S.L., Matchar, D.B., Meta-analysis: The detection of pancreatic malignancy with positron emission tomography. *Aliment Pharmacol Therapeut*, 2004. **20**(10): 1063–70.
70. Hisanaga, K., Hisanaga, A., Nagata, K., Ichie, Y., High speed rotating scanner for transgastric sonography. *Am J Roentgenol*, 1980. **135**(3): 627–9.
71. Ainsworth, A.P., Rafaelsen, S.R., Wamberg, P.A., Durup, J., Pless, T.K., Mortensen, M.B., Is there a difference in diagnostic accuracy and clinical impact between endoscopic ultrasonography and magnetic resonance cholangiopancreatography? *Endoscopy*, 2003. **35**(12): 1029–32.
72. Gress, F.G., Hawes, R.H., Savides, T.J., Ikenberry, S.O., Cummings, O., Kopecky, K. *et al.*, Role of EUS in the preoperative staging of pancreatic cancer: A large single-center experience. *Gastrointest Endosc*, 1999. **50**(6): 786–91.
73. Muller, M.F., Meyenberger, C., Bertschinger, P., Schaer, R., Marincek, B., Pancreatic tumors: Evaluation with endoscopic, U.S., CT, and MR imaging. *Radiology*, 1994. **190**(3): 745–51.
74. Akahoshi, K., Chijiiwa, Y., Nakano, I., Nawata, H., Ogawa, Y., Tanaka, M. *et al.*, Diagnosis and staging of pancreatic cancer by endoscopic ultrasound. *Brit J Radiol*, 1998. **71**(845): 492–6.

75. Rosch, T., Dittler, H.J., Lorenz, R., Braig, C., Gain, T., Feuerbach, S. *et al.*, The endosonographic staging of pancreatic carcinoma. *Deutsche medizinische Wochenschrift (1946)*, 1992. **117**(15): 563–9.
76. Bhutani, M.S., Hawes, R.H., Hoffman, B.J., A comparison of the accuracy of echo features during endoscopic ultrasound (EUS) and EUS-guided fine-needle aspiration for diagnosis of malignant lymph node invasion. *Gastrointest Endosc*, 1997. **45**(6): 474–9.
77. Nguyen, P., Feng, J.C., Chang, K.J., Endoscopic ultrasound (EUS) and EUS-guided fine-needle aspiration (FNA) of liver lesions. *Gastrointest Endosc*, 1999. **50**(3): 357–61.
78. tenBerge, J., Hoffman, B.J., Hawes, R.H., Van Enckevort, C., Giovannini, M., Erickson, R.A. *et al.*, EUS-guided fine needle aspiration of the liver: Indications, yield, and safety based on an international survey of 167 cases. *Gastrointest Endosc*, 2002. **55**(7): 859–62.
79. Hawes, R.H., Paul, F., Shyam, V., Endosonography: Elsevier Saunders; 2011. Available from: http: //site.ebrary.com/id/10493400 Materials specified: Ebraryhttp: //site.ebrary.com/id/10493400.
80. Buscail, L., Pages, P., Berthelemy, P., Fourtanier, G., Frexinos, J., Escourrou, J., Role of EUS in the management of pancreatic and ampullary carcinoma: A prospective study assessing resectability and prognosis. *Gastrointest Endosc*, 1999. **50**(1): 34–40.
81. Mertz, H.R., Sechopoulos, P., Delbeke, D., Leach, S.D., EUS, PET, and CT scanning for evaluation of pancreatic adenocarcinoma. *Gastrointest Endosc*, 2000. **52**(3): 367–71.
82. Rosch, T., Braig, C., Gain, T., Feuerbach, S., Siewert, J.R., Schusdziarra, V. *et al.*, Staging of pancreatic and ampullary carcinoma by endoscopic ultrasonography. Comparison with conventional sonography, computed tomography, and angiography. *Gastroenterology*, 1992. **102**(1): 188–99.
83. Hewitt, M.J., McPhail, M.J., Possamai, L., Dhar, A., Vlavianos, P., Monahan, K.J., EUS-guided FNA for diagnosis of solid pancreatic neoplasms: A meta-analysis. *Gastrointest Endosc*, 2012. **75**(2): 319–31.
84. Micames, C., Jowell, P.S., White, R., Paulson, E., Nelson, R., Morse, M. *et al.*, Lower frequency of peritoneal carcinomatosis in patients with pancreatic cancer diagnosed by EUS-guided FNA vs. percutaneous FNA. *Gastrointest Endosc*, 2003. **58**(5): 690–5.

85. Horwhat, J.D., Paulson, E.K., McGrath, K., Branch, M.S., Baillie, J., Tyler, D. *et al.*, A randomized comparison of EUS-guided FNA versus CT or US-guided FNA for the evaluation of pancreatic mass lesions. *Gastrointest Endosc*, 2006. **63**(7): 966–75.
86. Mertz, H., Gautam, S., The learning curve for EUS-guided FNA of pancreatic cancer. *Gastrointest Endosc*, 2004. **59**(1): 33–7.
87. Othman, M.O., Wallace, M.B., The role of endoscopic ultrasonography in the diagnosis and management of pancreatic cancer. *Gastroenterol Clin North Am*, 2012. **41**(1): 179–88.
88. Lee, W.J., Endoscopic ultrasound elastography for pancreatic cancer diagnosis: A step forward? *Clin Endoscopy*, 2013. **46**(2): 116–7.
89. Saftoiu, A., Vilmann, P., Gorunescu, F., Janssen, J., Hocke, M., Larsen, M. *et al.*, Efficacy of an artificial neural network-based approach to endoscopic ultrasound elastography in diagnosis of focal pancreatic masses. *Clinical Gastroenterol Hepatol*, 2012. **10**(1): 84–90.e1.
90. Iglesias-Garcia, J., Larino-Noia, J., Abdulkader, I., Forteza, J., Dominguez-Munoz, J.E., Quantitative endoscopic ultrasound elastography: An accurate method for the differentiation of solid pancreatic masses. *Gastroenterology*, 2010. **139**(4): 1172–80.
91. Xu, W., Shi, J., Zeng, X., Li, X., Xie, W.F., Guo, J. *et al.*, EUS elastography for the differentiation of benign and malignant lymph nodes: A meta-analysis. *Gastrointest Endosc*, 2011. **74**(5): 1001–9; quiz 115.e1–4.
92. Cote, G.A., Smith, J., Sherman, S., Kelly, K., Technologies for imaging the normal and diseased pancreas. *Gastroenterology*, 2013. **144**(6): 1262–71.e1.
93. Kitano, M., Kudo, M., Sakamoto, H., Komaki, T., Endoscopic ultrasonography and contrast-enhanced endoscopic ultrasonography. *Pancreatology*, 2011. **11**(Suppl 2): 28–33.
94. Kitano, M., Kudo, M., Yamao, K., Takagi, T., Sakamoto, H., Komaki, T. *et al.*, Characterization of small solid tumors in the pancreas: The value of contrast-enhanced harmonic endoscopic ultrasonography. *Am J Gastroenterol*, 2012. **107**(2): 303–10.
95. Ahualli, J., The double duct sign. *Radiology*, 2007. **244**(1): 314–5.
96. Anderson, M.A., Fisher, L., Jain, R., Evans, J.A., Appalaneni, V., Ben-Menachem, T. *et al.*, Complications of ERCP. *Gastrointest Endosc*, 2012. **75**(3): 467–73.

97. de Bellis, M., Sherman, S., Fogel, E.L., Cramer, H., Chappo, J., McHenry, L., Jr. *et al.*, Tissue sampling at ERCP in suspected malignant biliary strictures (Part 2). *Gastrointest Endosc*, 2002. **56**(5): 720–30.
98. Iacono, C., Ruzzenente, A., Campagnaro, T., Bortolasi, L., Valdegamberi, A., Guglielmi, A., Role of preoperative biliary drainage in jaundiced patients who are candidates for pancreatoduodenectomy or hepatic resection: Highlights and drawbacks. *Ann Surg*, 2013. **257**(2): 191–204.
99. Rumstadt, B., Schwab, M., Schuster, K., Hagmuller, E., Trede, M., The role of laparoscopy in the preoperative staging of pancreatic carcinoma. *J Gastrointestinal Sur*, 1997. **1**(3): 245–50.
100. Bemelman, W.A., de Wit, L.T., van Delden, O.M., Smits, N.J., Obertop, H., Rauws, E.J. *et al.*, Diagnostic laparoscopy combined with laparoscopic ultrasonography in staging of cancer of the pancreatic head region. *Brit J Surg*, 1995. **82**(6): 820–4.
101. John, T.G., Greig, J.D., Carter, D.C., Garden, O.J., Carcinoma of the pancreatic head and periampullary region. Tumor staging with laparoscopy and laparoscopic ultrasonography. *Ann Surg*, 1995. **221**(2): 156–64.
102. Pisters, P.W., Lee, J.E., Vauthey, J.N., Charnsangavej, C., Evans, D.B., Laparoscopy in the staging of pancreatic cancer. *Brit J Surg*, 2001. **88**(3): 325–37.
103. Allen, V.B., Gurusamy, K.S., Takwoingi, Y., Kalia, A., Davidson, B.R., Diagnostic accuracy of laparoscopy following computed tomography (CT) scanning for assessing the resectability with curative intent in pancreatic and periampullary cancer. *Cochrane Database Systematic Rev*, 2013. **11**: Cd009323.
104. Barabino, M., Santambrogio, R., Pisani Ceretti, A., Scalzone, R., Montorsi, M., Opocher, E., Is there still a role for laparoscopy combined with laparoscopic ultrasonography in the staging of pancreatic cancer? *Surg Endoscopy*, 2011. **25**(1): 160–5.
105. Barreiro, C.J., Lillemoe, K.D., Koniaris, L.G., Sohn, T.A., Yeo, C.J., Coleman, J. *et al.*, Diagnostic laparoscopy for periampullary and pancreatic cancer: What is the true benefit? *J Gastrointestinal Surg*, 2002. **6**(1): 75–81.
106. Soriano, A., Castells, A., Ayuso, C., Ayuso, J.R., de Caralt, M.T., Gines, M.A. *et al.*, Preoperative staging and tumor resectability assessment of pancreatic cancer: Prospective study comparing endoscopic

ultrasonography, helical computed tomography, magnetic resonance imaging, and angiography. *Am J Gastroenterol*, 2004. **99**(3): 492–501.

107. Tierney, W.M., Francis, I.R., Eckhauser, F., Elta, G., Nostrant, T.T., Scheiman, J.M., The accuracy of EUS and helical CT in the assessment of vascular invasion by peripapillary malignancy. *Gastrointest Endosc*, 2001. **53**(2): 182–8.
108. Ahmad, N.A., Lewis, J.D., Siegelman, E.S., Rosato, E.F., Ginsberg, G.G., Kochman, M.L., Role of endoscopic ultrasound and magnetic resonance imaging in the preoperative staging of pancreatic adenocarcinoma. *Am J Gastroenterol*, 2000. **95**(8): 1926–31.
109. *AJCC Cancer Staging Handbook. 7th ed.* Frederick, L., Greene, M.D., Andy Trotti I.M.D., April, G., Fritz C.T.R.R.H.I.T., Carolyn, C., Compton, M.D PD, David, R., Byrd, M.D FACS, Stephen, B., Edge, M.D FACS, editors. Chicago, IL: American Joint Committee on Cancer. 2010.
110. Appel, B.L., Tolat, P., Evans, D.B., Tsai, S., Current staging systems for pancreatic cancer. *Cancer J*, 2012. **18**(6): 539–49.
111. Halperin, D.M., Varadhachary, G.R., Resectable, borderline resectable, and locally advanced pancreatic cancer: What does it matter? *Curr Oncol Reports*, 2014. **16**(2): 366.
112. Fesinmeyer, M.D., Austin, M.A., Li, C.I., De Roos, A.J., Bowen, D.J., Differences in survival by histologic type of pancreatic cancer. *Cancer Epidemiol Biomarkers Prev*, 2005. **14**(7): 1766–73.
113. Capella, C., Heitz, P.U., Hofler, H., Solcia, E., Kloppel, G., Revised classification of neuroendocrine tumours of the lung, pancreas and gut. *Virchows Archiv*, 1995. **425**(6): 547–60.
114. Oberg, K., Pancreatic endocrine tumors. *Semin Oncol*, 2010. **37**(6): 594–618.
115. Metz, D.C., Jensen, R.T., Gastrointestinal neuroendocrine tumors: Pancreatic endocrine tumors. *Gastroenterology*, 2008. **135**(5): 1469–92.
116. Bosman, F.T., *WHO Classification of Tumours of the Digestive System. 4th ed.* Lyon: International Agency for Research on Cancer. 2010. 417 pp.
117. Kimura, W., Kuroda, A., Morioka, Y., Clinical pathology of endocrine tumors of the pancreas. Analysis of autopsy cases. *Digest Dis Sci*, 1991. **36**(7): 933–42.
118. Yao, J.C., Hassan, M., Phan, A., Dagohoy, C., Leary, C., Mares, J.E. *et al.*, One hundred years after "carcinoid": Epidemiology of and prognostic factors

for neuroendocrine tumors in 35,825 cases in the United States. *J Clinical Oncol*, 2008. **26**(18): 3063–72.

119. Yao, J.C., Eisner, M.P., Leary, C., Dagohoy, C., Phan, A., Rashid, A. *et al.*, Population-based study of islet cell carcinoma. *Anna Surg Oncol*, 2007. **14**(12): 3492–500.
120. Lawrence, B., Gustafsson, B.I., Chan, A., Svejda, B., Kidd, M., Modlin, I.M., The epidemiology of gastroenteropancreatic neuroendocrine tumors. *Endocrinol Metabolism Clinics North Am*, 2011. **40**(1): 1–18, vii.
121. Vagefi, P.A., Razo, O., Deshpande, V., McGrath, D.J., Lauwers, G.Y., Thayer, S.P. *et al.*, Evolving patterns in the detection and outcomes of pancreatic neuroendocrine neoplasms: The Massachusetts General Hospital experience from 1977 to 2005. *Arch Surg*, 2007. **142**(4): 347–54.
122. Cheema, A., Weber, J., Strosberg, J.R., Incidental detection of pancreatic neuroendocrine tumors: An analysis of incidence and outcomes. *Ann Surg Oncol*, 2012. **19**(9): 2932–6.
123. Madura, J.A., Cummings, O.W., Wiebke, E.A., Broadie, T.A., Goulet, R.L., Jr., Howard, T.J., Nonfunctioning islet cell tumors of the pancreas: A difficult diagnosis but one worth the effort. *Am Surgeon*, 1997. **63**(7): 573–7; discussion 7–8.
124. Matthews, B.D., Heniford, B.T., Reardon, P.R., Brunicardi, F.C., Greene, F.L. Surgical experience with nonfunctioning neuroendocrine tumors of the pancreas. *Am Surgeon*, 2000. **66**(12): 1116–22; discussion 22–23.
125. Service, F.J., McMahon, M.M., O'Brien, P.C., Ballard, D.J., Functioning insulinoma — incidence, recurrence, and long-term survival of patients: A 60-year study. *Mayo Clinic Proceed*, 1991. **66**(7): 711–9.
126. Placzkowski, K.A., Vella, A., Thompson, G.B., Grant, C.S., Reading, C.C., Charboneau, J.W. *et al.*, Secular trends in the presentation and management of functioning insulinoma at the Mayo Clinic, 1987–2007. *J Clinical Endocrinol Metabolism*, 2009. **94**(4): 1069–73.
127. Vortmeyer, A.O., Huang, S., Lubensky, I., Zhuang, Z., Non-islet origin of pancreatic islet cell tumors. *J Clinical Endocrinol Metabolism*, 2004. **89**(4): 1934–8.
128. Harrington, M.G., McGeorge, A.P., Ballantyne, J.P., Beastall, G., A prospective survey for insulinomas in a neurology department. *Lancet*, 1983. **1**(8333): 1094–5.

129. Norton, J.A., Neuroendocrine tumors of the pancreas and duodenum. *Curr Prob Surg*, 1994. **31**(2): 77–156.
130. Berna, M.J., Hoffmann, K.M., Serrano, J., Gibril, F., Jensen, R.T., Serum gastrin in Zollinger-Ellison syndrome: I. Prospective study of fasting serum gastrin in 309 patients from the National Institutes of Health and comparison with 2229 cases from the literature. *Medicine*, 2006. **85**(6): 295–330.
131. Roy, P.K., Venzon, D.J., Shojamanesh, H., Abou-Saif, A., Peghini, P., Doppman, J.L. *et al.*, Zollinger-Ellison syndrome. Clinical presentation in 261 patients. *Medicine*, 2000. **79**(6): 379–411.
132. Norton, J.A., Alexander, H.R., Fraker, D.L., Venzon, D.J., Gibril, F., Jensen, R.T., Possible primary lymph node gastrinoma: Occurrence, natural history, and predictive factors: A prospective study. *Ann Surg*, 2003. **237**(5): 650–7; discussion 7–9.
133. Gibril, F., Doppman, J.L., Reynolds, J.C., Chen, C.C., Sutliff, V.E., Yu, F. *et al.*, Bone metastases in patients with gastrinomas: A prospective study of bone scanning, somatostatin receptor scanning, and magnetic resonance image in their detection, frequency, location, and effect of their detection on management. *J Clinical Oncol*, 1998. **16**(3): 1040–53.
134. Meko, J.B., Norton, J.A., Management of patients with Zollinger-Ellison syndrome. *Ann Rev Med*, 1995. **46**: 395–411.
135. Zollinger, R.M., Ellison, E.H., Primary peptic ulcerations of the jejunum associated with islet cell tumors of the pancreas. 1955. *CA*, 1989. **39**(4): 231–47.
136. Friesen, S.R., Update on the diagnosis and treatment of rare neuroendocrine tumors. *Surg Clinics North Am*, 1987. **67**(2): 379–93.
137. Lecorguille, M., Hammel, P., Couvelard, A., O'Toole, D., Ratouis, A., Belghiti, J. *et al.* Jejunal vipoma. *Gastroenterologie clinique et biologique*, 2004. **28**(8–9): 797–800.
138. Perry, R.R., Vinik, A.I., Clinical review 72: Diagnosis and management of functioning islet cell tumors. *J Clinical Endocrinol Metabolism*, 1995. **80**(8): 2273–8.
139. Smith, S.L., Branton, S.A., Avino, A.J., Martin, J.K., Klingler, P.J., Thompson, G.B. *et al.*, Vasoactive intestinal polypeptide secreting islet cell tumors: A 15-year experience and review of the literature. *Surgery*, 1998. **124**(6): 1050–5.

140. Meriney, D.K., Pathophysiology and management of VIPoma: A case study. *Oncol Nursing Forum*, 1996. **23**(6): 941–8; quiz 9–50.
141. Bloom, S.R., Yiangou, Y., Polak, J.M., Vasoactive intestinal peptide secreting tumors. Pathophysiological and clinical correlations. *Ann New York Acad Sci*, 1988. **527**: 518–27.
142. Verner, J.V., Morrison, A.B., Islet cell tumor and a syndrome of refractory watery diarrhea and hypokalemia. *Am J Med*, 1958. **25**(3): 374–80.
143. Kon, T., Wada, R., Suzuki, R., Nakayama, Y., Ebina, Y., Yagihashi, S., VIP and calcitonin-producing pancreatic neuroendocrine tumor with watery diarrhea: Clinicopathological features and the effect of somatostatin analogue. *JOP*, 2012. **13**(2): 226–30.
144. Boden, G., Glucagonomas and insulinomas. *Gastroenterol Clinics North Am*, 1989. **18**(4): 831–45.
145. Stacpoole, P.W., The glucagonoma syndrome: Clinical features, diagnosis, and treatment. *Endocrine Rev*, 1981. **2**(3): 347–61.
146. Pujol, R.M., Wang, C.Y., el-Azhary, R.A., Su, W.P., Gibson, L.E., Schroeter, A.L., Necrolytic migratory erythema: Clinicopathologic study of 13 cases. *Internat J Dermatol*, 2004. **43**(1): 12–8.
147. Wermers, R.A., Fatourechi, V., Wynne, A.G., Kvols, L.K., Lloyd, R.V., The glucagonoma syndrome. Clinical and pathologic features in 21 patients. *Medicine*, 1996. **75**(2): 53–63.
148. Wilkinson, D.S., Necrolytic migratory erythema with carcinoma of the pancreas. *Trans St John's Hospital Dermatological Soc*, 1973. **59**(2): 244–50.
149. Fenkci, S.M., Fidan Yaylali, G., Sermez, Y., Akdam, H., Sabir, N., Kirac, S., Malign cystic glucagonoma presented with diabetic ketoacidosis: Case report with an update. *Endocrine-related Cancer*, 2005. **12**(2): 449–54.
150. Harris, G.J., Tio, F., Cruz, A.B., Jr. Somatostatinoma: A case report and review of the literature. *J Surgical Oncol*, 1987. **36**(1): 8–16.
151. Soga, J., Yakuwa, Y., Somatostatinoma/inhibitory syndrome: A statistical evaluation of 173 reported cases as compared to other pancreatic endocrinomas. *J Exp Clinical Cancer Res*, 1999. **18**(1): 13–22.
152. Yamada, T.A.D.H., *Textbook of Gastroenterology*: Hoboken, NJ; 2009. Available from: http://site.ebrary.com/id/10300962 Materials specified: ebraryhttp://site.ebrary.com/id/10300962.
153. Ehehalt, F., Saeger, H.D., Schmidt, C.M., Grutzmann, R., Neuroendocrine tumors of the pancreas. *Oncologist*, 2009. **14**(5): 456–67.

154. Filippella, M., Davi, M.V., Doveri, G., Lillaz, E., Ciccarelli, A., Massimetti, E. *et al.*, Hyperinsulinemic hypoglycemia associated with ectopic Cushing's syndrome due to a pancreatic endocrine tumor in a Type 2 diabetes mellitus patient: Clinical implications of a rare association. *J Endocrinological Invest*, 2011. **34**(3): 175–9.
155. Papazachariou, I.M., Virlos, I.T., Williamson, R.C., Parathyroid hormone-related peptide in pancreatic neuroendocrine tumours associated with hypercalcaemia. *HPB*, 2001. **3**(3): 221–5.
156. Wu, T.J., Lin, C.L., Taylor, R.L., Kvols, L.K., Kao, P.C., Increased parathyroid hormone-related peptide in patients with hypercalcemia associated with islet cell carcinoma. *Mayo Clinic Proceed*, 1997. **72**(12): 1111–5.
157. Ardill, J.E., O'Dorisio, T.M., Circulating biomarkers in neuroendocrine tumors of the enteropancreatic tract: Application to diagnosis, monitoring disease, and as prognostic indicators. *Endocrinol Metabolism Clinics North Am*, 2010. **39**(4): 777–90.
158. Nikou, G.C., Marinou, K., Thomakos, P., Papageorgiou, D., Sanzanidis, V., Nikolaou, P. *et al.*, Chromogranin a levels in diagnosis, treatment and follow-up of 42 patients with non-functioning pancreatic endocrine tumours. *Pancreatology*, 2008. **8**(4–5): 510–9.
159. Baudin, E., Gigliotti, A., Ducreux, M., Ropers, J., Comoy, E., Sabourin, J.C. *et al.*, Neuron-specific enolase and chromogranin A as markers of neuroendocrine tumours. *Brit J Cancer*, 1998. **78**(8): 1102–7.
160. Modlin, I.M., Gustafsson, B.I., Moss, S.F., Pavel, M., Tsolakis, A.V., Kidd, M., Chromogranin A — biological function and clinical utility in neuro endocrine tumor disease. *Ann Surgical Oncol*, 2010. **17**(9): 2427–43.
161. Nehar, D., Lombard-Bohas, C., Olivieri, S., Claustrat, B., Chayvialle, J.A., Penes, M.C. *et al.*, Interest of Chromogranin A for diagnosis and follow-up of endocrine tumours. *Clinical Endocrinol*, 2004. **60**(5): 644–52.
162. Kouvaraki, M.A., Ajani, J.A., Hoff, P., Wolff, R., Evans, D.B., Lozano, R. *et al.*, Fluorouracil, doxorubicin, and streptozocin in the treatment of patients with locally advanced and metastatic pancreatic endocrine carcinomas. *J Clinical Oncol*, 2004. **22**(23): 4762–71.
163. Bajetta, E., Ferrari, L., Martinetti, A., Celio, L., Procopio, G., Artale, S. *et al.*, Chromogranin, A., neuron specific enolase, carcinoembryonic antigen, and hydroxyindole acetic acid evaluation in patients with neuroendocrine tumors. *Cancer*, 1999. **86**(5): 858–65.

164. Friesen, S.R., Tomita, T., Kimmel, J.R., Pancreatic polypeptide update: Its roles in detection of the trait for multiple endocrine adenopathy syndrome, type I and pancreatic polypeptide-secreting tumors. *Surgery*, 1983. **94**(6): 1028–37.
165. Rockall, A.G., Reznek, R.H., Imaging of neuroendocrine tumours (CT/MR/US). *Best Pract Res Clinical Endocrinol Metabolism*, 2007. **21**(1): 43–68.
166. Gouya, H., Vignaux, O., Augui, J., Dousset, B., Palazzo, L., Louvel, A. *et al.*, CT, endoscopic sonography, and a combined protocol for preoperative evaluation of pancreatic insulinomas. *Am J Roentgenol*, 2003. **181**(4): 987–92.
167. Khashab, M.A., Yong, E., Lennon, A.M., Shin, E.J., Amateau, S., Hruban, R.H. *et al.*, EUS is still superior to multidetector computerized tomography for detection of pancreatic neuroendocrine tumors. *Gastrointest Endosc*, 2011. **73**(4): 691–6.
168. Ichikawa, T., Peterson, M.S., Federle, M.P., Baron, R.L., Haradome, H., Kawamori, Y. *et al.*, Islet cell tumor of the pancreas: Biphasic CT versus MR imaging in tumor detection. *Radiology*, 2000. **216**(1): 163–71.
169. Dromain, C., de Baere, T., Lumbroso, J., Caillet, H., Laplanche, A., Boige, V. *et al.*, Detection of liver metastases from endocrine tumors: A prospective comparison of somatostatin receptor scintigraphy, computed tomography, and magnetic resonance imaging. *J Clinical Oncol*, 2005. **23**(1): 70–8.
170. Reidy-Lagunes, D.L., Gollub, M.J., Saltz, L.B., Addition of octreotide functional imaging to cross-sectional computed tomography or magnetic resonance imaging for the detection of neuroendocrine tumors: Added value or an anachronism? *J Clinical Oncol*, 2011. **29**(3): e74–5.
171. Fjallskog, M.L., Ludvigsen, E., Stridsberg, M., Oberg, K., Eriksson, B., Janson, E.T., Expression of somatostatin receptor subtypes 1 to 5 in tumor tissue and intratumoral vessels in malignant endocrine pancreatic tumors. *Medical Oncol*, 2003. **20**(1): 59–67.
172. Kimura, N., Pilichowska, M., Date, F., Kimura, I., Schindler, M., Immunohistochemical expression of somatostatin type 2A receptor in neuroendocrine tumors. *Clinical Cancer Res*, 1999. **5**(11): 3483–7.
173. Abboud, B., Boujaoude, J., Occult sporadic insulinoma: Localization and surgical strategy. *World J Gastroenterol*, 2008. **14**(5): 657–65.

174. Jensen, R.T., Cadiot, G., Brandi, M.L., de Herder, W.W., Kaltsas, G., Komminoth, P. *et al.*, ENETS Consensus Guidelines for the management of patients with digestive neuroendocrine neoplasms: Functional pancreatic endocrine tumor syndromes. *Neuroendocrinology*, 2012. **95**(2): 98–119.
175. Klimstra, D.S., Modlin, I.R., Coppola, D., Lloyd, R.V., Suster, S., The pathologic classification of neuroendocrine tumors: A review of nomenclature, grading, and staging systems. *Pancreas*, 2010. **39**(6): 707–12.
176. Ramage, J.K., Ahmed, A., Ardill, J., Bax, N., Breen, D.J., Caplin, M.E. *et al.*, Guidelines for the management of gastroenteropancreatic neuroendocrine (including carcinoid) tumours (NETs). *Gut*, 2012. **61**(1): 6–32.
177. Reid, M.D., Balci, S., Saka, B., Adsay, N.V., Neuroendocrine tumors of the pancreas: Current concepts and controversies. *Endocrine Pathol*, 2014. **25**(1): 65–79.
178. Travis, W.D., Rush, W., Flieder, D.B., Falk, R., Fleming, M.V., Gal, A.A. *et al.*, Survival analysis of 200 pulmonary neuroendocrine tumors with clarification of criteria for atypical carcinoid and its separation from typical carcinoid. *Am J Surgical Pathol*, 1998. **22**(8): 934–44.
179. Strosberg, J.R., Cheema, A., Weber, J.M., Ghayouri, M., Han, G., Hodul, P.J. *et al.*, Relapse-free survival in patients with nonmetastatic, surgically resected pancreatic neuroendocrine tumors: An analysis of the AJCC and ENETS staging classifications. *Ann Surg*, 2012. **256**(2): 321–5.
180. Strosberg, J.R., Cheema, A., Weber, J., Han, G., Coppola, D., Kvols, L.K., Prognostic validity of a novel American Joint Committee on Cancer Staging Classification for pancreatic neuroendocrine tumors. *J Clin Oncol*, 2011. **29**(22): 3044–9.
181. Klimstra, D.S., Nonductal neoplasms of the pancreas. *Modern Pathol*, 2007. **20**(Suppl 1): S94–112.
182. Papavramidis, T., Papavramidis, S., Solid pseudopapillary tumors of the pancreas: Review of 718 patients reported in English literature. *J Am College Surgeons*, 2005. **200**(6): 965–72.
183. Mortenson, M.M., Katz, M.H., Tamm, E.P., Bhutani, M.S., Wang, H., Evans, D.B. *et al.*, Current diagnosis and management of unusual pancreatic tumors. *Am J Surg*, 2008. **196**(1): 100–13.
184. Yao, X., Ji, Y., Zeng, M., Rao, S., Yang, B., Solid pseudopapillary tumor of the pancreas: Cross-sectional imaging and pathologic correlation. *Pancreas*, 2010. **39**(4): 486–91.

185. Madan, A.K., Weldon, C.B., Long, W.P., Johnson, D., Raafat, A., Solid and papillary epithelial neoplasm of the pancreas. *J Surgical Oncol*, 2004. **85**(4): 193–8.
186. Holen, K.D., Klimstra, D.S., Hummer, A., Gonen, M., Conlon, K., Brennan, M. *et al.*, Clinical characteristics and outcomes from an institutional series of acinar cell carcinoma of the pancreas and related tumors. *J Clin Oncol*, 2002. **20**(24): 4673–8.
187. Chiou, Y.Y., Chiang, J.H., Hwang, J.I., Yen, C.H., Tsay, S.H., Chang, C.Y., Acinar cell carcinoma of the pancreas: Clinical and computed tomography manifestations. *J Comp Assisted Tomography*, 2004. **28**(2): 180–6.
188. Tatli, S., Mortele, K.J., Levy, A.D., Glickman, J.N., Ros, P.R., Banks, P.A. *et al.*, CT and MRI features of pure acinar cell carcinoma of the pancreas in adults. *Am J Roentgenol*, 2005. **184**(2): 511–9.
189. Wisnoski, N.C., Townsend, C.M., Jr., Nealon, W.H., Freeman, J.L., Riall, T.S., 672 patients with acinar cell carcinoma of the pancreas: A population-based comparison to pancreatic adenocarcinoma. *Surgery*, 2008. **144**(2): 141–8.
190. Saif, M.W., Primary pancreatic lymphomas. *JOP*, 2006. **7**(3): 262–73.
191. Merkle, E.M., Bender, G.N., Brambs, H.J., Imaging findings in pancreatic lymphoma: Differential aspects. *Am J Roentgenol*, 2000. **174**(3): 671–5.
192. Roland, C.F., van Heerden, J.A., Nonpancreatic primary tumors with metastasis to the pancreas. *Surg Gynecol Obstetrics*, 1989. **168**(4): 345–7.
193. Ghavamian, R., Klein, K.A., Stephens, D.H., Welch, T.J., LeRoy, A.J., Richardson, R.L. *et al.*, Renal cell carcinoma metastatic to the pancreas: Clinical and radiological features. *Mayo Clinic Proceed*, 2000. **75**(6): 581–5.
194. de Juan, C., Sanchez, M., Miquel, R., Pages, M., Ayuso, J.R., Ayuso, C., Uncommon tumors and pseudotumoral lesions of the pancreas. *Curr Probl Diag Radiol*, 2008. **37**(4): 145–64.
195. Montemarano, H., Lonergan, G.J., Bulas, D.I., Selby, D.M., Pancreatoblastoma: Imaging findings in 10 patients and review of the literature. *Radiology*, 2000. **214**(2): 476–82.
196. Klimstra, D.S., Wenig, B.M., Adair, C.F., Heffess, C.S., Pancreatoblastoma. A clinicopathologic study and review of the literature. *Am J Surgical Pathol*, 1995. **19**(12): 1371–89.
197. Cavallini, A., Falconi, M., Bortesi, L., Crippa, S., Barugola, G., Butturini, G., Pancreatoblastoma in adults: A review of the literature. *Pancreatology*, 2009. **9**(1–2): 73–80.

198. Iodice, S., Gandini, S., Maisonneuve, P., Lowenfels, A.B., Tobacco and the risk of pancreatic cancer: A review and meta-analysis. *Langenbeck's Arch Surg/Deutsche Gesellschaft fur Chirurgie*, 2008. **393**(4): 535–45.
199. Genkinger JM, Spiegelman, D., Anderson, K.E., Bergkvist, L., Bernstein, L., van den Brandt, P.A. *et al.*, Alcohol intake and pancreatic cancer risk: A pooled analysis of fourteen cohort studies. *Cancer Epidemiol, Biomarkers Prev*, 2009. **18**(3): 765–76.
200. Tramacere, I., Scotti, L., Jenab, M., Bagnardi, V., Bellocco, R., Rota, M. *et al.*, Alcohol drinking and pancreatic cancer risk: A meta-analysis of the dose-risk relation. *Internat J Cancer*, 2010. **126**(6): 1474–86.
201. Genkinger, J.M., Spiegelman, D., Anderson, K.E., Bernstein, L., van den Brandt, P.A., Calle, E.E. *et al.*, A pooled analysis of 14 cohort studies of anthropometric factors and pancreatic cancer risk. *Internat J Cancer*, 2011. **129**(7): 1708–17.
202. Larsson, S.C., Wolk, A., Red and processed meat consumption and risk of pancreatic cancer: Meta-analysis of prospective studies. *Brit J Cancer*, 2012. **106**(3): 603–7.
203. Rohrmann, S., Linseisen, J., Nothlings, U., Overvad, K., Egeberg, R., Tjonneland, A. *et al.*, Meat and fish consumption and risk of pancreatic cancer: Results from the European Prospective Investigation into Cancer and Nutrition. *Internat J Cancer*, 2013. **132**(3): 617–24.
204. Singh, S., Singh, P.P., Singh, A.G., Murad, M.H., McWilliams, R.R., Chari, S.T., Anti-diabetic medications and risk of pancreatic cancer in patients with diabetes mellitus: A systematic review and meta-analysis. *Am J Gastroenterol*, 2013. **108**(4): 510–9; quiz 20.
205. Klein, A.P., Lindstrom, S., Mendelsohn, J.B., Steplowski, E., Arslan, A.A., Bueno-de-Mesquita, H.B. *et al.*, An absolute risk model to identify individuals at elevated risk for pancreatic cancer in the general population. *PloS One*, 2013. **8**(9): e72311.
206. Andreotti, G., Silverman, D.T., Occupational risk factors and pancreatic cancer: A review of recent findings. *Mol Carcinogenesis*, 2012. **51**(1): 98–108.
207. Duell, E.J., Lucenteforte, E., Olson, S.H., Bracci, P.M., Li, D., Risch, H.A. *et al.*, Pancreatitis and pancreatic cancer risk: A pooled analysis in the International Pancreatic Cancer Case-Control Consortium (PanC4). *Ann Oncol*, 2012. **23**(11): 2964–70.

Chapter 15

Borderline Resectable Adenocarcinoma of the Pancreas

Sarah B. Fisher, Michael C. Lowe and David A. Kooby

What is New

- The term "borderline resectable" is used to describe patients with tumors at high risk for margin-positive resection or treatment failure when treated with surgery alone.
- The limits of surgical resection are evolving as improvements in preoperative imaging, neoadjuvant therapy, operative techniques, and perioperative care have allowed oncologic teams to push the envelope regarding potentially curative resection of pancreatic adenocarcinoma.

Introduction

Pancreatic adenocarcinoma (PAC) remains a devastating diagnosis as the eighth most common major-organ cancer diagnosis and the fourth leading cause of cancer-related death in North America.[1] Surgical resection offers the only possibility for cure. Even with aggressive multimodality therapy the median survival of patients with resected PAC remains a disappointing

18 to 22 months[2–4] as a result of the high incidence of local and distant disease failures following treatment.[4–8] Careful selection of surgical candidates is necessary to maximize therapeutic benefit and avoid unnecessary morbidity. Patients with borderline resectable pancreas adenocarcinoma (BRPAC) are a particularly challenging subset, as it is difficult to identify the particular patients from this group who will benefit from the complex and potentially morbid therapy.

Plagued with conflicting definitions, BRPAC describes tumors involving the superior mesenteric-portal vein (SMV-PV) confluence or encroaching upon the mesenteric arterial axis. This class of tumors falls between the categories of resectable PAC and locally advanced/technically PAC, and is the main target of increased use of neoadjuvant therapy and aggressive surgical vascular resections. This chapter will review the definition and management of BRPAC with attention to patient selection, neoadjuvant therapy, vascular resection, and clinical outcomes measures such as complications and patient survival.

Defining Borderline Resectable Adenocarcinoma of the Pancreas

Patients with BRPAC are at higher risk for margin-positive resection when treated with surgery *de novo* than their resectable counterparts,[9] and it is established that margin-negative resection provides the best potential for long-term survival.[4–7] Presumably, these patients represent a cohort of patients with more aggressive tumor biology at increased risk for radiographically occult distant metastases.[9–11] Proper identification of patients with BRPAC is necessary to ensure delivery of appropriate multimodality therapy. One existing limitation in the use of the term BRPAC is that the definition lacks standardization, making it challenging for communication between clinicians and enrollment in clinical trials.

Historically, surgical resection of PAC with major vessel involvement was associated with prohibitive morbidity and mortality as well as high rates of margin-positive resection, influencing many clinicians to consider tumors involving the SMV-PV or mesenteric arterial axis locally advanced/unresectable.[12,13] A early series describing successful resection and reconstruction of the SMV-PV confluence was initially published in the 1970s[14] and then more reports surfaced in the 1990s,[15–17] leading surgeons to re-evaluate vascular involvement as a contraindication to resection. In 2001, using multimodality therapy, Mehta *et al.*[18] reported a median survival of 30 months for 9 patients with "marginally resectable" PAC treated with neoadjuvant chemoradiation and pancreaticoduodenectomy, as compared to 8 months for the 6 patients who completed neoadjuvant therapy but remained unresectable. In 2006, the National Comprehensive Cancer Network (NCCN) used the term "borderline resectable" to describe patients with tumors at high risk for margin-positive resection or treatment failure when treated with surgery alone.[19]

A uniformly accepted set of reliable and reproducible criteria to define patients with BRPAC does not exist. Current definitions use potentially ambiguous terms such as abutment, impingement, encasement, and occlusion to describe varying amounts of actual interface between the tumor and vessels (Fig. 1). Four major definitions of BRPC have been published (Table 1, reprinted with permission[9]); all of which base resectability on the tumor's relationship with the superior mesenteric vein-portal vein confluence (SMV-PV), the superior mesenteric artery (SMA), the common hepatic artery (CHA) and the celiac axis (CA).

The M.D. Anderson Cancer Center (MDACC) definition states that tumors are borderline resectable if they have short segment occlusion of the SMV-PV with appropriate vasculature to allow for venous reconstruction; tumor abutment of the SMA less than 180°, and/or short segment

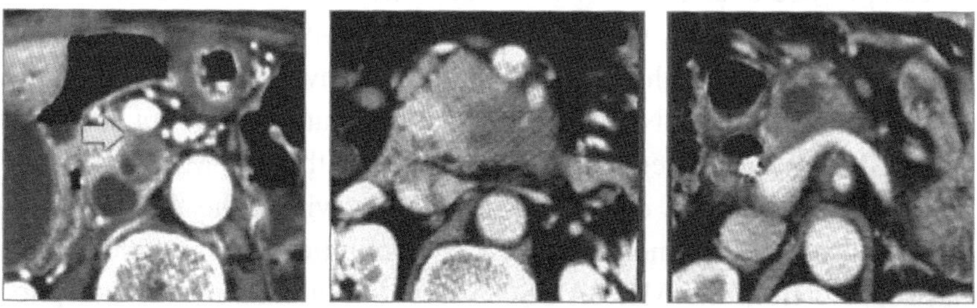

(a) (b) (c)

Fig. 1. Radiographic representations of vessel involvement with pancreatic cancer. Tumors can cause vessel abutment (a), partial encasement less than 180° (b), or complete encasement (c). The definitions of these terms are currently inconsistent.

Table 1. Four published definitions of borderline resectable pancreatic cancer. SMV-PV = superior mesenteric vein-portal vein, SMA = superior mesenteric artery, CHA = common hepatic artery.

—	AHPBA	MD Anderson	NCCN	Alliance
SMV-PV	Abutment, encasement or occlusion	Occlusion	Abutment with impingement or narrowing	Interface measuring ≥180°
SMA	Abutment	Abutment	Abutment	Interface measuring ≤180°
CHA	Abutment or short-segment encasement	Abutment or short-segment encasement	Abutment or short-segment encasement	Reconstructable short segment interface
Celiac	No abutment or encasement	Abutment	No abutment or encasement	Interface measuring <180°

encasement of the CHA amenable to resection and reconstruction without evidence of celiac axis involvement.[20,21] By contrast, the Americas Hepato-Pancreato-Biliary Association (AHPBA)/Society of Surgical Oncology (SSO)/Society for Surgery of the Alimentary Tract (SSAT) consensus definition deems a tumor borderline resectable when it abuts, encases, or occludes the SMV-PV over a short distance with vasculature amenable to resection and reconstruction; involves the gastroduodenal artery (GDA) even with short segment CHA involvement; or abuts the SMA less than 180°.[22] Notably patients with abutment but not occlusion of the SMV-PV are categorized as resectable within the MDACC definition, whereas they are considered borderline within the AHPBA/SSO/SSAT consensus. The most recent NCCN definition is nearly identical to and adapted from the AHPBA/SSO/SSAT definition, with the exception that SMV-PV involvement is defined as either occlusion or impingement/distortion of the vessel due to tumor.[23]

The degree of SMV-PV involvement, from minimal abutment to complete occlusion, likely represents a key factor in identifying patients with borderline resectable tumors.[24] A recent multi-institutional study of 70 patients undergoing margin-negative SMV-PV resection with varying degrees of radiologic SMV-PV involvement demonstrated equivalent survival without neoadjuvant therapy as compared to patients with categorically resectable PAC,[25] suggesting that simple SMV-PV involvement does not necessarily represent a different phenotype of patients.

A newer definition of BRPAC established in the context of the Alliance A021101 trial defines borderline resectable as the presence of any one of the following: 180° or greater interface between tumor and SMV-PV, short-segment *occlusion* of the SMV-PV with remnant vein amenable to reconstruction, short-segment interface of any degree between tumor and CHA with remnant artery amenable to reconstruction, and/or less than 180° interface between the SMA or the CA.[26] The results of this single-arm multi-institutional pilot study examining survival for patients with BRPAC after neoadjuvant modified FOLFIRINOX (5-fluorouracil, oxaliplatin, irinotecan, and leucovorin), capecitabine-radiotherapy, surgical resection, and adjuvant gemcitabine are pending.

One less commonly used classification system that highlights the importance of the degree of venous involvement is that developed by Ishikawa and colleagues.[27] In this system, patients are divided into five categories of venous involvement based on morphology at preoperative angiography. Patients with bilateral narrowing of the SMV-PV confluence (classes IV and V depending on the absence or presence of collaterals respectively) undergoing resection demonstrated worse overall survival than patients in whom operative intervention was not possible.[27] The relevance of this classification system is minimized in Western countries where preoperative angiography is not routinely performed.

It is important to note that the term “borderline resectable” may also apply to patients with anatomically resectable tumors but questionable disease biology (i.e. radiographic suspicion but not confirmation of extra-pancreatic disease) or physiology (i.e. limited performance status and/or significant comorbidity) in studies examining neoadjuvant therapy has added an additional layer of ambiguity to the definition of BRPAC as well as the interpretation of outcomes of studies.[11]

In 2008, researchers at MDACC described three classifications of BRPAC based on: (1) anatomy (as described previously); (2) suspicion but not confirmation of extra-pancreatic disease; or (3) limited performance status.[21] In a study of 138 patients with anatomically *resectable* PAC including 41 patients with questionable extra-pancreatic disease and 38 separate patients with poor performance status treated with neoadjuvant therapy, Tzeng *et al.*[28] demonstrated that these "borderline" patients had similar overall survival to that of patients with resectable disease and preserved performance status provided they were able to undergo resection. However, only 37% to 46% of these patients were able to achieve definitive resection, compared to 75% of patients with completely resectable disease and preserved performance status undergoing neoadjuvant therapy.[28] When used to describe patients with questionable tumor biology or impaired performance status, the term borderline should be regarded as a marker for patients at high risk of progression.

The heterogeneous definition of BRPAC promotes inconsistency among treating institutions and hinders interpretation and comparison of existing clinical trials. One review of response and resection percentages after neoadjuvant therapy for initially resectable, borderline, and locally advanced PAC noted that 59 of 111 studies (53.2%) failed to clearly state resectability criteria, making conclusions difficult to apply to specific populations.[29] Another review specific to BRPAC noted that of 23 identified reports, 2 used the MDACC definition, 5 used the AHPBA definition, 5 used the NCCN definition, and the remaining studies used various other definitions or did not define BRPAC at all.[24] Development of a reliable, reproducible, and uniformly accepted definition of BRPAC should be a focus of future research efforts.

Neoadjuvant Therapy

Multimodality therapy for PAC is widely accepted to improve survival, and some advocate for neoadjuvant therapy for patients with both resectable and borderline resectable disease.[10,30,31] Proponents of neoadjuvant therapy cite several reasons, of which perhaps the most important is the ability to test tumor biology, offering a window in which radiographically occult metastatic disease may declare. In a series of 228 patients with resectable PAC, Barugola *et al.*[32] noted that almost 20% of patients died within 12 months of resection, suggesting inadequate patient selection due to occult micrometastatic disease or aggressive tumor biology. Although not specifically analyzed, similar trends can be identified in other larger series,[33,34] indicating that significant limitations in the ability to detect micrometastatic disease exist and our ability to select whom surgery will benefit remains imperfect. In addition to aiding in patient selection and providing up front treatment of micrometastatic disease, neoadjuvant therapy offers a way to provide systemic therapy to all patients, circumventing the postoperative morbidity that prevents up to 25% of patients from receiving adjuvant therapy.[35–37]

In contrast, critics of neoadjuvant therapy argue that delaying resection allows for potential progression of disease and may result in systemic toxicities that may increase morbidity and mortality after a major operation. Depending on the study, the proportion of patients progressing on therapy is significant. One meta-analysis of patients undergoing neoadjuvant therapy that grouped patients with BRPAC and locally advanced PAC together demonstrated a progression rate of 20.8%.[29] When disease progression does occur during neoadjuvant therapy, it is most often distant metastases. In a phase II trial at MDACC of 86 patients with potentially resectable disease undergoing gemcitabine based neoadjuvant chemoradiation, 24% of patients progressed during the neoadjuvant period either due to decline in performance status ($n = 4$) or development of distant metastases ($n = 17$); none developed prohibitive local tumor advancement.[38] It is difficult to assess whether decline in preoperative performance status is due to neoadjuvant therapy or to the disease process itself, but it appears that tumor progression is more common than functional deterioration.

For the patient with BRPAC who does achieve resection, concerns exist regarding the contribution of neoadjuvant therapy to development of postoperative complications. Postoperative morbidity is multifactorial and the root cause is difficult to study. One case matched retrospective review compared 29 patients with initially unresectable or borderline resectable PAC who successfully underwent resection after neoadjuvant chemoradiation to patients with resectable disease. Rates of 90-day postoperative morbidity (55% versus 41%), major morbidity (21% for both groups), pancreatic fistulae (7% versus 10%), and 90-day mortality (0% versus 1.7%) were similar between the groups ($p > 0.05$ for all).[39] These studies highlights the importance of surgical standardization in medical oncology trials, as differing surgical approaches can influence trial results.

Although histological confirmation of PAC is not required for surgical resection, it must be obtained prior to initiation of neoadjuvant therapy.[40] Endoscopic ultrasonography (EUS) guided fine needle aspiration is the preferred method of tissue diagnosis with the highest sensitivity and specificity, although brushings obtained during endoscopic retrograde cholangiopancreatography or computed tomography (CT) guided fine needle aspiration are also possible.[9] For patients with BRPAC, EUS has the additional advantage of characterizing the surrounding vasculature.[41]

If immediate operation is not pursued, biliary decompression should be considered, particularly when using chemotherapeutics cleared by the biliary system.[42] Ideally, cross sectional imaging should be obtained prior to endoscopic drainage as decompression eliminates a visual transition point and the possibility of post-procedure pancreatitis can obscure tumor delineation.[43] The choice between the more expensive but larger diameter covered metal stent versus a plastic stent should be made based on expectation of duration of therapy prior to surgical intervention, or in the setting of unresectable disease, the patient's life expectancy, as plastic stents typically occlude in 3–4 months.[44,45] A prospective study of patients with resectable or borderline resectable PAC undergoing neoadjuvant therapy showed stent malfunction (occlusion or migration) in 3/27 patients who underwent pancreaticoduodenectomy and 5/21 patients with disease progression, and concluded that the use of self-expandable metal stents produced a safe and durable biliary decompression that did not interfere with surgical intervention.[46]

Regimen and duration of neoadjuvant therapy

Current neoadjuvant strategies are based on data from trials of patients treated for unresectable disease.[47–49] These often incorporate chemoradiation and include continuous infusion 5-FU, cisplatin or gemcitabine-based chemoradiation with or without induction chemotherapy.[50–54] Phase III trials are lacking in the neoadjuvant setting,[55] and many phase II trials include patients with locally advanced disease (LAPC) as well as BRPAC. Recent retrospective and phase II trials of neoadjuvant therapy specific to BPRAC are summarized in Table 2.[56–71] One of the few *randomized* phase

Table 2. Selected phase II trials of neoadjuvant chemotherapy and/or chemoradiation for borderline resectable pancreas adenocarcinoma.

Author Year [Ref]	n	Study population (n)	BRPAC definition	Study Design	Resected (%)	Margin negative resection (%)	Vein resection (%)	30-day surgical morbidity (%)	30-day surgical mortality (%)	Median overall survival (months)	Median overall survival resected patients (months)
Pipas 2005 [55]	24	RPAC (4) BRPAC (7) LAPC (13)	Unique	Gem + Docetaxel followed by Gem-RT	71	76	—	—	0*	14	—
Small 2008 [56]	39	RPAC (16) BRPAC (9) LAPC (14)	NCCN	Full dose Gem and concurrent RT	44 (33 BRPAC)	—	—	—	—	—	—
Landry 2010 [57]	21	BRPAC LAPC	Unique	Full dose Gem + Cis+ 5-FU followed by 5-FU-RT (A) versus Gem-RT (B)	24	60	0	—	—	19.4 (A) 13.4 (B)	26.3
Sahora 2011 [58]	25	BRPAC (12) LAPC (13)	AHPBA	Gem + Docetaxel	32	87	25	38	12.5	13.5	16

(*Continued*)

Table 2. (*Continued*)

Author Year [Ref]	n	Study Population (n)	BRPAC Definition	Study Design	Resected (%)	Margin Negative Resection (%)	Vein Resection (%)	30-day Surgical Morbidity (%)	30-day Surgical Mortality (%)	Median Overall Survival (months)	Median Overall Survival Resected Patients (months)
Sahora 2011 [59]	33	BRPAC (15) LAPC (18)	AHPBA	Gem + Ox	39	69	38	30	15.4	16	22
Small 2011 [60]	29	RPAC (7) BRPAC (10) LAPC (12)	NCCN	Full dose Gem + Bevacizumab and concurrent RT	21	—	—	67	0	11.8	—
Stokes 2011 [61]	40	BRPAC	MDACC	Capecitabine-XRT in either accelerated fractions or standard doses	46	75	25	38	6.3	12	23
Lee 2012 [62]	43	BRPAC (18) LAPC (25)	NCCN	Gem + Capecitabine (with additional chemo, chemo-RT if unresectable)	40 (61 BRPAC)	82	—	29	0	16.6	23.1

Chakra-borty 2013 [63]	13	BRPAC	MDACC	IMRT with Capecitabine versus 3D conformal RT with Capecitabine	38	80	—	—	20	9.1	Not reached
Jensen 2013 [64]	23	BRPAC LAPC	Unique	5-FU + Cis + Interferon-α with concurrent RT	30	86	—	—	—	11.5	22.6
Kim 2013 [65]	68	RPAC (23) BRPAC (39) LAPC (6)	NCCN	Full dose Gem + Ox with concurrent RT	63	84	40	—	0	18.2	27.1
Leone 2013 [66]	39	BRPAC (15) LAPC (24)	Unique	Full dose Gem + Ox followed by Gem-RT	36	64	—	—	—	16.7	31.5
Motoi 2013 [67]	35	RPAC (19) BRPAC (16)	NCCN	Gem + S-1	87	87	—	40	3.3	19.7	34.7
Christians 2014 [68]	18	BRPAC	Unique	FOLFIRINOX followed by Gem or capecitabine RT	67	100	83	17	0	—	Not reached

(*Continued*)

Table 2. *(Continued)*

Author Year [Ref]	n	Study Population (n)	BRPAC Definition	Study Design	Resected (%)	Margin Negative Resection (%)	Vein Resection (%)	30-day Surgical Morbidity (%)	30-day Surgical Mortality (%)	Median Overall Survival (months)	Median Overall Survival Resected Patients (months)
Esnaola 2014 [69]	37	BRPAC (13) LAPC (24)	Unique	Gem + Ox + Cetuximab (with additional capecitabine IMRT if unresectable)	30 (69 BRPAC)	100	45	—	—	11.8	Not reached
Sahora 2014 [70]	30	BRPAC (11) LAPC (19)	AHPBA	Gem + bevacizumab versus Gem alone	37	91	27	72	27	13	13

BRPAC: Borderline resectable pancreas adenocarcinoma; RPAC: resectable pancreas adenocarcinoma; LAPC: locally advanced pancreas adenocarcinoma; Gem: Gemcitabine; RT: Radiotherapy; NCCN: National Comprehensive Cancer Network; AHPBA: Americas Hepatopancreatobiliary Association; Ox: Oxaliplatin; IMRT: Intensity modulated radiotherapy; Cis: Cisplatin; FOLFIRINOX: 5-fluorouracil, leucovorin, irinotecan, oxaliplatin; —: not reported

*90-day mortality 15%

II clinical trials to examine neoadjuvant therapy in patients with BRPAC was terminated early due to low patient accrual. This multi-institutional study included 21 patients with BRPAC and LAPC and compared either gemcitabine-based chemoradiation to induction chemotherapy (gemcitabine, cisplatin and 5-FU) followed by 5-FU-based chemoradiation. Five of 21 patients (24%) underwent resection with 3 of 5 achieving R0 resection.[72] Both neoadjuvant regimens were well-tolerated and resectability rates were similar between the groups, suggesting safety and utility of either regimen. Recently Sahora *et al.* reported on the addition of bevacizumab to neoadjuvant gemcitabine in a randomized phase II trial of 30 patients. Unfortunately the addition of bevacizumab did not appear to impact survival and may have contributed to an unusually high operative morbidity and mortality in the 11 patients (37%) who underwent resection. The optimal regimen of neoadjuvant therapy requires further study.

While most regimens are gemcitabine-based, the success of FOLFIRINOX in the advanced and metastatic patient population[47] has prompted interest in the neoadjuvant setting. Recently Christians *et al.*[69] demonstrated that of 18 patients with BRPAC, 83% were able to complete neoadjuvant therapy with FOLFIRINOX followed by chemoradiation. Two thirds of the patients successfully underwent resection with most requiring portal vein resection (10 of 12) and all achieving a margin negative resection. At a median of 22 months from diagnosis, 7 patients (58.3%) are alive including 5 who are disease free, indicating that induction therapy with an aggressive multimodality regimen is likely to be beneficial in highly selected patients with preserved performance status.

Duration of therapy is also controversial. In one retrospective review of 56 patients with BRPAC or locally advanced PAC treated with chemoradiation followed by variable duration of chemotherapy, Chen *et al.*[73] demonstrated that patients with the longest interval between radiation and resection had the greatest pathologic response and the longest survival. These results are difficult to interpret as the longer duration of therapy may have simply allowed presentation of occult metastases in patients with aggressive disease, or the pathologic response may be attributed effects of additional chemotherapy as opposed to time interval from radiation.

In addition to the previously mentioned Alliance A021101 trial,[24] there are three phase II trials examining FOLFIRINOX with or without radiation therapy (NCT01992705, NCT0189945, NCT01688336) and two others are investigating the combination of gemcitabine and radiotherapy with bevacizumab and paclitaxel (NCT00557492 and NCT01470417 respectively).[74] The results of these trials are anticipated, as are future well-designed trials investigating additional agents.

Assessing response to neoadjuvant therapy

The capacity to characterize response to therapy in an objective and reproducible format is essential to the multidisciplinary treatment of all malignancies, yet response criteria for patients with BRPAC undergoing neoadjuvant therapy is not well-developed. In a recent meta-analysis of 111 studies with 4,394 patients with resectable, borderline, and locally advanced disease who received neoadjuvant chemotherapy, only 40% of studies reported criteria used to measure treatment response.[29] One such criteria, the Response Evaluation Criteria in Solid Tumors (RECIST) represents a commonly applied scale for assessing response to therapy based on radiographic tumor size.[75] Unfortunately, RECIST may not be effective in assessing patients with PAC. Katz *et al.*[76] showed that of 122 patients with BRPAC undergoing neoadjuvant therapy, the majority of patients had either no change radiographically (69%) or had disease progression (19%), yet 85 patients (66%) underwent successful resection with a median overall survival of 33 months. Change in standardized uptake value (SUV) on positron emission tomography is an alternative radiographic criteria that has been used to assess response to neoadjuvant therapy in PAC;[77] it is most sensitive in diagnosing distant metastases.[78,79]

Others have used pathologic response on biopsy to guide decisions about response to therapy, as complete pathologic response in surgical specimens has been correlated with improved survival in patients with resectable and borderline PAC.[80–82] One series demonstrated near complete tumor fibrosis (>95%) in surgical specimens from 21 of 135 patients treated with neoadjuvant chemoradiation and complete resection; the median overall survival of these patients was 66 months.[83] Use of pathologic response in the preoperative setting requires an additional invasive procedure and is subject to sampling error. Regardless, pathologic response on EUS guided biopsy has been used in combination with other assessments to assist in determining response to therapy.[77]

When elevated initially, serum cancer antigen 19-9 (CA 19-9) is useful in guiding decisions about treatment response and selection for surgery. Among 141 patients with resectable, borderline, and locally advanced PAC and elevated CA 19-9 prior to neoadjuvant therapy, Tzeng *et al.*[84] showed that normalization of CA 19-9 after neoadjuvant therapy correlated with longer overall survival in both resected and nonresected populations (38 versus 26 months, and 15 versus 11 months, respectively, $p = 0.02$ for both). Conversely, patients with an increase in CA 19-9 upon completion of neoadjuvant chemotherapy were rarely able to undergo resection.[84]

Surgical Considerations

Radiographic differentiation between true tumor-vessel invasion and inflammatory fibrosis is imperfect,[13,43,85] and downstaging after neoadjuvant therapy is uncommon (0.8% in one well-defined study of 122 patients with BRPAC) and may not correlate with resectability.[76] Surgical resection should therefore be attempted for all patients with BRPAC completing neoadjuvant therapy in the absence of metastatic disease, clear disease progression, or severely impaired functional status.[9–11,13]

Diagnostic laparoscopy

Patients with BRPAC are at increased risk of harboring either occult metastatic disease or technically unresectable disease. Diagnostic laparoscopy (DL) has been proposed to decrease the nontherapeutic laparotomy rate for patients with hepatobiliary cancers but remains controversial, with some groups documenting reduced nontherapeutic laparotomy rates[86] and others showing only minimal benefit.[87] The differences are likely due to patient selection. Although DL is unlikely to identify nonresectable tumors due to extensive vascular involvement, the authors believe DL to be particularly useful in patients with "type C" BRPAC — those in whom extra-pancreatic disease is suspected but cannot be clearly identified.

Cancer antigen 19–9 levels have also been shown to aid in selection for DL with subsequent decrease in the nontherapeutic laparotomy rate in patients with patients with both resectable and BRPAC.[88,89]

Vascular resection

When contemplating vascular resection for PAC, the motivating factor should be the ability to obtain complete margin negative resection. An extended resection to clear second-order lymph nodes and peripancreatic connective tissue is more representative of "extended pancreatectomy," which has not been associated with improved survival.[90–92] Improvements in imaging techniques have allowed for knowledge of potential vascular involvement preoperatively,[43] but the need to perform vascular resection often is not clear until after the pancreatic neck has been transected and the operating team is committed. Recently, the International Study Group of Pancreatic Surgery (ISGPS) released a consensus statement strongly recommending venous resection when necessary to obtain an R0 resection in the setting of an appropriate target for reconstruction for all patients with BRPAC due to venous involvement and operative exploration for resectability in the setting of arterial involvement. Such technically advanced procedures should only be managed in high-volume centers with experienced surgical and multidisciplinary teams.[13]

Venous involvement: Technical considerations and outcomes

When necessary, there are several reconstruction options available depending upon the extent of venous resection. In the simplest cases a lateral venorraphy may be performed, with the defect closed primarily without vessel narrowing (Fig. 2a) or with patch angioplasty (Fig. 2b). It may be necessary to ligate the splenic vein in order to achieve a tension-free anastomosis. If complete resection is required, proximal and distal targets must be verified prior to transecting the vein. Reconstruction options after vein resection include primary anastomosis (Fig. 2c) and vein graft interposition (Fig. 2d). Options for interposition vein grafts include the internal jugular, left renal, splenic and gonadal veins.[92,93]

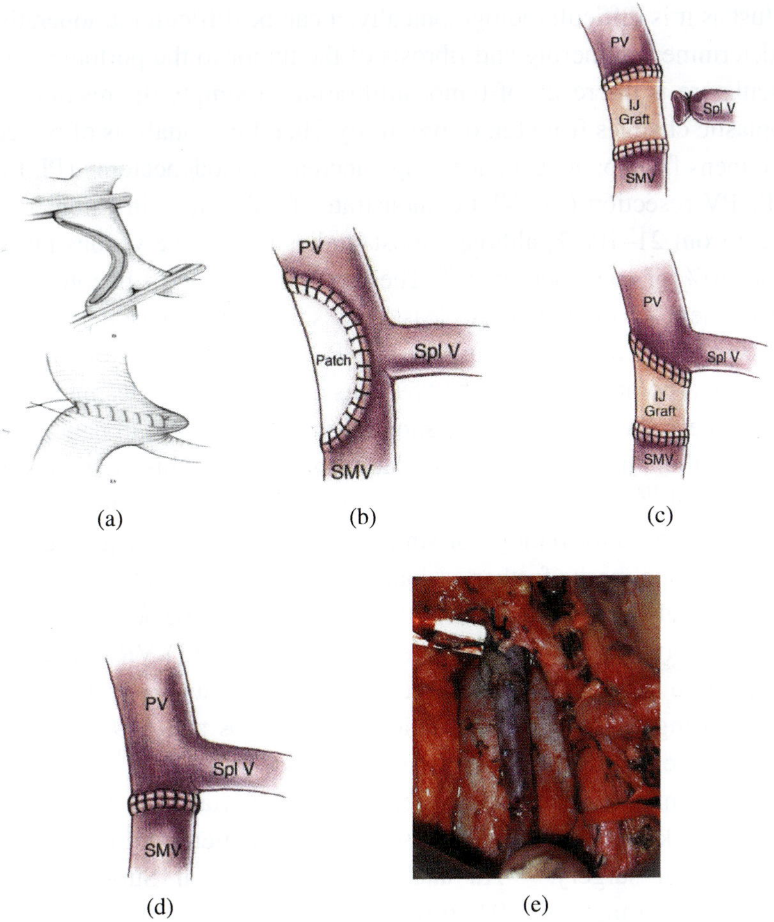

Fig. 2. Vascular reconstruction following venous resection with pancreaticoduodenectomy for BRPC. Options include primary repair without patch (a), patch angioplasty (b), primary repair (c), or interposition graft with vein conduit (d). (e) *In vivo* example of internal jugular interposition graft repair. PV=portal vein, Spl V = splenic vein, SMV = superior mesenteric vein, IJ = internal jugular.

Although concern for decreased patency rates exists, synthetic grafts such as polytetrafluoroethylene (PTFE) have also been used successfully.[94,95] Currently, heterogeneity between extent and method of venous resection and reconstruction makes identification of an optimal methodology difficult if not impossible.

Just as it is difficult radiographically, it can be difficult intraoperatively to determine if tethering and fibrosis of the tumor to the portomesenteric vasculature is the result of tumor infiltration or simply the result of desmoplastic changes from tumor proximity. Histologic analysis of resection specimens from patients undergoing pancreaticoduodenectomy (PD) with SMV-PV resection (PD-VR) demonstrates frank tumor invasion in anywhere from 21–100%, although most studies report true venous invasion in 60–70% of specimens.[25,95–98] The prognostic value of histologic vein involvement is unknown. At least one small study has demonstrated longer survival for patients undergoing PD-VR without histologic tumor invasion as compared to matched patients undergoing PD, leading them to query whether venous resection should be considered for all patients with PAC.[99] Others have not shown a relationship between histologic invasion and survival.[100,101] Whether the degree of venous involvement is a marker of aggressive tumor biology or simply a mechanical consequence due to tumor location merits further evaluation, but as this cannot be determined preoperatively or intraoperatively the true value may be academic.

An important consideration when contemplating PD-VR is the potential increase in morbidity and mortality of the procedure over that of cases not requiring PD-VR. Initial studies in the 1980s and 1990s suggested increased perioperative morbidity without survival benefit,[12,17,102] with a later systemic meta-analysis concluding that portal vein invasion was likely a marker of aggressive disease biology in patients unlikely to derive benefit from surgery.[103] An analysis of a National Surgical Quality Improvement sample of 10,206 patients from 2000 to 2009 also showed increased perioperative complications in patients undergoing PD-VR as compared to PD, although median hospital stay and perioperative mortality were similar.[104] In a retrospective multi-institution comparison of 70 patients undergoing PD-VR versus 422 patients undergoing PD, Kelly *et al.*[25] demonstrated increased overall morbidity (51 vs 33%, respectively, $p<0.01$). However, more patients in the PD-VR group required preoperative stent placement suggesting an unequal distribution of patients with significant jaundice, which is associated with postoperative infectious complications. After accounting for stent placement in a multivariate model the relationship between PD-VR and morbidity dimished.[25] In a large multi-institutional series of patients with BRPAC (n = 1,588),

Ravikumar *et al.*[105] demonstrated similar morbidity and mortality between the 230 patients undergoing PD-VR and the 840 undergoing PD; the remaining 518 were explored and underwent palliative surgical bypass with less morbidity and similar perioperative mortality. Other reports, including guidelines from the NCCN, have suggested similar morbidity and mortality as well as overall survival between patients undergoing PD-VR or PD.[42,92,106–110] It is plausible that patients undergoing a small lateral venorraphy do not have the same disease biology and perioperative or oncologic outcomes as do those undergoing long segment reconstruction such that the heterogeneity has obscured any relationship between vein resection and postoperative morbidity, mortality, and survival benefit. To facilitate future comparisons the ISGPS has proposed a classification of venous resections (Table 3).[13]

Arterial resection

Initially associated with prohibitive morbidity and mortality, major arterial tumor involvement has historically been considered a contraindication to resection. However, limited therapeutic options have pushed surgeons to develop more radical techniques, and in concept arterial resection may be necessary to achieve an R0 resection. En bloc mesenteric arterial resection was initially described by Appleby[111] in 1953 for treatment of locally advanced gastric cancer and later adapted to PDAC.[14] Over the past decade several retrospective single institution retrospective series have

Table 3. ISGPS proposed classification of venous resections.[13]

Type	Description
1	Venorraphy with primary suture closure
2	Venorrhaphy with patch closure
3	Segmental resection with primary venovenous anastomosis
4	Segmental resection with conduit

ISGPS: International Study Group of Pancreatic Surgery

documented experience with arterial resection and reconstruction in highly selected patients. A meta-analysis of 366 patients undergoing arterial resection with PD showed that while arterial resection was associated with improved survival as compared to patients not undergoing resection, arterial resection was also associated with increased perioperative morbidity and mortality and poor survival at 1 and 3 years (median 49% and 8.3% respectively) compared to patients undergoing conventional PD or PD-VR.[112] The conglomerate of studies in this meta-analysis included patients undergoing resection (and reconstruction) of the SMA, CA, left or right hepatic or common hepatic arteries. It is the authors' belief that SMA involvement should be considered a contraindication to resection whereas hepatic artery resection may be considered in appropriately selected patients.

Surgical margin assessment

Margin assessment for all patients with resected PAC is plagued by variable definitions, which contribute to a wide range of rates of margin positive resection (0–83%).[13] Using specific (and unique) algorithms for histopathologic assessment, several groups have demonstrated that patients with R0 margins less than 1 mm have an overall survival comparable to patients with R1 resections, which is suboptimal compared to patients with margins greater than 1 mm.[7,113,114] Others have proposed an ideal margin distance of 1.5 mm.[115] Additionally, the location of the positive margin may impact prognosis, with patients with tumor involvement along the portomesenteric vasculature having decreased survival when compared to those with positive retroperitoneal margins in at least one study.[116] Recently, two independent groups have demonstrated that intraoperative assessment of the pancreatic neck margin is prognostic for overall survival regardless of further parenchymal resection.[117,118] In one multicenter analysis of 1,399 patients, 14% of patients had positive frozen section neck margins, of which half were successfully converted to R0 resection with additional parenchymal resection. Unfortunately the converted patients had survival similar to that of patients undergoing R1 resection (11.9 months versus 13.7 months, respectively, $p < 0.001$).[117] This suggests that tumor at the pancreas neck at the time of initial transection may be a marker of tumor biology rather than a factor controlled by the surgeon.

Neoadjuvant therapy has been proposed as a mechanism by which to sterilize margins and thus impact survival. Although some studies focusing on neoadjuvant therapy in patients with potentially resectable and borderline resectable PAC do show higher rates of R0 resections,[11,20,119] other studies specific to BRPAC (with variable utilization of neoadjuvant therapy) suggest a higher risk of margin positive resection.[120] For example, one multicenter French study of 150 patients including 36 who underwent SMV-PV resection used a prospective protocol to designate margins for histologic analysis. Thirty-five patients had microscopically positive margins (R1), and the SMV-PV margin was the most frequently involved. Vein resection was the only risk factor for R1 resection, which negatively impacted progression free survival.[116]

Adjuvant Therapy

For patients with resectable PAC, it is well-established that additional chemotherapy and possibly chemoradiotherapy provide a survival advantage after complete resection,[121–129] but studies supporting adjuvant therapy for patients with borderline disease, an often heavily pre-treated population, are less defined. While specific data pertaining to patients with BRPAC is lacking,[9,10] it is conceivable that patients who successfully undergo neoadjuvant therapy and surgical resection for BRPAC can be considered for adjuvant therapy. If considered, restaging imaging to exclude residual tumor or early progression should be obtained prior to initiation of any adjuvant regimen.[43] In the absence of randomized data, the choice of post-operative chemotherapy should reflect individual responses to neoadjuvant regimens. Adjuvant radiation therapy remains a controversial topic. An analysis of the National Cancer Data Base (NCDB) revealed that patients receiving adjuvant chemoradiotherapy following resection for PAC had improved overall survival compared to patients receiving only adjuvant chemotherapy or no adjuvant treatment.[130] It remains conceptually advantageous for patients with BRPAC and preserved performance status to undergo additional therapy, however there is currently limited data to guide the decision.

Unresectable Non-metastatic Pancreas Cancer

For the patient with unresectable PAC identified outside of the operating room, multiple options for palliation exist, including endoscopic stenting and operative bypass. The pros and cons to each approach are outside of the scope of this chapter. In the 10–30% of patients who are identified as unresectable at the time of laparotomy, palliative surgical bypass remains a viable therapeutic option with a morbidity rate between 28% and 50% and should be considered in select patients.[131] When trained appropriately the surgeon should also consider celiac plexus neurolysis, which has been associated with improved quality of life and can be performed during laparoscopy[132] or at the time of laparotomy.[133] Additionally it is the authors' practice to place radio-opaque clips identifying the tumor bed to facilitate future palliative radiotherapy.

The definition of unresectable PAC is ever evolving and the classification of any single patient with PAC may change throughout his or her natural history. In 2010 MDACC researchers described a series of 88 patients who presented after an aborted resection, including 20 in whom reimaging demonstrated borderline resectable disease, many of whom underwent palliative bypass. After a neoadjuvant chemoradiation approach in the majority of patients, 66 patients underwent resection, with acceptable major morbidity (20%) and mortality (4.5%) and a clear survival benefit for those reaching resection (29.6 months versus 10.6 months for patients with locally advanced disease).[134] The multidisciplinary setting facilitates frequent communication between medical, radiation, and surgical oncologists and re-evaluation should be routine for all patients with BRPAC and LAPC.

Conclusion

Ultimately, there are three questions that must be addressed when considering surgical therapy for patients with BRPAC: (1) Can the operation be performed safely? (2) Will the patient tolerate the procedure? (3) Is there a true potential survival benefit for the patient? The answer to the first question depends on both the tumor characteristics, i.e. visceral vessel involvement, and the surgeon's experience. The answer to the second question depends mostly on the patient's performance status and comorbidities, which may negatively impact his or her recovery from the operation. The third question addresses the presence of findings concerning for but not diagnostic of metastatic disease as well as the extent to which tumor biology limits operative success. Even in the absence of a universally agreed upon definition of resectability, answering these three questions for each patient will guide clinicians through the process of patient selection such that surgical resection is offered to patients with a reasonable chance of benefit.

Borderline resectable pancreas cancer represents a gray area along the continuum of early stage, clearly resectable disease and infiltrative, locally advanced disease and is a result of aggressive multidisciplinary collaboration. The limits of surgical resection are evolving as improvements in preoperative imaging, neoadjuvant therapy, operative techniques, and perioperative care have allowed oncologic teams to push the envelope regarding potentially curative resection of PAC. Questions remain regarding exact definitions of terms, the degree of vascular resection and method of reconstruction, and the duration and regimen of adjunct therapies.

Take Home Messages

- Borderline resectable pancreas adenocarcinoma (BRPAC) describes tumors involving the superior mesenteric-portal vein (SMV-PV) confluence or encroaching upon the mesenteric arterial axis.
- The consideration of surgical therapy for patients with BRPAC depends on the tumor characteristics, the surgeon's experience, and also the patient's performance status.
- Additional chemotherapy and/or chemoradiotherapy may provide a survival advantage after resection for the patients with BRPAC.

References

1. Siegel, R., Ma, J., Zou, Z., Jemal, A., Cancer statistics, 2014. *CA*, 2014. **64**: 9–29.
2. Thomas, R.M., Ahmad, S.A., Current concepts in the surgical management of pancreatic cancer. *Surgical Oncol Clinics North Am,* 2010. **19**: 335–58.

3. Hilbig, A., Oettle, H., Adjuvant therapy of pancreatic cancer. *Exp Rev Anticancer Ther*, 2010. **10**: 485–91.
4. Mayo, S.C., Nathan, H., Cameron, JL. *et al.,* Conditional survival in patients with pancreatic ductal adenocarcinoma resected with curative intent. *Cancer,* 2012. **118**: 2674–881.
5. Katz, M.H., Wang, H., Fleming, J.B. *et al.,* Long-term survival after multidisciplinary management of resected pancreatic adenocarcinoma. *Ann Surgical Oncol*, 2009. **16**: 836–47.
6. Neoptolemos, J.P., Stocken, DD., Dunn, J.A. *et al.,* Influence of resection margins on survival for patients with pancreatic cancer treated by adjuvant chemoradiation and/or chemotherapy in the ESPAC-1 randomized controlled trial. *Ann Surg,* 2001. **234**: 758–68.
7. Konstantinidis, I.T., Warshaw, A.L., Allen, J.N. *et al.,* Pancreatic ductal adenocarcinoma: is there a survival difference for R1 resections versus locally advanced unresectable tumors? What is a "true" R0 resection? *Ann Surg,* 2013. **257**: 731–6.
8. Kimbrough, C.W., St Hill, C.R., Martin, R.C., McMasters, K.M,, Scoggins, C.R., Tumor-positive resection margins reflect an aggressive tumor biology in pancreatic cancer. *J Surgical Oncol,* 2013. **107**: 602–7.
9. Katz, M.H., Crane, C.H., Varadhachary, G., Management of borderline resectable pancreatic cancer. *Semin Radiation Oncol*, 2014. **24**: 105–12.
10. Cooper, A.B., Tzeng, C.W., Katz, M.H., Treatment of borderline resectable pancreatic cancer. *Curr Treatment Options Oncol*, 2013. **14**: 293–310.
11. Papavasiliou, P., Chun, Y.S., Hoffman, J.P., How to define and manage borderline resectable pancreatic cancer. *Surgical Clinics North Am*, 2013. **93**: 663–74.
12. Sindelar, W.F., Clinical experience with regional pancreatectomy for adenocarcinoma of the pancreas. *Arch Surgery*, 1989. **124**: 127–32.
13. Bockhorn, M., Uzunoglu, F.G., Adham, M. *et al.,* Borderline resectable pancreatic cancer: a consensus statement by the International Study Group of Pancreatic Surgery (ISGPS). *Surgery*, 2014. **155**: 977–88.
14. Fortner, J.G., Kim, D.K., Cubilla, A., Turnbull, A., Pahnke, L.D., Shils, M.E., Regional pancreatectomy: en bloc pancreatic, portal vein and lymph node resection. *Ann Surg,* 1977. **186**: 42–50.
15. Harrison, L.E., Klimstra, D.S., Brennan, M.F., Isolated portal vein involvement in pancreatic adenocarcinoma. A contraindication for resection? *Ann Surgery,* 1996. **224**: 342–7; discussion 7–9.

16. Fuhrman, G.M., Leach, S.D., Staley, C.A. *et al.,* Rationale for en bloc vein resection in the treatment of pancreatic adenocarcinoma adherent to the superior mesenteric-portal vein confluence. Pancreatic Tumor Study Group. *Ann Surg,* 1996. **223**: 154–62.
17. Allema, J.H., Reinders, M.E., van Gulik, T.M. *et al.,* Portal vein resection in patients undergoing pancreatoduodenectomy for carcinoma of the pancreatic head. *Brit J Surg,* 1994. **81**: 1642–6.
18. Mehta, V.K., Fisher, G., Ford, J.A. *et al.,* Preoperative chemoradiation for marginally resectable adenocarcinoma of the pancreas. *J Gastrointestinal Surg*, 2001. **5**: 27–35.
19. Tempero, M.A., Behrman, S., Ben-Josef, E. *et al.,* Pancreatic adenocarcinoma: Clinical Practice Guidelines in Oncol. *J Nat Comprehensive Cancer Network,* JNCCN 2005. **3**: 598–626.
20. Varadhachary, G.R., Tamm, E.P., Abbruzzese, J.L. *et al.,* Borderline resectable pancreatic cancer: definitions, management, and role of preoperative therapy. *Ann Surg Oncol,* 2006. **13**: 1035–46.
21. Katz, M.H., Pisters, P.W., Evans, D.B. *et al.,* Borderline resectable pancreatic cancer: the importance of this emerging stage of disease. *J Am College Surgeons*, 2008. **206**: 833–46; discussion 46–8.
22. Callery, M.P., Chang, K.J., Fishman, E.K., Talamonti, M.S., William, Traverso, L., Linehan, D.C., Pretreatment assessment of resectable and borderline resectable pancreatic cancer: expert consensus statement. *Ann Surgical Oncol*, 2009. **16**: 1727–33.
23. Tempero, M.A., Arnoletti, J.P., Behrman, S. *et al.,* Pancreatic adenocarcinoma. *J Nat Comprehensive Cancer Network*, 2010. **8**: 972–1017.
24. Katz, M.H., Marsh, R., Herman, J.M. *et al.,* Borderline resectable pancreatic cancer: need for standardization and methods for optimal clinical trial design. *Ann Surgical Oncol*, 2013. **20**: 2787–95.
25. Kelly, K.J., Winslow, E., Kooby, D. *et al.,* Vein involvement during pancreaticoduodenectomy: is there a need for redefinition of "borderline resectable disease"? *J Gastrointestinal Surg*, 2013. **17**: 1209–17; discussion 17.
26. Katz, M.H., Marsh, R., Herman, J.M. *et al.,* Borderline resectable pancreatic cancer: need for standardization and methods for optimal clinical trial design. *Ann Surgical Oncol*, 2013. **20**: 2787–95.
27. Ishikawa, O., Ohigashi, H., Imaoka, S. *et al.,* Preoperative indications for extended pancreatectomy for locally advanced pancreas cancer involving the portal vein. *Ann Surg*, 1992. **215**: 231–6.

28. Tzeng, C.W., Fleming, J.B., Lee, J.E. *et al.,* Defined clinical classifications are associated with outcome of patients with anatomically resectable pancreatic adenocarcinoma treated with neoadjuvant therapy. *Ann Surgical Oncol*, 2012. **19**: 2045–53.
29. Gillen, S., Schuster, T., Meyer, Zum, Buschenfelde, C., Friess, H., Kleeff, J., Preoperative/neoadjuvant therapy in pancreatic cancer: a systematic review and meta-analysis of response and resection percentages. *PLoS Medi*, 2010. **7**: e1000267.
30. Breslin, T.M., Hess, K.R., Harbison, D.B. *et al.,* Neoadjuvant chemoradiotherapy for adenocarcinoma of the pancreas: treatment variables and survival duration. *Ann Surgical Oncol*, 2001. **8**: 123–32.
31. Abrams, R.A., Lowy, A.M., O'Reilly, E.M., Wolff, R.A., Picozzi, V.J., Pisters, P.W., Combined modality treatment of resectable and borderline resectable pancreas cancer: expert consensus statement. *Ann Surg Oncol*, 2009. **16**: 1751–6.
32. Barugola, G., Partelli, S., Marcucci, S. *et al.,* Resectable pancreatic cancer: who really benefits from resection? *Ann Surgical Oncol*, 2009. **16**: 3316–22.
33. Schmidt, C.M., Powell, E.S., Yiannoutsos, C.T. *et al.,* Pancreaticoduodenectomy: a 20-year experience in 516 patients. *Arch Surg*, 2004. **139**: 718–25; discussion 25–7.
34. Winter, J.M., Cameron, J.L., Campbell, K.A. *et al.,* 1423 pancreaticoduodenectomies for pancreatic cancer: A single-institution experience. *J Gastrointestinal Surg,* 2006. **10**: 1199–210; discussion 210–1.
35. Rose, J.B., Rocha, F.G., Alseidi, A. *et al.,* Extended neoadjuvant chemotherapy for borderline resectable pancreatic cancer demonstrates promising postoperative outcomes and survival. *Ann Surgical Oncol,* 2014. **21**: 1530–7.
36. Sohn, T.A., Yeo, C.J., Cameron, J.L. *et al.,* Resected adenocarcinoma of the pancreas-616 patients: results, outcomes, and prognostic indicators. *J Gastrointestinal Surg,* 2000. **4**: 567–79.
37. Aloia, T.A., Lee, J.E., Vauthey, J.N. *et al.,* Delayed recovery after pancreaticoduodenectomy: a major factor impairing the delivery of adjuvant therapy? *J Am College Surgeons*, 2007. **204**: 347–55.
38. Evans, D.B., Varadhachary, G.R., Crane, C.H. *et al.,* Preoperative gemcitabine-based chemoradiation for patients with resectable adenocarcinoma of the pancreatic head. *J clinical Oncol*, 2008. **26**: 3496–502.

39. Araujo, R.L., Gaujoux, S., Huguet, F. *et al.,* Does pre-operative chemoradiation for initially unresectable or borderline resectable pancreatic adenocarcinoma increase post-operative morbidity? A case-matched analysis. *HPB,* 2013. **15**: 574–80.
40. Asbun, H.J., Conlon, K., Fernandez-Cruz, L. *et al.,* When to perform a pancreatoduodenectomy in the absence of positive histology? A consensus statement by the International Study Group of Pancreatic Surgery. *Surgery,* 2014. **155**: 887–92.
41. Yang, R., Lu, M., Qian, X. *et al.,* Diagnostic accuracy of EUS and CT of vascular invasion in pancreatic cancer: a systematic review. *J Cancer Res Clin Oncol*, 2014.
42. Tempero, M.A., Arnoletti, J.P., Behrman, S.W. *et al.,* Pancreatic Adenocarcinoma, version 2. **2012**: featured updates to the NCCN Guidelines. *J Nat Comprehensive Cancer Network*, 2012. **10**: 703–13.
43. Tamm, E.P., Balachandran, A., Bhosale, P.R. *et al.,* Imaging of pancreatic adenocarcinoma: update on staging/resectability. *Radiologic Clin North Am*, 2012. **50**: 407–28.
44. Kullman, E., Frozanpor, F., Soderlund, C. *et al.,* Covered versus uncovered self-expandable nitinol stents in the palliative treatment of malignant distal biliary obstruction: results from a randomized, multicenter study. *Gastrointestinal Endoscopy*, 2010. **72**: 915–23.
45. Soderlund, C., Linder, SCINGEJ, Pmid. Covered metal versus plastic stents for malignant common bile duct stenosis: a prospective, randomized, controlled trial. *Gastrointestinal Endoscopy*, 2006. **63**: 986–95.
46. Aadam, A.A., Evans, D.B., Khan, A., Oh, Y., Dua, K., Efficacy and safety of self-expandable metal stents for biliary decompression in patients receiving neoadjuvant therapy for pancreatic cancer: a prospective study. *Gastrointestinal Endoscopy*, 2012. **76**: 67–75.
47. Conroy, T., Desseigne, F., Ychou, M. *et al.,* FOLFIRINOX versus gemcitabine for metastatic pancreatic cancer. *N Eng J Med*, 2011. **364**: 1817–25.
48. Heinemann, V., Boeck, S., Hinke, A., Labianca, R., Louvet, C., Meta-analysis of randomized trials: evaluation of benefit from gemcitabine-based combination chemotherapy applied in advanced pancreatic cancer. *BMC Cancer*, 2008. **8**: 82.
49. Louvet, C., Labianca, R., Hammel, P. *et al.,* Gemcitabine in combination with oxaliplatin compared with gemcitabine alone in locally advanced or

metastatic pancreatic cancer: results of a GERCOR and GISCAD phase III trial. *J Clinical Oncol*, 2005. **23**: 3509–16.

50. Evans, D.B., Varadhachary, G.R., Crane, C.H. *et al.,* Preoperative gemcitabine-based chemoradiation for patients with resectable adenocarcinoma of the pancreatic head. *J Clin Oncol*, 2008. **26**: 3496–502.
51. Le Scodan, R., Mornex, F., Girard, N. *et al.,* Preoperative chemoradiation in potentially resectable pancreatic adenocarcinoma: feasibility, treatment effect evaluation and prognostic factors, analysis of the SFRO-FFCD 9704 trial and literature review. *Ann Oncol*, 2009. **20**: 1387–96.
52. Varadhachary, G.R., Wolff, R.A., Crane, C.H. *et al.,* Preoperative gemcitabine and cisplatin followed by gemcitabine-based chemoradiation for resectable adenocarcinoma of the pancreatic head. *J Clin Oncol*, 2008. **26**: 3487–95.
53. White, R.R., Hurwitz, H.I., Morse, M.A. *et al.,* Neoadjuvant chemoradiation for localized adenocarcinoma of the pancreas. *Ann Surgical Oncol,* 2001. **8**: 758–65.
54. Talamonti, M.S., Small, W., Jr., Mulcahy, M.F. *et al.,* A multi-institutional phase II trial of preoperative full-dose gemcitabine and concurrent radiation for patients with potentially resectable pancreatic carcinoma. *Ann Surg Oncol,* 2006. **13**: 150–8.
55. Kang, C.M., Hwang, H.K., Choi, S.H., Lee, W.J., Controversial issues of neoadjuvant treatment in borderline resectable pancreatic cancer. *Surgical Oncol,* 2013. **22**: 123–31.
56. Pipas, J.M., Barth, R.J., Jr., Zaki, B. *et al.,* Docetaxel/Gemcitabine followed by gemcitabine and external beam radiotherapy in patients with pancreatic adenocarcinoma. *Ann Surg Oncol,* 2005. **12**: 995–1004.
57. Small, W., Jr., Berlin, J., Freedman, G.M. *et al.,* Full-dose gemcitabine with concurrent radiation therapy in patients with nonmetastatic pancreatic cancer: a multicenter phase II trial. *J Clin Oncol,* 2008. **26**: 942–7.
58. Landry, J., Catalano, P.J., Staley, C. *et al.,* Randomized phase II study of gemcitabine plus radiotherapy versus gemcitabine, 5-fluorouracil, and cisplatin followed by radiotherapy and 5-fluorouracil for patients with locally advanced, potentially resectable pancreatic adenocarcinoma. *J Surgical Oncol,* 2010. **101**: 587–92.
59. Sahora, K., Kuehrer, I., Schindl, M., Koelblinger, C., Goetzinger, P., Gnant, M., NeoGemTax: gemcitabine and docetaxel as neoadjuvant

treatment for locally advanced nonmetastasized pancreatic cancer. *World J Surg,* 2011. **35**: 1580–9.

60. Sahora, K., Kuehrer, I., Eisenhut, A. *et al.,* NeoGemOx: Gemcitabine and oxaliplatin as neoadjuvant treatment for locally advanced, nonmetastasized pancreatic cancer. *Surgery,* 2011. **149**: 311–20.
61. Small, W., Jr., Mulcahy, M.F., Rademaker, A. *et al.,* Phase II trial of full-dose gemcitabine and bevacizumab in combination with attenuated three-dimensional conformal radiotherapy in patients with localized pancreatic cancer. *Int J Radiat Oncol Biol Phys,* 2011. **80**: 476–82.
62. Stokes, J.B., Nolan, N.J., Stelow, E.B. *et al.,* Preoperative capecitabine and concurrent radiation for borderline resectable pancreatic cancer. *Ann Surgical Oncol,* 2011. **18**: 619–27.
63. Lee, J.L., Kim, S.C., Kim, J.H. *et al.,* Prospective efficacy and safety study of neoadjuvant gemcitabine with capecitabine combination chemotherapy for borderline-resectable or unresectable locally advanced pancreatic adenocarcinoma. *Surgery,* 2012. **152**: 851–62.
64. Chakraborty, S., Morris, M.M., Bauer, T.W. *et al.,* Accelerated fraction radiotherapy with capecitabine as neoadjuvant therapy for borderline resectable pancreatic cancer. *Gastrointest Cancer,* Res 2014. **7**: 15–22.
65. Jensen, E.H., Armstrong, L., Lee, C. *et al.,* Neoadjuvant interferon-based chemoradiation for borderline resectable and locally advanced pancreas cancer: a Phase II pilot study. *HPB,* 2014. **16**: 131–9.
66. Kim, E.J., Ben-Josef, E., Herman, J.M. *et al.,* A multi-institutional phase 2 study of neoadjuvant gemcitabine and oxaliplatin with radiation therapy in patients with pancreatic cancer. *Cancer,* 2013. **119**: 2692–700.
67. Leone, F., Gatti, M., Massucco, P. *et al.,* Induction gemcitabine and oxaliplatin therapy followed by a twice-weekly infusion of gemcitabine and concurrent external-beam radiation for neoadjuvant treatment of locally advanced pancreatic cancer: a single institutional experience. *Cancer,* 2013. **119**: 277–84.
68. Motoi, F., Ishida, K., Fujishima, F. *et al.,* Neoadjuvant chemotherapy with gemcitabine and S-1 for resectable and borderline pancreatic ductal adenocarcinoma: results from a prospective multi-institutional phase 2 trial. *Ann Surg Oncol,* 2013. **20**: 3794–801.
69. Christians, K.K., Tsai, S., Mahmoud, A. *et al.,* Neoadjuvant FOLFIRINOX for borderline resectable pancreas cancer: a new treatment paradigm? *Oncologist,* 2014. **19**: 266–74.

70. Esnaola, N.F., Chaudhary, U.B., O'Brien, P. *et al.,* Phase 2 trial of induction gemcitabine, oxaliplatin, and cetuximab followed by selective capecitabine-based chemoradiation in patients with borderline resectable or unresectable locally advanced pancreatic cancer. *Int J Radiat Oncol Biol, Phys* 2014. **88**: 837–44.
71. Sahora, K., Schindl, M., Kuehrer, I. *et al.,* A phase II trial of two durations of Bevacizumab added to neoadjuvant gemcitabine for borderline and locally advanced pancreatic cancer. *Anticancer Res,* 2014. **34**: 2377–84.
72. Landry, J., Catalano, P.J., Staley, C. *et al.,* Randomized phase II study of gemcitabine plus radiotherapy versus gemcitabine, 5-fluorouracil, and cisplatin followed by radiotherapy and 5-fluorouracil for patients with locally advanced, potentially resectable pancreatic adenocarcinoma. *J surgical Oncol,* 2010. **101**: 587–92.
73. Chen, K.T., Devarajan, K., Milestone, B.N. *et al.,* Neoadjuvant chemoradiation and duration of chemotherapy before surgical resection for pancreatic cancer: does time interval between radiotherapy and surgery matter? *Ann Surgical Oncol,* 2014. **21**: 662–9.
74. Health USNIo. 2014.
75. Eisenhauer, E.A., Therasse, P., Bogaerts, J. *et al.,* New response evaluation criteria in solid tumours: revised RECIST guideline (version 1.1). *Eur J Cancer,* 2009. **45**: 228–47.
76. Katz, M.H., Fleming, J.B., Bhosale, P. *et al.,* Response of borderline resectable pancreatic cancer to neoadjuvant therapy is not reflected by radiographic indicators. *Cancer,* 2012. **118**: 5749–56.
77. Patel, M., Hoffe, S., Malafa, M. *et al.,* Neoadjuvant GTX chemotherapy and IMRT-based chemoradiation for borderline resectable pancreatic cancer. *J surgical Oncol,* 2011. **104**: 155–61.
78. Picchio, M., Giovannini, E., Passoni, P. *et al.,* Role of PET/CT in the clinical management of locally advanced pancreatic cancer. *Tumori,* 2012. **98**: 643–51.
79. Bang, S., Chung, H.W., Park, S.W. *et al.,* The clinical usefulness of 18-fluorodeoxyglucose positron emission tomography in the differential diagnosis, staging, and response evaluation after concurrent chemoradiotherapy for pancreatic cancer. *J Clin Gastroenterol,* 2006. **40**: 923–9.
80. Chatterjee, D., Katz, MH., Rashid, A. *et al.,* Histologic grading of the extent of residual carcinoma following neoadjuvant chemoradiation in pancreatic

ductal adenocarcinoma: a predictor for patient outcome. *Cancer,* 2012. **118**: 3182–90.

81. Chun, Y.S., Cooper, H.S., Cohen, S.J. *et al.,* Significance of pathologic response to preoperative therapy in pancreatic cancer. *Ann Surgical Oncol,* 2011. **18**: 3601–7.
82. Zhao, Q., Rashid, A., Gong, Y. *et al.,* Pathologic complete response to neoadjuvant therapy in patients with pancreatic ductal adenocarcinoma is associated with a better prognosis. *Ann Diagn Pathol*, 2012. **16**: 29–37.
83. Chun, Y.S., Cooper, H.S., Cohen, S.J. *et al.,* Significance of pathologic response to preoperative therapy in pancreatic cancer. *Ann Surgical Oncol,* 2011. **18**: 3601–7.
84. Tzeng, C.W., Balachandran, A., Ahmad, M. *et al.,* Serum carbohydrate antigen 19–9 represents a marker of response to neoadjuvant therapy in patients with borderline resectable pancreatic cancer. *HPB*, 2014. **16**: 430–8.
85. Porembka, M.R., Hawkins, W.G., Linehan, D.C. *et al.,* Radiologic and intraoperative detection of need for mesenteric vein resection in patients with adenocarcinoma of the head of the pancreas. *HPB*, 2011. **13**: 633–42.
86. Callery, M.P., Strasberg, S.M., Doherty, G.M., Soper, N.J., Norton, J.A., Staging laparoscopy with laparoscopic ultrasonography: optimizing resectability in hepatobiliary and pancreatic malignancy. *J Am College Surgeons,* 1997. **185**: 33–9.
87. Barreiro, C.J., Lillemoe, K.D., Koniaris, L.G. *et al.,* Diagnostic laparoscopy for periampullary and pancreatic cancer: what is the true benefit? *J Gastroint Surg*, 2002. **6**: 75–81.
88. Maithel, S.K., Maloney, S., Winston, C. *et al.,* Preoperative CA 19–9 and the yield of staging laparoscopy in patients with radiographically resectable pancreatic adenocarcinoma. *Ann Surgical Oncol,* 2008. **15**: 3512–20.
89. Satoi, S., Yanagimoto, H., Toyokawa, H. *et al.,* Selective use of staging laparoscopy based on carbohydrate antigen 19–9 level and tumor size in patients with radiographically defined potentially or borderline resectable pancreatic cancer. *Pancreas*, 2011. **40**: 426–32.
90. Riall, T.S., Cameron, J.L., Lillemoe, K.D. *et al.,* Pancreaticoduodenectomy with or without distal gastrectomy and extended retroperitoneal lymphadenectomy for periampullary adenocarcinoma — part **3**: update on 5-year survival. *J Gastroint Surg*, 2005. **9**: 1191–204; discussion 204–6.

91. Jang, J.Y., Kang, M.J., Heo, J.S. *et al.,* A prospective randomized controlled study comparing outcomes of standard resection and extended resection, including dissection of the nerve plexus and various lymph nodes, in patients with pancreatic head cancer. *Ann Surg*, 2014. **259**: 656–64.
92. Christians, K.K., Lal, A., Pappas, S., Quebbeman, E., Evans, D.B., Portal vein resection. *Surgical Clin North Am,* 2010. **90**: 309–22.
93. Katz, M.H., Fleming, J.B., Pisters, P.W., Lee, J.E., Evans, D.B., Anatomy of the superior mesenteric vein with special reference to the surgical management of first-order branch involvement at pancreaticoduodenectomy. *Ann Surg*, 2008. **248**: 1098–102.
94. Chu, C.K., Farnell, M.B., Nguyen, J.H. *et al.,* Prosthetic graft reconstruction after portal vein resection in pancreaticoduodenectomy: a multicenter analysis. *J Am College Surgeons*, 2010. **211**: 316–24.
95. Chua, T.C., Saxena, A., Extended pancreaticoduodenectomy with vascular resection for pancreatic cancer: a systematic review. *J Gastroint Surg*, 2010. **14**: 1442–52.
96. Harrison, L.E., Klimstra, D.S., Brennan, M.F., Isolated portal vein involvement in pancreatic adenocarcinoma. A contraindication for resection? *Ann Surg,* 1996. **224**: 342–7; discussion 7–9.
97. Riediger, H., Makowiec, F., Fischer, E., Adam, U., Hopt, U.T., Postoperative morbidity and long-term survival after pancreaticoduodenectomy with superior mesenterico-portal vein resection. *J Gastroint Surg*, 2006. **10**: 1106–15.
98. Tseng, J.F., Raut, C.P., Lee, J.E. *et al.,* Pancreaticoduodenectomy with vascular resection: margin status and survival duration. *J Gastrointestinal Surg*, 2004. **8**: 935–49; discussion 49–50.
99. Turrini, O., Ewald, J., Barbier, L., Mokart, D., Blache, J.L., Delpero, J.R., Should the portal vein be routinely resected during pancreaticoduodenectomy for adenocarcinoma? *Ann Surg*, 2013. **257**: 726–30.
100. Ouaissi, M., Hubert, C., Verhelst, R. *et al.,* Vascular reconstruction during pancreatoduodenectomy for ductal adenocarcinoma of the pancreas improves resectability but does not achieve cure. *World J Surg*, 2010. **34**: 2648–61.
101. Yekebas, E.F., Bogoevski, D., Cataldegirmen, G. *et al.,* En bloc vascular resection for locally advanced pancreatic malignancies infiltrating major

blood vessels: perioperative outcome and long-term survival in 136 patients. *Ann Surg*, 2008. **247**: 300–9.

102. Al-Haddad, M., Martin, J.K., Nguyen, J. *et al.,* Vascular resection and reconstruction for pancreatic malignancy: a single center survival study. *J Gastrointestinal Surg*, 2007. **11**: 1168–74.
103. Siriwardana, H.P., Siriwardena, A.K., Systematic review of outcome of synchronous portal-superior mesenteric vein resection during pancreatectomy for cancer. *Brit J Surg,* 2006. **93**: 662–73.
104. Worni, M., Castleberry, A.W., Clary, B.M. *et al.,* Concomitant vascular reconstruction during pancreatectomy for malignant disease: a propensity score-adjusted, population-based trend analysis involving 10,206 patients. *JAMA Surg,* 2013. **148**: 331–8.
105. Ravikumar, R., Sabin, C., Abu, Hilal, M. *et al.,* Portal vein resection in borderline resectable pancreatic cancer: a United Kingdom multicenter study. *J Am College Surgeons*, 2014. **218**: 401–11.
106. Bachellier, P., Rosso, E., Fuchshuber, P. *et al.,* Use of a temporary intraoperative mesentericoportal shunt for pancreatic resection for locally advanced pancreatic cancer with portal vein occlusion and portal hypertension. *Surgery*, 2014. **155**: 449–56.
107. Martin, R.C., 2nd, Scoggins, C.R., Egnatashvili, V., Staley, C.A., McMasters, K.M., Kooby, D.A., Arterial and venous resection for pancreatic adenocarcinoma: operative and long-term outcomes. *Arch Surg*, 2009. **144**: 154–9.
108. Riediger, H., Makowiec, F., Fischer, E., Adam, U., Hopt, U.T., Postoperative morbidity and long-term survival after pancreaticoduodenectomy with superior mesenterico-portal vein resection. *J Gastrointestinal Surg*, 2006. **10**: 1106–15.
109. Tseng, J.F., Raut, C.P., Lee, J.E. *et al.,* Pancreaticoduodenectomy with vascular resection: margin status and survival duration. *J Gastroint Surg*, 2004. **8**: 935–49; discussion 49–50.
110. Yekebas, E.F., Bogoevski, D., Cataldegirmen, G. *et al.,* En bloc vascular resection for locally advanced pancreatic malignancies infiltrating major blood vessels: perioperative outcome and long-term survival in 136 patients. *Ann Surg*, 2008. **247**: 300–9.
111. Appleby, L.H., The coeliac axis in the expansion of the operation for gastric carcinoma. *Cancer*, 1953. **6**: 704–7.

112. Mollberg, N., Rahbari, N.N., Koch, M. *et al.,* Arterial resection during pancreatectomy for pancreatic cancer: a systematic review and meta-analysis. *Ann Surg*, 2011. **254**: 882–93.
113. Rau, B.M., Moritz, K., Schuschan, S., Alsfasser, G., Prall, F., Klar, E., R1 resection in pancreatic cancer has significant impact on long-term outcome in standardized pathology modified for routine use. *Surgery*, 2012. **152**: S103–11.
114. Verbeke, C.S., Leitch, D., Menon, K.V., McMahon, M.J., Guillou, P.J., Anthoney, A., Redefining the R1 resection in pancreatic cancer. *Brit J Surg*, 2006. **93**: 1232–7.
115. Jamieson, N.B., Chan, N.I., Foulis, A.K., Dickson, E.J., McKay, C.J., Carter, C.R., The prognostic influence of resection margin clearance following pancreaticoduodenectomy for pancreatic ductal adenocarcinoma. *J Gastroint Surg*, 2013. **17**: 511–21.
116. Delpero, J.R., Bachellier, P., Regenet, N. *et al.,* Pancreaticoduodenectomy for pancreatic ductal adenocarcinoma: a French multicentre prospective evaluation of resection margins in 150 evaluable specimens. *HPB,* 2014. **16**: 20–33.
117. Lad, N.L., Squires, M.H., Maithel, S.K. *et al.,* Is it time to stop checking frozen section neck margins during pancreaticoduodenectomy? *Ann Surgical Oncol*, 2013. **20**: 3626–33.
118. Mathur, A., Ross, S.B., Luberice, K. *et al.,* Margin status impacts survival after pancreaticoduodenectomy but negative margins should not be pursued. *Am Surgeon*, 2014. **80**: 353–60.
119. Kang, C.M., Chung, Y.E., Park, J.Y. *et al.,* Potential contribution of preoperative neoadjuvant concurrent chemoradiation therapy on margin-negative resection in borderline resectable pancreatic cancer. *J Gastroint Surg*, 2012. **16**: 509–17.
120. Wang, J., Estrella, J.S., Peng, L. *et al.,* Histologic tumor involvement of superior mesenteric vein/portal vein predicts poor prognosis in patients with stage II pancreatic adenocarcinoma treated with neoadjuvant chemoradiation. *Cancer*, 2012. **118**: 3801–11.
121. Kalser, M.H., Ellenberg, S.S., Pancreatic cancer. Adjuvant combined radiation and chemotherapy following curative resection. *Arch Surg*, 1985. **120**: 899–903.
122. Further evidence of effective adjuvant combined radiation and chemotherapy following curative resection of pancreatic cancer. Gastrointestinal Tumor Study Group. *Cancer*, 1987. **59**: 2006–10.

123. Klinkenbijl, J.H., Jeekel, J., Sahmoud, T. *et al.,* Adjuvant radiotherapy and 5-fluorouracil after curative resection of cancer of the pancreas and periampullary region: phase III trial of the EORTC gastrointestinal tract cancer cooperative group. *Ann Surg*, 1999. **230**: 776–82; discussion 82–4.
124. Neoptolemos, J.P., Stocken, D.D., Friess, H. *et al.,* A randomized trial of chemoradiotherapy and chemotherapy after resection of pancreatic cancer. *N Eng J Med*, 2004. **350**: 1200–10.
125. Oettle, H., Neuhaus, P., Hochhaus, A. *et al.,* Adjuvant chemotherapy with gemcitabine and long-term outcomes among patients with resected pancreatic cancer: the CONKO-001 randomized trial. *JAMA*, 2013. **310**: 1473–81.
126. Oettle, H., Post, S., Neuhaus, P. *et al.,* Adjuvant chemotherapy with gemcitabine vs observation in patients undergoing curative-intent resection of pancreatic cancer: a randomized controlled trial. *JAMA*, 2007. **297**: 267–77.
127. Van Laethem, J.L., Hammel, P., Mornex, F. *et al.,* Adjuvant gemcitabine alone versus gemcitabine-based chemoradiotherapy after curative resection for pancreatic cancer: a randomized EORTC-40013–22012/FFCD-9203/GERCOR phase II study. *J Clin Oncol*, 2010. **28**: 4450–6.
128. Smeenk, H.G., van Eijck, C.H., Hop, W.C. *et al.,* Long-term survival and metastatic pattern of pancreatic and periampullary cancer after adjuvant chemoradiation or observation: long-term results of EORTC trial 40891. *Ann Surg*, 2007. **246**: 734–40.
129. Regine, W.F., Winter, K.A., Abrams, R.A. *et al.,* Fluorouracil vs gemcitabine chemotherapy before and after fluorouracil-based chemoradiation following resection of pancreatic adenocarcinoma: a randomized controlled trial. *JAMA*, 2008. **299**: 1019–26.
130. Kooby, D.A., Gillespie, T.W., Liu, Y. *et al.,* Impact of adjuvant radiotherapy on survival after pancreatic cancer resection: an appraisal of data from the national cancer data base. *Ann Surgical Oncol*, 2013. **20**: 3634–42.
131. Spanheimer, P.M., Cyr, A.R., Liao, J. *et al.,* Complications and survival associated with operative procedures in patients with unresectable pancreatic head adenocarcinoma. *J surgical Oncol*, 2014. **109**: 697–701.
132. Allen, P.J., Chou, J., Janakos, M., Strong, V.E., Coit, D.G., Brennan, M.F., Prospective evaluation of laparoscopic celiac plexus block in patients with unresectable pancreatic adenocarcinoma. *Ann Surgical Oncol*, 2011. **18**: 636–41.

133. Lillemoe, K.D., Cameron, J.L., Kaufman, H.S., Yeo, C.J., Pitt, H.A., Sauter, P.K., Chemical splanchnicectomy in patients with unresectable pancreatic cancer. A prospective randomized trial. *Ann Surg*, 1993. **217**: 447–55; discussion 56–7.
134. Truty, M.J., Thomas, R.M., Katz, M.H. *et al.,* Multimodality therapy offers a chance for cure in patients with pancreatic adenocarcinoma deemed unresectable at first operative exploration. *J Am College Surgeons*, 2012. **215**: 41–51; discussion 2.

Chapter 16

Treatment of Advanced Pancreatic Cancer

Hemchandra Mahaseth, Bassel El-Rayes and Philip A. Philip

What is New

- Ductal pancreatic adenocarcinoma is a lethal disease with median overall survival of less than six months without treatment. Gemcitabine single agent has been the only standard treatment for advanced pancreatic cancer until recently.
- FOLFIRINOX became a new standard of treatment for advanced pancreatic cancer in 2010 for patients with excellent performance status and otherwise healthy. FOLFIRINOX improved the median overall survival to 11 months.
- Nab-Paclitaxel was approved in 2013 for treatment of pancreatic cancer in combination with gemcitabine.
- MM-398, a nanoliposomal encapsulated Irinotecan in combination with 5-FU seems active in randomized phase III study and may become one of the standard treatment regimens in advanced pancreatic camcer.
- Drugs targeting the stroma, inflammation, immune system etc. are in different stages of development.

Introduction

Ductal pancreatic adenocarcinoma (PDAC) is the fourth leading cause of cancer-related mortality after lung, prostate, breast and colorectum.[1] The American Cancer Society estimates 46,420 new cases of PDAC will be diagnosed annually in the United States. Approximately 40,000 patients will die of PDAC in 2014.[1] Estimated annual incidence and mortality from PDAC are closely suggesting the high degree of lethality associated with this disease. Surgery is the only potentially curative therapeutic option. However, only 15–20% of patients meet the criteria for surgical resection at diagnosis. The rest of the patients present with advanced disease defined as either locally advanced unresectable or metastatic disease. This chapter will focus on the use of systemic chemotherapy in the management of advanced PDAC.

Risk Factors and Genetic Predisposition

Although the increase in risk is small, several environmental factors, such as cigarette smoking,[2] occupational exposure to beta-naphthylamine and benzidine,[3] consumption of red or processed meat[4,5] or dairy products,[4] obesity,[6] heavy alcohol consumption,[7] chronic pancreatitis[8] and vitamin D deficiency[9] are linked with PDAC. True cases of familial pancreatic cancer are rare. Approximately 5% of pancreatic cancer patients have family history of the disease and may have genetic predisposition. Risk of developing pancreatic cancer for an individual with aggregation of this disease in family is higher than general population. Germline mutations in CDKN2A (p16),[10] BRCA2,[11] PALB2,[12] MSH2[13] and ATM[14] are associated with higher risk of developing this disease. Individuals with family history of Peutz-Jeghers syndrome[15] (germline mutation in STK11 gene) or Lynch syndrome[16] (germline mutations in DNA mismatch repair genes, i.e. MLH1, MSH2, MSH6 or PMS2) are also at high risk for developing PDAC. An international Cancer of Pancreas Screening (CAPS) Consortium guidelines[17] recommend screening with endoscopic ultrasound (EUS) or magnetic resonance cholangiopancreatography (MRCP) for individuals with first-degree relative with PDAC, carriers of mutated p16 and STK11 (Peutz-Jeghers syndrome). Screening for pancreatic cancer is not recommended for individuals at average risk.

Clinical Manifestations and Diagnosis

Common presenting symptoms of PDAC include weight loss, jaundice, abdominal pain, steatorrhea, dyspepsia, nausea, new onset diabetes or worsening of existing diabetes, depression or thromboembolism. Multiple sub-specialties, including radiology, gastroenterology, pathology, medical, surgical and radiation oncology are involved in management of PDAC. Diagnostic work-up includes a CT or MRI with pancreas protocol. Typical findings on cross sectional imaging include presence of a hypo-enhancing mass. An elevated level of biomarker, CA-19-9 strengthens the suspicion. If the patient is thought to have resectable early stage pancreatic cancer, surgical resection as described in Chapter 15 should be considered without biopsy confirmation of cancer. For patients with unresectable or borderline resectable disease, the diagnosis of pancreatic ductal adenocarcinoma should be confirmed with biopsy of primary pancreatic or metastatic lesion prior to any treatment. The biopsy of pancreatic tumor can be performed by endoscopic ultrasonography (EUS) or under CT guidance. Once the diagnosis is made, staging should be completed with chest CT scan.

Prognosis

Advanced PDAC is incurable and objective of therapy is palliative. Without treatment, the median overall survival of a patient with metastatic pancreatic cancer is less than six months. The last decade has made milestones in treatment of metastatic pancreatic cancer. Among patients treated with FOLFIRINOX, median survival is approximately 11 months.[18]

Treatment of Advanced Pancreatic Ductal Adenocarcinoma

Systemic chemotherapy is the mainstay of treatment in advanced PDAC. A vast majority of pancreatic cancer patients are symptomatic and initiation of supportive treatment for symptom palliation is an important part of management of this disease. Historically, single agent 5-FU was the most frequently used treatment regimen in metastatic pancreatic cancer. In mid-1990s, single agent gemcitabine became the standard of treatment. The past decade has witnessed remarkable improvement in treatment of pancreatic cancer with approval of erlotinib, nab-paclitaxel and FOLFIRINOX regimen. The most commonly used regimens can be divided as gemcitabine-based or 5-FU-based. Gemcitabine-based regimens include gemcitabine single agent, gemcitabine plus nab-paclitaxel or gemcitabine plus erlotinib. 5-FU-based regimens include single agent 5-FU or capecitabine, FOLFIRINOX, FOLFOX or CapeOX. Whether a patient should be treated with gemcitabine- or fluoropyrimidine-based chemotherapy is not well-defined and practically depends on the physicians' preference. Gemcitabine combination is usually considered in the second-line setting, if patient had fluoropyrimidine-based treatment in the first-line or vice versa.

Gemcitabine-based chemotherapy

In early 1990, Burris and colleagues[19] randomized 126 patients with advanced symptomatic pancreatic cancer to receive either gemcitabine 1000 mg/m^2 per week for seven weeks followed by one week of rest, then weekly for three weeks every four weeks or 5-FU 600 mg/m^2 once weekly. The primary endpoint was clinical benefit response, which included a composite measurement of pain, Karnofsky performance status and weight. In order to be considered a clinical benefit response, a clinical benefit required sustained improvement for more than four weeks without worsening in other symptoms. The secondary endpoint was time to progressive disease and overall survival. The clinical benefit response was noted in 23.8% of gemcitabine-treated patients compared to 4.8% of 5-FU-treated patients (p = 0.0022). Median overall survival was 5.65 months for gemcitabine-treated patients and 4.41 months for 5-FU-treated patients ($p = 0.0025$). Median time to progression was 9 weeks in gemcitabine arm compared with 4 weeks in 5-FU arms. Patients with clinical benefit response had longer median survival (10.7 vs. 4.8 months) and time to disease progression (3.7 months vs. 1.6 months) than those who did not have a clinical benefit response. Both gemcitabine and 5-FU were well-tolerated with acceptable toxicity. Improvement in clinical benefit as well as survival in this study led to the approval of gemcitabine for first-line treatment of metastatic pancreatic cancer and it has been the only standard of treatment until recently.

Gemcitabine in the above study was administered as a 30-minute i.v. infusion. The intracellular activation of gemcitabine occurs by its conversion to gemcitabine triphosphate by deoxycytidine kinase, which is saturated at infusion rates of 10 mg/m^2 per minute. Using the fixed dose rate infusion, the maximum tolerated dose of gemcitabine is higher.[20] Initially it was thought that with fixed dose rate infusion, higher dose of gemcitabine can be administered, which was expected to provide better outcome. A large randomized phase III trial by the Eastern Cooperative Oncology Group[21] tested this hypothesis. In this study, 832 patients with metastatic or locally advanced pancreatic cancer were randomized into three arms, standard gemcitabine arm (weekly gemcitabine 1000 mg/m^2 as 30 minute infusion), fixed dose rate gemcitabine (weekly gemcitabine 1500 mg/m^2 over 150 minutes) or GEMOX (gemcitabine 1000 mg/m^2 over 100 minutes on day 1 plus oxaliplatin 100 mg/m^2 on day 2 every two weeks). Median survival was not substantially different between standard and fixed dose rate gemcitabine arms (4.9 months vs. 6.2 months, HR = 0.83, $p = 0.04$). In addition, more grade ¾ thrombocytopenia and neutropenia were observed with fixed dose rate gemcitabine administration. Gemcitabine 1000 mg/m^2 administered as 30-minute i.v. infusion remains the standard.

Human epidermal growth factor receptor type 1 (HER1/EGFR) is frequently overexpressed in PDAC. Tumors with overexpression of EGFR tend to be more aggressive. In order to target EGFR, the National Cancer Institute of Canada Clinical Trials Group (NCICCTG) in cooperation with Australasian Gastrointestinal Tumor Group (AGITG) randomly assigned 569 patients with previously untreated locally advanced unresectable or metastatic pancreatic cancer into two arms, gemcitabine plus placebo vs. gemcitabine plus erlotinib arm in 1:1 ratio.[22] Erlotinib is an oral EGFR tyrosine kinase inhibitor. In gemcitabine plus placebo arm, gemcitabine was administered at the dose of 1000 mg/m^2 as 30 minute intravenous infusion on days 1, 8, 15, 22, 29, 36 and 43 followed by one week of rest in first cycle (8 weeks) and on days 1, 8 and 15 followed by one week of rest in all subsequent cycles (4 weeks) until disease progression or unacceptable toxicity. Placebo was administered orally once a day. In gemcitabine plus erlotinib arm, gemcitabine was administered once a week as in gemcitabine plus placebo arm. Erlotinib was administered orally at 100 or

150 mg/day. The primary endpoint was overall survival. Secondary end points included progression-free survival, response rate, response duration, toxicity, quality of life and correlation of baseline tissue EGFR level with outcome. Median overall survival was significantly longer in gemcitabine and erlotinb arm, 6.24 months vs. 5.91 months (HR = 0.82, 95% CI: 0.69 to 0.99; $p = 0.038$). Median progression-free survival was 3.75 months in gemcitabine plus erlotinib arm and 3.55 in gemcitabine and placebo arm (HR = 0.77, 95% CI: 0.64 to 0.92, $p = 0.004$). The overall disease control rate (complete response plus partial response plus stable disease) or global quality of life was not significantly different. EGFR expression in pancreatic tumors did not correlate with outcome. Development of rash in erlotinib treated patients was associated with better outcome. Median overall survival was respectively 5.3, 5.8 and 10.5 months for patients with grade 0, 1 and 2+ rashes. Treatment was generally well-tolerated in both arms. Patients in gemcitabine plus erlotinib arm had more rash, diarrhea, infection and stomatitis, but they were generally grade 1 or 2. Based on this study, erlotinib in combination with gemcitabine was approved for treatment of advanced pancreatic cancer. However, the improvement in outcome attributable to addition of erlotinib was very small and not considered clinically meaningful by most pancreatic cancer experts. Despite FDA approval of erlotinib in pancreatic cancer, the enthusiasm to use it has been low among clinicians.

Several randomized trials compared gemcitabine to gemcitabine plus a second agent. The second agent ranged from chemotherapeutic agents (irinotecan, 5FU, cisplatin, oxaliplatin, pemetrexed), EGFR inhibitor (cetuximab), antiangiogenic agent (bevacizumab, axitinib) or targeted agents (matrix metallopotenase inhibitors or farnysl transferase inhitors). These trials had negative results and consequently, gemcitabine was considered the standard of care for pancreatic cancer for over a decade.

Recently approved nab-Paclitaxel is a 130-nm albumin bound paclitaxel. In a phase I/II trial by Von Hoff *et al.*,[23] nab-Paclitaxel showed synergistic activity with gemcitabine in pancreatic cancer. In addition, nab-Paclitaxel increased the intra-tumor bioavailability of gemcitabine. The concentration of gemcitabine inside the pancreatic tumor was higher when subjects were treated with nab-Paclitaxel and gemcitabine than gemcitabine alone. The natural next step was a randomized phase III study comparing the efficacy of gemcitabine plus nab-Paclitaxel with gemcitabine alone. Von Hoff and colleagues[24] randomized 861 newly diagnosed advanced pancreatic cancer patients from 151 centers in 11 countries into two arms in 1:1 ratio, gemcitabine plus nab-Paclitaxel arm and gemcitabine alone arm. In gemcitabine and nab-Paclitaxel arm, each patient received 30–40 minute intravenous infusion of nab-Paclitaxel 125 mg/m^2 and 30 minute intravenous infusion of gemcitabine 1000 mg/m^2 on days 1, 8, and 15 every 4 weeks until disease progression or development of unacceptable toxicity. Patients in gemcitabine alone arm received 30 minute intravenous infusion of gemcitabine 1000 mg/m^2 on days 1, 8, 15, 22, 29, 36, and 43 followed by 1 week of rest in first cycle (8 weeks) and days 1, 8, and 15 of subsequent cycles every 4 weeks until disease progression or unacceptable toxicity. The primary end point was overall survival and secondary end points were progression-free survival and response rate. Median overall survival was respectively 8.5 and 6.7 months in gemcitabine plus nab-Paclitaxel and gemcitabine alone arms (HR = 0.72, 95% CI: 0.62–0.83, $p < 0.001$). Median progression-free survival was respectively 5.5 and 3.7 months in gemcitabine plus nab-Paclitaxel and gemcitabine alone arms (HR = 0.69; 95% CI: 0.58–0.82, $p < 0.001$). The response rate was 23% in gemcitabine plus nab-Paclitaxel and 7% in gemcitabine alone arm ($p < 0.001$). Gemcitabine and nab-Paclitaxel combination was more toxic than gemcitabine alone. More grade 3 or 4 neutropenia, neutropenic fever, fatigue and peripheral neuropathy were noted among patients treated with gemcitabine and nab-Paclitaxel. Peripheral neuropathy was cumulative and rapidly reversible with temporary discontinuation of nab-Paclitaxel and subsequent dose reduction. Based on this study's result, nab-Paclitaxel was approved for treatment of advanced pancreatic cancer in combination with gemcitabine in early 2014. Gemcitabine and nab-paclitaxel combination has been rapidly accepted in treatment of pancreatic cancer. It has also been frequently used as the backbone in currently ongoing clinical trials.

Gemcitabine and fluoropyrimidines both have clinical activity in pancreatic cancer. In order to study the efficacy of gemcitabine plus capecitabine together, Cunningham and colleagues[25] randomized 533 patients with advanced pancreatic cancer without any prior systemic treatment into two groups, gemcitabine alone and gemcitabine plus capecitabine.

In gemcitabine arm, patients were treated with gemcitabine 1000 mg/m^2 intravenously over 30 minutes on days 1, 8, 15, 22, 29, 36 and 43 of first cycle followed by days 1, 8 and 15 of subsequent cycles (4 weeks each). Patients randomized to gemcitabine plus capecitabine arm received gemcitabine 1000 mg/m^2 intravenously on days 1, 8 and 15 every 4 weeks and capecitabine 830 mg/m^2 by mouth twice daily for 3 weeks followed by one week of rest. Treatment was administered until disease progression or unacceptable toxicities. Primary endpoint was overall survival. Secondary endpoints were progression-free survival and response rate. The results of this study were pooled with other two randomized studies in a meta-analysis. Objective response rate was higher in gemcitabine plus capecitabine arm (19.1% vs. 12.4%, $p = 0.03$). Median progression-free survival was longer in gemcitabine plus capecitabine arm (5.3 vs. 3.8 months, HR = 0.78, 95% CI: 0.66–0.93; $p = 0.004$). Patients treated with gemcitabine plus capecitabine trended to have longer median overall survival compared to patients in gemcitabine alone arm, however it was not statistically significant (7.1 vs. 6.2 months, HR = 0.86, 95% CI: 0.72–1.02; $p = 0.08$). In a pooled meta-analysis of this study with another two randomized trials comparing gemcitabine with gemcitabine plus capecitabine (pooled number of patients 935), there was significant improvement in overall survival in favor of gemcitabine plus capecitabine (HR = 0.86, 95% CI: 0.75–0.98; $p = 0.02$). All the three randomized studies included in the meta-analysis consistently showed better survival in patients treated with gemcitabine and capecitabine. Treatment in both arms was well-tolerated. Patients getting capecitabine with gemcitabine did have increased incidence of hand-foot syndrome. Based on these findings, the combination of gemcitabine and capecitabine should be considered an option for treatment of advanced pancreatic cancer.

A retrospective study from Johns Hopkins group[26] suggested that pancreatic adenocarcinomas in patients with a family history of breast, ovarian or pancreatic cancers were sensitive to platinum. They had substantial improvement in median overall survival when they were treated with platinum-based regimen. If patients with advanced pancreatic cancer have a strong family history of breast, ovarian or pancreatic cancer, they should be considered for treatment with gemcitabine plus cisplatin. However, several randomized phase III studies[27–29] failed to demonstrate superiority of gemcitabine plus cisplatin over gemcitabine alone in advanced pancreatic cancer in general. Gemcitabine has also been studied with 5-FU,[30] S-1,[31] irinotecan,[32] oxaliplatin[21] and bevacizumab,[33] but the addition of these agents to gemcitabine did not improve the clinical outcome.

5-FU-based chemotherapy

As noted earlier, 5-FU has been the mainstay of treatment for advanced pancreatic cancer until the approval of gemcitabine in mid-1990. Capecitabine is an oral form, which gets converted to 5-FU in the body. It is more convenient than 5-FU for patients. We are not aware of a randomized non-inferiority study comparing 5-FU with capecitabine in advanced pancreatic cancer. However, by extrapolation of data from colorectal cancer, it is frequently used as single agent to treat pancreatic cancer, particularly if a patient is unable to tolerate the combination chemotherapy. Combination chemotherapies with 5-FU/capecitabine backbone are preferred over single agent fluoropyrimidines, if patients are expected to tolerate them. In countries where S-1 is available, single agent S-1 can also be used to treat metastatic pancreatic cancer.[31]

5-FU has been used to treat metastatic pancreatic cancer for the last 5–6 decades. Oxaliplatin is effective in pancreatic cancer when combined with 5-FU.[34] Irinotecan also has its clinical activity in pancreatic cancer[35] and if administered before 5-FU, it is synergistic.[36] Oxaliplatin and Irinotecan show synergy *in vitro*.[37] In addition, there is no overlapping toxicity among 5-FU, Leucovorin, Oxaliplatin and Irinotecan. In a phase I study,[38] toxicity of FOLFIRINOX (a combination of 5-FU, Leucovorin, Oxaliplatin and Irinotecan) was acceptable and its efficacy in pancreatic cancer was encouraging. Conroy and colleagues[18] randomized 342 advanced pancreatic cancer patients with no prior treatment into FOLFIRINOX and gemcitabine arms in 1:1 ratio. In FOLFIRINOX arm, patients were treated with FOLFIRINOX (5-FU 400 mg/m^2 as bolus followed by 2400 mg/m^2 as 46 hour infusion, Leucovorin 400 mg/m^2, Oxaliplatin 85 mg/m^2 and Irinotecan 180 mg/m^2) every 2 weeks. In gemcitabine arm, they were treated with gemcitabine 1000 mg/m^2 as 30-minute infusion on days 1, 8, 15, 22, 29, 36 and 43 of 1st cycle (8 weeks) and days 1, 8, 15 of subsequent cycles (4 weeks). Patients in both arms were treated for six months if they had their disease in control. It was a randomized phase II/III study. For phase III study, the primary end point was overall survival and secondary end points were progression-free survival, response rate, safety and quality of life. In FOLFIRINOX and gemcitabine arm, median overall survival was 11.1 and 6.8 months (HR = 0.57, 95% CI: 0.45–0.73; $p < 0.001$), median progression-free survival was 6.4 and 3.3 months (HR = 0.47, 95% CI: 0.37–0.59; $p < 0.001$) and objective response rate 31.6 and 9.4% ($p < 0.001$) respectively. FOLFIRINOX was more toxic. The grade 3 or 4 neutropenia, febrile neutropenia, thrombocytopenia, diarrhea, sensory neuropathy as well as grade 2 alopecia were significantly more frequent in FOLFIRINOX group. Quality of life was better in FOLFIRINOX-treated patients. At six months, 31% of patients in FOLFIRINOX arm had a definitive degradation of the quality of life compared to 66% in gemcitabine arm (HR = 0.47, 95% CI: 0.30–0.70; $p < 0.001$).

FOLFIRINOX provides a groundbreaking improvement in overall survival over gemcitabine. However, it is a toxic regimen. Many patients with borderline performance status at presentation are unable to tolerate this regimen. In order to make FOLFIRINOX more tolerable, different modifications are introduced, i.e. no bolus 5-FU, obligatory primary prophylaxis with myeloid growth factor or dropping either Oxaliplatin or Irinotecan.[39] Critics are concerned that this study may not represent the advanced pancreatic cancer population in general as only 38% of participating patients had primary tumor in head of the pancreas unlike 50–70% in other randomized clinical trials. The reason for decreased participation of patients with pancreatic head mass was strict exclusion criteria that disqualified patients with bilirubin more than 1.5 times normal. However, retrospective studies confirm that FOLFIRINOX is equally effective in patients with lesions in pancreatic head with or without stent.[40] In general, FOLFIRINOX treatment should be considered for patients with good performance status and otherwise healthy.

FOLFOX (5-FU, Leucovorin and Oxaliplatin) and CAPOX (Capecitabine and Oxaliplatin) are frequently used in treatment of pancreatic cancer. Randomized phase III studies confirming the superior efficacy of FOLFOX or CAPOX compared to gemcitabine or Fluoropyrimidines are lacking. In a phase II study of 30 eligible locally advanced or metastatic pancreatic cancer patients with no prior treatments, FOLFOX was clinically active with disease control rate of 62%, median progression-free survival of 4 and overall survival of 7.5 months.[41] The combination of capecitabine and Oxaliplatin was explored in second line setting in metastatic pancreatic cancer refractory to gemcitabine. Xiong and colleagues[42] studied CAPOX (capecitabine 1000 mg/m^2 twice a day for 14 days and Oxaliplatin 130 mg/m^2 given on day 1 of each cycle repeated every 3 weeks) in 39 patients with metastatic pancreatic cancer refractory to gemcitabine in a prospective phase II study. One patient had a partial response and 10 stable diseases. Median overall and progression-free survival respectively were 23 and 9.9 weeks. In general, CAPOX was well-tolerated. 5-FU and Oxaliplatin combination was superior to best supportive care in second-line treatment of pancreatic cancer refractory to gemcitabine.[43] In this phase III study from the German CONKO-study group, Pelzer and colleagues randomized 46 patients with advanced pancreatic cancer with documented disease progression on gemcitabine into two groups, treatment group and best supportive care group. In the treatment group, patients were treated with OFF (folinic acid 200 mg/m^2 followed by 5-FU 2000 mg/m^2 over 24 hours on days 1, 8, 15 and 22; and Oxaliplatin 85 mg/m^2 on days 8 and 22 followed by 3 weeks of rest). The primary endpoint was overall survival. It should be noted that best supportive care was not well-accepted by patients as well as treating physicians and the study was prematurely terminated due to poor accrual. OFF regimen was well-tolerated. Median overall survival from randomization was 4.82 months in OFF treatment group and 2.3 months in best supportive care group. Although terminated prematurely, this study confirms the clinical activity of 5-FU and Oxaliplatin in second-line setting in pancreatic cancer. These studies support the use of FOLFOX or CAPOX in treatment of metastatic pancreatic cancer. Although evidence from randomized phase III studies for efficacy of FOLFOX or CAPOX in first-line treatment of pancreatic cancer is lacking, they are frequently used to treat metastatic pancreatic cancer at several institutions. They are labeled as 2B by NCCN.

Emerging treatment regimens in pancreatic cancer

Many cytotoxic and targeted regimens are in development for pancreatic cancer. It is beyond the scope of this chapter to discuss all the new drugs in development. However, we will briefly discuss a few drugs with high potential. MM-398 is a nanoliposomal encapsulated Irinotecan with improved pharmacokinetics compared to classic Irinotecan in pipeline of Merrimack Pharmaceuticals. In a phase II study,[44] MM-398 was found to have moderate activity in advanced pancreatic cancer patients refractory to gemcitabine with median OS of 5.2 months. A randomized phase III study, NAPOLI-1 comparing MM-398 plus 5-FU to 5-FU alone in gemcitabine refractory patients recently met its primary endpoint. Median overall survival was longer by 1.9 month with addition of MM-398 to 5-FU.[45] An application for registration of MM-398 with FDA is planned in 2014. The microenvironment inside a pancreatic tumor is hypoxic. TH-302 is a prodrug that is activated only under hypoxic conditions. Inside the hypoxic environment of pancreatic tumor, TH-302 is metabolized to bromo isophosphoramide mustard, which forms DNA crosslinks rendering the cancer cells unable to replicate. In a randomized phase II study[46] in untreated advanced pancreatic cancer, addition of TH-302 to gemcitabine improved the median progression-free survival to six months ($HR = 0.589$, $p = 0.008$). Median overall survival trended to be better, although not statistically significant. A randomized phase III MAESTRO trial assessing the efficacy and safety of TH-302 in combination with gemcitabine in previously untreated advanced pancreatic adenocarcinoma is currently ongoing.[47] Addition of bevacizumab[33] and other antiangiogenic compounds to standard cytotoxic chemotherapy did not improve the outcome in pancreatic cancer. Interestingly, sunitinib maintenance after first-line systemic chemotherapy improved the overall survival in a randomized phase II study.[48]

Pancreatic tumors have highly desmoplastic stroma that creates high interstitial fluid pressure. It induces a vascular collapse and presents a substantial barrier to bioavailability of drugs in pancreatic tumor. Hyaluronan is the basic component of desmoplastic stroma. Enzymatic agents, such as PEGPH20 targeting hyaluronan remodels the stroma increasing bioavailability of chemotherapy in pancreatic tumors.[49] In a phase I study, a combination of gemcitabine and PEGPH20 was well-tolerated in patients with metastatic pancreatic adenocarcinoma and response rate was 33%.[50] Phase II studies with PEGPH20 in advanced pancreatic cancer in combination with gemcitabine plus nab-paclitaxel and FOLFIRINOX are ongoing.[47] Inflammation is the hallmark of pancreatic cancer and adversely affects prognosis. JAK/STAT signaling pathway is intricately involved in inflammation. Ruxolitinib, a JAK1 and JAK2 inhibitor is approved for treatment of inflammatory reaction in myelofibrosis. In a randomized phase II study in patients with advanced pancreatic cancer after first-line chemotherapy, addition of ruxolitinib to capecitabine significantly improved median overall survival in patients with elevated CRP[51] and a phase III study is currently ongoing.

Multiple immune checkpoints are targeted in treatment of pancreatic cancer. Le, D and colleagues presented the results of a randomized phase II study in GI symposium of ASCO in 2014.[52] Previously treated metastatic pancreatic ductal adenocarcinoma patients were randomized 2:1 to receive CY/GVAX followed by CRS-207 or CY/GVAX arms. In CY/GVAX → CRS-207 arm, patients received cyclophosphamide to inhibit regulatory T cells, then GVAX intradermally (irradiated GM-CSF secreting allogenic pancreatic cells to elicit broad antigenic response), followed by CRS-207 (live attenuated Listeria monocytogenes which expresses mesothelin and stimulates innate and adaptive immunity). In CY/GVX arm, patients received cyclophosphamide followed by GVAX. The primary endpoint was overall survival. In per protocol analysis, median OS was 9.7 months in Cy/GVAX → CRS-207 arm and 4.6 months in Cy/GVAX arm ($HR = 0.529$, $p = 0.0167$). A three-arm phase 2b randomized study comparing CY/GVAX plus CRS-207, CRS-207 and chemotherapy is ongoing. phase I studies targeting PD1 and PDL1 are also ongoing in pancreatic cancer. Radioimmunotherapy for advanced pancreatic ductal adenocarcinoma is studied in phase III trial. Humanized clivatuzumab tetraxetan (hPAM4) antibody selectively targets pancreatic ductal carcinoma. ^{90}Yttrium labeled humanized clivatuzumab tetraxetan demonstrated promising activity and manageable toxicity in a phase I study of patients with advanced pancreatic cancer refractory to standard chemotherapy.[53] A phase III study (PANCRIT-I) comparing ^{90}Y-clivatuzumab tetraxetan plus low-dose gemcitabine to placebo plus low-dose gemcitabine in patients with metastatic pancreatic adenocarcinoma who received at least two prior treatments is ongoing.[47]

PARP (poly ADP-ribose polymerase) inhibitors are active in ovarian and breast tumors of BRCA mutated patients. Veliparib, a PARP inhibitor is being developed in combination with cisplatin and gemcitabine in a randomized phase II study in BRCA/PALB mutated pancreatic cancer. Hedgehog pathway is abnormally expressed in more than 70% of pancreatic cancer. Vismodegib, a small molecule antagonist to sonic hedgehog in combination with gemcitabine demonstrated encouraging activity in metastatic pancreatic cancer.[54] Similarly, notch 2/3 is activated in pancreatic cancer. OMP-59R5, a notch inhibitor is in Phase II trial with nab-Paclitaxel and gemcitabine.

Supportive treatment in advanced pancreatic ductal adenocarcinoma

As noted earlier, advanced PDAC is an incurable disease and goal of treatment is palliation. In addition, most pancreatic cancer patients are symptomatic and present with jaundice, pain, pancreatic insufficiency, depression, venous thromboembolism, weight loss, anorexia and cachexia. Providing excellent supportive treatment is of paramount importance. Patients with jaundice from obstructed biliary tree may also suffer pruritis or even cholangitis. They should be referred to gastroenterologist with expertise in ERCP (endoscopic retrograde cholangiopancreatography) for stent placement. Many patients with pancreatic cancer present with abdominal pain. Opioid analgesics should be generously used and tailored for patients' comfort. If they have nausea and vomiting, transdermal analgesics should be considered. Celiac neurolysis and radiation alleviate pain and should be considered if opioid analgesics are ineffective. Patients presenting with pancreatic insufficiency (steatorrhea or upset stomach) need pancreatic enzyme replacement. If venous thromboembolism develops in pancreatic cancer patients, lifelong subcutaneous low molecular weight heparin should be administered. Some patients suffer from depression. They should be treated with selective serotonin uptake inhibitors and referred for psychotherapy.

Ductal pancreatic adenocarcinoma (PDAC) is one of the most lethal malignancies. Majority of patients with PDAC present with unresectable locally advanced and metastatic adenocarcinomas. Systemic chemotherapy is the mainstay of treatment of advanced PDAC. Common presenting symptoms include abdominal or back pain, jaundice, weight loss, anorexia, cachexia, depression or diarrhea from pancreatic insufficiency. Objective of treatment in this group of patients is palliative and as such, treatment targeting the symptoms is an essential part of the management plan. The last decade has witnessed significant progress in treatment of metastatic pancreatic cancer. A newly diagnosed patient with advanced pancreatic cancer should be considered for treatment with single agent regimens (gemcitabine, 5-FU and leucovorin or capecitabine) or combination regimens (FOLFIRINOX, FOLFOX, CapOX, gemcitabine plus nab-paclitaxel or gemcitabine plus erlotinib). The decision to use single or combination chemotherapy depends on the patient's performance status and other co-morbidities. In general, patients with excellent performance status and are otherwise healthy should be treated with combination regimens.

Take Home Messages

- Ductal pancreatic adenocarcinoma is a lethal malignancy with median overall survival of less than six months without treatment.
- Patients usually are symptomatic at the time of diagnosis of pancreatic cancer. Supportive treatment to alleviate symptoms should be emphasized.
- The objective of treatment for advanced pancreatic cancer is palliative and mainstay of treatment is chemotherapy. Patients could be considered for gemcitabine- or fluoropyrimidine-based chemotherapy.
- The standard regimens for gemcitabine-based chemotherapy include gemcitabine single agent or gemcitabine plus nab-Paclitaxel or gemcitabine plus erlotinib. Gemcitabine plus capecitabine could also be considered.
- The standard regimens for fluoropyrimidine-based chemotherapy include single agent 5-FU or capecitabine or combination regimens, such as FOLFIRINOX, FOLFOX or CAPOX.

References

1. Siegel, R. *et al.*, Cancer statistics, 2014. *CA Cancer J Clin*, 2014. **64**(1): 9–29.
2. Bosetti, C. *et al.*, Cigarette smoking and pancreatic cancer: An analysis from the International Pancreatic Cancer Case-Control Consortium (Panc4). *Ann Oncol*, 2012. **23**(7): 1880–8.

3. Mancuso, T.F., and el-Attar, A.A., Cohort study of workers exposed to beta-naphthylamine and benzidine. *J Occup Med*, 1967. **9**(6): 277–85.
4. Thiebaut, A.C. *et al.*, Dietary fatty acids and pancreatic cancer in the NIH-AARP diet and health study. *J Natl Cancer Inst*, 2009. **101**(14): 1001–11.
5. Larsson, S.C. and Wolk, A., Red and processed meat consumption and risk of pancreatic cancer: meta-analysis of prospective studies. *Br J Cancer*, 2012. **106**(3): 603–7.
6. Li, D. *et al.*, Body mass index and risk, age of onset, and survival in patients with pancreatic cancer. *JAMA*, 2009. **301**(24): 2553–62.
7. Lucenteforte, E. *et al.*, Alcohol consumption and pancreatic cancer: A pooled analysis in the International Pancreatic Cancer Case-Control Consortium (PanC4). *Ann Oncol*, 2012. **23**(2): 374–82.
8. Lowenfels, A.B. *et al.*, Pancreatitis and the risk of pancreatic cancer. International Pancreatitis Study Group. *N Engl J Med*, 1993. **328**(20): 1433–7.
9. Wolpin, B.M. *et al.*, Plasma 25-hydroxyvitamin D and risk of pancreatic cancer. *Cancer Epidemiol Biomarkers Prev*, 2012. **21**(1): 82–91.
10. Whelan, A.J., Bartsch, D., Goodfellow, P.J., Brief report: a familial syndrome of pancreatic cancer and melanoma with a mutation in the CDKN2 tumor-suppressor gene. *N Engl J Med*, 1995. **333**(15): 975–7.
11. Iqbal, J. *et al.*, The incidence of pancreatic cancer in BRCA1 and BRCA2 mutation carriers. *Br J Cancer*, 2012. **107**(12): 2005–9.
12. Slater, E.P. *et al.*, PALB2 mutations in European familial pancreatic cancer families. *Clin Genet*, 2010. **78**(5): 490–4.
13. Lindor, N.M. *et al.*, Pancreatic cancer and a novel MSH2 germline alteration. *Pancreas*, 2011. **40**(7): 1138–40.
14. Roberts, N.J. *et al.*, ATM mutations in patients with hereditary pancreatic cancer. *Cancer Discov*, 2012. **2**(1): 41–6.
15. Giardiello, F.M. *et al.*, Very high risk of cancer in familial Peutz-Jeghers syndrome. *Gastroenterology*, 2000. **119**(6): 1447–53.
16. Win, A.K. *et al.*, Colorectal and other cancer risks for carriers and noncarriers from families with a DNA mismatch repair gene mutation: A prospective cohort study. *J Clin Oncol*, 2012. **30**(9): 958–64.
17. Canto, M.I. *et al.*, International Cancer of the Pancreas Screening (CAPS) Consortium summit on the management of patients with increased risk for familial pancreatic cancer. *Gut*, 2013. **62**(3): 339–47.
18. Conroy, T. *et al.*, FOLFIRINOX versus gemcitabine for metastatic pancreatic cancer. *N Eng J Med*, 2011. **364**(19): 1817–25.

19. Burris, H.A. 3rd, *et al.*, Improvements in survival and clinical benefit with gemcitabine as first-line therapy for patients with advanced pancreas cancer: a randomized trial. *J Clin Oncol*, 1997. **15**(6): 2403–13.
20. Touroutoglou, N. *et al.*, Clinical results of a pharmacodynamically-based strategy for higher dosing of gemcitabine in patients with solid tumors. *Ann Oncol*, 1998. **9**(9): 1003–8.
21. Poplin, E. *et al.*, Phase III, randomized study of gemcitabine and oxaliplatin versus gemcitabine (fixed-dose rate infusion) compared with gemcitabine (30-minute infusion) in patients with pancreatic carcinoma E6201: A trial of the Eastern Cooperative Oncology Group. *J Clin Oncol*, 2009. **27**(23): 3778–85.
22. Moore, M.J. *et al.*, Erlotinib plus gemcitabine compared with gemcitabine alone in patients with advanced pancreatic cancer: A phase III trial of the National Cancer Institute of Canada Clinical Trials Group. *J Clin Oncol*, 2007. **25**(15): 1960–6.
23. Von Hoff, D.D. *et al.*, Gemcitabine plus nab-paclitaxel is an active regimen in patients with advanced pancreatic cancer: A phase I/II trial. *J Clin Oncol*, 2011. **29**(34): 4548–54.
24. Von Hoff, D.D. *et al.*, Increased survival in pancreatic cancer with nab-paclitaxel plus gemcitabine. *N Engl J Med*, 2013. **369**(18): 1691–703.
25. Cunningham, D., *et al.*, Phase III randomized comparison of gemcitabine versus gemcitabine plus capecitabine in patients with advanced pancreatic cancer. *J Clin Oncol*, 2009. **27**(33): 5513–8.
26. Oliver, G.R., Laheru, D., Sugar, E., Diaz, L.A., Family history of cancer and sensitivity to platinum chemotherapy in pancreatic adenocarcinoma. *2010 Gastrointestinal Cancers Symposium*, 2010: Abstract no. 180.
27. Heinemann, V. *et al.*, Randomized phase III trial of gemcitabine plus cisplatin compared with gemcitabine alone in advanced pancreatic cancer. *J Clin Oncol*, 2006. **24**(24): 3946–52.
28. Colucci, G. *et al.*, Randomized phase III trial of gemcitabine plus cisplatin compared with single-agent gemcitabine as first-line treatment of patients with advanced pancreatic cancer: The GIP-1 study. *J Clin Oncol*, 2010. **28**(10): 1645–51.
29. Chao, Y. *et al.*, A randomized controlled trial of gemcitabine plus cisplatin versus gemcitabine alone in the treatment of metastatic pancreatic cancer. *Cancer Chemother Pharmacol*, 2013. **72**(3): 637–42.
30. Berlin, J.D. *et al.*, Phase III study of gemcitabine in combination with fluorouracil versus gemcitabine alone in patients with advanced pancreatic

carcinoma: Eastern Cooperative Oncology Group Trial E2297. *J Clin Oncol*, 2002. **20**(15): 3270–5.

31. Ueno, H. *et al.*, Randomized phase III study of gemcitabine plus S-1, S-1 alone, or gemcitabine alone in patients with locally advanced and metastatic pancreatic cancer in Japan and Taiwan: GEST study. *J Clin Oncol*, 2013. **31**(13): 1640–8.
32. Stathopoulos, G.P. *et al.*, A multicenter phase III trial comparing irinotecan-gemcitabine (IG) with gemcitabine (G) monotherapy as first-line treatment in patients with locally advanced or metastatic pancreatic cancer. *Br J Cancer*, 2006. **95**(5): 587–92.
33. Kindler, H.L. *et al.*, Gemcitabine plus bevacizumab compared with gemcitabine plus placebo in patients with advanced pancreatic cancer: Phase III trial of the Cancer and Leukemia Group B (CALGB 80303). *J Clin Oncol*, 2010. **28**(22): 3617–22.
34. Ducreux, M. *et al.*, Randomized phase II study evaluating oxaliplatin alone, oxaliplatin combined with infusional 5-FU, and infusional 5-FU alone in advanced pancreatic carcinoma patients. *Ann Oncol*, 2004. **15**(3): 467–73.
35. Ueno, H. *et al.*, A phase II study of weekly irinotecan as first-line therapy for patients with metastatic pancreatic cancer. *Cancer Chemother Pharmacol*, 2007. **59**(4): 447–54.
36. Azrak, R.G. *et al.*, Therapeutic synergy between irinotecan and 5-fluorouracil against human tumor xenografts. *Clin Cancer Res*, 2004. **10**(3): 1121–9.
37. Zeghari-Squalli, N. *et al.*, Cellular pharmacology of the combination of the DNA topoisomerase I inhibitor SN-38 and the diaminocyclohexane platinum derivative oxaliplatin. *Clin Cancer Res*, 1999. **5**(5): 1189–96.
38. Ychou, M. *et al.*, An open phase I study assessing the feasibility of the triple combination: oxaliplatin plus irinotecan plus leucovorin/5-fluorouracil every 2 weeks in patients with advanced solid tumors. *Ann Oncol*, 2003. **14**(3): 481–9.
39. Bekaii-Saab, T. and Goldberg, R.M., FOLFIRINOX in locally advanced pancreas adenocarcinoma: back to the future? *Oncologist*, 2013. **18**(5): 487–9.
40. Mahaseth, H. *et al.*, Modified FOLFIRINOX regimen with improved safety and maintained efficacy in pancreatic adenocarcinoma. *Pancreas*, 2013. **42**(8): 1311–5.
41. Ghosn, M. *et al.*, FOLFOX-6 combination as the first-line treatment of locally advanced and/or metastatic pancreatic cancer. *Am J Clin Oncol*, 2007. **30**(1): 15–20.

42. Xiong, H.Q. *et al.*, Phase 2 trial of oxaliplatin plus capecitabine (XELOX) as second-line therapy for patients with advanced pancreatic cancer. *Cancer*, 2008. **113**(8): 2046–52.
43. Pelzer, U. *et al.*, Best supportive care (BSC) versus oxaliplatin, folinic acid and 5-fluorouracil (OFF) plus BSC in patients for second-line advanced pancreatic cancer: A phase III-study from the German CONKO-study group. *Eur J Cancer*, 2011. **47**(11): 1676–81.
44. Ko, A.H. *et al.*, A multinational phase 2 study of nanoliposomal irinotecan sucrosofate (PEP02, MM-398) for patients with gemcitabine-refractory metastatic pancreatic cancer. *Br J Cancer*, 2013. **109**(4): 920–5.
45. http://www.marketwatch.com/story/merrimack-pharmaceuticals-announces-mm-398-achieves-primary-endpoint-of-overall-survival-in-phase-3-trial-in-post-gemcitabine-metastatic-pancreatic-cancer-2014-05-01.
46. Borad, MJ, Reddy, S., Bahary, N., Uronis, H., Sigal, D.S., Cohn, A.L., Schelman, W.R., Stephenson, J., Chiorean, E.G., Rosen, P.J., Ulrich, B., Dragovich, T., Prete, S.D., TH-302 plus gemcitabine vs. gemcitabine in patients with untreated advanced pancreatic adenocarcinoma. *ESMO 2012 Congress (Abstract 6660)*, 2012.
47. www.clinicaltrials.gov (accessed July 21, 2014).
48. Reni, M. *et al.*, Maintenance sunitinib or observation in metastatic pancreatic adenocarcinoma: A phase II randomised trial. *Eur J Cancer*, 2013. **49**(17): 3609–15.
49. Provenzano, P.P. *et al.*, Enzymatic targeting of the stroma ablates physical barriers to treatment of pancreatic ductal adenocarcinoma. *Cancer Cell*, 2012. **21**(3): 418–29.
50. Hingorani, S.R., Harris, W.P., Beck, J.T., Berdov, B.A., Wanger, S.A., Pshevlotsky, E.M., Tjulandin, S., Gladkov, O., Holcombe, R.F., Jiang, P., Maneval, D.C., Zhu, J., Devoe, C.E., A phase Ib study of gemcitabine plus PEGPH20 (pegylated recombinant human hyaluronidase) in patients with stage IV previously untreated pancreatic cancer. *J Clin Oncol* 31, 2013 (suppl; abstr 4010).
51. Hurwitz, H., Uppal, N., Wagner, S.A., Bendell, J.C., Beck, J.T., Wade, S., Nemunaitis, J.J., Stella, P.J., Pipas, J.M., Clark, J., Leopold, L., Levy, R.S., Sandor, V., A randomized double-blind phase 2 study of ruxolitinib (RUX) or placebo (PBO) with capecitabine (CAPE) as second-line therapy in

patients (pts) with metastatic pancreatic cancer (mPC). *J Clin Oncol* 32:5s, 2014 (suppl; abstr 4000).

52. Le, D.T., Wang-Gillam, A., Picozzi Jr, V., Greten, T.F., Crocenzi, T.S., Springett, G.M., Morse, M., Zeh, H., Cohen, D.J., Fine, R.L., Onners, B., Uram, J.N., Laheru, D., Murphy, A., Skoble, J., Lemmens, E., Grous, J.J., Dubensky, T., Brockstedt, D.G., Jaffee, E.M., A phase 2, randomized trial of GVAX pancreas and CRS-207 immunotherapy versus GVAX alone in patients with metastatic pancreatic adenocarcinoma: Updated results. *J Clin Oncol* 32, 2014 (suppl 3; abstr 177).
53. Ocean, A.J. *et al.*, Fractionated radioimmunotherapy with (90) Y-clivatuzumab tetraxetan and low-dose gemcitabine is active in advanced pancreatic cancer: A phase I trial. *Cancer*, 2012. **118**(22): 5497–506.
54. Catenacci, D.V.T., Bahary, N., Edelman, M.J., Nattam, S.R., Marsh, R.W., Kaubisch, A., Wallace, J.A., Cohen, D.J., Stiff, P.J., Sleckman, B.G., Thomas, S.P., Lenz, H.-J., Henderson, L., Zagaya, C., Vannier, M., Karrison, T., Stadler, W.M., Kindler, H.L., A phase IB/randomized phase II study of gemcitabine (G) plus placebo (P) or vismodegib (V), a hedgehog (Hh) pathway inhibitor, in patients (pts) with metastatic pancreatic cancer (PC): Interim analysis of a University of Chicago phase II consortium study. *J Clin Oncol* 30, 2012 (suppl; abstr 4022), 2012.

Chapter 17

Diagnosis of Hepatobiliary Malignancies

Xu Shu, Xu Guo, Viginia O. Shaffer,
Jinghua Hao and Qiang Cai

What is New

- Growing evidence indicates that metabolic conditions, such as diabetes and obesity, are associated with the rising incidence of hepatocellular carcinoma.
- When conventional staining for the sample of liver lesion is not conclusive, two immunoreactive markers (out of glypican-3, heat-shock protein-70 and glutamine synthetase) are recommended as useful diagnostic combination for hepatocellular carcinoma detection.
- If other imaging examinations cannot give a diagnosis of cholangiocarcinoma, the combination use of endoscopic ultrasonography (EUS) and the cholangioscopy (SpyGlass) can provide a conclusive diagnosis for a majority of patients and minimize the incidences of adverse events.

Hepatobiliary malignancies include hepatocellular carcinoma and biliary tract cancer (gallbladder and cholangiocarcinoma). Due to the high morbidity and mortality, hepatobiliary malignancies are important health issues. In 2014, about 33,190 people will be diagnosed with liver cancer and intrahepatic cholangiocarcinoma and 10,310 people with gallbladder cancer or other biliary tract cancer in the United States. There will be about 23,000 deaths from liver cancer or intrahepatic cholangiocarcinoma, and 3,630 deaths from gallbladder cancer or other biliary tract cancer.[1]

Hepatocellular Carcinoma

Hepatocellular carcinoma (HCC) refers to cancer cells from the liver cells and is the most common form of primary liver cancer. Because of insidious onset, most patients have advanced stage or distant metastasis when diagnosed HCC. Annually, HCC is diagnosed in more than half a million people all over the world. HCC ranks as fifth most common carcinoma in men and seventh in women.[2] HCC is the third leading cause of cancer-related mortality worldwide and the ninth leading cause of cancer deaths with the fastest growing in the United States.[3,4] By region, the incidence of HCC is divided into three main geographic subgroups: (1) sub-Saharan Africa; (2) eastern Asia; and (3) North and South America, northern Europe, and Oceania.[5] About 85% of the patients were in developing countries. HCC ordinarily occurs after 40 years of age. The mean age of diagnosis is approximately 65 years in the United States. The worldwide male to female incidence ratio is usually between 2:1 and 4:1.[5–7]

Etiology and risk factors

The following factors are related to the incidence of HCC according to epidemiological surveys and studies of molecular biology.

Viral infections

Chronic viral infections are the most important risk factors of HCC, including hepatitis B virus (HBV) and hepatitis C virus (HCV) infection. HBV and HCV infection account for estimated 78% of liver cancer cases worldwide.[8] About 0.1% to 2% of patients with chronic hepatitis B can develop cirrhosis each year, depending on the duration of HBV replication and other coexisting risks. In those patients who have developed cirrhosis, the risk of developing HCC annually is about 2–10%.[9] Hepatitis B e antigen (HBeAg) and hepatitis B surface antigen (HBsAg)-positive increase the risk of HCC in patients with chronic HBV infection.[10] The risk of HCC can be better predicted with the combination of detection of HBsAg and HBV-DNA level.[11] The incidence of HCC is significantly increased in the patients with HCV infection. Compared with HCV-negative controls, HCC risk is increased approximately 17-fold in those infected with HCV.[12] The annual incidence of HCC is from 2% to 8% in patients with HCV-related cirrhosis. The risk of HCC is particularly high with the infection of HBV and HCV at the same time.[13] However, there are regional differences between the dominant viral infections for HCC. In Asia and Africa, HBV infection is a major cause, while in Europe and South America, the major cause is mainly HCV infection.[14]

Aflatoxin

Dietary exposure to fungal aflatoxin increases the risk for development of HCC. The incidence of HCC is high in the areas where food is severely polluted by aflatoxin according to epidemiological survey.[15] The metabolite aflatoxin B1 has a strong carcinogenic effect. So far, aflatoxin is known to be the strongest natural carcinogens. It can make a variety of animals liver cancer, suggesting that aflatoxin may be a risk factor of HCC. In addition, the aflatoxin are synergistic with chronic HBV infection for the development of HCC.[16]

Cirrhosis

Cirrhosis from any cause, including chronic viral hepatitis, alcohol, nonalcoholic fatty liver disease, genetics and metabolic diseases (such as hemochromatosis or α-1 antitrypsin deficiency), is closely associated with HCC. Overall, 1/3 patients with cirrhosis progress to HCC.[17] The cumulative risk at five years for patients with cirrhosis to develop HCC is between 5% and 30%, depending on the cause, with the greatest risk among those viral hepatitis and lower risk among those autoimmune hepatitis.[13,18]

Nonalcoholic fatty liver disease

Growing evidence indicates that the majority of "cryptogenic" HCC in the United States is attributed to NAFLD.[19] Some HCC patients, without chronic HBV or HCV infection, have clinical or biochemical alterations in accordance with NAFLD, such as obesity or metabolic syndrome.[20] In population-based cohort studies, HCC is 1.5 to 2.0 times more frequent in obese than in non-obese patients.[21,22] Diabetes also appears to increase the risk of HCC, which is independent of alcohol use or viral hepatitis, and such risk is correlated with a long duration of diabetes.[23,24] NAFLD, which is present in most obese individuals and individuals with type 2 diabetes, appears to increase HCC risk predominantly in individuals with cirrhosis.[25,26] There is a growing metabolic syndrome epidemic in the United States, which will lead to large increases in the incidence of HCC over the next decades.[19]

Surveillance for hepatocellular carcinoma

Surveillance for HCC consists of the regular application of a diagnostic test to target population at risk for developing HCC. The purpose of screening test is to detect early the presence of HCC in an asymptomatic individual. Consequently, patients who get an early diagnosis have more treatment choices and a better prognosis. A randomized controlled trial from China indicated that biannual screening reduced HCC mortality by 37%.[27] Based on the risk factors of HCC, patients with chronic hepatitis B and C and non-viral liver cirrhosis are defined as high-risk populations for HCC in The American Association for the Study of Liver Diseases (AASLD) guidelines. Patients with liver cirrhosis types B and C are defined as a super-high-risk population (Table 1). Risk factors other than hepatitis virus or liver cirrhosis are also proposed (Table 1).[28]

The serum alpha-fetoprotein (AFP) level testing and liver ultrasonography examination are the most commonly used methods for screening HCC. Serum AFP is often elevated in patients with HCC, but its sensitivity is estimated at 41% to 65%, which diminish the utility for detecting early-stage tumors.[29,30] AFP alone should not be used for screening unless ultrasound is not available. Other later serum tumor markers, including

Table 1. Definition of populations at high risk for HCC and other risks for HCC.

A. Super-high-risk population
• Hepatitis B-related liver cirrhosis
• Hepatitis C-related liver cirrhosis
B. High-risk population
• Chronic hepatitis B
• Chronic hepatitis C
• Liver cirrhosis (causes other than HBV or HCV)
C. Other risks
• Older age
• Male gender
• Diabetes mellitus
• High body mass index (BMI)
• High AST
• High ALT
• Low platelet count (PLT)
• Heavy alcohol drinker
• High viral load (HBV carrier)

the AFP-L3 isoform and the des-gamma-carboxyprothrombin (DCP), have not shown the superiority compared with AFP for the diagnosis of early and very early stage HCC, but may be useful when utilized in combination with ultrasonography and AFP.[31] Ultrasonography is relatively inexpensive, noninvasive, and accurate in the detection of early stage HCC. One study indicates that ultrasonography is a better way for screening HCC than AFP testing.[32] Nevertheless, since ultrasonography is highly operator dependent, the addition of AFP can enhance the probability of detecting HCC in a screening program. Although computed tomography (CT) and magnetic resonance imaging (MRI) are effective imaging modalities for the diagnosis of HCC, they are not recommended for routine surveillance but may be preferred if adequate ultrasound images cannot be obtained because of technical reasons or body habitus. The 2010

AASLD guidelines recommend that surveillance be performed using US at 6-month intervals, while National Comprehensive Cancer Network guidelines recommend periodic screening with ultrasound and AFP testing every 6 to 12 months for patients at risk for HCC.[28,33]

Clinical manifestations of hepatocellular carcinoma

Subclinical HCC is typically asymptomatic and difficult to diagnose. Patients with early stage HCC are usually detected in the surveillance program. A small number of patients may have abdominal distension and pain, fatigue, anorexia and other symptoms associated with chronic underlying liver disease. Therefore, those who have above symptoms with HCC risk factors should be taken into account the likelihood of liver cancer. The patients are usually diagnosed as advanced liver cancer once they have typical symptoms.

Right upper quadrant pain is the most common and important symptom of HCC. The pain often appears intermittent, persistent, dull, tenderness and severe with increasing progression of the disease. The pain location is closely related to the lesion location. Right upper quarter rib pain is present with the lesion in the right lobe of liver, while xiphoid pain with left lobe. The main reason for pain is the tension of liver capsule caused by the growth of tumor. Acute severe abdominal pain and peritoneal irritation are associated with spontaneous rupture of liver subcapsular cancer nodules.

HCC fever is generally about 37.5–38°C and appears intermittently or persistently. It has a similar presentation of a liver abscess, but there are no chills and antibiotics is ineffective. The fever may be related to the absorption of tumor necrosis, cholangitis or other infections. In contrast to fever, night sweats are quite common in advanced HCC and indicate a poor prognosis.

Some symptoms, such as anorexia, indigestion, nausea, fatigue, vomiting and diarrhea, are easily overlooked due to the lack of specificity. Some patients with advanced HCC can present with jaundice, cachexia, bleeding tendency (gums, nose bleeding and subcutaneous ecchymosis, etc.), upper gastrointestinal bleeding, or hepatic encephalopathy.

Normally, metastatic complications of HCC are similar to the metastatic complications of other neoplastic diseases. Corresponding clinical symptoms can appear according to the metastatic sites, such as coughing caused by pulmonary metastases, chest pain and bloody pleural effusion caused by pleural metastasis, headache caused by pituitary metastases, and pathologic fractures caused by bone metastases.

Paraneoplastic syndromes in HCC are rare but include hypoglycemia, hypercalcemia, erythrocytosis, thrombophlebitis migrans, arterial hypertension, and the syndrome of watery diarrhea, hypokalemia, and achlorhydria.[34] One of the important syndromes is hypoglycemia, which occurs in less than 5% of patients, appears as severe hypoglycemia early in the course of HCC, and is considered to be mediated by insulin-like growth factors.[35,36] Patients with HCC may present with hypercalcemia in the absence of osteolytic metastases. The probable cause is secretion of parathyroid hormone–related protein (PTHrP) by the tumor. Erythrocytosis is due to the generation of erythropoietin or an erythropoietin-like substance by malignant hepatic cells.

In the early stage of HCC, most patients have no obvious signs. Hepatomegaly and jaundice commonly appear in advanced HCC.[37] If HCC patients have the background of cirrhosis, signs of portal hypertension, such as varicosity of abdominal wall, splenomegaly and ascites can be found.

Symptoms and signs of hepatocellular carcinoma are shown in Fig. 1.

Blood tests

Liver cancer (HCC) can demonstrate abnormalities in the aspartate aminotransferase (AST or GOT) and glutamic acid aminotransferase (alanine aminotransferase, ALT or GPT), serum alkaline phosphatase (AKP), lactate dehydrogenase (LDH) or elevated bilirubin. The positive results in the Hepatitis B surface antigen or five quantitative examination, including HBsAg, HBeAg, HbsAb, HBeAb and anti-HBc or hepatitis C antibodies (anti-HCV IgG, anti-HCVst, anti-HCVns and anti-HCV IgM) are also important symbols of hepatitis virus infection; while HBV-DNA and HCV-mRNA can reflect hepatitis viral load. However, these tests do not distinguish HCC from other hepatic mass lesions or cirrhosis.

Serum AFP is a specific tumor marker of HCC and commonly used in liver cancer screening, early diagnosis, postoperative monitoring and

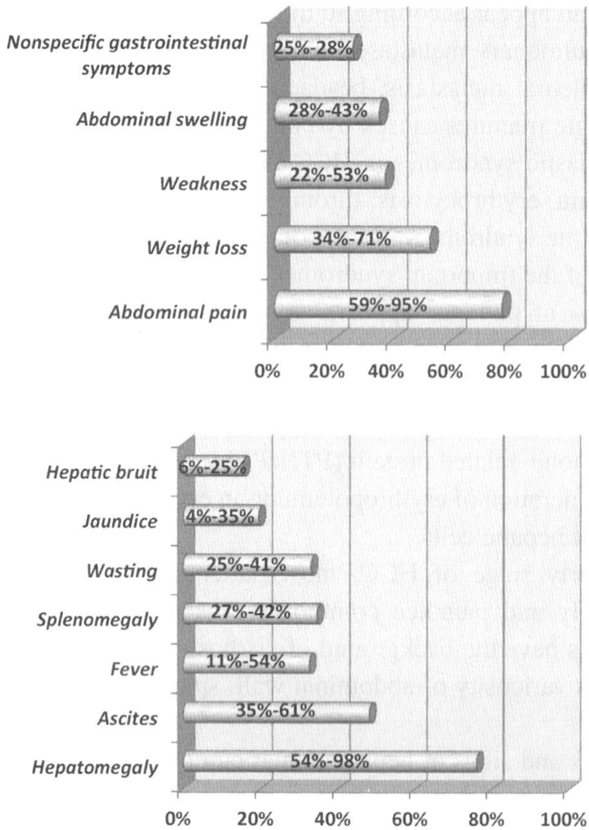

Fig. 1. Symptoms and signs of hepatocellular carcinoma.

follow-up. High serum levels of AFP strongly suggests the presence of HCC especially in Chinese and black African patients in whom HCC is most prevalent.[38,39] An AFP level higher than 200μg/L is highly suggestive of HCC.[38,40] Although AFP has been widely used as a serum tumor marker for HCC, its sensitivity and specificity are not high.[41] False-positive and false-negative results limit the usefulness of AFP. AFP is increased in patients with hepatitis and chronic liver disease without HCC.[42] In addition, it is less likely to increase in some 30–40% of HCC, including well-differentiated or poorly differentiated HCC, small size or liquefaction necrosis HCC. Therefore, the search for an ideal marker continues. Lens culinaris agglutinin-reactive AFP (AFP-L3), an isoform of AFP, appears to be highly specific with low serum AFP levels.[43–45] Another tumor marker being used is Des-gamma-carboxyprothrombin (DCP), an abnormal form of prothrombin, has also shown promise in the diagnosis of HCC.[46] However, it seems none of these biomarkers is considered optimal and is not recommended by the AASLD.[31,40,47] The latter studies show the accuracy of AFP, AFP-L3, DCP in combination was higher than that of any test in isolation.[30,48,49]

Imaging

Abdominal ultrasonography (US)

Because abdominal ultrasonography (US) examination is simple, direct, non-invasive and inexpensive, US examination has become the most important method in the liver surveillance. This method can determine the presence or absence of liver occurrence lesions, suggest its nature, identify if it is liquid or a substantive lesions, make clear foci in the liver specific location and its relationship with major hepatic blood vessels and help to understand the spread and invasion of liver lesions in adjacent tissues and other organs. It also has significant value in the differential diagnosis of liver cancer, liver cysts, liver hemangiomas, and other hepatic diseases.[50] However, the sensitivity and accuracy of abdominal US can be affected by the equipment used, anatomical site, techniques and experience of the operator and other factors. A systematic review has shown that US has 60% (95% CI 44–76) sensitivity, 97% (95% CI 95–98) specificity in detection of liver cancer.[51] About two thirds of symptomatic HCC are uniformly hyperechoic, whereas the others are partially hyperechoic and partially hypoechoic.[52] Real-time US imaging (ultrasound contrast CEUS) can dynamically observe the hemodynamics of the lesion and help to improve the accuracy of diagnosis. On the other hand intraoperative US directly from the surface of the liver during laparotomy exploration can avoid abdominal US attenuation and interference from ribs, which can be used to detected small hepatic lesions undiscovered in preoperative imaging process.

Computer tomography (CT)

Currently, CT scan is the most important imaging method for the diagnosis and differential diagnosis of liver cancer and can be used in detecting the morphology and blood supply, staging, evaluation after treatment of liver cancer. Multi-slice spiral CT is of high-resolution and can complete the whole liver scan within a few seconds to avoid respiratory motion artifacts. It is capable of performing multi-phase dynamic enhanced scanning with a minimum slice thickness of 0.5 mm, which can significantly improve the sensitivity and accuracy of detecting the small lesions of HCC. CT is used to characterize the nature of the lesion and identify whether there are foci in the surrounding liver tissues and organs, which is helpful for localization in radiotherapy. Enhanced CT scan can clearly show the number, size, shape and characteristics of the lesion, the relationship of the lesion with the major blood vessels, the existence of the enlargement lymph nodes in peritoneal cavity and the invasion of adjacent organs. Liver examinations in the diagnosis of HCC should include four phases: one phase without and three phases with contrast enhancement — one in the arterial phase (30 to 35 seconds after starting the injection), one in the portal phase (75 to 90 seconds) and one in the late phase (3 minutes).[53] HCC is usually detected to be a hypodense mass with clear or fuzzy edges, a central necrosis with liquefaction in large lesions. The most common form is single or a small number (3 to 4) of nodular lesions. The typical diagnostic pattern for HCC is a combination of enhancement in the arterial phase (with the uninvolved liver lacking enhancement), loss of central nodule enhancement compared with the uninvolved liver (washout), and capsular enhancement in the portal-venous and delayed phases.[47] This characteristic appearance is increasingly common in lesions over 2 cm in size.

Magnetic resonance imaging (MRI)

The advantages of MRI are non-radioactive and high tissue resolution. MRI is superior to CT and US in detecting the internal changes in the organizational structure of liver lesions, such as hemorrhage and necrosis, fatty degeneration and envelope existence, and very useful in the discrimination of benign and malignant liver lesions, especially for hepatic hemangioma. MRI is the best examination to detect and characterize different nodules in cirrhosis.[54] With growing popularity and development of high-field MRI equipment, MRI has been significantly improved in scan speed and can complete thin-layer, multi-phase, dynamic contrast-enhanced scans to fully display the features of lesions in minutes. Furthermore, functional imaging techniques and the application of hepatocyte-specific contrast agent can provide valuable additional information to improve HCC foci detection and improve the diagnostic sensitivity and accuracy. The pooled estimate of sensitivity and specificity for detecting HCC by MRI is 80.6% (95% CI, 70% to 91%) and 84.8% (95% CI, 77% to 93%), respectively.[51] MRI is slightly superior overall to CT.

Selective hepatic artery digital subtraction angiography (DSA)

The significance of hepatic artery DSA lies not only in the diagnosis and differential diagnosis of HCC, but also in providing valuable information to evaluate the possibility of surgical successful resection and other reasonable treatments. Hepatic artery DSA can clearly demonstrate small hepatic lesions and their blood supplies. The major Hepatic artery DSA findings in HCC are: (1) tumor blood vessels; (2) tumor staining; (3) displacement and distortion of intrahepatic arteries in larger tumors; (4) intrahepatic arteries being serrated and beaded due to the invasion of HCC; and (5) arteriovenous fistula.[50] Because Hepatic artery DSA is an invasive examination, its diagnostic role in HCC has decreased since the advent and development of CT and MRI. However, Hepatic artery DSA is essential for delineating the hepatic arterial anatomy in planning embolization of the lesion or infusion of cytotoxic drugs directly into the hepatic artery or its branches.

Positron emission tomography (PET-CT)

PET-CT is a blend made of PET and CT imaging systems. PET functional imaging can reflect the biochemical metabolic information of the hepatic tumor, and CT imaging can be performed to locate precisely the lesion. A whole body scan can elucidate the situation and assess the metastasis for the purpose of early detection of lesions. PET-CT scan is also valuable before and after cancer treatment.[55] 18F-Fluorodeoxyglucose (18F-FDG) is the most common clinical PET tracer, but it is not critical for the diagnosis of HCC. Studies show that 18F-FDG PET detection of HCC is mainly limited to tumor size. For lesions less than 5 cm the detection rate is 25%, compared to 100% for lesions greater than or equal to 5 cm.[56] The clinical diagnostic sensitivity and specificity of PET-CT for HCC needs to be improved. Because PET-CT is very expensive and low sensitivity in smaller liver lesions, it is not recommended as a routine examination for liver cancer. However, PET-CT scan can be used not only for staging but also as a tool for preoperative prediction of cellular differentiation in patients with HCC.[57] It is also useful to assess whether there is distant metastases prior to liver transplantation and can be served as a complement to other methods.

Liver biopsy

Imaging has a crucial role in the diagnosis of HCC. If a lesion in a cirrhotic patient does not have the typical feature of HCC in CT or MRI scan, then liver biopsy is necessary. US-guided percutaneous core needle biopsy (Core biopsy) and fine-needle aspiration (FNA) are used for histological or cytological examination of liver cancers. FNA has the advantage of a lower complication rate, especially when sampling tumors located deeply or near major blood vessels. Although a core biopsy is a more invasive procedure, it is capable of providing pathologic information of both tissue architecture and cell morphology. Moreover, immunohistochemical tests can be taken on the paraffin wax embedded sample.[30] Undoubtedly, histopathology and/or cytology diagnosis of HCC is the gold standard. However, the value of biopsy to diagnose HCC is limited by tumor size.[14] A study reported only 60% positive result for the first liver biopsy on a tumor less than or equal to 2 cm.[58] Also, it is very difficult to distinguish well-differentiated HCC from dysplastic nodules by biopsy.[59] Therefore, when conventional staining is not conclusive, two immunoreactive markers (out of glypican-3, heat-shock protein-70 and glutamine synthetase) are recommended as the most useful diagnostic combination for HCC detection.[60] Early liver tumors are vaguely nodular and are characterized by major histologic features such as increased cell density (>x2) with increased nuclear/cytoplasm ratio and irregular thin-trabecular pattern, varying numbers of portal tracts within the nodule, pseudoglandular pattern, diffuse fatty change, varying number of unpaired arteries, and stromal invasion.[59] Liver biopsy should be performed with great caution to prevent needle tract bleeding and spreading of cancer cells. Contraindications include a clear tendency to bleed, suffering from severe heart, lung, brain or kidney diseases.

Diagnosis modalities

HCC is the only type of cancer that can be diagnosed with clinical criteria, which is accepted widely. AFP level are not recommended as a tool for HCC diagnosis in America while it is still recommended by the latest guidelines of China and Japan.[28,47,50] Diagnostic HCC imaging involves the use of one or more of the following modalities: 4-phase helical CT; 4-phase dynamic contrast-enhanced MRI; or contrast-enhanced US (CEUS).[61] Typical HCC imaging profile is characterized by intense arterial uptake or enhancement followed by contrast washout in the venous/delayed phase at CT or MRI.[58,61] For liver lesions <1 cm, if the lesions are enlarging according to size, CT or MRI should be used to evaluate every 3 to 6 months.[62] Patients with lesions stable in size should be followed with ultrasound at intervals from 3–6 months, then returning to routine surveillance program after two years of stability. For liver nodules larger than 1 cm, a single dynamic imaging examination with typical findings is sufficient for HCC diagnosis. If appearances are not characteristic or if the vascular pattern is not typical, a second contrast enhanced imaging technique should be performed, or the lesion should be biopsied.[63] Biopsies of small lesions should be evaluated by expert pathologists. If the biopsy is negative, a follow-up plan must be established that includes ultrasonography every 3 months. If the lesion enlarges but remains atypical for HCC, a repeat biopsy should be performed. The diagnostic algorithm for hepatocellular carcinoma is shown in Fig. 2.

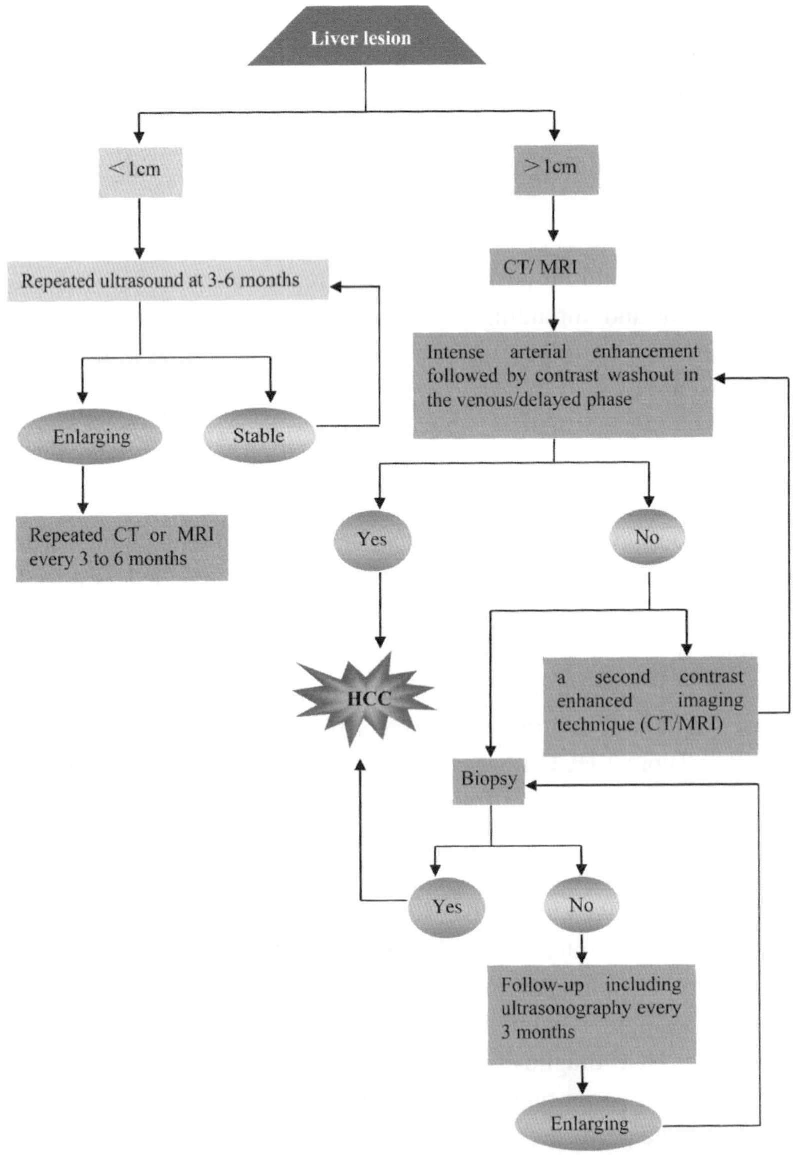

Fig 2. Diagnostic algorithm for hepatocellular carcinoma.

Pathology

The gross morphologic types of HCC can be classified as nodular, massive and diffuse. HCC may develop a large solitary mass with or without satellite nodules in the surrounding liver. It may consist of multiple nodules spread throughout the liver, or it may infiltrate the liver diffusely without forming nodules. In microscopic examination, HCC is graded as well, moderately, or poorly differentiated types.[64] Both cytologic and architectural features are helpful in diagnostic of HCC.

Staging

Cancer classification is intended to establish prognosis and enable the selection of the adequate treatment for the best candidates. Several staging systems have been proposed to provide a clinical classification of HCC.[65] In oncology, the standard classification of cancer is based on the TNM staging. which mainly based on tumor size, number, vascular invasion, lymph node involvement and distant metastasis. TNM staging are divided into stages from low to high to reflect the severity of the tumor. The detailed descriptions for the development of HCC are the advantages of TNM staging; however, it does not provide information on liver functional status or health status, which is essential to the options of treatment and prognosis prediction. Barcelona Clínic Liver Cancer (BCLC) staging includes prognostic variables related to tumor status, liver function, health performance status and links with treatment principles supported by evidence-based medicine.[66,67] It has been adopted by the AASLD and EASL–EORTC for use in its practice guidelines on management of HCC.[47,68] BCLC classification is showed in Table 2.[53]

Cholangiocarcinoma

Cholangiocarcinoma refers to malignant neoplasm of bile duct epithelium. According to the site, it can be divided into intrahepatic cholangiocarcinoma (ICC) and extrahepatic cholangiocarcinoma (ECC). ICC originates from the epithelium of intrahepatic bile duct and its branches to fine biliary tree; ECC is divided into hilarcholangiocarcinoma and distal

Table 2. Barcelona Clinic Liver Cancer (BCLC) classification.

BCLC stages	PS	Tumor features	Liver functions
Early HCC			
A1	0	Single, < 5 cm	No portal hypertension and normal bilirubin
A2	0	Single, < 5 cm	Portal hypertension and normal bilirubin
A3	0	Single, < 5 cm	Portal hypertension and abnormal bilirubin
A4	0	3 tumors < 3 cm	Child-Pugh A–B
Intermediate			
B	0	Large multinodular	Child-Pugh A–B
Advanced			
C	1–2	Vascular invasion or metastases	Child-Pugh A–B
End stage			
D	3–4	Any	Child-Pugh C

HCC: hepatocellular carcinoma. PS: performance status
A and B stages: all the criteria. C and D stages: one of the criteria.

ECC by the confluence point of cystic duct and the common hepatic duct. ECC is more common than the ECC, and hilar cholangiocarcinoma is the most common type of ECC.

Epidemiology

Cholangiocarcinoma is commonly considered to be a rare disease. However, in recent years, studies have shown that incidence and mortality rates are increasing in United States and other countries.[69–72] The cause of the rise in cholangiocarcinoma is unknown and is not explained by improvements in diagnosis.[73,74] In the United States, incidence rates has been reported to be 0.95 per 100,000 population for ICC and 0.82 per 100,000 for ECC.[74,75] There are regional differences in the incidence of cholangiocarcinoma. Southeast Asia has the highest incidence, while the lowest incidence is observed in Australia.[76] The incidences also vary in different racial and ethnic groups, with highest in Hispanics and the lowest in African Americans.[77,78]

Risk factors

In the majority of patients with cholangiocarcinoma, the risk factors are unknown. A number of different risk factors have been identified in a minority of patients.[79,80] The established risk factors are characterized by their association with inflammation and cholestasis, including parasitic infections, biliary tree disorders, primary sclerosing cholangitis, bile duct stones, and toxins.[81]

Pathology

According to WHO classification of biliary malignancies, premalignant lesions of intrahepatic bile ducts include biliary intraepithelial neoplasia, intraductal papillary neoplasm and mucinous cystic neoplasm. Premalignant lesions of extrahepatic bile ducts include adenoma, biliary intraepithelial neoplasia, intraductal papillary neoplasm and mucinous cystic neoplasm. Macroscopically, ICC can be described according to its growth characteristics as mass forming, periductal-infiltrating, and intraductal growth type, while extrahepatic bile duct cancers are divided into three types of polypoid or nodular masses, sclerosing, and diffusely infiltrating. The prognosis of intraductal growth type is usually the best compared to the others, and is also suitable for surgical resection. Nodular type and sclerosis type tend to invade surrounding tissues whereas diffuse infiltrative type tend to spread along the bile duct. Histologically, 90% of cholangiocarcinomas are adenocarcinomas. Other histologic types, such as intestinal-type adenocarcinoma, clear cell adenocarcinoma, signet-ring cell carcinoma, adenosquamous carcinoma, squamous cell carcinoma, and small cell carcinoma are also included.[82]

Diagnosis

Unlike other types of gastrointestinal cancer, diagnosis of biliary tract tumors can be a challenge. The diagnostic methods of cholangiocarcinomas are described in the following sections. Methods in combination and in conjunction with the appropriate clinical context are helpful for achieving diagnostic accuracy.

Clinical presentations

Clinical manifestations of cholangiocarcinoma vary due to location and size of the tumor. In the early stage of ICC, patients often show no specific clinical symptoms. As the disease progresses, there may be abdominal discomfort, abdominal pain, fatigue, nausea, abdominal mass, jaundice and fever. Jaundice is rare to ICC patients, but quite common to hilar or ECC patients. Jaundice will gradually deepen with time and other clinical manifestations appear such as gray, light color stool, deep yellow urine, and itching. Systemic manifestations, such as fatigue, weakness, weight loss are often present. Right hypochondrial region pain, chills and fever are usually associated with cholangitis.[83]

Blood tests

When biliary obstruction occurs, liver function test shows increased bilirubin, alkaline phosphatase and γ-glutamyl transpeptidase. Transaminases may rise, especially when accompanied by cholangitis. Long term biliary obstruction can result in the reduction of lipid-soluble vitamins A, D, E and K and prolonged prothrombin time. As the disease progresses, albumin, hemoglobin, and lactate dehydrogenase levels can be decreased.

Serum tumor markers

There is no specific tumor marker for the diagnosis of cholangiocarcinoma. Carbohydrate antigen (CA) 19-9, CA-125 and carcinoembryonic antigen (CEA) are often used in the diagnosis. Though they have some limitations, they may be useful in conjunction with other diagnostic modalities. CA19-9 is the most commonly used marker, its sensitivity and specificity for the diagnosis of cholangiocarcinoma is 79% and 98% respectively in patients with PSC.[84] Most of patients with cholangiocarcinoma have elevated serum CA19-9.[85] The increase of serum CA19-9 can also be seen in other causes of obstructive jaundice. If CA19-9 level continues to rise after biliary decompression, cholangiocarcinoma is highly suggested. Pancreas, gastric cancer and severe hepatic injury may also be associated with elevated CA19-9. Besides, 10% of patients with a negative Lewis antigen status cannot produce CA19-9.[85–87] CA125 and CEA are also increased in some patients with cholangiocarcinoma. However, they have limited value for the detection of cholangiocarcinoma.

Imaging

Imaging is the main diagnostic modality for cholangiocarcinoma.[88] Reasonable application of imaging examination can be helpful for the localization and qualitative diagnosis and tumor staging.

US

US is the preferred imaging modality for the evaluation of cholestasis or liver dysfunction. It has only limited value in identification of cholangiocarcinomas.[89] US may miss small lesions and cannot accurately identify tumor extent. Findings of ICC may only show imitated hepatic tumors. In hilar tumors there is a intrahepatic bile duct dilatation, but no extrahepatic hepatic duct dilatation. The advantages of US are that it can reliably discriminate tumors and stones, and initially identify the site of obstruction based on the dilatation of intrahepatic or extrahepatic bile duct. In addition, US can show the bile duct and its surrounding lesions, and evaluate the degree of portal vein invasion. However, US seldom identifies ECC tumor masses. Overall, the sensitivity and specificity of US is not high in the diagnosis of cholangiocarcinoma.

CT

Dynamic spiral CT can show the unique signs of ICC: dilatated bile duct and enlarged lymph nodes. However, it usually cannot define the extent of cholangiocarcinoma. Contrast CT has higher sensitivity for detection of cholangiocarcinoma than US, and provides good images of intrahepatic tumors, dilated intrahepatic ducts and extrahepatic metastases. Enhanced CT scan can better show the relationship between hilar tumor and hepatic artery or portal vein. Chest CT is helpful in evaluating distant metastasis. Thin layer of small field image is valuable to evaluate the extent of biliary involvement.

MRI

MRI is the best way to diagnose cholangiocarcinoma. MRI can show the anatomy and the scope of the liver and bile duct cancer, and whether there is liver metastasis. Magnetic resonance cholangio-pancreatography (MRCP) may preferably show the biliary branches, bile duct involvement, and has especially a high sensitivity in biliary obstruction. After the initial identification of the site of obstruction with US, MRCP should be used to conduct a comprehensive assessment of the bile duct involvement. MR vascular imaging can show cases of hilar vascular involvement.[90,91]

PET-CT

PET-CT can be used for assessing the benign and malignant tumors. However, biliary mucinous adenocarcinoma may show false negative. Comparing CT or MRI, PET-CT exhibits no advantage for cholangiocarcinoma diagnosis but has higher accuracy for detecting distant metastases. However, it is not suitable for detection of regional lymph node metastases.[92]

Endoscopic retrograde cholangiopancreatography (ERCP) and percutaneous transhepatic cholangiography (PTC)

ERCP and PTC have their advantages in the diagnosis of cholangiocarcinoma. Typically, ERCP is used to evaluate bile duct anatomy distal to the obstruction site, and PTC is applied to explore the morphology of bile duct proximal to the obstruction site. If necessary, a combination of both can help evaluate the whole biliary tract. Bile samples can be collected for cytology through ERCP or PTC. Combined brushing biopsy and biopsy can increase the positive rate, but negative cytology result does not rule out a tumor. ERCP/PTC should not be routinely recommended for the diagnosis of cholangiocarcinoma, since this is an invasive procedure with risks of complications.

Endoscopic ultrasonography (EUS) and choledochoscope SpyGlass

EUS can provide a better observation of the distal extrahepatic bile duct, regional lymph nodes and blood vessels. For biliary obstruction caused by distal bile duct tumors, if other imaging examinations cannot confirm the diagnosis, EUS can be used for guiding fine needle biopsy of lesions and lymph nodes. For most hard-to-diagnose patients with biliary stricture (60%), EUS examination is a feasible, safe and economical method. If EUS examination is invalid, choledochoscope SpyGlass examination can be used as a supplement. It is more valuable in differentiating benign or malignant biliary stricture. The combination use of EUS examination and the SpyGlass can provide a correct clinical diagnosis for a majority of 94% patients, and minimize the incidence of adverse events.[93]

Cytologic and histologic diagnosis

Pathological diagnosis of cholangiocarcinoma is very important for planning clinical treatment. But for patients suitable for radical resection of the tumor biopsy, it is generally not recommended due to the risk of tumor seeding. Different histological types of cholangiocarcinoma vary in mechanism and biological behavior. Thus, accurate histological type is very important in pathological diagnosis. Many pathological features may affect the prognosis, such as lymph node metastasis, nerve tissue and microvascular invasion, intrahepatic satellite lesions or metastases, surgical margin, histological type and grade as well as the merger of bile duct precancerous lesions (especially neoplasia degree of the biliary epithelial). Those features should be described in detail in pathology reports to help clinicians develop individualized treatment plan and prognosis. Cholangiocarcinoma is mainly adenocarcinoma, but we need to pay attention to the pseudoglandular hepatocellular carcinoma and hepatic metastasis from gastrointestinal adenocarcinoma, immunohistochemistry may help differential diagnosis when necessary.

Staging

TNM system is generally used for the staging of ICC, hilar cholangiocarcinoma and distal ECC. Unlike HCC, tumor size is not considered important because it has no effect on survival in patients undergoing surgery, but tumor number, vascular invasion, and lymph node metastasis are associated with survival.[94,95]

Gallbladder Carcinoma

Gallbladder carcinoma is the most common and aggressive type of all the biliary tract tumors. The incidence of gallbladder carcinoma varies by geographic location with high incidence rates in South America, Asia, and certain Eastern European countries.[96] Gallbladder carcinoma often occurs after age 65. The incidence is higher for women than men, especially higher in white women.[97]

Risk factors

Risk factors of gallbladder carcinoma are associated with chronic inflammation. The most common risk factor is gallstones and the risk increases with the stone size.[98,99] Calcification of gallbladder (magnetic gallbladder) is the result of chronic inflammation of the gallbladder, which is also related to gallbladder cancer, but the risk is much lower than anticipated. Chronic typhus infection patients are susceptible to gallbladder cancer.

Clinical presentations

The clinical symptoms of gallbladder cancer, gallstone and chronic cholecystitis are similar. Gallbladder cancer is often accidentally discovered during cholecystectomy. This is mainly because most of the patients have concomitant gallstones and its symptoms are largely caused by stones. Upper abdominal pain is the most common symptom. About 80% patients have varying degrees of pain. When patients with long asymptomatic stones begin to present abdominal pain or chronic cholecystitis, the possibility of cancer should be considered. Nearly half of the patients have jaundice, which are primarily caused by malignant bile duct obstruction, and other accompanying symptoms, such as nausea, vomiting and weight loss.

Early stage patients generally lack typical signs. In advanced patients, ascites may appear. According to statistics, about one of two patients who come to see a doctor has metastasis. High metastasis rate and partial rapid progress make the prognosis poor.

Pathology and staging

Sixty percent of gallbladder carcinoma is found in the fundus, 30% in the body, and 10% in the neck of the gallbladder. They can spread to the entire gallbladder by separating or diffusion in the wall. Approximately 80% of gallbladder cancer is adenocarcinoma. Gallbladder cancer often shows early lymph node and blood transfer. Tumor stage is closely related to survival. The TNM staging system of the American Joint Committee on Cancer is preferred. Survival is related to tumor stage and pathological type.

Diagnosis

Patients with gallstones in the history and emergence of the clinical manifestations mentioned above should be suspected gallbladder carcinoma. Since most patients have varying degrees of jaundice when coming for treatment, the laboratory tests mainly show the features of obstructive jaundice, including elevated serum alkaline phosphatase, total bilirubin and direct bilirubin. In patients with liver cell damage, serum ALT may show mild to moderate elevation; Patients with secondary biliary infection may present with cholangitis. Some patient's serum CEA and CA19-9 can also be increased, but these markers are not specific for gallbladder cancer. Imaging is an important means of diagnosis of gallbladder carcinoma, especially B-US, in which substantial hyperechoic mass followed by no shadow can be found in the gallbladder, or localized or diffuse thickening of gallbladder wall. CT can help find out not only the lesions of gallbladder and liver, but also the relationship between the tumor and surrounding blood vessels, which can be used to determine whether a radical treatment will be successful. For patients with obstructive jaundice, ERCP or PTC can be helpful in finding out the hilar cholangiocarcinoma.

Take Home Messages

- Hepatobiliary malignancies are significant health threats, and the incidences of hepatocellular carcinoma and cholangiocarcinoma are increasing in many countries, including the United States.
- Predisposing conditions of hepatocellular carcinoma include hepatitis B, hepatitis C with or without cirrhosis, and metabolic conditions, such as diabetes and obesity.
- Current surveillance programs for early detection of hepatocellular carcinoma use abdominal US with or without α-fetoprotein every 6–12 months.
- Diagnosis of hepatobiliary malignancies depends largely on imaging examination in clinical practice, especially in CT or MRI. However, serum biomarkers and biopsy are also utilized.

References

1. Siegel, R., Ma, J., Zou, Z., Jemal, A., Cancer statistics, 2014. *CA Cancer J Clin*, 2014. **64**(1): 9–29.
2. Jemal, A., Bray, F., Center, M.M., Ferlay, J., Ward, E., Forman, D., Global cancer statistics. *CA Cancer J Clin*, 2011. **61**(2): 69–90.
3. El-Serag, H.B., Epidemiology of hepatocellular carcinoma in USA. *Hepatol Res*, 2007. **37** Suppl 2: S88–94.
4. Hepatocellular carcinoma — United States, 2001–2006. *MMWR Morb Mortal Wkly Rep*. 2010. **59**(17): 517–20.
5. Augustine, M.M., Fong, Y., Epidemiology and risk factors of biliary tract and primary liver tumors. *Surg Oncol Clin N Am*, 2014. **23**(2): 171–88.
6. Gomes, M.A., Priolli, D.G., Tralhao, J.G., Botelho, M.F., Hepatocellular carcinoma: Epidemiology, biology, diagnosis, and therapies. *Rev Assoc Med Bras*, 2013. **59**(5): 514–24.
7. El-Serag, H.B., Rudolph, K.L., Hepatocellular carcinoma: Epidemiology and molecular carcinogenesis. *Gastroenterology*, 2007. **132**(7): 2557–76.

8. Perz, J.F., Armstrong, G.L., Farrington, L.A., Hutin, Y.J., Bell, B.P., The contributions of hepatitis B virus and hepatitis C virus infections to cirrhosis and primary liver cancer worldwide. *J Hepatol*, 2006. **45**(4): 529–38.
9. Chu, C.M., Natural history of chronic hepatitis B virus infection in adults with emphasis on the occurrence of cirrhosis and hepatocellular carcinoma. *J Gastroenterol Hepatol*, 2000. **15** Suppl: E25–30.
10. Yang, H.I., Lu, S.N., Liaw, Y.F. *et al.*, Hepatitis B e antigen and the risk of hepatocellular carcinoma. *N Engl J Med*, 2002. **347**(3): 168–74.
11. Tseng, T.C., Liu, C.J., Chen, C.L. *et al.*, Risk stratification of hepatocellular carcinoma in hepatitis B virus e antigen-negative carriers by combining viral biomarkers. *J Infect Dis*, 2013. **208**(4): 584–93.
12. Donato, F., Tagger, A., Gelatti, U. *et al.*, Alcohol and hepatocellular carcinoma: the effect of lifetime intake and hepatitis virus infections in men and women. *Am J Epidemiol*, 2002. **155**(4): 323–31.
13. Fattovich, G., Stroffolini, T., Zagni, I., Donato, F., Hepatocellular carcinoma in cirrhosis: incidence and risk factors. *Gastroenterology*, 2004. **127**(5 Suppl 1): S35–50.
14. Volk, M.L., Marrero, J.A., Early detection of liver cancer: Diagnosis and management. *Curr Gastroenterol Rep*, 2008. **10**(1): 60–6.
15. Groopman, J.D., Johnson, D., Kensler, T.W., Aflatoxin and hepatitis B virus biomarkers: a paradigm for complex environmental exposures and cancer risk. *Cancer Biomark*, 2005. **1**(1): 5–14.
16. Lutwick, L.I., Relation between aflatoxin, hepatitis-B virus, and hepatocellular carcinoma. *Lancet*, 1979. **1**(8119): 755–7.
17. Sangiovanni, A., Prati, G.M., Fasani, P., *et al.*, The natural history of compensated cirrhosis due to hepatitis C virus: A 17-year cohort study of 214 patients. *Hepatology*, 2006. **43**(6): 1303–10.
18. Park, S.Z., Nagorney, D.M., Czaja, A.J., Hepatocellular carcinoma in autoimmune hepatitis. *Dig Dis Sci*, 2000. **45**(10): 1944–8.
19. Siegel, A.B., Zhu, A.X., Metabolic syndrome and hepatocellular carcinoma: Two growing epidemics with a potential link. *Cancer*, 2009. **115**(24): 5651–61.
20. Stickel, F., Hellerbrand, C., Non-alcoholic fatty liver disease as a risk factor for hepatocellular carcinoma: Mechanisms and implications. *Gut*, 2010. **59**(10): 1303–7.

21. Calle, E.E., Kaaks, R., Overweight, obesity and cancer: epidemiological evidence and proposed mechanisms. *Nat Rev Cancer*, 2004. **4**(8): 579–91.
22. Calle, E.E., Rodriguez, C., Walker-Thurmond, K., Thun, M.J., Overweight, obesity, and mortality from cancer in a prospectively studied cohort of U.S. adults. *N Engl J Med*, 2003. **348**(17): 1625–38.
23. El-Serag, H.B., Hampel, H., Javadi, F., The association between diabetes and hepatocellular carcinoma: a systematic review of epidemiologic evidence. *Clin Gastroenterol Hepatol*, 2006. **4**(3): 369–80.
24. Hassan, M.M., Curley, S.A., Li, D. *et al.*, Association of diabetes duration and diabetes treatment with the risk of hepatocellular carcinoma. *Cancer*, 2010. **116**(8): 1938–46.
25. Neuschwander-Tetri, B.A., Caldwell, S.H., Nonalcoholic steatohepatitis: summary of an AASLD Single Topic Conference. *Hepatology*, 2003. **37**(5): 1202–19.
26. White, D.L., Kanwal, F., El-Serag, H.B., Association between nonalcoholic fatty liver disease and risk for hepatocellular cancer, based on systematic review. *Clin Gastroenterol Hepatol*, 2012. **10**(12): 1342–59.e2.
27. Zhang, B.H., Yang, B.H., Tang, Z.Y., Randomized controlled trial of screening for hepatocellular carcinoma. *J Cancer Res Clin Oncol*, 2004. **130**(7): 417–22.
28. Kudo, M., Izumi, N., Kokudo, N. *et al.*, Management of hepatocellular carcinoma in Japan: Consensus-Based Clinical Practice Guidelines proposed by the Japan Society of Hepatology (JSH) 2010 updated version. *Dig Dis*, 2011. **29**(3): 339–64.
29. Gupta, S., Bent, S., Kohlwes, J., Test characteristics of alpha-fetoprotein for detecting hepatocellular carcinoma in patients with hepatitis C. A systematic review and critical analysis. *Ann Intern Med*, 2003. **139**(1): 46–50.
30. Lok, A.S., Sterling, R.K., Everhart, J.E. *et al.*, Des-gamma-carboxy prothrombin and alpha-fetoprotein as biomarkers for the early detection of hepatocellular carcinoma. *Gastroenterology*, 2010. **138**(2): 493–502.
31. Marrero, J.A., Feng, Z., Wang, Y. *et al.*, Alpha-fetoprotein, des-gamma carboxyprothrombin, and lectin-bound alpha-fetoprotein in early hepatocellular carcinoma. *Gastroenterology*, 2009. **137**(1): 110–8.
32. Zhang, B., Yang, B., Combined alpha fetoprotein testing and ultrasonography as a screening test for primary liver cancer. *J Med Screen*, 1999. **6**(2): 108–10.

33. Crissien, A.M., Frenette, C., Current management of hepatocellular carcinoma. *Gastroenterol Hepatol (N Y)*, 2014. **10**(3): 153–61.
34. Yamada, T., Alpers, D.H., Kalloo, A.N. *et al.*, eds. *Textbook of Gastroenterology, Vol 2. 5th*. Philadelphia: Blackwell Publishing, 2009. 2386–2405 .
35. Kew, M.C., Paterson, A.C., Unusual clinical presentations of hepatocellular carcinoma. *Trop Gastroenterol*, 1985. **6**(1): 10–22.
36. Zapf, J., Futo, E., Peter, M., Froesch, E.R., Can "big" insulin-like growth factor II in serum of tumor patients account for the development of extrapancreatic tumor hypoglycemia. *J Clin Invest*, 1992. **90**(6): 2574–84.
37. Mark, Feldman., Lawrence, S., Friedman. *et al.*, eds. Sleisenger and Fordtran's *Gastrointestinal and Liver Disease: Pathophysiology, Diagnosis, Management. vol 2. 9th*, Philadelphia, PA: Saunders Elsevier, 2010. 1569–80.
38. Nguyen, M.H., Garcia, R.T., Simpson, P.W., Wright, T.L., Keeffe, E.B., Racial differences in effectiveness of alpha-fetoprotein for diagnosis of hepatocellular carcinoma in hepatitis C virus cirrhosis. *Hepatology*, 2002. **36**(2): 410–7.
39. Marrero, J.A., Screening tests for hepatocellular carcinoma. *Clin Liver Dis*, 2005. **9**(2): 235–51, vi.
40. Bruix, J., Sherman, M., Management of hepatocellular carcinoma. *Hepatology*, 2005. **42**(5): 1208–36.
41. Sherman, M., Serological surveillance for hepatocellular carcinoma: time to quit. *J Hepatol*, 2010. **52**(4): 614–5.
42. Sherman, M., Screening for hepatocellular carcinoma. *Hepatol Res*, 2007. **37**(Suppl 2): S152–65.
43. Sterling, R.K., Jeffers, L., Gordon, F. *et al.*, Clinical utility of AFP-L3% measurement in North American patients with HCV-related cirrhosis. *Am J Gastroenterol*, 2007. **102**(10): 2196–205.
44. Leerapun, A., Suravarapu, S.V., Bida, J.P. *et al.*, The utility of Lens culinaris agglutinin-reactive alpha-fetoprotein in the diagnosis of hepatocellular carcinoma: evaluation in a United States referral population. *Clin Gastroenterol Hepatol*, 2007. **5**(3): 394–402; quiz 267.
45. Sterling, R.K., Jeffers, L., Gordon, F. *et al.*, Utility of Lens culinaris agglutinin-reactive fraction of alpha-fetoprotein and des-gamma-carboxy prothrombin, alone or in combination, as biomarkers for hepatocellular carcinoma. *Clin Gastroenterol Hepatol*, 2009. **7**(1): 104–13.

46. Yamamoto, K., Imamura, H., Matsuyama, Y. *et al.*, AFP, AFP-L3, DCP, and GP73 as markers for monitoring treatment response and recurrence and as surrogate markers of clinicopathological variables of HCC. *J Gastroenterol*, 2010. **45**(12): 1272–82.
47. Bruix, J., Sherman, M., Management of hepatocellular carcinoma: an update. *Hepatology*, 2011. **53**(3): 1020–2.
48. Tateishi, R., Yoshida, H., Matsuyama, Y., Mine, N., Kondo, Y., Omata, M., Diagnostic accuracy of tumor markers for hepatocellular carcinoma: a systematic review. *Hepatol Int*, 2008. **2**(1): 17–30.
49. Hu, B., Tian, X., Sun, J., Meng, X., Evaluation of individual and combined applications of serum biomarkers for diagnosis of hepatocellular carcinoma: a meta-analysis. *Int J Mol Sci*, 2013. **14**(12): 23559–80.
50. People's Republic of China Ministry of Health, Primary hepatic cancer diagnostic and treatment practices (2011 Edition). *J Clin Oncol (Chinese)*, 2011. **16**(10): 929–46.
51. Colli, A., Fraquelli, M., Casazza, G. *et al.*, Accuracy of ultrasonography, spiral CT, magnetic resonance, and alpha-fetoprotein in diagnosing hepatocellular carcinoma: a systematic review. *Am J Gastroenterol*, 2006. **101**(3): 513–23.
52. Yu, S.C., Yeung, D.T., So, N.M., Imaging features of hepatocellular carcinoma. *Clin Radiol*, 2004. **59**(2): 145–56.
53. Cartier, V., Aube, C., Diagnosis of hepatocellular carcinoma. *Diagn Interv Imaging*, 2014. **95**(7–8): 709–19.
54. Luciani, A., Allice, O., Zegai, B. *et al.*, Imaging nodules within cirrhotic liver: how do I do it? *J Radiol*, 2007. **88**(7–8 Pt 2): 1073–90.
55. Ma, W., Jia, J., Wang, S. *et al.*, The prognostic value of 18F-FDG PET/CT for hepatocellular carcinoma treated with transarterial chemoembolization (TACE). *Theranostics*, 2014. **4**(7): 736–44.
56. Wolfort, R.M., Papillion, P.W., Turnage, R.H., Lillien, D.L., Ramaswamy, M.R., Zibari, G.B., Role of FDG-PET in the evaluation and staging of hepatocellular carcinoma with comparison of tumor size, AFP level, and histologic grade. *Int Surg*, 2010. **95**(1): 67–75.
57. Pant, V., Sen, I.B., Soin, A.S., Role of (1)(8)F-FDG PET CT as an independent prognostic indicator in patients with hepatocellular carcinoma. *Nucl Med Commun*, 2013. **34**(8): 749–57.

58. Forner, A., Vilana, R., Ayuso, C. *et al.*, Diagnosis of hepatic nodules 20 mm or smaller in cirrhosis: Prospective validation of the noninvasive diagnostic criteria for hepatocellular carcinoma. *Hepatology*, 2008. **47**(1): 97–104.
59. Pathologic diagnosis of early hepatocellular carcinoma: A report of the international consensus group for hepatocellular neoplasia. *Hepatology*, 2009. **49**(2): 658–64.
60. Di, T.L., Destro, A., Seok, J.Y. *et al.*, The application of markers (HSP70 GPC3 and GS) in liver biopsies is useful for detection of hepatocellular carcinoma. *J Hepatol*, 2009. **50**(4): 746–54.
61. Miller, G., Schwartz, L.H., D'Angelica, M., The use of imaging in the diagnosis and staging of hepatobiliary malignancies. *Surg Oncol Clin N Am*, 2007. **16**(2): 343–68.
62. NCCN clinical practice guidelines in oncology, hepatobiliary cancers. National Comprehensive Cancer Network. http://www.nccn.org/professionals/physician_gls/f_guidelines.asp.Version 2.2014 .
63. Mendez-Sanchez, N., Ridruejo, E., de Mattos, A.A. *et al.*, Latin American Association for the Study of the Liver (LAASL) Clinical Practice Guidelines: Management of Hepatocellular Carcinoma. *Ann Hepatol*, 2014. **13** Suppl 1: 4–40.
64. Kojiro, M., Histopathology of liver cancers. *Best Pract Res Clin Gastroenterol*, 2005. **19**(1): 39–62.
65. Dohmen, K., Many staging systems for hepatocellular carcinoma: evolution from Child-Pugh, Okuda to SLiDe. *J Gastroenterol Hepatol*, 2004. **19**(11): 1227–32.
66. Cillo, U., Vitale, A., Grigoletto, F. *et al.*, Prospective validation of the Barcelona Clinic Liver Cancer staging system. *J Hepatol*, 2006. **44**(4): 723–31.
67. Guglielmi, A., Ruzzenente, A., Pachera, S. *et al.*, Comparison of seven staging systems in cirrhotic patients with hepatocellular carcinoma in a cohort of patients who underwent radiofrequency ablation with complete response. *Am J Gastroenterol*, 2008. **103**(3): 597–604.
68. EASL-EORTC clinical practice guidelines: management of hepatocellular carcinoma. *Eur J Cancer*, 2012. **48**(5): 599–641.
69. Welzel, T.M., McGlynn, K.A., Hsing, A.W., O'Brien, T.R., Pfeiffer, R.M., Impact of classification of hilar cholangiocarcinomas (Klatskin tumors) on

the incidence of intra- and extrahepatic cholangiocarcinoma in the United States. *J Natl Cancer Inst*, 2006. **98**(12): 873–5.

70. Ustundag, Y., Bayraktar, Y., Cholangiocarcinoma: a compact review of the literature. *World J Gastroenterol*, 2008. **14**(42): 6458–66.
71. Mosconi, S., Beretta, G.D., Labianca, R., Zampino, M.G., Gatta, G., Heinemann, V., Cholangiocarcinoma. *Crit Rev Oncol Hematol*, 2009. **69**(3): 259–70.
72. Khan, S.A., Thomas, H.C., Davidson, B.R., Taylor-Robinson, S.D., Cholangiocarcinoma. *Lancet*, 2005. **366**(9493): 1303–14.
73. Khan, S.A., Emadossadaty, S., Ladep, N.G. *et al.*, Rising trends in cholangiocarcinoma: is the ICD classification system misleading us. *J Hepatol*, 2012. **56**(4): 848–54.
74. Khan, S.A., Toledano, M.B., Taylor-Robinson, S.D., Epidemiology, risk factors, and pathogenesis of cholangiocarcinoma. *HPB (Oxford)*, 2008. **10**(2): 77–82.
75. Shaib, Y.H., Davila, J.A., McGlynn, K., El-Serag, H.B., Rising incidence of intrahepatic cholangiocarcinoma in the United States: a true increase. *J Hepatol*, 2004. **40**(3): 472–7.
76. Shaib, Y., El-Serag, H.B., The epidemiology of cholangiocarcinoma. *Semin Liver Dis*, 2004. **24**(2): 115–25.
77. McLean, L., Patel, T., Racial and ethnic variations in the epidemiology of intrahepatic cholangiocarcinoma in the United States. *Liver Int*, 2006. **26**(9): 1047–53.
78. Hammill, C.W., Wong, L.L., Intrahepatic cholangiocarcinoma: a malignancy of increasing importance. *J Am Coll Surg*, 2008. **207**(4): 594–603.
79. Aljiffry, M., Walsh, M.J., Molinari, M., Advances in diagnosis, treatment and palliation of cholangiocarcinoma: 1990–2009. *World J Gastroenterol*, 2009. **15**(34): 4240–62.
80. Yachimski, P., Pratt, D.S., Cholangiocarcinoma: natural history, treatment, and strategies for surveillance in high-risk patients. *J Clin Gastroenterol*, 2008. **42**(2): 178–90.
81. Khan, S.A., Davidson, B.R., Goldin, R.D. *et al.*, Guidelines for the diagnosis and treatment of cholangiocarcinoma: an update. *Gut*, 2012. **61**(12): 1657–69.
82. Blechacz, B.R., Gores, G.J., Cholangiocarcinoma. *Clin Liver Dis*, 2008. **12**(1): 131–50, ix.

83. Diagnosis and treatment of cholangiocarcinoma — consensus of surgery expert (Chinese). *Chinese J Pract Surg*, 2014. (01): 1–5.
84. Levy, C., Lymp, J., Angulo, P., Gores, G.J., Larusso, N., Lindor, K.D., The value of serum CA 19-9 in predicting cholangiocarcinomas in patients with primary sclerosing cholangitis. *Dig Dis Sci*, 2005. **50**(9): 1734–40.
85. Gores, G.J., Early detection and treatment of cholangiocarcinoma. *Liver Transpl*, 2000. **6**(6 Suppl 2): S30–4.
86. Abbas, G., Lindor, K.D., Cholangiocarcinoma in primary sclerosing cholangitis. *J Gastrointest Cancer*, 2009. **40**(1–2): 19–25.
87. Hultcrantz, R., Olsson, R., Danielsson, A. *et al.*, A 3-year prospective study on serum tumor markers used for detecting cholangiocarcinoma in patients with primary sclerosing cholangitis. *J Hepatol*, 1999. **30**(4): 669–73.
88. Aljiffry, M., Walsh, M.J., Molinari, M., Advances in diagnosis, treatment and palliation of cholangiocarcinoma: 1990–2009. *World J Gastroenterol*, 2009. **15**(34): 4240–62.
89. Khan, S.A., Davidson, B.R., Goldin, R. *et al.*, Guidelines for the diagnosis and treatment of cholangiocarcinoma: consensus document. *Gut*, 2002. **51**(Suppl 6): VI1–9.
90. Maccioni, F., Martinelli, M., Al, A.N. *et al.*, Magnetic resonance cholangiography: past, present and future: a review. *Eur Rev Med Pharmacol Sci*, 2010. **14**(8): 721–5.
91. Kaltenthaler, E.C., Walters, S.J., Chilcott, J., Blakeborough, A., Vergel, Y.B., Thomas, S., MRCP compared to diagnostic ERCP for diagnosis when biliary obstruction is suspected: a systematic review. *BMC Med Imaging*, 2006. **6**: 9.
92. Kluge, R., Schmidt, F., Caca, K. *et al.*, Positron emission tomography with [(18)F]fluoro-2-deoxy-D-glucose for diagnosis and staging of bile duct cancer. *Hepatology*, 2001. **33**(5): 1029–35.
93. Nguyen, N.Q., Schoeman, M.N., Ruszkiewicz, A., Clinical utility of EUS before cholangioscopy in the evaluation of difficult biliary strictures. *Gastrointest Endosc*, 2013. **78**(6): 868–74.
94. Nathan, H., Aloia, T.A., Vauthey, J.N. *et al.*, A proposed staging system for intrahepatic cholangiocarcinoma. *Ann Surg Oncol*, 2009. **16**(1): 14–22.
95. de Jong, M.C., Nathan, H., Sotiropoulos, G.C. *et al.*, Intrahepatic cholangiocarcinoma: an international multi-institutional analysis of prognostic factors and lymph node assessment. *J Clin Oncol*, 2011. **29**(23): 3140–5.

96. Randi, G., Franceschi, S., La Vecchia, C., Gallbladder cancer worldwide: geographical distribution and risk factors. *Int J Cancer*, 2006. **118**(7): 1591–602.
97. Levy, A.D., Murakata, L.A., Rohrmann, C.A. Jr., Gallbladder carcinoma: radiologic-pathologic correlation. *Radiographics*, 2001. **21**(2): 295–314; questionnaire, 549–55.
98. Sheth, S., Bedford, A., Chopra, S., Primary gallbladder cancer: recognition of risk factors and the role of prophylactic cholecystectomy. *Am J Gastroenterol*, 2000. **95**(6): 1402–10.
99. Tazuma, S., Kajiyama, G., Carcinogenesis of malignant lesions of the gall bladder. The impact of chronic inflammation and gallstones. *Langenbecks Arch Surg*, 2001. **386**(3): 224–9.

Chapter 18

Non-Surgical Management of Hepatobiliary Malignancies

Anne M. Noonan and Tanios Bekaii-Saab

What is New

- A meta-analysis assessing adjuvant treatment of biliary tract neoplasms performed with curative intent reported a possible benefit for post-surgery patients with positive lymph node and R1 resections.
- Results of the STORM trial showed positive role of adjuvant treatment with sorafenib in patients post resection or ablation of hepatocellular carcinoma treated with curative intent.

Introduction

Hepatobiliary malignancies comprise malignancies of the liver, bile ducts and gallbladder. Usually, biliary tract cancers have been difficult to diagnose at an early stage due to anatomical considerations leading to late presentation. While they can be initially chemosensitive, traditional systemic therapies offer little hope for cure and chemoresistance eventually develops. Gemcitabine, platinums and fluorpyrimidines comprise the backbone of most traditional chemotherapeutic regimens for biliary tract malignancies. In the past, similar chemotherapy regimens and doxorubicin have been tried in hepatocellular carcinoma with limited benefit. However, elucidation of key signaling mechanisms offer promise for more targeted approaches to the treatment of these malignancies. A good example of this is the switch to sorafenib as the mainstay of treatment for advanced and metastatic hepatocellular carcinoma. There are some reports of limited sequencing of biliary tract tumors in small cohorts of patients. In one report, whole genome sequencing of six patients with advanced intrahepatic cholangiocarcinoma revealed recurrent translocation events involving the FGFR2 locus in 3 of 6 assessed patients.[1] Treatment with pazopanib resulted in limited anti-tumor activity. Treatment with erlotinib in patient with an ERRFI1 mutation resulted in tumor response in this series. Table 1 shows a list of mutations currently identified in biliary tract

Table 1. Frequency of mutations in cholangiocarcinoma (*cohort associated with liver fluke, #cohort not associated with liver fluke) and hepatocellular carcinoma.

Gene	Cholangiocarcinoma $n = 62$, $n = 6$*, $n = 111$#	Hepatocellular Carcinoma $n = 149$ (%)
BAP1	16.7%*	0
CSPG4	33.3%*	0.7
CTNNB1	0%	34.9
ERRFI1	16.7%*	0.7
GRIN3A	33.3%*	0
IDH1	13%	0
IDH2	16.7%*	0
KRAS	16.7%#	1.3
LAMA2	16.7%*	0
MLL3	16.7%*, 14.8%#	0
NLRP1	16.7%*	0
NOTCH1	16.7%*	0
PLXNB3	33.3%*	0
PTK2	16.7%*	0
SMAD4	16.7%#	0
TP53	33.3%*, 44.4%#	19.5

cancers and hepatocellular carcinoma.[2,3] The Cancer Genome Atlas project is a large scale tumor sequencing project sponsored by the United States National Cancer Institute which aims to profile a large selection of tumor types.[4] The collection and sequencing of tissue from cholangiocarcinomas and hepatocellular carcinomas is ongoing. The results may help to define subtypes of these cancers and pinpoint specific mutations which may enable more tailored therapies to be developed. In recent years there has been a renewed interest in immune therapies in solid tumors, with particular interest in manipulation of immune tolerance seen in the liver as a means of treating hepatocellular carcinoma. Inhibitors of immune checkpoint receptors such as CTLA-4 and PD-1 are in development for hepatocellular carcinoma, with several phase I and II trials currently in progress.[5]

Adjuvant Treatment of Biliary Tract Cancers

Despite complete surgical resection, local recurrence is common and is more common in cholangiocarcinomas than with gallbladder cancer where distant metastases are more common.[6,7] All patients with carcinomas of the gallbladder, intrahepatic or extrahepatic cholangiocarcinomas should undergo multidisciplinary review to determine the best treatment options. Participation in clinical trials when available should be encouraged. Unfortunately due to the rarity of these tumors, there is a paucity of evidence to define standard regimens. Many studies examining the role of adjuvant chemotherapy and/or radiotherapy are retrospective in nature or have small numbers of the individual subtypes of cancer thus limiting the statistical power and validity of the conclusions that can be drawn. If clinical trials are not available, treatment decisions for adjuvant therapy should be made based on the best available evidence. Factors associated with adverse survival include R1 resection, lymph node positivity, lymphovascular invasion.

Adjuvant treatment of gallbladder carcinomas

The role of adjuvant chemoradiotherapy for resected gallbladder cancer is controversial but is generally recommended except for T1a or T1b N1 tumors as it has been associated with improvement in regional control and survival in retrospective studies.[8] Numerous studies have been performed assessing adjuvant therapy in gallbladder cancer.[9] Balachandran *et al.* performed a retrospective review of 117 patients with gallbladder cancer resected between 1989 and 2002. In this study, T status and adjuvant chemoradiotherapy were independent predictors of long-term survival (>2 years). Eighty of these patients had simple cholecystectomies and adjuvant chemoradiotherapy was associated with improved survival in this group ($p = 0.008$) but not in the group that had extended surgery ($n = 37$). Adjuvant chemoradiotherapy was also associated with significant benefit in patients with stage III ($p = 0.001$) and node-positive disease ($p = 0.0005$). In a retrospective study of 73 patients from the Mayo Clinic, no significant difference was seen in the group receiving 5-fluouracil (5-FU) and radiotherapy versus those treated with surgery alone. However, when analyzed by stage, those patients with higher stage and node positivity appeared to derive a significant benefit.[10]

A large retrospective SEER database study of 2,325 patients showed an overall survival advantage for radiotherapy alone, particularly in patients with gallbladder cancer that is node positive disease or with invasion into the liver.[11] No overall survival advantage was seen in patients with disease limited to the gallbladder.

Takada *et al.* performed a prospective phase III study to assess the role of adjuvant mitomycin C and 5-FU versus surgery alone in patients with pancreatic, bile duct, gallbladder and ampulla of Vater carcinomas. The study included 112 patients with gallbladder cancer. Mitomycin C was given at a dose of 6 mg/kg by rapid intravenous infusion at the time of surgery, followed by 5-FU 350 mg/m^2 by slow intravenous infusion in two courses of treatment over five consecutive days each in postoperative weeks 1 and 3, followed by 5-FU 100 mg/m^2 orally daily from postoperative week 5 until disease recurrence.[12] Only the patients with gallbladder carcinoma appeared to benefit from adjuvant therapy. The five-year survival rate was 26% in the mitomycin C and 5-FU group compared to 14% in the surgery alone group ($p = 0.0367$). In addition, there was a statistically significant difference in the five-year disease free survival rate for patients with gallbladder carcinoma in the mitomycin and 5-FU group with the rate being 20.3% versus 11.6% in the surgery alone control group. Interestingly, patients with gallbladder carcinoma in this study reported increased weight on therapy.

Adjuvant therapy for intrahepatic and extrahepatic cholangiocarcinomas

There are no randomized prospective studies assessing the role of adjuvant radiotherapy or chemoradiotherapy in patients with completely resected intra- and extra-hepatic cholangiocarcinoma. Several retrospective studies and a few small phase II studies suggest a benefit for adjuvant fluoropyrimidine-based chemoradiotherapy, although in some of these studies, the populations included patients within incomplete resections. The prospective phase III study of mitomycin C and 5-FU by Takada *et al.* described above included 118 patients with biliary tract cancers.[12] No statistically significant difference in survival was seen in the chemotherapy arm compared to the control group in patients with cholangiocarcinoma. In the ESPAC-3 trial of 428 patients with periampullary cancers including 297 patients with periampullary, 96 bile duct and 35 other cancers, patients were randomized to observation alone, 6 months of modulated 5-FU or 6 months of gemcitabine.[13] While there was a trend towards an overall survival benefit in the adjuvant chemotherapy arms, it was not statistically significant. A subgroup analysis of the 96 patients with bile duct cancers showed no difference between the three arms with survival times of 27, 18 and 20 months respectively.

Meta-analysis of adjuvant therapy trials for biliary tract cancers and gallbladder cancers

A meta-analysis by Horgan *et al.* examined two SEER registries, the phase III study by Takada *et al.*, and 17 retrospective studies, giving a total of 6,712 patients with gallbladder or cholangiocarcinoma, of whom 1,797 were treated with adjuvant therapy — either chemotherapy alone (three studies), radiotherapy alone (nine studies) or combined chemoradiotherapy (eight studies).[14] The studies required patients to have curative-intent surgery (either negative R0 or microscopically positive R1 resection margins). When the results for extrahepatic biliary tract cancers and gallbladder were pooled, there was a non-significant benefit for adjuvant therapy in unselected patients. When the two registry analyses were excluded, the association between adjuvant therapy and improved survival became significant (OR, 0.53; 95% CI, 0.39 to 0.72; $p < 0.001$). When analyzed by subgroup, high-risk patients (node positive or margin positive) there was a significant benefit for any adjuvant therapy in node-positive disease (OR, 0.49, 95% CI, 0.30 to 0.80; $p = 0.004$). Similarly, there was a significant benefit for adjuvant therapy in patients with R1 resection (OR, 0.36, 95% CI, 0.19 to 0.68; $p = 0.002$). Regarding modality of adjuvant treatment, 63% of patients with R1 resections received radiotherapy alone, while the majority of R0 patients received chemoradiotherapy, and most of these studies included node-positive patients. Of interest, in patients with R0 resection, treatment with radiation was associated with a non-significant odds of harm (OR, 1.26; 95% CI, 0.88 to 1.79; $p = 0.2$). There were insufficient numbers of patients with node negative disease to make an accurate estimate of benefit for adjuvant therapy. The authors thus concluded that radiotherapy should be reserved for patients with margin-positive disease, and chemotherapy reserved for patients with node-positive disease, a combined modality approach being favored if both of these adverse features are present.

A retrospective study by the same group who looked at 296 patients with biliary tract cancers at Princess Margaret Hospital showed a significant improvement in overall survival in patients receiving adjuvant therapy.[15] Once again, patients with R1 resection and node positive disease derived the most overall survival advantage. For those with node positive disease, median overall survival was 37.7 months in those receiving adjuvant therapy versus 21 months in those who did not ($p = 0.07$). For patients with R1 resection, the benefit associated with adjuvant therapy was significantly increased compared to R0 resection ($p = 0.02$).

Wang and colleagues used data from 1,137 patients with resected gallbladder cancer from the SEER-Medicare Database who were diagnosed between 1995 and 2005, to generate a nomogram to assist in decision-making adjuvant therapies.[16] The nomogram takes into consideration the patient's age, sex, race, T stage and N stage, and offers figures for predicted median survival and overall survival (http://skynet.ohsu.edu/nomograms).

Neoadjuvant therapy for biliary tract cancers

Data for neoadjuvant therapy for biliary tract cancers is obtained mainly from small retrospective or phase II studies. In one study from MD Anderson, neoadjuvant gemcitabine chemotherapy was associated with worse survival compared to surgery alone.[17] Another small non-randomized study of 45 patients compared adjuvant vs. neoadjuvant fluouropyrimidine based chemoradiotherapy. Twelve patients were treated with neoadjuvant therapy and had a numerical but non-significant longer survival (five-year survival of 53% vs 23%, $p = 0.16$) and similar rates of grade 2–3 surgical morbidity compared to those treated in the postoperative setting.[18] Another study assessed the outcome of 22 patients treated with neoadjuvant therapy with gemcitabine 1000 mg/m^2 on days 1,8 and 15 of a 28-day schedule. Nine patients responded and eight had successful surgical resection, with an R0 resection in four patients and R1 resection in four. The survival rate at five-years for the 22 patients treated with neoadjuvant therapy was similar to the 249 patients treated with surgery upfront.[19] Another retrospective analysis looked at 91 patients with extrahepatic cholangiocarcinoma. Forty of these patients had unresectable disease. Nine underwent preoperative chemoradiation, with three patients achieving a complete pathologic response at the time of surgery. Negative margins were achieved in all patients ($n = 9$) that have undergone preoperative chemoradiation compared to only 54% of patients who did not.[20]

Based on all of the above evidence, neoadjuvant therapy for clearly resectable disease cannot be considered a standard treatment strategy. However, in patients whose disease is initially thought to be borderline resectable, it is reasonable to consider a trial of chemotherapy as the initial option with the intent of conversion to resection.

Locally advanced biliary tract cancers

The prognosis for locally advanced unresectable or locally recurrent biliary tract cancers is generally poor and is measured in months. Patients often have biliary obstruction and the aims of therapy include relief of biliary obstruction and amelioration of quality of life in addition to prolongation of survival. Palliative radiotherapy may offer symptomatic relief. Few small studies have reported the use of external beam radiotherapy with or without fluoropyrimidine based chemotherapy with evidence of limited benefit in outcome.[21] In some instances, intrahepatic arterial infusion of chemotherapy was given with radiation therapy with historically similar outcomes to systemic therapy.[22,23]

There are emerging data on the role of hepatic arterial infusion for treatment of advanced biliary tract cancers. A recent update on two prospective phase II clinical trials from the Memorial Sloan Kettering cancer center assessed the use of hepatic arterial infusion of floxuridine with or without systemic bevacizumab in patients with locally advanced unresectable intrahepatic cholangiocarcinoma. Median survival was 29.3 months in the floxuridine alone trial and 28.5 months in the floxuridine/bevacizumab trial. When data from the two trials were combined 48% of patients had a partial response lasting over a median time of 11.4 months (range 3.2–37.9 months) and 50% achieved stable disease over a median of 7 months (range 2–11 months).[24] Three patients (7%) were dowstaged and able to undergo hepatic resection. Another recent study of hepatic arterial infusion of cisplatin, 5-FU and isovorin with systemic gemcitabine in seven advanced intrahepatic cholangiocarcinoma patients resulted in a response rate of 57% and a median overall survival of 22.3 months. The main toxicities were hematolgic.[25]

Metastatic biliary tract cancer

The ABC-02 trial carried out in the United Kingdom was a landmark trial in metastatic biliary tract cancers. This pivotal trial established what most would regard as the current standard regimen. The trial randomized 410 patients with locally advanced unresectable or metastatic cholangiocarcinoma, gallbladder cancer and ampullary cancer to either cisplatin 25 mg/m^2 IV followed by gemcitabine 1000 mg/m^2 IV each on days 1 and 8 every three weeks for 8 cycles, or gemcitabine alone 1000 mg/m^2 on days 1, 8 and 15, every 4 weeks for 6 cycles. The median overall survival was 11.7 months in the cisplatin-gemcitabine arm versus 8.1 months in the gemcitabine alone arm.[26] The same regimen was tested in a Japanese population in the BT-22 trial, except the chemotherapy was given until disease progression. The median overall survival was 11.2 months in the cisplatin-gemcitabine arm compared to 7.7 months in the gemcitabine alone arm.[27] A meta-analysis of the two trials reported an improvement of PFS to 8.8 months with the combination versus 6.7 months with gemcitabine alone; HR = 0.64 (95% CI 0.53–0.76, $p < 0.001$).[28] The median overall survival was reported as 11.6 months versus 8.0 months; HR = 0.65 (95% CI 0.54–0.78), $p < 0.001$. Other first-line treatment options explored in phase II trials include CAPOX (capectitabine 1000 mg/m^2 orally BID days 1–14, and oxaliplatin 130 mg/m^2 IV day 1, every 3 weeks).[29] Response rates were stratified by location of the primary. In the gallbladder cancer/extrahepatic cholangiocarcinoma group was 27% (including 4% complete responses), and in the intrahepatic cholangiocarcinomas stable disease was the best response seen in 33%. Median overall survival was 8.2 months in gallbladder cancer (95% CI, 4.2–11.7), 16.8 months in extrahepatic cholangiocarcinoma (95% CI, 12.7–20.5) and 5.2 months in intrahepatic cholangiocarcinoma (95% CI, 0.6–9.8). Several studies including a large meta-analysis of phase II trials, have also shown that the combination of gemcitabine and oxaliplatin has activity in biliary tract cancers.[30] The addition of erlotinib[31] or cetuximab[32] to the combination of gemcitabine and oxaliplatin did not show any improvement in survival. A phase II trial of gemcitabine, irinotecan and panitumumab showed encouraging results with an overall survival of 12.9 months.[33] A phase II trial of bevacizumab 5 mg/kg on days 1 and 15 and erlotinib 150 mg daily on days 1–28, in the first-line treatment of unresectable or metastatic cholangiocarcinoma showed promising results with a median overall survival of 9.9 months and a time to progression of 4.4 months. Nine (12%) of the 49 patients evaluable for response achieved a partial response. Molecular profiling suggested that patients whose tumors have mutations in EGFRvIII, or who have non-wild-type KRAS may be less likely to respond to erlotinib therapy.[34]

A meta-analysis of the role of second-line therapy for biliary tract cancers showed that there was a survival benefit for second-line salvage treatment; the cohort of patients who stand to benefit most are those who maintain a good performance status after progression on first-line therapy.[35] Fornaro *et al.* developed a model to predict individual patient risk associated with second-line therapy for advanced biliary tract cancers.[36] The model was derived from a retrospective review of 300 patients with advanced biliary tract cancers treated with second-line chemotherapy at

10 Italian institutions between 2004 and 2013. Data on first- and second-line therapies was compiled. The population was enriched for patients who received a platinum and gemcitabine combination first-line (either gemcitabine and oxaliplatin from 2004–2010 or gemcitabine and cisplatin from 2010 onwards when ABC-02 and BT trials were published) as this was the standard approach. The primary endpoint of the analysis was overall survival. On univariate analysis, four independent favorable prognostic factors were found: an ECOG PS of 0 ($p < 0.001$; HR, 0.348; 95% CI 0.215–0.562), Ca19.9 ≤152 Uml-1 ($p = 0.013$; HR, 0.574; 95% CI. 0.370–0.891), previous surgery on primary tumor ($p = 0.027$; HR, 0.609; 95% CI, 0.392–0.945) and PFS after first-line chemotherapy ≥6 months ($p = 0.027$; HR, 0.633; 95% CI, 0.422–0.949). A multivariate prognosis model was devised by combining these four independent prognostic factors according to the following criteria: good-risk group included patients with zero to one negative prognostic factors; intermediate-risk group included patients with two negative prognostic factors; poor-risk group which included patients with three to four negative prognostic factors. Curves were constructed using the 249 patients in the study who received second-line therapy with 98, 73 and 78 patients in the good-, intermediate- and poor-risk groups respectively. The median overall survival for the good-, intermediate- and poor-risk groups were 13.1 months (95% CI, 9.0–17.2), 6.6 months (95% CI, 5.2–8.0) and 3.7 months (95% CI, 3.0–4.4), respectively, and the survival differences were statistically significantly different ($p < 0.001$). This model has not yet been validated in other studies but provides an interesting starting point to help determine who will benefit from second-line therapy for advanced and metastatic biliary tract cancers.

Novel and targeted agents in metastatic biliary tract cancers

Insights from molecular profiling of biliary tract cancers have informed the design of several phase II trials of novel and targeted agents. These trials unfortunately suffer from the same problems as older trials in that all subtypes of biliary tract cancers are lumped together because of the rarity of these cancers. Agents targeting the EGFR, VEGF, Her-2 and MEK signaling have been assessed in clinical trials (Table 2).[37–46] MEK

Table 2. Complete phase II trials in biliary tract cancer (BTC).

Agent	Disease	Number of patients	Study type	Treatment line	ORR	Comments	Reference
Bevacizumab & Erlotinib	BTC	53	Phase II	First	17%		37
Bevacizumab & Erlotinib	Upper GI cancers	102 (16 had BTC)	Phase II	Second line or beyond	6%	2 patients with BTC had a response	38
Sorafenib	BTC	46	Phase II	Any line	2%		39
Sorafenib	BTC	31	Phase II	First	6%	Terminated early due to failure to meet minimum of 1 confirmed PR	40
Sunitinib	BTC	56	Phase II	Second	9%		41
Lapatinib	HCC or BTC	57 (17 BTC)	Phase II	First and second	0% in BTC		42
Lapatinib	HCC or BTC	9	Phase II	Any	0%	Terminated early for futility. No evidence of HER-2 overexpression	43
Bortezomib	BTC	20	Phase II	First, second, third	5%	Trial stopped early for futility	44
Selumetinib	BTC	29	Phase II	Second	10%		45
Sorafenib & Erlotinib	BTC	34	Phase II	First	6%	2 unconfirmed PRs. Terminated early for futility	46

inhibitors seem to hold significant promise leading the way for a number of trials across the globe with single agent studies and combination studies with other agents such as PIK3CA inhibitors or standard chemotherapy.

Cetuximab and bevacizumab have also been added to gemcitabine and oxaliplatin based regimens with nine patients in one study achieving a good enough response to allow resection.[32,47–49]

Hepatocellular Carcinoma

Adjuvant therapy in resected or ablated hepatocellular carcinoma

Sorafenib is an oral multikinase inhibitor targeting VEGFR-2/PDGFR-beta signaling cascade thereby blocking angiogenesis, and it also blocks RAF kinase, a critical component of the RAF/MEK/ERK signaling pathway that controls cell division and proliferation and Flt-3 and RET. The STORM trial reported at the ASCO Annual Meeting, 2014 was a phase III, randomized, double blind, placebo-controlled trial of adjuvant sorafenib to prevent recurrence after resection or ablation of hepatocellular carcinoma. The trial randomized 1,114 patients treated with surgical resection or ablation with curative intent, intermediate to high risk of recurrence and Child Pugh Score 5–7 to sorafenib 400 mg BID p.o. vs. placebo for a maximum of four years. There was no difference in recurrence-free survival, time-to-recurrence or overall survival was observed.[50] Based on these results, adjuvant therapy is not recommended following surgery or ablation with curative intent.

Locally advanced and metastatic hepatocellular carcinoma

Two studies established sorafenib as the standard of care for the systemic treatment of locally advanced unresectable and metastatic hepatocellular carcinoma. The SHARP trial was a multinational trial that enrolled 602 patients and randomized in 1:1 ratio to sorafenib 400 mg BID p.o. vs. placebo on a day 1–28 schedule.[51] The primary endpoint was overall survival. The majority (95%) of the patients had Child's Pugh Class A liver dysfunction as intended by the trial. The trial was prematurely stopped at the second interim analysis when a significant survival advantage was observed in the intervention arm. The median overall survival was 10.7 months in the sorafenib group vs. 7.9 months in the observation arm (HR, 0.69 [95% CI, 0.55–0.87]. $p < 0.001$). The Asia-Pacific trial was another Asian confirmatory phase III trial of sorafenib vs. placebo in advanced or metastatic HCC.[52] The median overall survival was 6.5 months in the sorafenib arm versus 4.2 months in the placebo arm (HR, 0.68 [95% CI, 0.50–0.93]; $p = 0.014$). The difference in survival may be explained by the fact that the two trials enrolled different populations: the patients in the SHARP trial were mainly of Caucasian ethnicity and had a high prevalence of hepatitis C infection; patients enrolled in the Asia-Pacific trial had a higher prevalence of hepatitis B virus, but also had worse liver function and presented with a more advanced stage of HCC. However, the HR for survival, which some would argue can be regarded as a measure of sorafenib efficacy, was similar in both studies (0.69 and 0.68, respectively).[13] Exploratory subgroup analyses in both studies showed that sorafenib consistently improved median overall survival rate and disease control rate, irrespective of disease etiology, baseline tumor burden, performance status, tumor stage or prior therapy. The most common reasons for discontinuing sorafenib were diarrhea, fatigue and liver dysfunction. Subsequent follow on studies of sorafenib in a real-life setting such as GIDEON (Global Investigation of therapeutic Decisions in hepatocellular carcinoma and Of its treatment[53] with sorafeNib) and SOFIA[54] have attempted to assess the performance of sorafenib in patients who were excluded from randomized clinical trials, including Child-Pugh B patients. The second interim analysis of the observational phase IV GIDEON study reported safety data for 1,571 patients.[53] Sixty-one percent had Child-Pugh A status, 32% had Child-Pugh B and 2% had Child-Pugh C status with the status unknown for the remaining patients. Seventy-four percent of patients received the approved 800 mg/day initial sorafenib dose, regardless of Child-Pugh status; however, median duration of therapy was shorter in the Child-Pugh B patients vs. Child-Pugh A patients (8.6 weeks vs. 13.7 weeks) . There was a similar incidence of drug-related adverse events in both groups, but a higher percentage of severe drug-related adverse events, and a higher rate of discontinuation of treatment due to adverse events in the Child-Pugh B patients. Safety profiles appeared similar regardless of initial dose. Efficacy has not yet been reported.

A field practice study led by SOFIA (SOraFenib Italian Assessment) is a prospective multicenter study in Italy which aimed to adequately assess the risks and benefits of sorafenib in daily practice.[54] Two hundred and ninety-six patients with advanced or intermediate HCC who were unfit, or failed to respond to ablative therapies, were commenced on 800 mg/day of sorafenib. Dose reductions or interruptions were performed according to the drug label recommendations. Treatment interruptions occurred in 40% of patients because of adverse events. The median survival time was 10.5 months in the overall cohort which was similar to the SHARP study. Median survival was 8.4 months in BCLC-C versus 20.6 months in BCLC-B patients ($p < 0.0001$). Of note, median survival in 77 patients treated for >70% of the time with 200 mg BID was 21.6 months versus 9.6 months in the 219 patients treated for >70% of the time with full dose (400 mg BID). The authors explained these unexpected results as being due to the ability of a targeted cytostatic molecule to retain anticancer activity at suboptimal dosing, and the prolonged exposure of down-dosed patients to sorafenib as it was better tolerated. Interestingly, a cost-effectiveness study led by the SOFIA group showed that dose-adjusted sorafenib, but not full-dose, sorafenib is a cost-effective treatment compared to best supportive care in intermediate and advanced hepatocellular carcinoma.[55] These interesting findings will need further validation in prospective randomized trials.

Elderly patients

A retrospective analysis of the outcomes and safety of sorafenib in elderly patients categorized patients into age ≥70 years (35 patients) and ≤70 years (137 patients).[56] The results were similar between the older and younger groups with median progression-free survival of 2.99 months vs. 3.09 months ($p = 0.275$) and median overall survival of 5.32 months vs. 5.16 months ($p = 0.310$) respectively. The adverse event profile was overall similar in both groups, but the authors called to attention that neutropenia, malaise and mucositis were more frequently reported in the elderly cohort.

Sorafenib combined with locoregional approaches

Sorafenib has been combined with locoregional approaches in advanced disease combined to the liver. While this approach is not considered standard of care at present, data from phase II studies show promising results. The rationale behind combining locoregional therapies with sorafenib is based on the hypothesis that tumor ischemia and hypoxia created following the locoregional therapy in the liver leads to upregulation of hypoxia inducible factor 1α and stimulation of expression of VEGF which results in neovascularization facilitating tumor regrowth and progression.[57] An early multicenter phase II study of radioembolization with yttrium-90 followed 14 days later by sorafenib 400 mg BID p.o. reported manageable toxicity profile.[58] Median survival was 20.3 months in BCLC-B patients and 8.6 months in BCLC-C patients. The START study (Study in Asia of the combination of Transcatheter Arterial Chemoembolization with sorafenib in patients with hepatocellular carcinoma) reported on 147 patients that were treated with transcatheter arterial chemoembolization (TACE) using an emulsion of lipiodol (5–20 ml) and doxorubicin (30–60 mg) followed 4 to 7 days later by oral sorafenib 400 mg BID, with TACE cycles repeated every 6–8 weeks.[59] Results from the first interim analysis reported a median progression free survival of 270 days, a time to progression of 280 days and an overall survival probability of >90% over the same time period. Almost 50% of patients achieved a partial or complete response after the first TACE cycle. However, two randomized placebo-controlled trials failed to show any survival benefit when sorafenib or placebo were administered following TACE. In a phase III trial in Japan and Korea, patients with unresectable HCC, Child-Pugh class A cirrhosis and ≥25% tumor necrosis/shrinkage 1–3 months after 1 or 3 TACE procedures were randomized 1:1 to sorafenib 400 mg BID po or placebo. Patients were treated until progression, recurrence or unacceptable toxicity. The study failed to meet its primary endpoint of TTP. Median TTP in sorafenib group was 5.4 months and in placebo group was 3.7 months (HR, 0.87; 95% CI, 0.70–1.09; $p = 0.252$). There was no difference in overall survival (HR 1.06, 95% CI 0.69–1.64; $p = 0.790$).[60] The SPACE trial randomized patients to sorafenib or placebo and after all patients had received the first dose of study drug, they proceeded to get TACE with drug-eluting beads with doxorubicin

(DEBDOX), and again on day 1 (±4days) of months 3,7 and 13, and every 6 months thereafter. This study has only been published in abstract form to date. According to authors of the abstract the study met its primary endpoint of time to radiologic progression (HR, 0.797, 95% CI 0.588–1.080, p=0.072). There was no difference in overall survival between the sorafenib and placebo arms (HR 0.898, 95% CI 0.606–1.330, p=0.295).[52] Thus, there is insufficient evidence at present to recommend combining TACE with sorafenib.

Other targeted agents for advanced HCC

Two randomized phase III trials of the selective VEGF and FGF receptor inhibitor brivanib failed to show any significant overall survival benefit in either the first-line metastatic setting vs. sorafenib or post-progression on sorafenib.[61,62] It also appeared to be less well-tolerated than sorafenib. In another randomized phase III trial (SUN1170) comparing another VEGF, PDGF and Kit inhibitor, sunitinib, vs. sorafenib, overall survival with sunitinib was not superior or equivalent to sorafenib but was significantly inferior to sorafenib. It was also associated with more toxicity.[63] Linifanib, a selective VEGFR and PDGFR tyrosine-kinase inhibitor, was also investigated in first-line treatment of HCC compared to sorafenib. Survival with linifinib was inferior to sorafenib (9.1 versus 9.8 months, HR 1.045, 95% CI, 0.896–1.221).[64] Ramucirumab is a fully human monoclonal antibody which specifically inhibits VEGFR2. Ramucirumab is currently being investigated in a phase III trial in patients with HCC after failure of sorafenib (http://clinicaltrials.gov/show/NCT01140347). Currently, there are a number of targeted agents undergoing phase III trial assessment in advanced and metastatic hepatocellular carcinoma (Table 3). MET is a protooncogene that encodes a protein known as hepatocyte growth-factor receptor.[65,66] C-MET inhibitors offer promise as MET may be overexpressed in HCC and aberrant MET signaling is frequently found.[67–69] Drugs such as tivantinib and cabozantanib (targeting Met and VEGFR2) are currently in clinical trials. Immune therapies such as the PD-1 inhibitors nivolumab and pembrolizumab, and CTLA4 inhibitors such as tremelimumab are also undergoing assessment in phase I and II trials.

Table 3. Ongoing phase III trials of novel and targeted agents in advanced and metastatic hepatocellular carcinoma.

Drug	Target	Setting	Clinicaltrials.gov identifier
Tivantinib	c-MET	Post progression on sorafenib	NCT02029157
Lenvatinib	VEGFR-2, VEGFR-3, FGFR, PDGFR	First line versus sorafenib	NCT01761266
Sorafenib and doxorubicin		First line versus sorafenib alone	NCT01015833
Ramucirumab	VEGFR-2	Post progression on sorafenib	NCT01140347
Cabozantinib	c-Met, VEGFR-2	Post progression on sorafenib	NCT01908426
ADI-PEG 20 (arginine deaminase with polyethylene glycol)	Arginine	Second line post progression on any prior systemic agent	NCT01287585

Second-line therapy beyond sorafenib

Continuation of sorafenib beyond progression is a strategy sometimes employed when no further treatment options are available. Two studies support this option compared with best supportive care, although the studies have been criticized for selection bias and failed to show an overall survival benefit.[70,71] Prior to the era of sorafenib, cytotoxic chemotherapies such as doxorubicin, gemcitabine, oxaliplatin, 5-FU and capecitabine have been used. If a clinical trial is not available, chemotherapy could be considered in a fit patient, although the evidence is based mainly on phase II data. One example is the PIAF regimen (cisplatin, interferon-α, doxorubicin and 5-FU) which has reported activity, including partial responses and some complete pathologic responses reported in phase II trials. However, the regimen is associated with significant toxicity.[64–66]

Take Home Messages

- Adjuvant chemotherapy +/– radiotherapy is recommended for resected biliary tract cancers with R1 (positive margins) and/or lymph node involvement.
- Cisplatin and gemcitabine are currently the recommended standard regimen for metastatic biliary tract cancers.
- There is no survival benefit associated with sorafenib in the adjuvant setting following resection or ablation of hepatocellular carcinoma with curative intent or following or combined with TACE.
- Sorafenib remains the standard first-line option for locally advanced unresectable and metastatic hepatocellular carcinoma.
- Whole exome sequencing of hepatobiliary tumors may enlighten the development of molecular targeted therapies.
- Mechanisms under circumvent immune tolerance in the liver through the use of immune checkpoint inhibitors offer promise treatment results in hepatocellular carcinoma.

References

1. Borad, M.J. *et al.*, Integrated genomic characterization reveals novel, therapeutically relevant drug targets in FGFR and EGFR pathways in sporadic intrahepatic cholangiocarcinoma. *PLoS Genet*, 2014. **10**(2): e1004135.
2. Ito, T. *et al.*, Genomic and transcriptional alterations of cholangiocarcinoma. *J Hepato-Biliary-Pancreatic Sci*, 2014. **21**(6): 380–7.
3. Hezel, A. & Noel, M., New and emerging treatment options for biliary tract cancer. *OncoTargets Ther*, 2013. 1545.
4. http://cancergenome.nih.gov *The Cancer Genome Atlas*. National Cancer Institute, 2014.
5. Hato, T., Goyal, L., Greten, T.F., Duda, D.G., Zhu, A.X., Immune checkpoint blockade in hepatocellular carcinoma: Current progress and future directions. *Hepatology*, 2014.
6. Jarnagin, W.R. *et al.*, Patterns of initial disease recurrence after resection of gallbladder carcinoma and hilar cholangiocarcinoma. *Cancer*, 2003. **98**(8): 1689–700.

7. Hasegawa, S., Ikai, I., Fujii, H., Hatano, E., Shimahara, Y., Surgical Resection of hilar cholangiocarcinoma: analysis of survival and postoperative complications. *World J Surg*, 2007. **31**(6): 1258–65.
8. Macdonald, O.K. & Crane, C.H., Palliative and postoperative radiotherapy in biliary tract cancer. *Surg Oncol Clinics North Am*, 2002. **11**(4): 941–54.
9. Williams, T.M., Majithia, L., Wang, S.J., Thomas, C.R., Defining the role of adjuvant therapy: cholangiocarcinoma and gall bladder cancer. *Semin Radiation Oncol*, 2014. **24**(2): 94-104.
10. Gold, D.G. *et al.*, Adjuvant therapy for gallbladder carcinoma: the mayo clinic experience. *Int J Rad Oncol Biol Phys*, 2009. **75**(1): 150–5.
11. Mojica, P., Smith, D., & Ellenhorn, J., Adjuvant radiation therapy is associated with improved survival for gallbladder carcinoma with regional metastatic disease. *J Surgical Oncol*, 2007. **96**(1): 8–13.
12. Takada, T. *et al.*, Is postoperative adjuvant chemotherapy useful for gallbladder carcinoma? *Cancer*, 2002. **95**(8): 1685–95.
13. Di Marco, V. *et al.*, Sorafenib: from literature to clinical practice. *Ann Oncol*, 2013. **24**(Suppl 2): ii30-7.
14. Horgan, A.M., Amir, E., Walter, T., Knox, J.J., Adjuvant therapy in the treatment of biliary tract cancer: a systematic review and meta-analysis. *J Clinical Oncol*, 2012. **30**(16): 1934–40.
15. McNamara, M.G. *et al.*, Outcome of adjuvant therapy in biliary tract cancers. *Am J Clinical Oncol*, 2013. 1.
16. Wang, S.J. *et al.*, Nomogram for predicting the benefit of adjuvant chemoradiotherapy for resected gallbladder cancer. *J Clinical Oncol*, 2011. **29**(35): 4627–32.
17. Glazer, E.S., Liu, P., Abdalla, E.K., Vauthey, J.-N., Curley, S.A., Neither neoadjuvant nor adjuvant therapy increases survival after biliary tract cancer resection with wide negative margins. *J Gastrointestinal Surg*, 2012. **16**(9): 1666–71.
18. Nelson, J.W. *et al.*, Concurrent chemoradiotherapy in resected extrahepatic cholangiocarcinoma. *Int J Radiat Oncol Biol Phys*, 2009. **73**(1):148–53.
19. Kato, A. *et al.*, Surgical resection after downsizing chemotherapy for initially unresectable locally advanced biliary tract cancer: a retrospective single-center study. *Ann Surgical Oncol*, 2012. **20**(1): 318–24.
20. McMasters, K.M. *et al.*, Neoadjuvant chemoradiation for extrahepatic cholangiocarcinoma. *Am J Surg*, 1997. **174**(6): 605–8; discussion 608–9.

21. Minsky, B.D., Kemeny, N., Armstrong, J.G., Reichman, B., Botet, J., Extrahepatic biliary system cancer: an update of a combined modality approach. *Am J Clin Oncol*, 1991. **14**(5): 433–7.
22. Robertson, J.M. *et al.*, Long-term results of hepatic artery fluorodeoxyuridine and conformal radiation therapy for primary hepatobiliary cancers. *Int J Radiat Oncol Biol Phys*, 1997. **37**(2): 325–30.
23. Ben-Josef, E. *et al.*, Phase II trial of high-dose conformal radiation therapy with concurrent hepatic artery floxuridine for unresectable intrahepatic malignancies. *J Clin Oncol*, 2005. **23**(34): 8739–47.
24. Konstantinidis, I.T. *et al.*, Regional chemotherapy for unresectable intrahepatic cholangiocarcinoma: a potential role for dynamic magnetic resonance imaging as an imaging biomarker and a survival update from two prospective clinical trials. *Annals of Surgical Oncology*, 2014.
25. Marumoto, M. *et al.*, Systemic gemcitabine combined with hepatic arterial infusion chemotherapy with cisplatin, 5-fluorouracil, and isovorin for the treatment of advanced intrahepatic cholangiocarcinoma: a pilot study. *Hepatogastroenterology*, 2014. **61**(129): 162–7.
26. Valle, J. *et al.*, Cisplatin plus gemcitabine versus gemcitabine for biliary tract cancer. *N Engl J Med*, 2010. **362**(14): 1273–81.
27. Okusaka, T. *et al.*, Gemcitabine alone or in combination with cisplatin in patients with biliary tract cancer: a comparative multicentre study in Japan. *Brit J Cancer*, 2010. **103**(4): 469–74.
28. Valle, J.W. *et al.*, Cisplatin and gemcitabine for advanced biliary tract cancer: a meta-analysis of two randomised trials. *Ann Oncol*, 2013. **25**(2): 391–8.
29. Nehls, O. *et al.*, Capecitabine plus oxaliplatin as first-line treatment in patients with advanced biliary system adenocarcinoma: a prospective multicentre phase II trial. *Brit J Cancer*, 2008. **98**(2): 309–15.
30. Eckel, F. & Schmid, R.M., Chemotherapy in advanced biliary tract carcinoma: a pooled analysis of clinical trials. *Brit J Cancer*, 2007. **96**(6): 896–902.
31. Lee, J. *et al.*, Gemcitabine and oxaliplatin with or without erlotinib in advanced biliary-tract cancer: a multicentre, open-label, randomised, phase 3 study. *Lancet Oncol*, 2012. **13**(2): 181–8.
32. Malka, D. *et al.*, Gemcitabine and oxaliplatin with or without cetuximab in advanced biliary-tract cancer (BINGO): a randomised, open-label, non-comparative phase 2 trial. *Lancet Oncol*, 2014.

33. Sohal, D.P.S. *et al.*, A phase II trial of gemcitabine, irinotecan and panitumumab in advanced cholangiocarcinoma. *Ann Oncol*, 2013. **24**(12): 3061–5.
34. Lubner, S.J. *et al.*, Report of a multicenter phase II trial testing a combination of biweekly bevacizumab and daily erlotinib in patients with unresectable biliary cancer: a phase II consortium study. *J Clin Oncol*, 2010. **28**(21): 3491–7.
35. Lamarca, A., Hubner, R.A., Ryder, W.D., Valle, J.W., Second-line chemotherapy in advanced biliary cancer: a systematic review. *Ann Oncol*, 2014.
36. Fornaro, L. *et al.*, Multivariate prognostic factors analysis for second-line chemotherapy in advanced biliary tract cancer. *Br J Cancer*, 2014. **110**(9): 2165–9.
37. Lubner, S.J. *et al.*, Report of a multicenter phase II trial testing a combination of biweekly bevacizumab and daily erlotinib in patients with unresectable biliary cancer: a phase II Consortium study. *J Clin Oncol*, 2010. **28**(21): 3491–7.
38. Rohrberg, K.S. *et al.*, Phase II trial of erlotinib and bevacizumab in patients with advanced upper gastrointestinal cancers. *Acta Oncol*, 2012. **51**(2): 234–42.
39. Bengala, C. *et al.*, Sorafenib in patients with advanced biliary tract carcinoma: a phase II trial. *Br J Cancer*, 2010. **102**(1): 68–72.
40. El-Khoueiry, A.B. *et al.*, SWOG 0514: a phase II study of sorafenib in patients with unresectable or metastatic gallbladder carcinoma and cholangiocarcinoma. *Invest New Drugs*, 2012. **30**(4): 1646–51.
41. Yi, J.H. *et al.*, A phase II study of sunitinib as a second-line treatment in advanced biliary tract carcinoma: a multicentre, multinational study. *Eur J Cancer*, 2012. **48**(2): 196–201.
42. Ramanathan, R.K. *et al.*, A phase II study of lapatinib in patients with advanced biliary tree and hepatocellular cancer. *Cancer Chemother Pharmacol*, 2009. **64**(4): 777–83.
43. Peck, J. *et al.*, HER2/neu may not be an interesting target in biliary cancers: results of an early phase II study with lapatinib. *Oncology*, 2012. **82**(3): 175–9.
44. Costello N.J.M, M. R., Denlinger, C. S., Engstrom, P. F., Wright, J. J., Li, T., Mclaughlin, S., Beard, M., Cimildoro R. and Cohen S. J., A phase II trial of the proteasome inhibitor bortezomib in patients with recurrent or metastatic adenocarcinoma of the bile duct or gallbladder (NCI #6135) *J Clini Oncol*, 2009. **27**(15S).

45. Bekaii-Saab, T. *et al.*, Multi-institutional phase II study of selumetinib in patients with metastatic biliary cancers. *J Clin Oncol*, 2011. **29**(17): 2357–63.
46. El-Khoueiry, A.B. *et al.*, S0941: a phase 2 SWOG study of sorafenib and erlotinib in patients with advanced gallbladder carcinoma or cholangiocarcinoma. *Br J Cancer*, 2014. **110**(4): 882–7.
47. Gruenberger, B. *et al.*, Cetuximab, gemcitabine, and oxaliplatin in patients with unresectable advanced or metastatic biliary tract cancer: a phase 2 study. *Lancet Oncol*, 2010. **11**(12): 1142–8.
48. Zhu, A.X., *et al.*, Efficacy and safety of gemcitabine, oxaliplatin, and bevacizumab in advanced biliary-tract cancers and correlation of changes in 18-fluorodeoxyglucose PET with clinical outcome: a phase 2 study. *Lancet Oncol*, 2010. **11**(1): 48–54.
49. Chen, L.-T., Chen, J.-S., Chao, Y., Tsai, C.-S., Shan, Y.-S., Hsu, C., Huang, S.-F., Tsou, H.-H., Lee, K.-D., Chiu, C.-F., Rau, K.-M., Ho., C.-L., Yu, M.-S., and Taiwan Cooperative Oncology Group, KRAS mutation status-stratified randomized phase II trial of GEMOX with and without cetuximab in advanced biliary tract cancer (ABTC): The TCOG T1210 trial. *J Clin Oncol*, 2013. **15**(Supplement May 20).
50. Bruix, J., Takayama, T., Mazzaferro, V., Chau, G.-Y., Yang, J., Kudo, M., Cai, J., Poon, R.T.-P., Han, K.-H., Tak, W.-Y., Lee, H.C., Song, T., Roayaie, S., Bolondi, L., Lee, K.S., Makuuchi, M., Souza, F., Le Berre, M.-A., Meishardt, G., Llovet, J.M., STORM Investigator, STORM: A phase III randomized, double-blind, placebo-controlled trial of adjuvant sorafenib after resection or ablation to prevent recurrence of hepatocellular carcinoma (HCC). *J Clin Oncol*, 2014. **32**(5s):Suppl; abst 4006.
51. Llovet, J.M. *et al.*, Sorafenib in advanced hepatocellular carcinoma. *N Engl J Med*, 2008. **359**(4): 378–90.
52. Lencioni, R., Llovet, J.M., Han, E., Tak, W.Y., Yang, J., Leberre, M.-A., Niv, W., Nicholson, K., Meinhardt, G., Bruix, J., Sorafenib or placebo in combination with transarterial chemoembolization (TACE) with doxorubicin-eluting beads (DEBDOX) for intermediate-stage hepatocellular carcinoma (HCC): Phase II, randomized, double-blind SPACE trial. *J Clin Oncol*, 2012. **30**(Suppl 4): Abstr LBA 154.
53. Lencioni, R. *et al.*, GIDEON (Global Investigation of therapeutic DEcisions in hepatocellular carcinoma and of its treatment with sorafeNib): second interim analysis. *Int J Clin Pract*, 2014. **68**(5): 609–17.

54. Iavarone, M. *et al.*, Field-practice study of sorafenib therapy for hepatocellular carcinoma: a prospective multicenter study in Italy. *Hepatology*, 2011. **54**(6): 2055–2063.
55. Camma, C. *et al.*, Cost-effectiveness of sorafenib treatment in field practice for patients with hepatocellular carcinoma. *Hepatology*, 2013. **57**(3): 1046–1054.
56. Wong, H. *et al.*, The outcomes and safety of single-agent sorafenib in the treatment of elderly patients with advanced hepatocellular carcinoma (HCC). *Oncologist*, 2011. **16**(12): 1721–8.
57. Liapi, E., Geschwind, J.F., Combination of local transcatheter arterial chemoembolization and systemic anti-angiogenic therapy for unresectable hepatocellular carcinoma. *Liver Cancer*, 2012. **1**(3–4): 201–15.
58. Chow, P.K. *et al.*, Multicenter phase II study of sequential radioembolization-sorafenib therapy for inoperable hepatocellular carcinoma. *PLoS ONE*, 2014. **9**(3): e90909.
59. Chung, Y.H. *et al.*, Interim analysis of START: Study in Asia of the combination of TACE (transcatheter arterial chemoembolization) with sorafenib in patients with hepatocellular carcinoma trial. *Int J Cancer*, 2013. **132**(10): 2448–58.
60. Kudo, M. *et al.*, Phase III study of sorafenib after transarterial chemoembolisation in Japanese and Korean patients with unresectable hepatocellular carcinoma. *Eur J Cancer*, 2011. **47**(14): 2117–27.
61. Johnson, P.J. *et al.*, Brivanib versus sorafenib as first-line therapy in patients with unresectable, advanced hepatocellular carcinoma: results from the randomized phase III BRISK-FL study. *J Clin Oncol*, 2013. **31**(28): 3517–24.
62. Llovet, J.M. *et al.*, Brivanib in patients with advanced hepatocellular carcinoma who were intolerant to sorafenib or for whom sorafenib failed: results from the randomized phase III BRISK-PS study. *J Clin Oncol*, 2013. **31**(28): 3509–16.
63. Cheng, A.L. *et al.*, Sunitinib versus sorafenib in advanced hepatocellular cancer: results of a randomized phase III trial. *J Clin Oncol*, 2013. **31**(32): 4067–75.
64. Cainap, C., Qin, S., Huang, W.-T., Chung, I.-J., Pan, H., Cheng, Y., Kudo, M., Kang, Y.-K., Chen, P.-J., Toh, H.C., Gorbunva, V., Eskens, F., Qian, J., Mckee, M.D., Ricker, J.L., Carlson, D.M., Nowiem, S.E., Phase III trial of linifanib versus sorafenib in patients with advanced hepatocellular carcinoma (HCC). *J Clin Oncol,* 2013. **31**(Suppl 4): Abst 249.

65. Christensen, J.G., Burrows, J., Salgia, R., c-Met as a target for human cancer and characterization of inhibitors for therapeutic intervention. *Cancer Lett*, 2005. **225**(1): 1–26.
66. Danilkovitch-Miagkova, A., Zbar, B., Dysregulation of Met receptor tyrosine kinase activity in invasive tumors. *J Clin Invest*, 2002. **109**(7): 863–7.
67. Kondo, S. *et al.*, Clinical impact of c-Met expression and its gene amplification in hepatocellular carcinoma. *Int J Clin Oncol*, 2013. **18**(2): 207–13.
68. Kaposi-Novak, P. *et al.*, Met-regulated expression signature defines a subset of human hepatocellular carcinomas with poor prognosis and aggressive phenotype. *J Clin Invest*, 2006. **116**(6): 1582–95.
69. Ueki, T., Fujimoto, J., Suzuki, T., Yamamoto, H., Okamoto, E., Expression of hepatocyte growth factor and its receptor, the c-met proto-oncogene, in hepatocellular carcinoma. *Hepatology*, 1997. **25**(3): 619–23.
70. Woo, H.Y., *et al.*, Clinical course of sorafenib treatment in patients with hepatocellular carcinoma. *Scand J Gastroenterol*, 2012. 47(7):809–19.
71. Rimassa, L. *et al.*, A phase II randomized dose escalation trial of sorafenib in patients with advanced hepatocellular carcinoma. *Oncologist*, 2013. **18**(4): 379–80.

Chapter 19

Surgical Treatment of Hepatobiliary Malignancies and Liver Transplantation

Jean-Sébastien Pelletier and David A. Geller

What is New

- Laparoscopic resection of hepatocellular carcinoma is comparable to open liver resection in case-cohort studies.

Introduction

Once associated with a high morbidity and mortality, liver surgery has become increasingly safe and feasible. Thanks to advances in surgical anatomy, operative techniques as well as pre- and post-operative care, the associated morbidity and mortality have decreased markedly.[1] While other modalities are commonly used in the treatment of hepatic tumors, including ablative techniques and intra-arterial chemotherapy, liver surgery — either by resection of by the use of liver transplantation — confers the only potential for cure in patients with primary liver cancer. As such, the potential for resection should be assessed in all patients prior to the consideration of other treatment modalities. It is therefore of utmost importance for patients to be evaluated by qualified surgeons as soon as possible in order to give patients the best chance for cure.

Hepatocellular Carcinoma

Introduction

Hepatocellular carcinoma (HCC) is a common form of cancer, being the sixth most common neoplasm worldwide.[2] The worldwide distribution of this cancer is not evenly distributed, and most of these occur in the developing world where hepatitis B is endemic.[3] Approximately 85% of all cases occur in East Asia and Sub-Saharan Africa.[4] The incidence of this cancer is markedly increasing in the western world, and it is the fastest-growing cause of cancer-related death in the United States.[3] Unfortunately, even in countries with advanced medical technologies, it is a particularly lethal form of cancer, second only to pancreatic adenocarcinoma in terms of five-year survival in the United States of America.[3,5]

Risk factors

worldwide, the most common cause of HCC is the hepatitis B virus, and an estimated 300 million people are infected worldwide.[6] However, thanks to successful vaccination programs, this is a rare etiological agent in developed countries. Rather, the hepatitis C virus is the most common cause of HCC in the western world and is the cause of 48% of cases in the United States.[6] Other important causes include alcohol abuse, non-alcoholic steatohepatitis (NASH), hemochromatosis, alpha-1 antitrypsin deficiency and certain environmental toxins such as aflatoxin.[7,8]

Clinical presentation

Most often, HCC is not associated with particular symptoms, which underlines the need for screening measures. In certain cases, acute decompensation of hepatic function may be the only clue. Therefore, in patients with previously well-controlled cirrhosis, the development of variceal bleeding, jaundice, ascites or encephalopathy should alert the clinician of the possibility of a malignancy as the cause. This occurs due to liver being replaced by tumor, invasion into major vascular structures or arterio-venous shunting caused by the tumor. Uncommonly, patients may present with symptoms of metastatic disease, such as bone pain or dyspnea, intra-peritoneal bleeding from tumor rupture or fever from central tumor necrosis.[9]

Screening

Screening for HCC is of utmost importance because, as noted above, it is usually clinically silent in the early stages and is only potentially curative in its early stages.[4] According to the American Association of Liver Diseases (AASLD), screening should be performed on anybody who has cirrhosis, as well as HBV carriers if they fall into one of the following four categories: (1) males of Asian descent over the age of 40; (2) females of Asian descent over the age of 50; (3) African or North American black men or women of any age; and (4) any patient with a family history of HCC.[10] In spite of these recommendations, it is clear that screening is not being performed appropriately, as evidenced by a large series from Veterans Affairs where only 22% of patients with cirrhosis were obtaining regular surveillance.[11]

According to the AASLD, screening for HCC should consist of abdominal ultrasounds every 6 months, which provides a sensitivity of 94% but only 63% for early HCC. If a nodule that is less than 1 cm is detected, an ultrasound should be repeated in three months time. If a nodule that is greater than 1 cm is detected, a four-phase contrast-enhanced computed tomography (CT) scan or a contrast-enhanced magnetic resonance imaging (MRI) scan should then be performed.[12] Routine CT scans or MRIs are not recommended for surveillance as they incur high false-positive rates, increase the cost and expose the patients to radiation (in the case of CTs). Additionally, while a serum alpha-fetoprotein (AFP) increases the detection rate by 6–8% when used in conjunction with ultrasound, it is not endorsed by the AASLD nor its European counterpart, the European Association for the Study of the Liver-European Organization for the Research and Treatment of Cancer (EASL-EORTC), for screening purposes due to the increased false-positive rate and the 80% increase in cost.[10]

Diagnosis

The diagnosis of HCC is often made radiologically, and a biopsy is only required for diagnostic uncertainty and if it would cause a change in management. Routine biopsies are avoided to decrease the risk of bleeding, rupture or tumor seeding.[12] HCC has a characteristic enhancement pattern on cross-sectional imaging, consisting of early arterial enhancement followed by portal venous or delayed phase washout.[13] Unfortunately, not all HCC will present with these characteristics, especially in smaller lesions, and as such a biopsy is warranted if clinical suspicion is high.[14]

Staging

Multiple systems are currently in use to stage HCC, which include the TNM, Okuda, Japan Integrated Staging (JIS), Cancer of the Liver Italian Program (CLIP) and the Barcelona Clinic Liver Cancer (BCLC) staging systems. All of these systems attempt to stratify patients based on their overall prognosis. As surgeons, the most clinically relevant and therefore most widely used is the American Liver Tumor Study Group Modified TNM classification and staging system (Table 1).[15] This system takes into

Table 1. American liver tumor study group modified TNM classification and staging system for hepatocellular carcinoma.

Primary tumor (T) stage		Regional lymph node (N) stage		Distant metastasis (M) stage	
TX	Not assessed	NX	Not assessed	MX	Not assessed
T0	None found	N0	None found	M0	None found
T1	One nodule ≤ 1.9 cm	N1	Regional nodal involvement	M1	Metastatic disease
T2	One nodule 2–5 cm or 2–3 nodules, all < 3 cm	—	—	—	—
T3	One nodule > 5 cm or 2–3 nodules, at least one > 3 cm	—	—	—	—
T4a	Four or more nodules	—	—	—	—
T4b	T2, T3 or T4a plus gross portal or hepatic venous involvement	—	—	—	—

(*Continued*)

Table 1. (*Continued*)

Stage	Primary tumor (T) stage	Regional lymph node (N) stage	Distant metastasis (M) stage
I	T1	N0	M0
II	T2	N0	M0
III	T3	N0	M0
IVA1	T4a	N0	M0
IVA2	T4b	N0	M0
IVB	Any T	N1	M0
	Any T	Any N	M1

account the Milan criteria, and thus simplifies the language when discussing the potential treatments for patients. As such, all patients whose tumor characteristics fall within Milan criteria are considered stage 2. Therefore, all patients that are stage 3 and above are not considered candidates for a liver transplantation for most organ allocation organizations.

Surgical management

The only cure for HCC is the surgical removal of the affected liver, either via resection or orthotopic liver transplantation (OLT). OLT is theoretically superior as it addresses the underlying cause of the cancer, the cirrhosis. There are however donor shortages with long waiting lists and high dropout rates. OLT also exposes the patient to the risks and side effects associated with immunosuppression. As such, both of these procedures present advantages and drawbacks. The direct comparison of these two treatment modalities are flawed and no randomized comparative trials comparing resection and transplantation have to date been performed. In either case, pre-operative planning is of utmost importance to ensure the successful completion of the procedure. A treatment algorithm for HCC is presented in Fig. 1.

Surgical resection for HCC

The safety and feasibility of liver resections has increased dramatically over the last few decades, due mainly to a better understanding of intrahepatic anatomy, improved surgical techniques, a better grasp of perioperative care

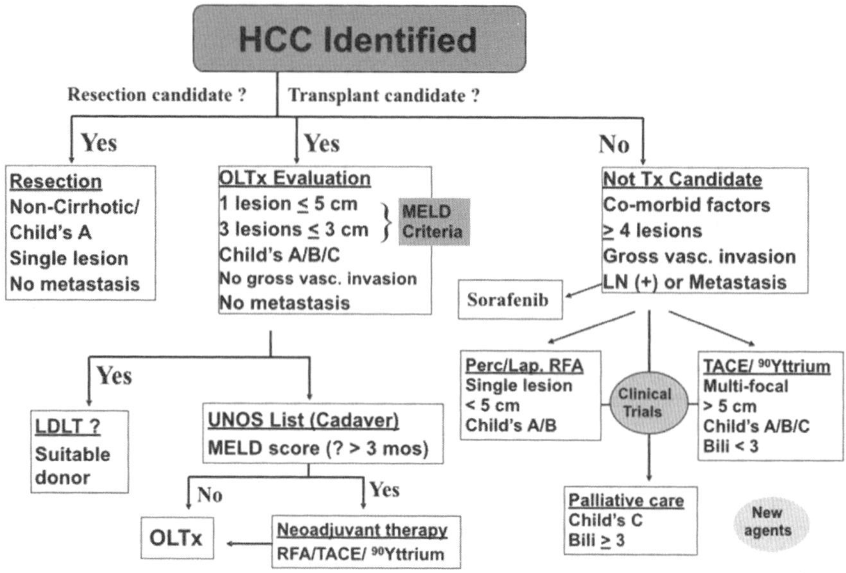

Fig. 1. Treatment algorithm for hepatocellular carcinoma.

and technological improvements in imaging modalities. The goal of surgical resection is to remove all viable tumors with negative surgical margins and an adequate functional liver remnant.

If a resection is planned, an evaluation of the potential for the patient to tolerate major surgery should be undertaken. In addition, an evaluation of hepatic function using the Child's-Turcotte-Pugh (CTP) or Model for End-Stage Liver Disease (MELD) score should be undertaken. An evaluation of the functional liver remnant should be performed as at least 25% should be left behind in patients with normal liver function,[16] 40% in high-grade steatosis and greater than 50% in patients with cirrhosis.[17] If there is any concern as to the size of the remaining liver, volumetric assessments using CT or MRI can be utilized for an objective measure and are invaluable tools to the operating surgeon.[18] In instances when a larger functional liver remnant is required, ipsilateral portal vein embolization can be utilized.[19]

The advantages of resection for HCC are that there are no wait times, no need for immunosuppression, lower morbidity and early mortality and it does not preclude from an OLT in the future.[20] While resection is associated with a higher rate of recurrence than OLT, it has been shown that five-year survival rates are similar,[21] although there are no prospective trials comparing these two techniques. As such, in spite of higher recurrence rates as compared to OLT, surgical resection of HCC is a reasonable option in patients without extensive medical comorbidities and who have early cirrhosis.[20]

Laparoscopic liver resections have been shown to be safe and feasible for a variety of benign and malignant surgical conditions and greater than 3,000 have been performed worldwide. Being that the most common indications for liver resections are malignant in nature, HCC was the most common indication for laparoscopic liver resections in a recent world review.[22] Patient selection is key, and care must be taken to avoid patients who have tumors near the transection line or major vessels.[23]

Multiple studies have compared laparoscopic and open resections for HCC in case-control matched studies, without a difference in overall survival found (Table 2).[24–36] Several systematic reviews have compared these two techniques, and found that certain important benefits were

Table 2. Comparison of five-year overall survival comparing laparoscopic liver resection (LLR) to open liver resection (OLR) for hepatocellular carcinoma (HCC) in case-cohort matched studies.

				Number of cases		Five-year overall survival (OS) (%)		
Authors	Year	Journal	Country	LLR	OLR	LLR	OLR	*p*-value
Shimada *et al.*[24]	2001	*Surg Endosc*	Japan	17	38	50	38	NS
Kaneko *et al.*[25]	2005	*Am J Surg*	Japan	30	28	61	62	NS
Cai *et al.*[26]	2008	*Surg Endosc*	China	31	31	50	51	NS
Sarpel *et al.*[27]	2009	*Ann Surg Onc*	USA	20	56	95	75	NS
Endo *et al.*[28]	2009	*Surg Lap Endo*	Japan	10	11	57	48	NS
Tranchart *et al.*[29]	2010	*Surg Endosc*	France	42	42	60	47	NS
Truant *et al.*[30]	2011	*Surg Endosc*	France	35	53	70	46	NS
Lee *et al.*[31]	2011	*World J Surg*	China	33	50	76	76	NS
Hu *et al.*[32]	2011	*World J Gastro*	China	30	30	50	53	NS
Kim *et al.*[33]	2011	*J Kor Surg Soc*	Korea	26	29	57	56	NS
Ker *et al.*[34]	2011	*Int J Hepatol*	Taiwan	116	208	62	72	NS
Cheung *et al.*[35]	2013	*Ann Surg*	China	32	64	77	57	NS
Kim *et al.*[36]	2014	*Surg Endosc*	Korea	29	29	92	88	NS

associated with the laparoscopic approach, including shorter hospital stay, less blood loss and less complications.[37–41] There may also be a cost benefit to perform these procedures laparoscopically,[42] although this may not be the case for more complex resections.[43]

Robotic hepatic resections have also been reported with some success. Surgical robotics were designed to assist with the limitations of laparoscopic surgery, and confers important advantages in visualization, dexterity, ergonomics and the elimination of the physiologic tremor.[44] While no randomized trials comparing the use of robotic technology with either open or laparoscopic surgery have been performed, recent systematic reviews have confirmed that robotic-assisted hepatectomies are safe, feasible, may overcome some of the limitations of laparoscopy, associated with good short-term outcomes and compare favorably to laparoscopic resections.[45] Additionally, it has been suggested that liver resections are more likely to be performed in a totally minimally invasive fashion when using the robot.[46] As such, minimally invasive resections for HCC are safe and effective and should be considered in the setting of local expertise and favorable patients and tumor factors.

OLT for HCC

OLT is the procedure of choice in patients with advanced cirrhosis (CTB B or C), early stage HCC (within Milan criteria) and acceptable operative candidates.[20] Pre-operative assessment for OLT is complex and requires a multidisciplinary team that will evaluate medical, surgical and socio-economic factors that will determine the patient's suitability for transplantation. Additionally, stringent tumor factors must be taken into account to ensure the best possible outcomes. In 1996, Mazzaferro *et al.* published guidelines known as the Milan criteria for OLT in the setting of HCC with tremendous results.[47] Prior to this, the results for OLT in the setting of HCC was quite disappointing with five-year survival rates as low as 18%.[48] These criteria, of a single tumor less than 5 cm or up to three tumors less than 3 cm in the absence of vascular involvement, are still in use today. Newer systems have been developed, the most commonly used being the University of California San Francisco (UCSF) criteria that allows for an expansion of tumor size (single tumor nodule up to 6.5 cm; or three or fewer tumors, the largest of which is ≤4.5 cm with the sum of the tumor diameters ≤8 cm).[49] Such expanded criteria have been adopted in certain areas, but there is some concern of a lower survival rate in patients within UCSF criteria but outside of Milan criteria.[50] Therefore, in the setting of increasing demand and worsening shortages, most regions elect to maintain adherence to the Milan criteria.

Cholangiocarcinoma

Introduction

Cholangiocarcinomas or bile duct cancers are the second most common primary liver cancer, represent 3% of all gastrointestinal malignancies, and originates in the biliary tree and are classified and surgically managed based on their anatomical location.[51] Intra-hepatic cholangiocarcinomas (iCCA), which represent only 10% of these cancers, are defined as being proximal to the second-degree bile duct tributaries. Perihilar cholangiocarcinoma or Klatskin tumors, the most common location for these tumors representing 50% of them, are located between the second-degree bile duct tributaries and the insertion of the cystic duct into the common bile duct. Distal bile duct cancers account for the remaining 40% and are found between the cystic duct insertion and the ampulla of Vater.[52,53] These last two may also be classified as extra-hepatic cholangiocarcinomas (eCCA). It has been proposed that the iCCA and eCCA should be considered separately as, in spite of some commonalties, they have important etiological, clinical and therapeutic differences.[54]

All of these tumors are aggressive and form a strong desmoplastic reaction making their involvement of surrounding structures likely and consequently their surgical management challenging. These remain uncommon tumors in the western world, and the incidences of eCCA are decreasing, while iCCA are increasing.[54] However, in spite of some activity to some chemotherapeutic regiments,[55] they are relatively resistant to non-surgical management and the only chance for cure is complete surgical extirpation.[56]

Risk factors

While most cholangiocarcinomas are sporadic without etiological agent identified, several risk factors have been associated with this type of tumor and are found in up 30% of patients.[57] These vary geographically, with primary sclerosing cholangitis (PSC) being the most common risk factor in western countries. It is thought that the increased risk of developing cancer with PSC is related to chronic inflammation, proliferation of progenitor cells and liver injury.[52] Cholangiocarcinoma develops in approximately 5–15% of patients with PSC,[58,59] and it seems to occur early in the disease process as 50% of patients will be diagnosed with cancer within one year of their diagnosis of PSC.[60,61]

In Asian countries, chronic inflammation from hepatolithiasis and hepatobiliary flukes are common risk factors, and are often found concurrently.[51] The presence or a history of choledochal cysts has been shown to have an association with cholangiocarcinomas, and are associated with a much earlier presentation as they present at an average age of 32, as compared to the general population where it typically presents after age 70.[62] While the malignant risk associated with choledochal cysts decrease after excision, these patients are still at a higher risk of developing cholangiocarcinoma as compared to the general population.[62] Other risk factors include thorotrast, a now banned contrast agent, cholelithiasis, choledocholithiasis, smoking, IBD independent of PSC and bilio-enteric drainage.[51,52,62]

The aforementioned risk factors may be classified as sources biliary stasis and/or inflammation, and are more often associated with eCCA. While it is true that sources of intrahepatic biliary inflammation, such as intrahepatic parasites and intrahepatic stones predispose to the development of iCCA, this is much less common and mostly limited to Asian countries.[63] It has recently been shown that iCCA are associated with a separate set of risk factors. Contrary to eCCA, iCCA may not only arise from biliary epithelial cells or peribiliary glands but also from hepatic stem cells found within canals of Hering that have the potential to differentiate into either hepatocytes or cholangiocytes. Cancers arising from these stem cells are found to have multiple different phenotypes ranging from iCCA to HCC to a mixture of both.[64] Supporting this, it has been shown that iCCA share multiple common risk factors with HCC. A recent meta-analysis has shown that iCCA are associated cirrhosis, hepatitis B, hepatitis C, obesity, type 2 diabetes mellitus and alcohol use.[63]

Diagnosis of iCCA

Much like HCC, the clinical presentation of iCCA is insidious and associated with only vague symptoms such as cachexia, malaise, fatigue abdominal pain and night sweats. Unfortunately, unlike HCC, they are not associated with specific radiological criteria, complicating their diagnosis.[65] Their diagnosis requires a high level of suspicion, in combination with radiological and biochemical data.[65] It is recommended that at a minimum, all patients require either a contrast-enhanced magnetic MRI or a contrast-enhanced high resolution CT scan.[51,57] These are used to determine resectability, which is defined as the ability to safely perform a liver resection with negative margins while preserving an adequate functional liver remnant with portal venous and hepatic arterial inflow and hepatic vein outflow as well as bilioenteric drainage.[66]

iCCA are further subclassified as mass-forming type (the most common), periductal-infiltrating type, intraductal growth type or mixed type,[67] all of which are associated with differing imaging characteristics. On contrast-enhanced CT or MRI, mass-forming cholangiocarcinomas are manifested by a homogenous mass with an irregular but well-defined margin, irregular peripheral enhancement with gradual centripedal filling, the presence of satellite nodules and vascular encasement and the absence of tumor thrombi.[68] The periductal-infiltrating type is manifested by dilated or narrowed bile ducts without clear mass formation, rather a speculated or branch-like abnormality. While challenging, these are differentiated from benign strictures by irregular margins, ductal enhancement and asymmetrical stricturing. The intra-ductal type, associated with a favorable prognosis, is characterized by a variety of imaging patterns which may be associated with moderate to severe ductal dilatation as well as visible papillary or polypoid mass or cast-like intraductal lesions.[68]

Carbohydrate antigen 19-9 (CA 19-9) is a commonly used biomarker for cholangiocarcinoma, but is only associated with a sensitivity and specificity of 62% and 63% respectively for iCCA. It is often elevated with biliary obstruction of any cause, but persistent elevation after decompression should suggest malignancy. CA 19-9 may also be elevated in pancreatic and gastric cancer as well as hepatic injury of any cause.[57] As such, it is often used as a confirmatory test as opposed to screening or diagnosis.[65] Cancer antigen 125 (CA-125), while more commonly associated with ovarian cancer, may also be elevated in cholangiocarcinoma, being found in up to 65% of patients, and is a negative prognostic factor for survival.[57,69] Carcinoembryonic antigen (CEA), a tumor marker commonly elevated in a variety of carcinomas including gastrointestinal, breast, urinary tract and lung primaries, may also be elevated in cholangiocarcinoma. Its elevation has also been shown to be associated with a more advanced stage and a poorer prognosis.[70,71]

iCCA is rarely conclusively diagnosed based on imaging or biochemical criteria and histological confirmation via biopsy is often utilized. If a diagnosis of adenocarcinoma is obtained, it has been suggested that iCCA must be differentiated from metastatic adenocarcinoma from another source. As such, in this clinical scenario, further investigations in the form of cross-sectional imaging of the chest, abdomen and pelvis, upper and lower endoscopy, mammography and gynecological examination may be performed as clinically indicated.[66]

Diagnosis of eCCA

The pattern of growth of eCCA can be either exophytic, which most commonly progresses in a periductal fashion, or intraductal.[51,65] Due to the early obstruction of the biliary tree, 90% of patients present with obstructive jaundice and 10% with cholangitis. Other non-specific symptoms include discomfort, malaise, weight loss and cachexia.[51]

For accurate pre-operative assessment and surgical planning of eCCA, cholangiographic examination via magnetic resonance cholangiopancreatography (MRCP) or endoscopic retrograde cholangiopancreatography (ERCP) are required in addition to high-resolution axial imaging with CT or MRI.[57] MRCP has the advantage of being a non-invasive examination of the biliary tree and can be performed at the same time as a standard MRI. However, a high-quality CT scan in conjunction with ERCP has been shown to be as accurate as MRI/MRCP, and an ERCP is often required for biliary decompression and brushings for cytology.[57,72] Due to the strong desmoplastic reaction that these tumors form, cytology from ERCP brushings is negative more than 50% of the time in eCC.[57] SpyGlass Direct Visualization System is a relatively new endoscopic technology that allows direct visualization within the biliary tree and may improve the diagnostic yield of biopsies.[73,74] Endoscopic ultrasound (EUS) allows for examination of the regional lymph nodes and vasculature and allows the obtaining of fine-needle aspiration (FNA) biopsies of the mass or of lymph nodes, which can increase the diagnostic yield of standard cytology to 40–70%.[57] Much like iCCA, CA 19-9, CEA and CA 125 are used in the diagnosis of eCC.[57] However, as CA 19-9 levels are elevated in the setting of biliary obstruction, it is a less specific marker for eCCA as opposed to iCCA.[51]

Staging

The staging of iCCA is based on a TNM classification, and the 7th edition is the first that separated iCCA from HCC (Table 3). The T stage is based on the number of lesions, the presence of vascular involvement, the number

Table 3. American Joint Commission on Cancer (AJCC) staging classification for intrahepatic cholangiocarcinoma.

Primary tumor (T) stage		Regional lymph node (N) stage		Distant metastasis (M) stage	
TX	Not assessed	NX	Not assessed	MX	Not assessed
T0	None found	N0	None found	M0	None found
T1	Solitary tumor, no vascular invasion	N1	Regional nodal involvement	M1	Metastatic disease
T2	Solitary tumor with vascular invasion	—	—	—	—
T3	Multiple tumors, ± vascular invasion	—	—	—	—
T4	Tumor with periductal invasion	—	—	—	—

(*Continued*)

Table 3. (*Continued*)

Stage	Primary tumor (T) stage	Regional lymph node (N) stage	Distant metastasis (M) stage
I	T1	N0	M0
II	T2	N0	M0
III	T3	N0	M0
IVA	T4	N0	M0
	Any T	N1	M0
IVB	Any T	Any N	M1

of lesions and the presence of invasion into the visceral peritoneum or adjacent organs.[74] Unlike HCC, the size of the primary tumor is not considered important as it has little prognostic significance on its own.[57]

As noted above, eCCAs include perihilar (Klatskin tumors) and distal cholangiocarcinomas. Klatskin tumors may be classified using the Bismuth-Corlette classification system, which gives an assessment of local spread. Type 1 tumors are found below the hepatic duct bifurcation, type 2 involve the bifurcation, type 3 involve the bifurcation and one of the major hepatic ducts and type 4 involves the confluence and extends to the second order biliary bifurcations bilaterally.[74] While commonly used and quoted, this classification system was found to be of low accuracy and of little prognostic significance, underlining the need for better staging systems.[75] More recent staging systems, namely the MSKCC (for perihilar cholangiocarcinomas) and the TNM classification (for all eCCA) systems were developed but were judged to lack in usefulness in the pre-operative setting.[76] Therefore, an international working group was created with the goal of designing a new classification system that was published in 2011. The consensus classification (European Hepato-Pancreato-Biliary Association) combines an evaluation of the biliary, portal venous and hepatic arterial involvement as well as tumor size, tumor form, liver remnant volume, underlying liver disease, lymph nodes and metastases.[77] While this staging system is certainly comprehensive, it remains to be seen if widespread adoption takes place considering its complexity.

Surgical management of iCCA

Surgical resection is the only chance for cure for patients with iCCA, although only 30% of patients will be candidates by the time of diagnosis.[58] The surgical management of iCCA is similar to that for HCC and requires that an adequately sized functional liver remnant remain following resection. This is determined by the pre-operative health of the liver (CTP status), hepatic arterial and portal venous inflow, hepatic venous outflow and bilioenteric drainage. If this can be achieved, surgical resections with negative margins may be associated with favorable outcomes, although five-year survival is still less than 50%. A recent large review examined 598 patients diagnosed with iCCA that underwent resection between 1988 and 2004.[78] The median overall survival after resection was 21 months. Three-year overall survival was 31%, and five-year overall survival was 18%. For those patients with negative lymph nodes and no metastatic disease (N0M0) at the time of surgery, five-year survival after resection was only 25%. Two other recent studies also report five-year survivals of 25% and 26%, respectively, after complete resection of intrahepatic cholangiocarcinoma.[79,80] In patients with negative margins, the most important prognostic factor is the lymph node status, and as such a lymphadenectomy for proper staging should be performed on all patients.[53] Additionally, multifocal disease is associated with high recurrence rates (>90%) and may preclude resection.[81] Other negative prognostic factors include vascular invasion and cirrhosis.[51]

While a much less common indication as compared to HCC, laparoscopic hepatic resections for iCCA have been reported.[22,82] As this is an uncommon indication, very little data exists and as such these resections should be limited to experienced centers.

Given the locally aggressive nature of iCCA, transplantation was previously thought to be an attractive treatment option. However, OLT for iCCA is associated with five-year recurrence rates as high as 70% and five-year survival around 40%,[51,83] and as such iCCA is not considered an indication for OLT. Long-term survivors have been reported however, and some have suggested that OLT should remain a potential treatment option for iCCA.[83] Currently however, the consideration of OLT for iCCA should only be in the context of a clinical trial.[66]

Surgical management of eCCA — Perihilar cholangiocarcinoma

Until recently, the only potential cure for perihilar cholangiocarcinoma was surgical excision and due to their proximity to multiple vital structures, resectability is determined by multiple factors. Factors that would render a lesion unresectable include: tumor involvement of second-degree biliary radicals bilaterally, encasement of the main portal vein proximal to its bifurcation, hepatic lobe atrophy with contralateral portal vein branch encasement or occlusion, hepatic lobe atrophy with contralateral tumor extension to secondary biliary radicles, unilateral tumor extension to secondary biliary radicles with contralateral portal-vein branch encasement or occlusion, lymph node metastases to distant basins and distant metastases.[84] Recently however, it has been shown that portal vein involvement should not be an absolute contraindication to resection, as portal vein resection and reconstruction can benefit certain patients.[85] In order to clear the tumor, the entire extra-hepatic biliary system must be resected, usually en bloc with a hemi-hepatectomy depending on the location of the tumor.[84] A caudate lobectomy is also routinely performed due to its propensity for recurrence.[57]

There is a very limited experience of minimally invasively resected perihilar cholangiocarcinomas with only two reported in the literature — one done with robotic assistance[86] and the other resected laparoscopically and reconstructed in an open fashion.[87] Needless to say, these resections should only be performed in very experienced centers at this time.

In spite of aggressive surgical therapy, perihilar cholangiocarcinomas were often found to be unresectable, even in early stages, due to its proximity to vital structures and the propensity for local invasion. To counter this, a protocol was developed at the Mayo clinic combining external beam radiation, brachytherapy, radiosensitizing therapy and chemotherapy followed by OLT.[88,89] Their results have been very promising and have since been adopted by other transplant centers. A recent analysis of the results of 12 US centers performing this technique found a five-year disease-free survival rate of 65%,[90,91] similar to the results from OLT performed for other indications.[58]

Surgical management of eCCA — Distal cholangiocarcinoma

Cholangiocarcinomas that are distal to the cystic duct insertion usually require a pancreaticoduodenectomy (Whipple procedure) in order to achieve negative margins, which is the most important prognostic factor.[58] Other important prognostic factors include lymph node and neural invasion.[92]

Take Home Messages

- Only chance for cure for hepatocellular carcinoma or cholangiocarcinoma is resection or transplantation.
- Referral of these patients to a multidisciplinary team is essential.

References

1. Reddy, S.K., Tsung, A., Geller, D.A., Laparoscopic liver resection. *World J Surg*, 2010. **35**(7): 1478–86.
2. Forner, A., Llovet, J.M., Bruix, J., Hepatocellular carcinoma. *Lancet*, 2012. **379**(9822): 1245–55.
3. El-Serag, H.B., Hepatocellular carcinoma. *New Engl J Med*, 2011. **365**(12): 1118–27.
4. van Meer, S., de Man, R.A., Siersema, P.D., van Erpecum, K.J., Surveillance for hepatocellular carcinoma in chronic liver disease: Evidence and controversies. *World J Gastroenterol*, 2013. **19**(40): 6744–56.
5. Farazi, P.A., DePinho, R.A., Hepatocellular carcinoma pathogenesis: From genes to environment. *Nat Rev Cancer*, 2006. **6**(9): 674–87.
6. El-Serag, H.B., Rudolph, K.L., Hepatocellular Carcinoma: Epidemiology and molecular carcinogenesis. *Gastroenterology*, 2007. **132**(7): 2557–76.
7. Bruix, J., Sherman, M., Management of hepatocellular carcinoma. *Hepatology*, 2005. **42**(5): 1208–36.
8. Altekruse, S.F., Henley, S.J., Cucinelli, J.E., McGlynn, K.A., Changing hepatocellular carcinoma incidence and liver cancer mortality rates in the United States. *Am J Gastroenterol*, 2014. **109**(4): 542–53.
9. Serag, EI, H.B., Marrero, J.A., Rudolph, L., Reddy, K.R., Diagnosis and treatment of hepatocellular carcinoma. *Gastroenterology*, 2008. **134**(6): 1752–63.

10. Ferenci, P., Fried, M., Labrecque, D. *et al.*, World Gastroenterology Organisation Global Guideline. Hepatocellular carcinoma (HCC): A global perspective. *J Gastrointestin Liver Dis*, 2010. **19**(3): 311–7.
11. Leykum, L.K., El-Serag, H.B., Cornell, J., Papadopoulos, K.P., Screening for hepatocellular carcinoma among veterans with hepatitis c on disease stage, treatment received, and survival. *Clin Gastroenterol H*, 2007. **5**(4): 508–12.
12. Asham, E.H., Kaseb, A., Ghobrial, R.M., Management of hepatocellular carcinoma. *Surg Clin North Am*, 2013. **93**(6): 1423–50.
13. Kim, T., Murakami, T., Takahashi, S. *et al.*, Optimal phases of dynamic CT for detecting hepatocellular carcinoma: Evaluation of unenhanced and triple-phase images. *Abdom Imaging*. **1999**. **24**(5): 473–80.
14. Bruix, J., Sherman, M., Management of hepatocellular carcinoma: An update. *Hepatology*, 2011. **53**(3): 1020–2.
15. Group ALTS, American Liver Tumor Study Group: A randomized prospective multi-institutional trial of orthotopic liver transplantation or partial hepatic resection with or without adjuvant chemotherapy for hepatocellular carcinoma. *United Network for Organ Sharing*, 1998; Investigators Booklet and Protocol.
16. Schindl, M.J., Redhead, D.N., Fearon, K.C.H., Garden, O.J., Wigmore, S.J., Edinburgh Liver Surgery and Transplantation Experimental Research Group (eLISTER), the value of residual liver volume as a predictor of hepatic dysfunction and infection after major liver resection. *Gut*, 2005. **54**(2): 289–96.
17. DuBray, B.J., Jr., Levy, R.V., Balachandran, P. *et al.*, Novel three-dimensional imaging technique improves the accuracy of hepatic volumetric assessment. *HPB*, 2011. **13**: 670–4.
18. Vauthey, J.N., Chaoui, A., Do, K.A., Bilimoria, M.M., Standardized measurement of the future liver remnant prior to extended liver resection: Methodology and clinical associations. *Surgery*, 2000. **127**(5): 512–9.
19. Shindoh, J., Vauthey, J.-N., Zimmitti, G. *et al.*, Analysis of the efficacy of portal vein embolization for patients with extensive liver malignancy and very low future liver remnant volume, including a comparison with the associating liver partition with portal vein ligation for staged hepatectomy approach. *J Am Coll Surgeons*, 2013. **217**(1): 126–33.
20. Facciuto, M.E., Rochon, C., Pandey, M. *et al.*, Surgical dilemma: Liver resection or liver transplantation for hepatocellular carcinoma and cirrhosis. *HPB*, 2009. **11**: 398–404.

21. Cha, C.H., Ruo, L., Fong, Y. *et al.*, Resection of hepatocellular carcinoma in patients otherwise eligible for transplantation. *Ann Surg*, 2003. **238**(3): 315–23.
22. Nguyen, K.T., Gamblin, T.C., Geller, D.A., World review of laparoscopic liver resection — 2,804 Patients. *Ann Surg*, 2009. **250**(5): 831–41.
23. Dagher, I., O'Rourke, N., Geller, D.A. *et al.*, Laparoscopic major hepatectomy. *Ann Surg*, 2009. **250**(5): 856–60.
24. Shimada, M., Hashizume, M., Maehara, S. *et al.*, Laparoscopic hepatectomy for hepatocellular carcinoma. *Surg Endosc*, 2001. **15**(6): 541–4.
25. Kaneko, H., Takagi, S., Otsuka, Y. *et al.*, Laparoscopic liver resection of hepatocellular carcinoma. *Am J Surg*, 2005. **189**(2): 190–4.
26. Cai, X.J., Yang, J., Yu, H. *et al.*, Clinical study of laparoscopic versus open hepatectomy for malignant liver tumors. *Surg Endosc*, 2008. **22**(11): 2350–6.
27. Sarpel, U., Hefti, M.M., Wisnievsky, J.P., Roayaie, S., Schwartz, M.E., Labow, D.M., Outcome for patients treated with laparoscopic versus open Resection of hepatocellular carcinoma: Case-matched analysis. *Ann Surg Oncol*, 2009. **16**(6): 1572–7.
28. Endo, Y., Ohta, M., Sasaki, A. *et al.*, A Comparative study of the long-term outcomes after laparoscopy-assisted and open left lateral hepatectomy for hepatocellular carcinoma. *Surg Laparo Endo Per*, 2009. **19**(5): e171–e174.
29. Tranchart, H., Di Giuro, G., Lainas, P. *et al.*, Laparoscopic resection for hepatocellular carcinoma: A matched-pair comparative study. *Surg Endosc*, 2010. **24**(5): 1170–6.
30. Truant, S., Bouras, A.F., Hebbar, M. *et al.*, Laparoscopic resection vs. open liver resection for peripheral hepatocellular carcinoma in patients with chronic liver disease: A case-matched study. *Surg Endosc*, 2011. **25**: 3668–77.
31. Lee, K.F., Chong, C.N., Wong, J., Cheung, Y.S., Wong, J., Lai, P., Long-term results of laparoscopic hepatectomy versus open hepatectomy for hepatocellular carcinoma: A case-matched analysis. *World J Surg*, 2011. **35**: 2268–74.
32. Hu, B.-S., Chen, K., Tan, H.-M., Ding, X.-M., Tan, J.-W., Comparison of laparoscopic vs open liver lobectomy (segmentectomy) for hepatocellular carcinoma. *World J Gastroenterol*, 2011. **17**(42): 4725.
33. Kim, K.-J., Jeong, C.-Y., Jeong, S.-H. *et al.*, Laparoscopic liver resection for hepatocellular carcinoma. *J Korean Surg Soc*, 2011. **80**(1): 51.

34. Ker, C.G., Chen, J.S., Kuo, K.K. *et al.*, Liver surgery for hepatocellular carcinoma: Laparoscopic versus open approach. *Int J Hepatol*, 2011. **2011**: 596792(Epub 2011 May 16).
35. Cheung, T.T., Poon, R.T.P., Yuen, W.K. *et al.*, Long-term survival analysis of pure laparoscopic versus open hepatectomy for hepatocellular carcinoma in patients with cirrhosis. *Ann Surg*, 2013. **257**(3): 506–11.
36. Kim, H., Suh, K.-S., Lee, K.-W. *et al.*, Long-term outcome of laparoscopic versus open liver resection for hepatocellular carcinoma: A case-controlled study with propensity score matching. *Surg Endosc*, 2014. **28**(3): 950–60.
37. Yin, Z., Fan, X., Ye, H., Yin, D., Wang, J., Short- and long-term outcomes after laparoscopic and open hepatectomy for hepatocellular carcinoma: A global systematic review and meta-analysis. *Ann Surg Oncol*, 2012. **20**(4): 1203–15.
38. Li, N., Wu, Y.-R., Wu, B., Lu, M.-Q., Surgical and oncologic outcomes following laparoscopic versus open liver resection for hepatocellular carcinoma: A meta-analysis. *Hepatol Res*, 2012. **42**(1): 51–9.
39. Zhou, Y.-M., Shao, W.-Y., Zhao, Y.-F., Xu, D.-H., Li, B., Meta-analysis of laparoscopic versus open resection for hepatocellular carcinoma. *Dig Dis Sci*, 2011. **56**(7): 1937–43.
40. Fancellu, A., Rosman, A.S., Sanna, V. *et al.*, Meta-analysis of trials comparing minimally-invasive and open liver resections for hepatocellular carcinoma. *J Surg Res*, 2011. **171**(1): e33–45.
41. Nguyen, K.T., Marsh, J.W., Tsung, A., Steel, J.J.L., Gamblin, T.C., Geller, D.A., Comparative benefits of laparoscopic vs open hepatic resection. *Arch Surg*, 2011. **146**(3): 348.
42. Vanounou, T., Steel, J.L., Nguyen, K.T. *et al.*, Comparing the clinical and economic impact of laparoscopic versus open liver resection. *Ann Surg Oncol*, 2009. **17**(4): 998–1009.
43. Cannon, R.M., Scoggins, C.R., Callender, G.G., Quillo, A., McMasters, K.M., Martin, R.C.G., Financial comparison of laparoscopic versus open hepatic resection using deviation-based cost modeling. *Ann Surg Oncol*, 2013. **20**: 2887–92.
44. Lanfranco, A.R., Castellanos, A.E., Desai, J.P., Meyers, W.C., Robotic surgery. *Ann Surg*, 2004. **239**(1): 14–21.
45. Pelletier, J.-S., Gill, R.S., Shi, X., Birch, D.W., Karmali, S., Robotic-assisted hepatic resection: A systematic review. *Int J Med Robot Comp*, 2013.

46. Tsung, A., Geller, D.A., Sukato, D.C. *et al.*, Robotic versus laparoscopic hepatectomy. *Ann Surg*, 2014. **259**(3): 549–55.
47. Mazzaferro, V., Regalia, E., Doci, R. *et al.*, Liver transplantation for the treatment of small hepatocellular carcinomas in patients with cirrhosis. *New Engl J Med*, 1996. **334**(11): 693–9.
48. Mazzaferro, V., Chun, Y.S., Poon, R.T.P. *et al.*, Liver transplantation for hepatocellular carcinoma. *Ann Surg Oncol*, 2008. **15**(4): 1001–7.
49. Yao, F.Y., Ferrell, L., Bass, N.M. *et al.*, Liver transplantation for hepatocellular carcinoma: Expansion of the tumor size limits does not adversely impact survival. *Hepatology*, 2001. **33**(6): 1394–403.
50. Decaens, T., Thoraval, F.R., Hadni-Bresson, S. *et al.*, Impact of UCSF criteria according to pre- and post-OLT tumor features: Analysis of 479 patients listed for HCC with a short waiting time. *Liver Transplant*, 2006. **12**: 1761–9.
51. Rizvi, S., Gores, G.J., Pathogenesis, diagnosis, and management of cholangiocarcinoma. *Gastroenterology*, 2013. **145**(6): 1215–29.
52. Razumilava, N., Gores, G.J., Cholangiocarcinoma. *Lancet*, 2014. [Epub ahead of print].
53. DeOliveira, M.L., Cunningham, S.C., Cameron, J.L. *et al.*, Cholangiocarcinoma. *Ann Surg*, 2007. **245**(5): 755–62.
54. Shaib, Y., El-Serag, H.B., The epidemiology of Cholangiocarcinoma. Berk, P.D., Gores, G., eds. *Semin Liver Dis*, 2004. **24**(2): 115–25.
55. Razumilava, N., Gores, G.J., Combination of gemcitabine and cisplatin for biliary tract cancer: A platform to build on. *J Hepatol*, 2011. **54**(3): 577–8.
56. Farges, O., Fuks, D., Le, Treut, Y.-P. *et al.*, AJCC 7th edition of TNM staging accurately discriminates outcomes of patients with resectable intrahepatic cholangiocarcinoma: By the AFC-IHCC-2009 study group. *Cancer*, 2011. **117**(10): 2170–7.
57. Khan, S.A., Davidson, B.R., Goldin, R.D. *et al.*, Guidelines for the diagnosis and treatment of cholangiocarcinoma: An update. *Gut*, 2012. **61**(12): 1657–69.
58. Razumilava, N., Gores, G.J., Classification, diagnosis, and management of cholangiocarcinoma. *Clin Gastroenterol Hepatol*, 2013. **11**(1): 13–21.
59. Chapman, R., Fevery, J., Kalloo, A. *et al.*, Diagnosis and management of primary sclerosing cholangitis. *Hepatology*, 2010. **51**(2): 660–78.
60. Boberg, K.M., Bergquist, A., Mitchell, S. *et al.*, Cholangiocarcinoma in primary sclerosing cholangitis: Risk factors and clinical presentation. *Scand J Gastroenterol*, 2002. **37**(10): 1205–11.

61. Chapman, M.H., Webster, G.J., Bannoo, S., Johnson, G., Wittmann, J., Pereira, S.P., Cholangiocarcinoma and dominant strictures in patients with primary sclerosing cholangitis. a 25 year single centre experience. *Eur J Gastroenterol Hepatol*, 2012. **24**(9): 1051–58.
62. Tyson, G.L., Serag, EI, H.B., Risk factors for cholangiocarcinoma. *Hepatology*, 2011. **54**(1): 173–84.
63. Palmer, W.C., Patel, T., Are common factors involved in the pathogenesis of primary liver cancers? A meta-analysis of risk factors for intrahepatic cholangiocarcinoma. *J Hepatol*, 2012. **57**: 69–76.
64. Cardinale, V., Carpino, G., Reid, L., Gaudio, E., Alvaro, D., Multiple cells of origin in cholangiocarcinoma underlie biological, epidemiological and clinical heterogeneity. *World J Gastrointest Oncol*, 2012. **4**(5): 94–102.
65. Blechacz, B., Komuta, M., Roskams, T., Gores, G.J., Clinical diagnosis and staging of cholangiocarcinoma. *Nat Rev Gastroenterol Hepatol*, 2011. **8**(9): 512–22.
66. Brown, K.M., Parmar, A.D., Geller, D.A., Intrahepatic cholangiocarcinoma. *Surg Oncol Clin N Am*, 2014. **23**(2): 231–46.
67. Yamasaki, S., Intrahepatic cholangiocarcinoma: Macroscopic type and stage classification. *J Hepatobiliary Pancreat Surg*, 2003. **10**(4): 288–91.
68. Chung, Y.E., Kim, M.-J., Park, Y.N. *et al.*, Varying appearances of cholangiocarcinoma: Radiologic-pathologic correlation1. *RadioGraphics*, 2009. **29**(3): 683–700.
69. Higashi, M., Yamada, N., Yokoyama, S. *et al.*, Pathobiological implications of MUC16/CA125 expression in intrahepatic cholangiocarcinoma-mass forming type. *Pathobiology*, 2012. **79**(2): 101–6.
70. Wirasorn, K., Ngamprasertchai, T., Chindaprasirt, J. *et al.*, Prognostic factors in resectable cholangiocarcinoma patients: Carcinoembryonic antigen, lymph node, surgical margin and chemotherapy. *World J Gastrointest Oncol*, 2013. **5**(4): 81–7.
71. Juntermanns, B., Radunz, S., Heuer, M. *et al.*, Tumor markers as a diagnostic key for hilar cholangiocarcinoma. *Eur J Med Res*, 2010. **15**(8): 357–61.
72. Park, H.S., Lee, J.M., Choi, J.-Y. *et al.*, Preoperative evaluation of bile duct cancer: MRI combined with MR cholangiopancreatography versus MDCT with direct cholangiography. *AJR Am J Roentgenol*, 2008. **190**(2): 396–405.

73. Draganov, P.V., Lin, T., Chauhan, S., Wagh, M.S., Hou, W., Forsmark, C.E., Prospective evaluation of the clinical utility of ERCP-guided cholangiopancreatoscopy with a new direct visualization system. *Gastrointest Endosc*, 2011. **73**(5): 971–9.
74. Brown, K.M., Geller, D.A., Proximal biliary tumors. *Surg Clin North Am*, 2014. **94**(2): 311–23.
75. Paul, A., Kaiser, G.M., Molmenti, E.P. *et al.*, Klatskin tumors and the accuracy of the Bismuth-Corlette classification. *Am Surg*, 2011. **77**(12): 1695–9.
76. Suarez-Munoz, M.A., Fernandez-Aguilar, J.L., Sanchez-Perez, B. *et al.*, Risk factors and classifications of hilar cholangiocarcinoma. *World J Gastrointest Oncol*, 2013. **5**(7): 132–8.
77. DeOliveira, M.L., Schulick, R.D., Nimura, Y. *et al.*, New staging system and a registry for perihilar cholangiocarcinoma. *Hepatology*, 2011. **53**(4): 1363–71.
78. Nathan, H., Aloia, T.A., Vauthey, J.-N. *et al.*, A proposed staging system for intrahepatic cholangiocarcinoma. *Ann Surg Oncol*, 2009. **16**(1): 14–22.
79. Konstadoulakis, M.M., Roayaie, S., Gomatos, I.P. *et al.*, Fifteen-year, single-center experience with the surgical management of intrahepatic cholangiocarcinoma: Operative results and long-term outcome. *Surgery*, 2008. **143**(3): 366–74.
80. Guglielmi, A., Ruzzenente, A., Campagnaro, T. *et al.*, Does intrahepatic cholangiocarcinoma have better prognosis compared to perihilar cholangiocarcinoma? *J Surg Oncol*, 2009. **101**(2): 111–5.
81. Endo, I., Gonen, M., Yopp, A.C. *et al.*, Intrahepatic cholangiocarcinoma. *Ann Surg*, 2008. **248**(1): 84–96.
82. Chan, F.K., Cheng, K.C., Yeung, Y.P., Laparoscopic liver resection: Lessons learnt after 100 cases. *Hong Kong Med J*, 2014. [Epub ahead of print].
83. Becker, N.S., Rodriguez, J.A., Barshes, N.R., O'Mahony, C.A., Goss, J.A., Aloia, T.A., Outcomes analysis for 280 patients with cholangiocarcinoma treated with liver transplantation over an 18-year period. *J Gastrointest Surg*, 2008. **12**(1): 117–22.
84. Jarnagin, W.R., Bowne, W., Klimstra, D.S. *et al.*, Papillary phenotype confers improved survival after resection of hilar cholangiocarcinoma. *Ann Surg*, 2005. **241**(5): 703–14.

85. Chen, W., Ke, K., Chen, Y.L., Combined portal vein resection in the treatment of hilar cholangiocarcinoma: A systematic review and meta-analysis. *Eur J Surg Oncol*, 2014. **40**(5): 489–95.
86. Giulianotti, P.C., Sbrana, F., Bianco, F.M., Addeo, P., Robot-assisted laparoscopic extended right hepatectomy with biliary reconstruction. *J Laparoendosc Adv Surg Tech A*, 2010. **20**(2): 159–63.
87. Machado, M.A.C., Makdissi, F.F., Surjan, R.C., Mochizuki, M., Laparoscopic resection of hilar cholangiocarcinoma. *J Laparoendosc Adv Surg Tech A*, 2012. **22**(10): 954–6.
88. De Vreede, I., Steers, J.L., Burch, P.A. *et al.*, Prolonged disease-free survival after orthotopic liver transplantation plus adjuvant chemoirradiation for cholangiocarcinoma. *Liver Transplant*, 2000. **6**(3): 309–16.
89. Heimbach, J.K., Gores, G.J., Haddock, M.G. *et al.*, Liver transplantation for unresectable perihilar cholangiocarcinoma. *Semin Liver Dis*, 2004. **24**(2): 201–7.
90. Darwish Murad, S., Kim, W.R., Harnois, D.M. *et al.*, Efficacy of neoadjuvant chemoradiation, followed by liver transplantation, for perihilar cholangiocarcinoma at 12 US centers. *Gastroenterology*, 2012. **143**(1): 88–98.
91. Gores, G.J., Darwish, Murad, S., Heimbach, J.K., Rosen, C.B., Liver transplantation for perihilar cholangiocarcinoma. *Dig Dis*, 2013. **31**(1): 126–9.
92. Tan, X., Xiao, K., Liu, W., Chang, S., Zhang, T., Tang, H., Prognostic factors of distal cholangiocarcinoma after curative surgery: A series of 84 cases. *Hepatogastroenterology*, 2013. **60**(128): 1892–5.

Chapter 20

Image-Guided Therapy of Liver Malignancy

Samdeep K. Mouli, Riad Salem
and Robert J. Lewandowski

What is New

- Minimally invasive image-guided cancer therapies have proven safe and effective in the treatment of unresectable primary and secondary hepatic malignancies.
- Image-guided ablative therapies have curative intent in the appropriately selected patients, while transcatheter intra-arterial therapies have typically been palliative while employed in more advanced patients. These therapies are more commonly being utilized in a multi-discipline fashion to facilitate more patients obtaining surgery.
- Advances in imaging techniques and guidance have improved safety and efficacy for both ablative and intra-arterial therapies.

Introduction

Hepatocellular carcinoma (HCC) is the third most common cause of cancer-related mortality worldwide, with a rising incidence in the United States.[1–3] Additionally, the liver is the most common solid organ site of cancer metastasis,[4–7] making metastatic disease the most common form of hepatic malignancy. Although surgery can potentially cure liver tumors, fewer than 20% of patients are surgical candidates due to advanced local disease or co-morbid medical conditions.[8,9] Given these circumstances, image-guided loco-regional therapies have been developed by interventional radiologists to treat patients with unresectable primary and secondary hepatic malignancies. These therapies broadly include ablation techniques employing chemical, thermal or electrical energy, and catheter-based approaches delivering high doses of local chemotherapy or radiotherapy. The ablation techniques may be curative in appropriately selected patients, while intra-arterial therapies often have a palliative intent, typically employed in more advanced patients. Intra-arterial therapies are more commonly being utilized to down-size tumors to surgical resectability.

Ablative Therapies

Percutaneous ablative therapies include both non-thermal and thermal techniques. Non-thermal techniques consist primarily of percutaneous ethanol ablation, and the newly developed irreversible electroporation (IRE). Most thermal ablative devices consist of a generator and probe system that delivers energy to tissue to induce cellular necrosis. Hyperthermic ablative techniques such as radiofrequency (RF) or microwave (MW) ablation raise the temperature within tissue to initiate a cascade of events leading towards cell death. At temperatures above 46° Celsius (C), microvascular thrombosis, ischemia, and hypoxia occur.[10] As temperature rises above 60°C, proteins denature, leading to coagulative necrosis. Hypothermic ablation, such as cryoablation, cools tissue to less than 40°C, resulting in breakdown of cellular metabolism, and ultimately extracellular ice formation. This leads to outflow of intracellular fluid due to an osmotic gradient, with cellular dehydration. This gradient is reversed upon tissue thawing, leading to influx of extracellular fluid, and irreversible cell membrane damage through osmotic shock.[10]

The goal of these therapies is to ablate the targeted lesion(s) with a circumferential margin of 0.5–1.0 cm, referred to as an A0 ablation, akin to R0 surgical resection.[11]

Percutaneous ethanol

Percutaneous ethanol injection (PEI) was one of the first methods developed to ablate liver tumors. In this procedure, imaging guidance is used to place a needle directly into the tumor and 95% ethanol is directly instilled into the tumor.[12] Ethanol injection leads to intracellular protein denaturing and tumor microvasculature thrombosis.[12] Early experience with this technique demonstrated five-year survival rates of 32–38% for small HCC tumors.[13–15] PEI is limited by high recurrence rates for lesions greater than 3 cm, intra-procedural pain, and the need for multiple treatment sessions. Additionally, uncertainty with regards to the ablation zone can result in high rates of local progression ranging from 17–38%.[16,17] Despite these limitations, PEI may be valuable in the treatment of lesions near key structures, such as bowel loops or the biliary tree, or in lesions adjacent to vasculature, as it avoids "heat-sink" effects seen with thermal ablative modalities (detailed below).[10,18] PEI is most useful for HCC less than 2 cm in diameter, where the risk of microvascular dissemination is low.[19]

Radiofrequency ablation

Radiofrequency (RF) ablation employs electrodes to generate a rapidly oscillating current, causing frictional heating and inducing coagulative necrosis/cell death in target tissue.[20] Tissues closest to the electrode encounter the highest current, and therefore experience the greatest rise in temperature,[10] while more distant tissues are heated via thermal conduction.[21] The electrodes may be inserted into a tumor percutaneously, under ultrasonography (US), computed tomography (CT), magnetic resonance imaging (MRI) or fluoroscopic guidance. Advances to this therapeutic modality include cooled-tip electrodes, expandable array designs, clustered electrodes, and saline perfused electrodes. These have enabled treatment of lesions ranging from 2–5 cm, by providing more uniform tissue heating, and minimizing "heat-sink" effects.[20] (Fig. 1). For lesions near critical structures, hydro-dissection,[22] instilling carbon dioxide,[23] or balloon interposition[24] can be utilized to separate and protect vital organs.

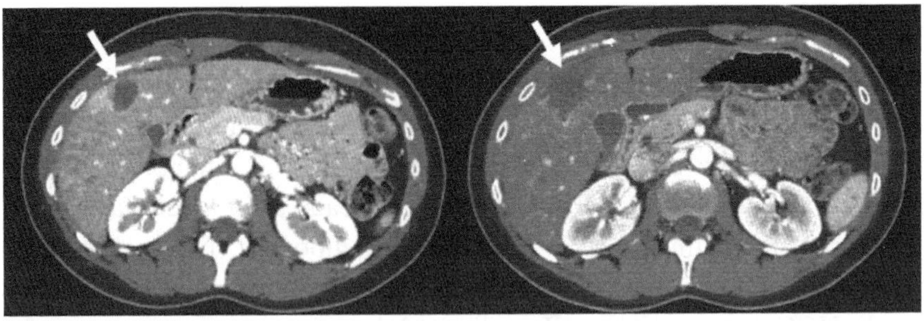

(a) (b)

Fig. 1. Radiofrequency ablation.

Radiofrequency ablation of mCRC. (a) Pretreatment CT scan demonstrates hypervascular tumor within left hepatic lobe (arrow). (b) CT images obtained post-RFA treatment demonstrate nonvisualization of the tumor, which is replaced by a wide nonenhancing ablation zone (arrow).

In patients with early-stage HCC (Child-Pugh A), several large series have demonstrated that RF ablation provides five-year survival rates of 50–64%.[25–28] The therapy is most beneficial for lesions less than 3 cm, with diminished local control for lesions exceeding 3 cm in size.[29] For HCC lesions less than 2 cm, five-year survival rates approach 70%, which is comparable to surgical resection.[30] Several prospective randomized studies have confirmed that for small, solitary, early stage HCC, RF ablation provides survival rates similar to surgical resection.[31,32]

For patients with isolated hepatic colorectal cancer metastasis (mCRC), five-year survival rates following RF ablation approach those for surgical resection for lesions smaller than 4 cm.[33]

Several well-described technical and anatomic factors limit RF ablation's applicability. As the mechanism of ablation relies on thermal conduction, the technique is susceptible to "heat-sink" effects. The presence of large vessels (>3 mm), with continuous flowing blood, adjacent to a lesion results in sub-lethal temperatures and limited tissue necrosis.[34–36] Lesions in a sub-capsular location are also associated with increased risk of incomplete ablation and resultant tumor progression.[37] In order to complete the electrical circuit needed to generate tissue heating, electrical grounding pads must be affixed to the patient's thighs or back, and may occasionally result in skin burns at these sites.[38]

Microwave ablation

Microwave (MW) ablation utilizes an interstitial antenna, which uses high frequency oscillating electromagnetic fields to agitate water molecules, and therefore induce frictional heating and tissue necrosis. Compared to RF ablation, microwave propagation is not limited by low electrical or thermal conductivity,[39] and generates a broader zone of active heating. This leads to higher temperatures within the target zone in a shorter time, and is therefore less susceptible to heat sink effects.[40,41] MW antennae may be positioned to generate overlapping fields to increase ablative zones.[39,42] Furthermore, grounding pads are not required.

Early experience with this modality in HCC demonstrates complete ablation rates of 89–94%, with five-year survival rates of 51–57%,[43–45] comparable to results with RF ablation. A large retrospective review of MW ablation in 452 patients demonstrated no significant difference in technical success, local progression, or survival rates when comparing lesions adjacent to large vessels (defined as >3 mm) versus those in more favorable locations. The authors reported overall five-year overall survival of 57–69%.[46]

While there is great enthusiasm for this treatment modality, data on outcomes remains limited when compared to RF ablation. Retrospective series have demonstrated comparable local control rates between MW and RF ablation.[47,48] A recent retrospective comparison of these two techniques for HCC less than 3 cm, in 198 patients, demonstrated no significant difference in local control rates between RF and MW ablation, with four-year survival rates of 77.8% and 77.6%, respectively.[49]

Early experience with mCRC demonstrated no significant difference in one-, two-, and three-year survival rates between patients treated with MW ablation and surgical resection.[50] A study by Ogata *et al.* of 102 patients with unresectable mCRC demonstrated a high local control rate of 95%; however, median survival was limited at 43 months.[51]

While evolved and improved compared to first generation systems, MW devices are still limited in their use. Rapid antennae shaft heating can occur, requiring cooling mechanisms to prevent thermal burns at the skin entry site.[42,52] Additionally, the size and shape of the ablative zone may be difficult to predict.[42] Given its potential benefits over RF ablation, continued technical advancements will likely expand the role of MW ablation in the treatment of hepatic malignancies.

Cryoablation

Cryoablation devices cyclically apply extremely cold temperatures to targeted tissue to induce cell death by ice ball formation and cell membrane destruction.[53] The advantage is that ice ball formation can be readily visualized intra-procedurally with imaging guidance.[54–57] The zone of ablation is considered to lie with the -20°C isotherm, which can be up to 1 cm within the boundaries of the ice ball.[58,59]

Despite these potential advantages, widespread adoption of cryoablation for the treatment of hepatic malignancies has not been observed, and data on outcomes is therefore limited. A study by Chen *et al.*[60] examined the outcomes in patients with unresectable and recurrent HCC (following resection). Complete ablation, after one or more sessions, was achieved in 75% of patients with unresectable HCC, and 76.9% of patients with recurrent HCC. Patients with unresectable HCC demonstrated one- and three-year survival rates of 81.4% and 60.3%, respectively, while patients with recurrent HCC experienced 1- and 3-year survival rates of 70.2% and 28.8%.[60]

The adoption of this modality for the treatment of hepatic malignancies has been limited for several reasons. Initial experience with the technique was complicated by hepatic hemorrhage secondary to ice ball fracture.[61,62] Due to uncertainty regarding the margins of the lethal zone within the ice ball boundaries, a larger amount of hepatic parenchyma must be treated to ensure adequate margins.[63,64] Similar to other thermal ablative techniques, adjacent vessels may induce a "cold sink" effect, limiting ablative zones.[36] Additionally, this technique is associated with the systemic release of cytokines, which can result in fever, tachycardia, acute lung injury, and acute tubular necrosis, termed "cryoshock."[61,62] Cryoshock has been observed in up to 1% of liver ablation procedures.[21] Finally, with regard to ablative therapies, ablation of the track is recommended to prevent tumor seeding, as well as to create hemostasis along the access tract.[65] However, this is not possible with cryoabalation.

Irreversible electroporation

Irreversible electroporation (IRE) is a non-thermal ablative technique that utilizes tissue electrodes to alter cell membrane potential via electrical pulses, inducing nano-size pores, and thus disrupting cellular integrity leading to cell death.[66] IRE creates ablation zones with sharp margins between treated and nonablated tissue, allowing precise control over the ablation zone.[67] Additionally, unlike thermal ablation techniques, IRE is not susceptible to heat sink from nearby vessels. The ablation zone leaves little scarring and damage to the underlying tissues, such as the adjacent vessels and bile ducts.[67]

IRE requires general anesthesia and muscle paralysis due to muscular twitching induced by electrical pulses. As this technique is the newest ablative therapy, data of its efficacy is limited. Initial experience with IRE in 33 patients with HCC demonstrated a progression-free survival of 11.6 months.[68] Future studies will likely focus on tumors in difficult locations, adjacent to vital structures, as IRE maybe useful in such settings.

Future directions

Improvements in navigation technology and multimodal image fusion may advance these techniques further, permitting the treatment of more complex lesions. These technologies may enhance accuracy and effectiveness, while reducing procedure time, radiation dose, and complications. Techniques such as image fusion permit co-display of images from multiple modalities together, facilitating real-time visualization of lesion targeting and therapy. For these strategies, cross-sectional images (CT/MRI) are acquired prior to ablation, and fused with real-time US images.[69] Early work by Salbiati *et al.* demonstrated that US-CT or US-MRI fusion systems permitted the ablation of 295 hepatic tumors in 175 patients which were not visible by conventional US alone. Within this cohort, incomplete ablation was observed in 16 lesions (5.4%), while 13 lesions were unable to be targeted (4.4%).[70] Future iterations of these techniques will be beneficial for improving tumor targeting.

Transarterial Therapies

Transarterial locoregional therapies involve placing angiographic catheters into the arteries perfusing the hepatic tumor(s) of interest and delivering therapeutic agents locally. The normal hepatic parenchyma derives its blood supply primarily from the portal vein (75%), while malignant cells derive their supply from the hepatic arteries.[71–74] Transarterial therapies exploit this concept to deliver cytotoxic therapies to the capillary beds of tumor cells, while limiting exposure to uninvolved hepatic tissue. These techniques have been widely utilized in the treatment of both HCC and metastatic disease with good outcomes.[75–79] Conventional transarterial chemoembolization (cTACE), utilizes a mixture of lipiodol and one or more chemotherapeutic agent (e.g., doxorubicin, cisplatin, mitomycin), which are injected within the target artery. Lipiodol acts as a delivery vehicle and emulsifying agent for the chemotherapeutics, and permits visualization under fluoroscopy with digital subtraction angiography (DSA).[80–83] Evolution of chemoembolization has led to the development of controlled release drug-eluting bead transarterial chemoembolization (DEB-TACE), where the chemotherapeutic drug is loaded into drug-eluting microspheres. Following delivery to the tumor arterial supply, a controlled therapeutic release occurs, providing anti-tumoral effects. Radioembolization involves the delivery of 30-micron sized microembolic particles into a tumor's arterial supply, which ultimately lodge within the tumor. This results in a low dose-rate local brachytherapy within the tumor. All three of these techniques have achieved promising clinical outcomes with regard to oncologic response, time-to-progression (TTP) and overall survival. While all of these treatments utilize a transarterial approach and are generally well-tolerated, there are differences in terms of patient selection, technique, and complications.

Following cTACE, almost all patients experience post-embolization syndrome, characterized by pain, nausea and vomiting. Symptoms are typically managed during the hospitalization (1–3 days), and can be seen in up to 10% of patients[84]. Additional complications may include: (1) biliary duct injury (up to 5.3%);[85,86] (2) liver abscesses in up to 25% of patients with biliary sphincterotomy;[84,85] (3) duodenal or gastric ulcers from off-target delivery of the chemotherapeutic agents(1.0%);[85] (4) vascular injury such as spasm/dissection from repeated chemotherapy injection in the arterial system (1.0%),[87] (5) and tumor rupture (<1%).[84,85]

Although the systemic chemotherapy exposure is limited with DEB-TACE compared to cTACE (detailed below), adverse events mirror conventional therapy, albeit in a lower frequency. These include pain, nausea, vascular injury, hepatic failure, abscess formation and tumor rupture.[88,89] Reported rates in the literature include post-embolization syndrome in up to 80%, and liver abscesses in up to 2%.[90–92] Given concerns of post-embolization, patients treated with either cTACE or DEB-TACE typically require inpatient admission for post-procedural pain control and symptom management.

Due to its unique properties, adverse events following radioembolization differ significantly from other transarterial therapies. The post-embolization syndrome occurs less commonly after radioembolization due to the small size of the particles, avoiding vessel occlusion. Radioembolization is an outpatient procedure; patients are discharged 2–6 hours following treatment. The predominant side effect is fatigue, with other adverse events including non-target deposition of microspheres (possibly leading to ulcer formation), fibrosis/scarring of the liver parenchyma and cholecystitis. Radiation-induced liver disease is rare, and seen in less than 4% of patients, when proper patient selection criteria are applied.[93,94]

Conventional transarterial chemoembolization

Employed since the 1980s, and the foundation of embolotherapy, cTACE involves the delivery of one or more chemotherapeutics directly to the tumor via hepatic arterial injection.[95–97] Common therapeutic regimens include doxorubicin alone or in combination with mitomycin C and/or cisplatin. Triple-drug therapy was the historically preferred regimen in the United States.[98] From a technical standpoint, however, several variations on this technique exist, with no uniform standard therapeutic protocol. Various reports have differed with regards to patient baseline characteristics, the choice of the embolic agent used, the choice and/or dose of the chemotherapeutic used, embolization end-points, and the schedule and interval of retreatment.[99]

cTACE is indicated in patients with preserved performance status and liver function without vascular invasion or extrahepatic disease. The common femoral artery is catheterized (similar to DEB-TACE and radioembolization), and the lipiodol/chemotherapy emulsion is administered to the hepatic artery perfusing the tumor(s).[100] Lipiodol, a poppy seed oil containing 38% iodine by weight, permits intra-procedural delivery visualization. Lipiodol also facilitates drug concentration within the tumor and is retained for weeks; normal hepatocytes excrete it within one week. To obtain an embolic effect and minimize drug washout, subsequent injection of 100–500 micron bland occlusive particles is typically performed.[101] Immediately following cTACE, a non-contrast CT can be obtained demonstrating the proper location of the chemotherapy/lipiodol combination (Fig. 2). Treatments can repeated at 2–4 month intervals, depending on the tumor burden and response.[102]

Two landmark prospective randomized studies from 2002 established the benefit of cTACE in patients in HCC by improving survival over supportive care.[78,103] Following the promising results of these initial studies, several groups explored the use of cTACE in patients with unresectable HCC. Takayasu *et al.* performed a phase II, cohort study in 8,510 HCC patients treated with cTACE. The authors identified significant prognosticators of survival including liver function, alpha-fetoprotein level, tumor size, number of lesions, and portal vein invasion.[104] Lewandowski *et al.*

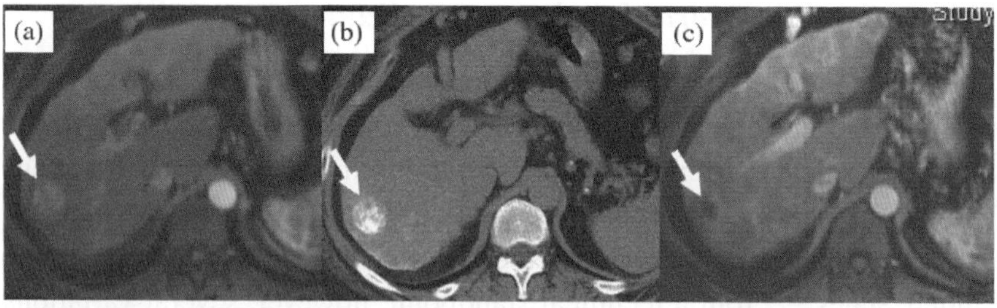

Fig. 2. Conventional chemoembolization.

Conventional cTACE for HCC. (a) Gadolinium-enhanced MR image reveals a hypervascular HCC (arrow) in the right hepatic lobe. (b) Nonenhanced CT scan immediately following conventional chemoembolization demonstrates dense lipiodol staining within the tumor (arrow). (c) Gadolinium-enhanced MR image 6 months after conventional chemoembolization reveals necrosis and tumor size reduction (arrow), which is consistent with a favorable response to therapy.

reported comprehensive imaging and long-term survival results of a cohort of 172 patients. The authors found that median survival differed significantly between patients with BCLC stages a, b and c (Stage a: 40.0 months; b: 17.4 months; c: 6.3 months; $p < 0.0001$). They concluded that chemoembolization was safe and effective in patients with HCC; however, time to progression (TTP) and survival was confounded by tumor biology and background cirrhosis (77). Another large cohort of 4,966 patients by Takayasu *et al.* demonstrated excellent results with a median survival of 3.3 years. The authors reported that Child-Pugh classification, tumor number, size, alpha-fetoprotein, and des-gamma carboxy-prothrombin levels were independent prognosticators of survival.[105] However, compared to the prior study by Lewandowski, the Japanese group excluded patients with vascular invasion, extrahepatic metastases and prior treatment. A meta-analysis of seven published randomized control trials corroborated these findings, concluding that cTACE is an effective palliative therapy for unresectable HCC.[106]

Chemoembolization has also successfully been utilized in the treatment of metastatic disease to the liver. Albert *et al.* examined response and survival following chemoembolization for 121 patients with mCRC.[107] The authors reported a 2% partial response rate (PR), a TTP of 3 months, and a median overall survival of 9 months from chemoembolization. Specifically, survival was significantly improved when chemoembolization was employed following first- or second-line chemotherapy rather than following third- to fifth-line therapies.[107] In a study involving 463 patients with mCRC who failed systemic chemotherapy, cTACE resulted in PR in 14.7% patients and 1–2-year survival rates of 62% and 28% respectively.[108] Tellez *et al.* performed a phase II trial examining chemoembolization in 30 patients with mCRC, who had failed prior systemic chemotherapy. A median survival of 8.6 months was seen.[109] These results were confirmed by Geschwind *et al.*, who demonstrated that cTACE can prolong survival of patients with colorectal metastases, including those patients who failed to respond to systemic chemotherapy.[110]

Drug-eluting bead chemoembolization

Drug-Eluting Bead Chemoembolization (DEB-TACE) represents an evolution of conventional chemoembolization that incorporates drug-eluting microspheres for therapeutic delivery. Through a drug-loading process, the microspheres are able to absorb the chemotherapeutic agent. Drug-elution is based on a strong drug-bead interaction that can be attributed to an ionic exchange process between anionic drug moieties and the hydrogel sulfonate or carboxyl counter ions.[111,112] The unique properties of the microspheres allow for controlled and sustained drug release, with a significant reduction of peak plasma concentration when compared to cTACE.[111,112] These characteristics suggest that a greater amount of the therapeutic agent is sequestered by the tumor versus dispersed within the systemic circulation. Data from explant studies demonstrate that drug-eluting beads provide a sustained delivery of drug for a period of one month within one millimeter of the treated vessel, and provide local tissue concentrations above cytotoxic threshold in HCC-bearing livers.[113]

DEB-TACE may be considered for intermediate BCLC B category patients with preserved performance status and liver function. However, ideally, patients should have a lesion that can be isolated angiographically, to permit selective (as opposed to lobar) arterial delivery (Fig. 3). Treatment guidelines for DEB-TACE recommend up to four treatments within 6 months to the entire treatment field.[114]

There is a growing body of literature examining the role of DEB-TACE in the treatment of unresectable HCC.[115,116] A randomized controlled trial (PRECISION V) of 212 patients comparing cTACE to DEB-TACE failed

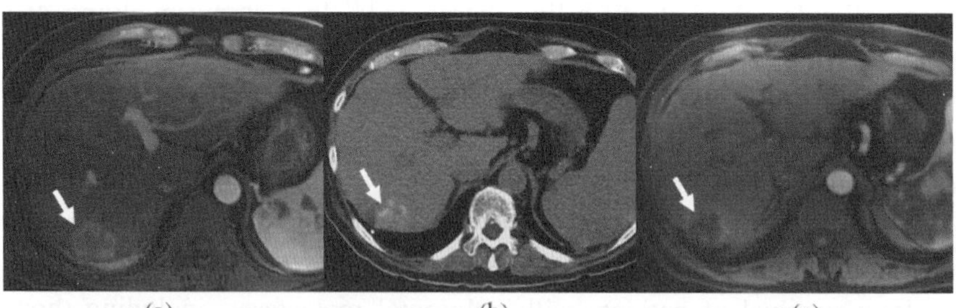

Fig. 3. Drug-eluting bead chemoembolization.

DEB-TACE for HCC. (a) Gadolinium-enhanced MR image reveals a hypervascular HCC (arrow) in the right hepatic lobe. (b) Nonenhanced CT scan immediately after DEB-TACE demonstrates contrast retention within the tumor (arrow). 1 month follow-up gadolinium-enhanced (c) MR images reveal necrosis (arrow), which is consistent with a favorable response to therapy.

to show an improvement in response with DEB-TACE (and failed to meet the study primary objective), despite the potential more controlled and sustained drug-release. However, subset analysis revealed that Childs Pugh B patients with bilobar or recurrent disease were better able to tolerate DEB-TACE compared with cTACE.[117] Based on these results, many now use DEB-TACE in patients with more advanced disease. A retrospective analysis by Dhanasekran *et al.* concluded that transcatheter therapy with DEB-TACE offered a survival benefit over cTACE in patients with unresectable HCC.[118] The authors reported fewer adverse events after DEB-TACE compared to cTACE, highlighting the safety profile of DEB-TACE. A study by Kalva *et al.* in 130 patients with HCC, reported a median overall survival of 14.7 months. Preserved liver function and performance status, lack of portal vein thrombus, and greater than 50% necrosis of the treated lesion on follow-up imaging were shown to be associated with improved survival.[119] A recent study in 121 patients with advanced HCC, BCLC C category, demonstrated DEB-TACE resulted in a median overall survival of 13.5 months, with the most therapeutic benefit seen in Child-Pugh A cirrhotics without portal vein thrombosis or metastatic disease.[120] A follow-up study by Kalva *et al.*, examining the role of DEB-TACE in 80 patients with advanced stage HCC (BCLC-C), demonstrated a median overall survival of 13.3 months following treatment, with Eastern Cooperative Oncology Group (ECOG) performance status and number of DEB-TACE procedures being significant prognosticators of survival.[121] An additional study involving a 104-patient cohort with preserved synthetic function and performance status, reported a median survival of 48 months;[122] however, these results may have been due to careful patient selection, and merits further investigation.

A prospective randomized trial comparing DEB-TACE to bland embolization demonstrated similar imaging response to therapy between the two groups. However, TTP was longer in the DEB-TACE arm, highlighting the benefit of the cytotoxic effects of chemotherapy when used in conjunction with embolization.[123] A five-year survival analysis in 173 patients demonstrated an overall survival of 43 months. However, this cohort included several patients with solitary lesions less than 5 cm in diameter, who were categorized as too high-risk for either surgical resection or ablative therapy. Furthermore, results of this study may be confounded by added treatments following the initial embolization, including RFA. While promising, these results warrant further study.[124]

The role of DEB-TACE in the treatment of mCRC has been explored, with limited initial results. In this subset of patients, irinotecan is the preferred chemotherapeutic of choice, although its elution from the therapeutic beads appears to be less optimal (more rapid) compared to doxorubicin.[125] Martin *et al.* examined the use of DEBIRI (Drug Eluting Bead, Irinotecan), in a multi-center series of 55 patients with mCRC treated with prior chemotherapy. The authors reported adverse events in 28%; response rates were 66% and 75% at 6 and 12 months; overall and progression-free survival was 19 and 11 months respectively.[126] DEBIRI has also been evaluated for possible surgical downstaging and as a neoadjuvant therapy for patients with metastatic colorectal cancer. Within this group, 20% of patients demonstrated a significant response to therapy and downstaging of disease, permitting resection. The authors concluded DEB-TACE was a safe and effective means of downstaging mCRC in select patients.[127] DEBIRI has also demonstrated favorable outcomes compared with systemic 5-FU/leucovorin/irinotecan (FOLFIRI) chemotherapy, the first-line treatment for stage IV disease. A randomized trial comparing DEBIRI versus systemic FOLFIRI demonstrated significantly prolonged overall survival, median survival, progression-free survival, and duration of quality of life improvement for patients in the DEBIRI group.[128]

Radioembolization

Radioembolization is a procedure that delivers micron-sized embolic particles loaded with a radioisotope via the hepatic arteries to hepatic tumor(s). Unlike external beam radiation therapy where dose limitations and hepatic radiosensitivity limit the amount of radiation that can be delivered to hepatic tissue before the development of radiation-induced liver disease (ascites, anicteric hepatomegaly, elevation of alkaline phosphatase), radioembolization permits selective delivery of high doses of radiation up to 170 Gy to hepatic tumors, with minimal toxicity to the surrounding liver.[129–131] In this therapy, 20–60 micron-sized radioactive particles are delivered to the tumor at the segmental or lobar level. This procedure is unlike cTACE/DEB-TACE in that it is intended to be micro-embolic; vessel occlusion is not desired with radioembolization.

Overall, radioembolization has been reserved for BCLC-B patients who are not candidates for cTACE due to the presence of multifocal bilobar disease, poor liver function or performance status, or portal vein thrombus (PVT). An initial study analyzing the long-term outcomes following radioembolization for HCC, demonstrated that patients with Child-Pugh A class disease, with or without PVT, benefited most from the treatment, as compared to Child-Pugh B patients with PVT. Time-to-progression was higher for Child-Pugh A and B patients without PVT than those with PVT. Overall survival for patients with Child–Pugh A and B disease was: CP-A, 17.2 months; CP-B, 7.7 months; ($p = 0.002$). Time-to-progression and overall survival varied by patient stage at baseline.[76] Several large phase 2 studies examining long-term outcomes following radioembolization have been published. An initial large 291-patient cohort from Salem *et al.* was the first to report toxicities, imaging and survival outcomes stratified by BCLC, United Network for Organ Sharing (UNOS), tumor stage and Child-Pugh score.[76] The authors confirmed that patients with Child-Pugh A disease with or without vascular invasion benefitted the most from radioembolization. Hilgard *et al.* corroborated these results in a 108-patient European cohort with advanced disease, which confirmed technical reproducibility and equivalent outcomes to cTACE/DEB-TACE.[132] These results were further validated with a 325-patient study describing long-term survival outcomes stratified by BCLC stages.[133] A recent Italian phase II study reported outcomes following radioembolization in intermediate/advanced patients. This study served to launch a randomized phase III trial comparing radioembolization to Sorafenib.[134]

Due to the inherent heterogeneity of patients with intermediate stage disease (BCLC-B), with prolonged survival in select sub-groups, comparison between radioembolization and cTACE is difficult. While there is no randomized study comparing radioembolization to chemoembolization, Salem *et al.* performed a comparative analysis at a single institution in a 245-patient cohort. When compared to cTACE, radioembolization demonstrated improved adverse event and toxicity profiles. The groups were well-balanced with regards to Child-Pugh, UNOS, and BCLC staging, with older patients seen in the radioembolization cohort ($p < 0.001$). When compared to cTACE, radioembolization demonstrated decreased abdominal pain and fewer transaminase elevations ($p < 0.05$). Radioembolization also demonstrated a longer TTP compared to cTACE, (13.3 months and 8.4 months, respectively; $p = 0.046$). However, overall survival was no different, likely as a result of competing risks of death from HCC and cirrhosis.[75] While there was no survival difference, these results demonstrate radioembolization provided better disease control (longer TTP) with less toxicity than cTACE. Lewandowski *et al.* confirmed the improvement in TTP, and also demonstrating that radioembolization was superior to cTACE in downstaging patients to transplantation.[135]

A prospective phase II study compared radioembolization to cTACE based on quality of life metrics. Although the treatment groups had comparable baseline Child-Pugh class and performance statuses, patients within the cTACE cohort had lower tumor burdens ($p = 0.018$) and less-advanced disease, based on UNOS and BCLC stage ($p = 0.03$ and $p = 0.02$, respectively). The greater tumor burden within the radioembolization cohort necessitated lobar therapeutic infusion (covering the entire lobe) as opposed to selective infusions during TACE (treating smaller tumors) ($p < 0.0001$). Despite the fact that radioembolization was used to treat more advanced disease, those who received this treatment had significant increases in several quality of life metrics, whereas patients who received cTACE had decreases in quality of life scores.[136]

Recent advances in dosimetry and selective therapy have led to the development of new treatment paradigms in radioembolization. The first is the concept of "radiation segmentectomy." This selective therapy involves delivering radiation doses to small sectors of liver tissue, 1,000 times greater than possible with external beam radiotherapy.[129] These segments of tumor bearing liver, not amenable to resection or ablation due to location, insufficient hepatic reserve, or comorbidities, can be effectively treated with radioembolization. Median survival in a cohort of 102 patients treated with this technique was 53.4 months.[137] This concept has been expanded to include "radiation lobectomy" for patients with right lobe disease. These patients can potentially be amenable to curative resection, but are excluded at time of presentation due to small future liver remnant. While portal vein embolization has been historically used in these patients to induce hepatic hypertrophy, results are suboptimal in the setting of cirrhosis. A study by Vouche *et al.* in 83 patients demonstrated that right lobe "radiation lobectomy" was able to treat the tumor while selectively inducing right hepatic lobe atrophy and lesion regression, with concomitant future liver remnant hypertrophy.[138]

Radioembolization has also been studied in the salvage setting for the treatment of hepatic metastatic disease. Mulcahy *et al.* presented results of 72 patients with mCRC treated with lobar radioembolization. The authors reported a PR rate of 40.3%, with median time to hepatic progression and overall survival from first treatment of 15.4 months and 14.5 months respectively.[139] A study by Kennedy *et al.* examined radioembolization in 208 patients who had failed irinotecan and/or oxaliplatin-based chemotherapy. The authors reported an imaging response of 35%, while PET response was 91%. Survival was 10.5 months for responders and 4.5 months for non-responders.[140] Jakobs *et al.* reported results on radioembolization in 41 salvage patients with unresectable hepatic colorectal metastases. The mean CEA decrease was 32% for the entire cohort of colorectal patients. By Response Evaluation Criteria In Solid Tumors (RECIST) criteria, partial response, stable disease and progressive disease were observed in 7, 25 and 4 patients, respectively. Median overall survival was 10.5 months; improved survival was observed for patients who demonstrated CEA and imaging response.[141]

Future directions

There are a few topics of future consideration in intra-arterial therapies worth discussing. The first concept is improving tumor targeting. Advances in imaging techniques can further expand the role of transcatheter therapies. Given the imaging limitations of DSA, several technologies have been developed to further aid in tumor targeting and therapeutic delivery. Cone beam CT involves the acquisition of 3D-CT-like data using a rotating C-arm apparatus in the fluoroscopy suite. Additionally, previously acquired cross-sectional imaging can be fused with procedural images, to enhance intraprocedural navigation.[142] These techniques have been successfully applied to superselective radioembolization (Fig. 4).[143] Several studies have demonstrated success with C-arm angiographic CT for chemoembolization and other transcatheter therapies.[144–146] Additional studies

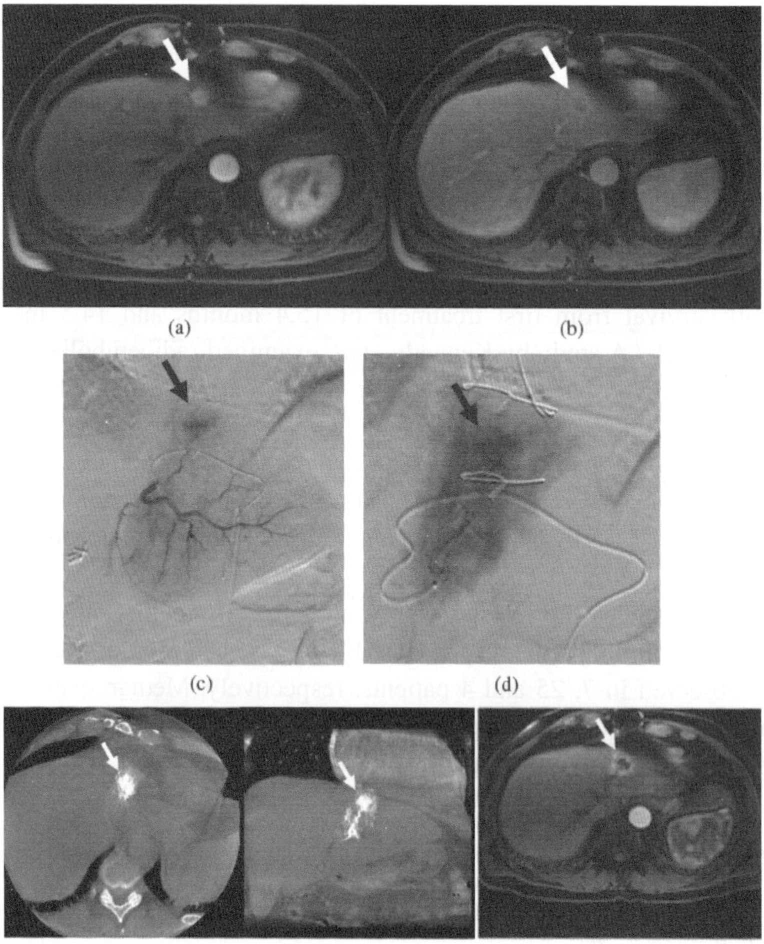

(a) (b) (c) (d) (e) (f) (g)

Fig. 4. Radioembolization.

Radioembolization with radiation segmentectomy for HCC, performed with the use of C-arm CT. Gadolinium enhanced MR images in (a) arterial and (b) portal venous phases reveals a hypervascular tumor within the left hepatic lobe demonstrating venous washout (white arrows), compatible with HCC. (c) Selective left hepatic angiogram depicts a small hypervascular tumor (black arrow) correlating with the pre-procedure MR imaging. (d) Distal segmental angiography demonstrates more selective tumor perfusion (black arrow). Axial (e) and coronal (f) C-arm CT images with the catheter selectively positioned in a tumor-feeding branch reveals marked tumor perfusion (white arrow) and minimal perfusion to the adjacent parenchyma. (g) 1 month follow-up gadolinium-enhanced MR image reveals complete tumor necrosis (white arrow), with adjacent parenchymal hyperemia, secondary to high-dose radiotherapy. These findings are consistent with a favorable response to therapy. This pattern of necrosis in a segmental distribution has been termed a "radiation segmentectomy."

have also examined combining DSA with MRI, resulting in catheter repositioning in 50% of cases, facilitating more complete tumor targeting, minimized non-target delivery, and increased operator confidence.[147,148]

There is much enthusiasm for combining systemic and locoregional therapies for patients with unresectable primary or secondary hepatic malignancies. In fact, systemic therapies may play a role in potentiating the effects of transcatheter therapies. An initial randomized trial by Gray *et al.* compared radioembolization in combination with floxuridine (FUDR) versus FUDR alone in 74 patients with unresectable bilobar mCRC. Patients within the combination therapy group demonstrated a longer TTP (12 vs. 7.6 months, $p = 0.04$), with a median survival of 15.9 months versus 9.7 months ($p = 0.001$).[149] A follow-up phase II randomized trial examined radioembolization in combination with 5-FU/levocorin versus 5-FU/levocorin alone in 21 treatment naïve patients. In the combination therapy group, TTP was significantly prolonged (18.6 vs. 3.6 months, $p < 0.0005$), with increased median survival (29.4 vs. 12.8 months, $p = 0.02$).[150] Hendlisz *et al.* compared intravenous fluorouracil (FU) alone with the combination of radioembolization and intravenous fluorouracil in a multicenter phase III randomized trial of 46 patients with unresectable mCRC. While median overall survival was not significantly different between combination therapy and FU alone (10 vs. 7.3 months, respectively, $p = 0.80$), median TTP was higher with combination therapy (4.5 vs. 2.1 months, respectively, $p = 0.03$).[151] Given its success in the salvage setting, with results comparing favorably to salvage chemotherapy, radioembolization is now being evaluated in combination with first- or second-line chemotherapy. In efforts to potentiate the effects of radiation, a recent phase I study by Hickey *et al.* examined the use of capecitabine in combination with escalating Y90 dosing in patients with metastatic disease. Doses of 170 Gy in the liver were obtained, with no dose limiting toxicities observed.[152]

Because transcatheter therapies such as TACE and DEB-TACE are associated with elevation in serum angiogenic growth factors,[153] which facilitate tumor proliferation, there has been increasing interest in the use of molecular targeted agents in the treatment of HCC, given the anti-angiogenic properties of agents such as sorafenib and bevacizumab (Bayer, Germany; Roche, Switzerland, respectively). Sorafenib was the first such agent to demonstrate survival benefit in patients with advanced HCC.[154] A recent study by Buijs *et al.* examined combination therapy with chemoembolization with bevacizumab in 25 patients with HCC. The authors reported an overall survival of 10.8 months.[155] Hu *et al.* compared chemoembolization and sorafenib with chemoembolization alone in 280 patients with BCLC stage C HCC. The authors reported greater OS in the combination therapy group versus the monotherapy group (7.0 vs. 4.9 months, $p = 0.003$), with longer TTP in the combination therapy group.[156] A few other studies revealed that while the combination of Sorafenib and locoregional therapies is safe, there does not appear to be an added benefit. Chow *et al.* examined the use of sorafenib following radioembolization in 29 patients with advanced HCC. The majority of patients experienced grade 1 toxicities (28/29), with 15 patients experiencing greater than grade 3 toxicities. The median survival for BCLC stage B and C were 20.3 and 8.6 months, respectively.[157] Results from a recent prospective trial by Kulik *et al.* examining the role of radioembolization combined with sorafenib in patients with HCC as a bridge to transplantation demonstrated that sorafenib did not potentiate radioembolization's effects. Compared to patients who received radioembolization alone, combination therapy with radioembolization and sorafenib resulted in no significant difference with regards to imaging response or pathologic outcomes.[158] Further trials examining the use of transcatheter therapies in combination with or comparison to sorafenib in patients with advanced HCC are ongoing. These trials are robust in their rationale, statistical design (international, multicenter, randomized phase III) and primary endpoints (survival).[159] Final results of these studies are expected within the next 3–5 years.

Conclusion

The available treatment strategies for the management of primary and secondary hepatic malignancies continue to evolve. Image-guided therapies, both percutaneous and transarterial, have demonstrated therapeutic effectiveness, while minimizing damage to normal hepatic parenchyma. As such, these techniques have provided compelling evidence demonstrating safety, minimal toxicity, efficacy, and improved survival in patients not amenable to surgical resection. Future studies examining the role of these therapies in conjunction with systemic treatments are ongoing. As advances in both techniques and therapeutics occur, the clinical indications and applicability of these interventions will continue to expand.

Take Home Messages

- Percutaneous ablative treatments deliver energy to tissue to induce cellular necrosis.
- Radiofrequency ablation is best applied to tumors less than 3 cm in diameter, with results approaching survival rates for surgical resection in select patients.
- Fewer data regarding outcomes is available for other percutaneous techniques including microwave ablation, cryoablation, and irreversible electroporation.
- Transcatheter therapies selectively deliver therapeutic agents to the hepatic artery supplying the targeted tumor, limiting off-target delivery and toxicity to normal hepatic parenchyma.
- Several studies have demonstrated improved survival following transcatheter therapy in patients not amenable to surgical resection.
- In select patients, treatment with transcatheter therapies may be used to downstage disease to surgical resection or transplantation.

References

1. Gramantieri, L., Fornari, F., Callegari, E., Sabbioni, S., Lanza, G., Croce, C.M. *et al.*, MicroRNA involvement in hepatocellular carcinoma. *J Cell Mol Med*, 2008. **12**(6A): 2189–204.
2. Parkin, D.M., Bray, F., Ferlay, J., Pisani, P., Global cancer statistics, 2002. *CA Cancer J Clin*, 2005. **55**(2): 74–108.
3. El-Serag, H.B., Mason, A.C., Rising incidence of hepatocellular carcinoma in the United States. *N Engl J Med*, 1999. **340**(10): 745–50.
4. Zavadsky, K.E., Lee, Y.T., Liver metastases from colorectal carcinoma: incidence, resectability, and survival results. *Am Surg*, 1994. **60**(12): 929–33.
5. Michalski, C.W., Erkan, M., Huser, N., Muller, M.W., Hartel, M., Friess, H. *et al.*, Resection of primary pancreatic cancer and liver metastasis: A systematic review. *Dig Surg*, 2008. **25**(6): 473–80.

6. Thomay, A.A., Charpentier, K.P., Optimizing resection for "responding" hepatic metastases after neoadjuvant chemotherapy. *J Surg Oncol*, 2010. **102**(8): 1002–8.
7. Davies, J.M., Goldberg, R.M., Optimum chemotherapy regimens for neoadjuvant therapy of hepatic colorectal metastases. *J Surg Oncol*, 2010. **102**(8): 946–54.
8. El-Serag, H.B., Rudolph, K.L., Hepatocellular carcinoma: epidemiology and molecular carcinogenesis. *Gastroenterology*, 2007. **132**(7): 2557–76.
9. Brown, D.B., Geschwind, J-F.H., Soulen, M.C., Millward, S.F., Sacks, D., Society of Interventional Radiology position statement on chemoembolization of hepatic malignancies. *J Vas Interv Radiol*, 2009. **20**(7 Suppl): S317–23.
10. Knavel, E.M., Brace, C.L., Tumor ablation: common modalities and general practices. *Tech Vasc Interv Radiol*, 2013. **16**(4): 192–200.
11. Hickey, R., Vouche, M., Sze, D.Y., Hohlastos, E., Collins, J., Schirmang, T. *et al.*, Cancer concepts and principles: primer for the interventional oncologist-part II. *J Vas Interv Radiol*, 2013. **24**(8): 1167–88.
12. Okuda, K., Intratumor ethanol injection. *J Surg Oncol Suppl*, 1993. **3**: 97–9.
13. Shiina, S., Tagawa, K., Niwa, Y., Unuma, T., Komatsu, Y., Yoshiura, K. *et al.*, Percutaneous ethanol injection therapy for hepatocellular carcinoma: results in 146 patients. *AJR Am J Roentgenol*, 1993. **160**(5): 1023–8.
14. Lencioni, R., Bartolozzi, C., Caramella, D., Paolicchi, A., Carrai, M., Maltinti, G. *et al.*, Treatment of small hepatocellular carcinoma with percutaneous ethanol injection. Analysis of prognostic factors in 105 Western patients. *Cancer*, 1995. **76**(10): 1737–46.
15. Livraghi, T., Giorgio, A., Marin, G., Salmi, A., de Sio, I., Bolondi, L. *et al.*, Hepatocellular carcinoma and cirrhosis in 746 patients: long-term results of percutaneous ethanol injection. *Radiology*, 1995. **197**(1): 101–8.
16. Hasegawa, S., Yamasaki, N., Hiwaki, T., Sako, K., Komorizono, Y., Baba, Y. *et al.*, Factors that predict intrahepatic recurrence of hepatocellular carcinoma in 81 patients initially treated by percutaneous ethanol injection. *Cancer*, 1999. **86**(9): 1682–90.
17. Koda, M., Murawaki, Y., Mitsuda, A., Ohyama, K., Horie, Y., Suou, T. *et al.*, Predictive factors for intrahepatic recurrence after percutaneous ethanol injection therapy for small hepatocellular carcinoma. *Cancer*, 2000. **88**(3): 529–37.

18. Livraghi, T., Lazzaroni, S., Meloni, F., Radiofrequency thermal ablation of hepatocellular carcinoma. *Eur J Ultrasound*, 2001. **13**(2): 159–66.
19. Chow, D.H., Sinn, L.H., Ng, K.K., Lam, C.M., Yuen, J., Fan, S.T. *et al.*, Radiofrequency ablation for hepatocellular carcinoma and metastatic liver tumors: a comparative study. *J Surg Oncol*, 2006. **94**(7): 565–71.
20. Goldberg, S.N., Gazelle, G.S., Mueller, P.R., Thermal ablation therapy for focal malignancy: a unified approach to underlying principles, techniques, and diagnostic imaging guidance. *AJR Am J Roentgenol*, 2000. **174**(2): 323–31.
21. Ahmed, M., Brace, C.L., Lee, F.T., Jr., Goldberg, S.N., Principles of and advances in percutaneous ablation. *Radiology*, 2011. **258**(2): 351–69.
22. Song, I., Rhim, H., Lim, H.K., Kim, Y.S., Choi, D., Percutaneous radiofrequency ablation of hepatocellular carcinoma abutting the diaphragm and gastrointestinal tracts with the use of artificial ascites: safety and technical efficacy in 143 patients. *Eur Radiol*, 2009. **19**(11): 2630–40.
23. Raman, S.S., Aziz, D., Chang, X., Sayre, J., Lassman, C., Lu, D., Minimizing diaphragmatic injury during radiofrequency ablation: efficacy of intraabdominal carbon dioxide insufflation. *AJR Am J Roentgenol*, 2004. **183**(1): 197–200.
24. Yamakado, K., Nakatsuka, A., Akeboshi, M., Takeda, K., Percutaneous radiofrequency ablation of liver neoplasms adjacent to the gastrointestinal tract after balloon catheter interposition. *J Vasc Interv Radiol*, 2003. **14**(9 Pt 1): 1183–6.
25. Choi, D., Lim, H.K., Rhim, H., Kim, Y.S., Lee, W.J., Paik, S.W. *et al.*, Percutaneous radiofrequency ablation for early-stage hepatocellular carcinoma as a first-line treatment: long-term results and prognostic factors in a large single-institution series. *Eur Radiol*, 2007. **17**(3): 684–92.
26. Lencioni, R., Cioni, D., Crocetti, L., Franchini, C., Pina, C.D., Lera, J. *et al.*, Early-stage hepatocellular carcinoma in patients with cirrhosis: long-term results of percutaneous image-guided radiofrequency ablation. *Radiology*, 2005. **234**(3): 961–7.
27. Tateishi, R., Shiina, S., Teratani, T., Obi, S., Sato, S., Koike, Y. *et al.*, Percutaneous radiofrequency ablation for hepatocellular carcinoma. An analysis of 1000 cases. *Cancer*, 2005. **103**(6): 1201–9.
28. N'Kontchou, G., Mahamoudi, A., Aout, M., Ganne-Carrie, N., Grando, V., Coderc, E. *et al.*, Radiofrequency ablation of hepatocellular

carcinoma: long-term results and prognostic factors in 235 Western patients with cirrhosis. *Hepatology*, 2009. **50**(5): 1475–83.

29. Livraghi, T., Goldberg, S.N., Lazzaroni, S., Meloni, F., Ierace, T., Solbiati, L. *et al.*, Hepatocellular carcinoma: radio-frequency ablation of medium and large lesions. *Radiology*, 2000. **214**(3): 761–8.
30. Livraghi, T., Meloni, F., Di Stasi, M., Rolle, E., Solbiati, L., Tinelli, C. *et al.*, Sustained complete response and complications rates after radiofrequency ablation of very early hepatocellular carcinoma in cirrhosis: Is resection still the treatment of choice? *Hepatology*, 2008. **47**(1): 82–9.
31. Huang, J., Yan, L., Cheng, Z., Wu, H., Du, L., Wang, J. *et al.*, A randomized trial comparing radiofrequency ablation and surgical resection for HCC conforming to the Milan criteria. *Ann Surg*, 2010. **252**(6): 903–12.
32. Chen, M.S., Li, J.Q., Zheng, Y., Guo, R.P., Liang, H.H., Zhang, Y.Q. *et al.*, A prospective randomized trial comparing percutaneous local ablative therapy and partial hepatectomy for small hepatocellular carcinoma. *Ann Surg*, 2006. **243**(3): 321–8.
33. Gillams, A.R., Lees, W.R., Five-year survival following radiofrequency ablation of small, solitary, hepatic colorectal metastases. *J Vasc Interv Radiol*, 2008. **19**(5): 712–7.
34. Kim, S.K., Rhim, H., Kim, Y.S., Koh, B.H., Cho, O.K., Seo, H.S. *et al.*, Radiofrequency thermal ablation of hepatic tumors: pitfalls and challenges. *Abdom Imaging*, 2005. **30**(6): 727–33.
35. Lu, D.S., Yu, N.C., Raman, S.S., Limanond, P., Lassman, C., Murray, K. *et al.*, Radiofrequency ablation of hepatocellular carcinoma: treatment success as defined by histologic examination of the explanted liver. *Radiology*, 2005. **234**(3): 954–60.
36. Bhardwaj, N., Strickland, A.D., Ahmad, F., Atanesyan, L., West, K., Lloyd, D.M., A comparative histological evaluation of the ablations produced by microwave, cryotherapy and radiofrequency in the liver. *Pathology (Phila)*, 2009. **41**(2): 168–72.
37. Komorizono, Y., Oketani, M., Sako, K., Yamasaki, N., Shibatou, T., Maeda, M. *et al.*, Risk factors for local recurrence of small hepatocellular carcinoma tumors after a single session, single application of percutaneous radiofrequency ablation. *Cancer*, 2003. **97**(5): 1253–62.
38. Gervais, D.A., Arellano, R.S., Percutaneous tumor ablation for hepatocellular carcinoma. *Am J Roentgenol*, 2011. **197**(4): 789–94.

39. Lubner, M.G., Brace, C.L., Hinshaw, J.L., Lee, F.T., Jr. Microwave tumor ablation: mechanism of action, clinical results, and devices. *J Vasc Interv Radiol*, 2010. **21**(8 Suppl): S192–203.
40. Wright, A.S., Sampson, L.A., Warner, T.F., Mahvi, D.M., Lee, F.T., Jr. Radiofrequency versus microwave ablation in a hepatic porcine model. *Radiology*, 2005. **236**(1): 132–9.
41. Yu, N.C., Raman, S.S., Kim, Y.J., Lassman, C., Chang, X., Lu, D.S., Microwave liver ablation: influence of hepatic vein size on heat-sink effect in a porcine model. *J Vasc Interv Radiol*, 2008. **19**(7): 1087–92.
42. Lubner, M.G., Brace, C.L., Ziemlewicz, T.J., Hinshaw, J.L., Lee, F.T., Microwave ablation of hepatic malignancy. *Semin Interv Radiol*, 2013. **30**(1): 56–66.
43. Dong, B., Liang, P., Yu, X., Su, L., Yu, D., Cheng, Z. *et al.*, Percutaneous sonographically guided microwave coagulation therapy for hepatocellular carcinoma: results in 234 patients. *AJR Am J Roentgenol*, 2003. **180**(6): 1547–55.
44. Liang, P., Dong, B., Yu, X., Yu, D., Wang, Y., Feng, L. *et al.*, Prognostic factors for survival in patients with hepatocellular carcinoma after percutaneous microwave ablation. *Radiology*, 2005. **235**(1): 299–307.
45. Lu, M.D., Chen, J.W., Xie, X.Y., Liu, L., Huang, X.Q., Liang, L.J. *et al.*, Hepatocellular carcinoma: US-guided percutaneous microwave coagulation therapy. *Radiology*, 2001. **221**(1): 167–72.
46. Huang, S., Yu, J., Liang, P., Yu, X., Cheng, Z., Han, Z. *et al.*, Percutaneous microwave ablation for hepatocellular carcinoma adjacent to large vessels: a long-term follow-up. *Eur J Radiol*, 2014. **83**(3): 552–8.
47. Lu, M.D., Xu, H.X., Xie, X.Y., Yin, X.Y., Chen, J.W., Kuang, M. *et al.*, Percutaneous microwave and radiofrequency ablation for hepatocellular carcinoma: a retrospective comparative study. *J Gastroenterol*, 2005. **40**(11): 1054–60.
48. Shibata, T., Iimuro, Y., Yamamoto, Y., Maetani, Y., Ametani, F., Itoh, K. *et al.*, Small hepatocellular carcinoma: comparison of radio-frequency ablation and percutaneous microwave coagulation therapy. *Radiology*, 2002. **223**(2): 331–7.
49. Ding, J., Jing, X., Liu, J., Wang, Y., Wang, F., Wang, Y. *et al.*, Comparison of two different thermal techniques for the treatment of hepatocellular carcinoma. *Eur J Radiol*, 2013. **82**(9): 1379–84.

50. Shibata, T., Niinobu, T., Ogata, N., Takami, M., Microwave coagulation therapy for multiple hepatic metastases from colorectal carcinoma. *Cancer*, 2000. **89**(2): 276–84.
51. Ogata, Y., Uchida, S., Hisaka, T., Horiuchi, H., Mori, S., Ishibashi, N. *et al.*, Intraoperative thermal ablation therapy for small colorectal metastases to the liver. *Hepatogastroenterology*, 2008. **55**(82–83): 550–6.
52. Knavel, E.M., Hinshaw, J.L., Lubner, M.G., Andreano, A., Warner, T.F., Lee, F.T., Jr. *et al.*, High-powered gas-cooled microwave ablation: shaft cooling creates an effective stick function without altering the ablation zone. *AJR Am J Roentgenol*, 2012. **198**(3): W260–5.
53. Erinjeri, J.P., Clark, T.W., Cryoablation: mechanism of action and devices. *J Vasc Interv Radiol*, 2010. **21**(8 Suppl): S187–91.
54. Orlacchio, A., Bazzocchi, G., Pastorelli, D., Bolacchi, F., Angelico, M., Almerighi, C. *et al.*, Percutaneous cryoablation of small hepatocellular carcinoma with US guidance and CT monitoring: initial experience. *Cardiovasc Intervent Radiol*, 2008. **31**(3): 587–94.
55. Morrison, P.R., Silverman, S.G., Tuncali, K., Tatli, S., MRI-guided cryotherapy. *J Magn Reson Imaging*, 2008. **27**(2): 410–20.
56. Shimizu, T., Sakuhara, Y., Abo, D., Hasegawa, Y., Kodama, Y., Endo, H. *et al.*, Outcome of MR-guided percutaneous cryoablation for hepatocellular carcinoma. *J Hepatobiliary Pancreat Surg*, 2009. **16**(6): 816–23.
57. Silverman, S.G., Sun, M.R., Tuncali, K., Morrison, P.R., vanSonnenberg, E., Shankar, S. *et al.*, Three-dimensional assessment of MRI-guided percutaneous cryotherapy of liver metastases. *AJR Am J Roentgenol*, 2004. **183**(3): 707–12.
58. Georgiades, C., Rodriguez, R., Azene, E., Weiss, C., Chaux, A., Gonzalez-Roibon, N. *et al.*, Determination of the nonlethal margin inside the visible "ice-ball" during percutaneous cryoablation of renal tissue. *Cardiovasc Intervent Radiol*, 2013. **36**(3): 783–90.
59. Littrup, P.J., Jallad, B., Vorugu, V., Littrup, G., Currier, B., George, M. *et al.*, Lethal isotherms of cryoablation in a phantom study: effects of heat load, probe size, and number. *J Vasc Interv Radiol*, 2009. **20**(10): 1343–51.
60. Chen, H.W., Lai, E.C., Zhen, Z.J., Cui, W.Z., Liao, S., Lau, W.Y., Ultrasound-guided percutaneous cryotherapy of hepatocellular carcinoma. *Int J Surg*, 2011. **9**(2): 188–91.

61. Sheen, A.J., Siriwardena, A.K. The end of cryotherapy for the treatment of nonresectable hepatic tumors? *Ann Surg Oncol*, 2005. **12**(3): 202–4.
62. Seifert, J.K., Morris, D.L. World survey on the complications of hepatic and prostate cryotherapy. *World J Surg*, 1999. **23**(2): 109–13; discussion 13–4.
63. Weber, S.M., Lee, F.T., Jr., Warner, T.F., Chosy, S.G., Mahvi, D.M., Hepatic cryoablation: US monitoring of extent of necrosis in normal pig liver. *Radiology*, 1998. **207**(1): 73–7.
64. Mala, T., Samset, E., Aurdal, L., Gladhaug, I., Edwin, B., Soreide, O., Magnetic resonance imaging-estimated three-dimensional temperature distribution in liver cryolesions: A study of cryolesion characteristics assumed necessary for tumor ablation. *Cryobiology*, 2001. **43**(3): 268–75.
65. Hong, K., Georgiades, C.S., Geschwind, J.-F.H., Technology insight: Image-guided therapies for hepatocellular carcinoma — intra-arterial and ablative techniques. *Nat Clin Pract Oncol*, 2006. **3**(6): 315–24.
66. Lencioni, R., Crocetti, L., Local-regional treatment of hepatocellular carcinoma. *Radiology*, 2012. **262**(1): 43–58.
67. Lee, E.W., Thai, S., Kee, S.T. Irreversible electroporation: a novel image-guided cancer therapy. *Gut Liver*, 2010. **4** Suppl 1: S99-S104.
68. Narayanan, G., Froud, T., Suthar, R., Barbery, K., Irreversible Electroporation of Hepatic Malignancy. *Semin Intervent Radiol*, 2013. **30**(1): 67–73.
69. Appelbaum, L., Mahgerefteh, S.Y., Sosna, J., Goldberg, S.N., Image-guided fusion and navigation: applications in tumor ablation. *Tech Vasc Interv Radiol*, 2013. **16**(4): 287–95.
70. Mauri, G., Cova, L., De Beni, S., Ierace, T., Tondolo, T., Cerri, A. *et al.*, Real-time US-CT/MRI image fusion for guidance of thermal ablation of liver tumors undetectable with US: results in 295 cases. *Cardiovasc Intervent Radiol*, 2014.
71. Breedis, C., Young, G., The blood supply of neoplasms in the liver. *Am J Pathol*, 1954. **30**(5): 969–77.
72. Liu, D.M., Salem, R., Bui, J.T., Courtney, A., Barakat, O., Sergie, Z. *et al.*, Angiographic considerations in patients undergoing liver-directed therapy. *J Vasc Interv Radiol*, 2005. **16**(7): 911–35.
73. Lewandowski, R.J., Sato, K.T., Atassi B, Ryu, R.K., Nemcek, A.A., Jr., Kulik, L. *et al.*, Radioembolization with (90)y microspheres: angiographic

and technical considerations. *Cardiovasc Intervent Radiol*, 2007. **30**(4): 571–92.

74. Salem, R., Lewandowski, R.J., Sato, K.T., Atassi, B., Ryu, R.K., Ibrahim, S. *et al.*, Technical aspects of radioembolization with 90Y microspheres. *Tech Vasc Interv Radiol*, 2007. **10**(1): 12–29.
75. Salem, R., Lewandowski, R.J., Kulik, L., Wang, E., Riaz, A., Ryu, R.K. *et al.*, Radioembolization results in longer time-to-progression and reduced toxicity compared with chemoembolization in patients with hepatocellular carcinoma. *Gastroenterology*, 2011. **140**(2): 497–507 e2.
76. Salem, R., Lewandowski, R.J., Mulcahy, M.F., Riaz, A., Ryu, R.K., Ibrahim, S. *et al.*, Radioembolization for hepatocellular carcinoma using Yttrium-90 microspheres: a comprehensive report of long-term outcomes. *Gastroenterology*, 2010. **138**(1): 52–64.
77. Lewandowski, R.J., Mulcahy, M.F., Kulik, L.M., Riaz, A., Ryu, R.K., Baker, T.B. *et al.*, Chemoembolization for hepatocellular carcinoma: comprehensive imaging and survival analysis in a 172-patient cohort. *Radiology*, 2010. **255**(3): 955–65.
78. Llovet, J.M., Real, M.I., Montana, X., Planas, R., Coll, S., Aponte, J. *et al.*, Arterial embolisation or chemoembolisation versus symptomatic treatment in patients with unresectable hepatocellular carcinoma: a randomised controlled trial. *Lancet*, 2002. **359**(9319): 1734–9.
79. Memon, K., Kulik, L., Lewandowski, R.J., Wang, E., Riaz, A., Ryu, R.K. *et al.*, Radiographic response to locoregional therapy in hepatocellular carcinoma predicts patient survival times. *Gastroenterology*, 2011. **141**(2): 526–35.e2.
80. Kan, Z., McCuskey, P.A., Wright, K.C., Wallace, S., Role of Kupffer cells in iodized oil embolization. *Invest Radiol*, 1994. **29**(11): 990–3.
81. Ohishi, H., Uchida, H., Yoshimura, H., Ohue, S., Ueda, J., Katsuragi, M. *et al.*, Hepatocellular carcinoma detected by iodized oil. Use of anticancer agents. *Radiology*, 1985. **154**(1): 25–9.
82. Kan, Z., Sato, M., Ivancev, K., Uchida, B., Hedgpeth, P., Lunderquist, A. *et al.*, Distribution and effect of iodized poppyseed oil in the liver after hepatic artery embolization: experimental study in several animal species. *Radiology*, 1993. **186**(3): 861–6.
83. Okayasu, I., Hatakeyama, S., Yoshida, T., Yoshimatsu, S., Tsuruta, K., Miyamoto, H. *et al.*, Selective and persistent deposition and gradual drainage

of iodized oil, Lipiodol in the hepatocellular carcinoma after injection into the feeding hepatic artery. *Am J Clin Pathol*, 1988. **90**(5): 536–44.

84. Brown, D.B., Cardella, J.F., Sacks, D., Goldberg, S.N., Gervais, D.A., Rajan, D. *et al.*, Quality improvement guidelines for transhepatic arterial chemoembolization, embolization, and chemotherapeutic infusion for hepatic malignancy. *J Vasc Interv Radiol*, 2006. **17**(2 Pt 1): 225–32.
85. Xia, J., Ren, Z., Ye, S., Sharma, D., Lin, Z., Gan, Y. *et al.*, Study of severe and rare complications of transarterial chemoembolization (TACE) for liver cancer. *Eur J Radiol*, 2006. **59**(3): 407–12.
86. Kim, H.K., Chung, Y.H., Song, B.C., Yang, S.H., Yoon, H.K., Yu, E. *et al.*, Ischemic bile duct injury as a serious complication after transarterial chemoembolization in patients with hepatocellular carcinoma. *J Clin Gastroenterol*, 2001. **32**(5): 423–7.
87. Belli, L., Magistretti, G., Puricelli, G.P., Damiani, G., Colombo, E., Cornalba, G.P., Arteritis following intra-arterial chemotherapy for liver tumors. *Eur Radiol*, 1997. **7**(3): 323–6.
88. Malagari, K., Pomoni, M., Spyridopoulos, T., Moschouris, H., Kelekis, A., Dourakis, S. *et al.*, Safety profile of sequential transcatheter chemoembolization with DC bead: results of 237 hepatocellular carcinoma (HCC) patients. *Cardiovas Inter Radiol*, 2011. **34**(4): 774–85.
89. Vogl, T.J., Lammer, J., Lencioni, R., Malagari, K., Watkinson, A., Pilleul, F. *et al.*, Liver, gastrointestinal, and cardiac toxicity in intermediate hepatocellular carcinoma treated with PRECISION TACE with drug-eluting beads: results from the PRECISION V randomized trial. *AJR Am J Roentgenol*, 2011. **197**(4): W562–70.
90. de Baere, T., Deschamps, F., Teriitheau, C., Rao, P., Conengrapht, K., Schlumberger, M. *et al.*, Transarterial chemoembolization of liver metastases from well differentiated gastroenteropancreatic endocrine tumors with doxorubicin-eluting beads: preliminary results. *J Vasc Interv Radiol*, 2008. **19**(6): 855–61.
91. Gaur, S.K., Friese, J.L., Sadow, C.A., Ayyagari, R., Binkert, C.A., Schenker, M.P. *et al.*, Hepatic arterial chemoembolization using drug-eluting beads in gastrointestinal neuroendocrine tumor metastatic to the liver. *Cardiovasc Intervent Radiol*, 2011. **34**(3): 566–72.
92. Bhagat, N., Reyes, D.K., Lin, M., Kamel, I., Pawlik, T.M., Frangakis, C. *et al.*, Phase II study of chemoembolization with drug-eluting beads in

patients with hepatic neuroendocrine metastases: high incidence of biliary injury. *Cardiovasc Intervent Radiol*, 2013. **36**(2): 449–59.
93. Riaz, A., Lewandowski, R.J., Kulik, L.M., Mulcahy, M.F., Sato, K.T., Ryu, R.K. *et al.*, Complications following radioembolization with yttrium-90 microspheres: a comprehensive literature review. *J Vasc Interv Radiol*, 2009. **20**(9): 1121–30; quiz 31.
94. Gil-Alzugaray, B., Chopitea, A., Inarrairaegui, M., Bilbao, J.I., Rodriguez-Fraile, M., Rodriguez, J. *et al.*, Prognostic factors and prevention of radioembolization-induced liver disease. *Hepatology*, 2012.
95. Brown, D.B., Gould, J.E., Gervais, D.A., Goldberg, S.N., Murthy, R., Millward, S.F. *et al.*, Transcatheter therapy for hepatic malignancy: standardization of terminology and reporting criteria. *J Vasc Interv Radiol*, 2009. **20**(7 Suppl): S425–34.
96. Ensminger, W. Hepatic arterial chemotherapy for primary and metastatic liver cancers. *Cancer Chemother Pharmacol*, 1989. **23** Suppl: S68–73.
97. Eksborg, S., Cedermark, B.J., Strandler, H.S., Intrahepatic and intravenous administration of adriamycin — a comparative pharmacokinetic study in patients with malignant liver tumours. *Med Oncol Tumor Pharmacother*, 1985. **2**(1): 47–54.
98. Solomon, B., Soulen, M.C., Baum, R.A., Haskal, Z.J., Shlansky-Goldberg, R.D., Cope C., Chemoembolization of hepatocellular carcinoma with cisplatin, doxorubicin, mitomycin-C, ethiodol, and polyvinyl alcohol: prospective evaluation of response and survival in a U.S. population. *J Vasc Interv Radiol*, 1999. **10**(6): 793–8.
99. Marelli, L., Stigliano, R., Triantos, C., Senzolo, M., Cholongitas, E., Davies, N. *et al.*, Transarterial therapy for hepatocellular carcinoma: which technique is more effective? A systematic review of cohort and randomized studies. *Cardiovas Interv Radiol*, 2007. **30**(1): 6–25.
100. Brown, D.B., Nikolic, B., Covey, A.M., Nutting, C.W., Saad, W.E., Salem, R. *et al.*, Quality improvement guidelines for transhepatic arterial chemoembolization, embolization, and chemotherapeutic infusion for hepatic malignancy. *J Vasc Interv Radiol*, 2012. **23**(3): 287–94.
101. Coldwell, D.M., Stokes, K.R., Yakes, W.F., Embolotherapy: agents, clinical applications, and techniques. *Radiographics*, 1994. **14**(3): 623–43; quiz 45–6.
102. Georgiades, C., Geschwind, J.F., Harrison, N., Hines-Peralta, A., Liapi, E., Hong, K. *et al.*, Lack of response after initial chemoembolization for

hepatocellular carcinoma: does it predict failure of subsequent treatment? *Radiology*, 2012. **265**(1): 115–23.

103. Lo, C.-M., Ngan, H., Tso, W.-K., Liu, C.-L., Lam, C.-M., Poon, R.T.-P. *et al.*, Randomized controlled trial of transarterial lipiodol chemoembolization for unresectable hepatocellular carcinoma. *Hepatology*, 2002. **35**(5): 1164–71.
104. Takayasu, K., Arii, S., Ikai, I., Omata, M., Okita, K., Ichida, T. *et al.*, Prospective cohort study of transarterial chemoembolization for unresectable hepatocellular carcinoma in 8510 patients. *Gastroenterology*, 2006. **131**(2): 461–9.
105. Takayasu, K., Arii, S., Kudo, M., Ichida, T., Matsui, O., Izumi, N. *et al.*, Superselective transarterial chemoembolization for hepatocellular carcinoma. Validation of treatment algorithm proposed by Japanese guidelines. *J Hepatol*, 2012. **56**(4): 886–92.
106. Llovet, J.M., Bruix J., Systematic review of randomized trials for unresectable hepatocellular carcinoma: Chemoembolization improves survival. *Hepatology*, 2003. **37**(2): 429–42.
107. Albert, M., Kiefer, M.V., Sun, W., Haller, D., Fraker, D.L., Tuite, C.M. *et al.*, Chemoembolization of colorectal liver metastases with cisplatin, doxorubicin, mitomycin C, ethiodol, and polyvinyl alcohol. *Cancer*, 2011. **117**(2): 343–52.
108. Vogl, T.J., Gruber, T., Balzer, J.O., Eichler, K., Hammerstingl, R., Zangos S., Repeated transarterial chemoembolization in the treatment of liver metastases of colorectal cancer: prospective study. *Radiology*, 2009. **250**(1): 281–9.
109. Tellez, C., Benson, A.B., 3rd, Lyster, M.T., Talamonti, M., Shaw, J., Braun, M.A. *et al.*, Phase II trial of chemoembolization for the treatment of metastatic colorectal carcinoma to the liver and review of the literature. *Cancer*, 1998. **82**(7): 1250–9.
110. Geschwind, J., Hong, K., Georgiades C., Utility of transcatheter arterial chemoembolization for liver dominant colorectal metastatic adenocarcinoma in the salvage setting. American Society of Clinical Oncology Gastrointestinal Cancers Symposium; January 26–28; San Francisco, CAJanuary 26–28, 2006.
111. Lencioni, R., Crocetti, L., Petruzzi, P., Vignali, C., Bozzi, E., Della Pina, C. *et al.*, Doxorubicin-eluting bead-enhanced radiofrequency ablation of

hepatocellular carcinoma: a pilot clinical study. *J Hepatol*, 2008. **49**(2): 217–22.

112. Liu, D.M., Kos, S., Buczkowski, A., Kee, S., Munk, P.L., Klass, D. *et al.*, Optimization of doxorubicin loading for superabsorbent polymer microspheres: *in vitro* analysis. *Cardiovas Interv Radiol*, 2012. **35**(2): 391–8.
113. Namur, J., Citron, S.J., Sellers, M.T., Dupuis, M.H., Wassef, M., Manfait, M. *et al.*, Embolization of hepatocellular carcinoma with drug-eluting beads: doxorubicin tissue concentration and distribution in patient liver explants. *J Hepatol*, 2011. **55**(6): 1332–8.
114. Lencioni, R., de Baere, T., Burrel, M., Caridi, J.G., Lammer, J., Malagari, K. *et al.*, Transcatheter treatment of hepatocellular carcinoma with Doxorubicin-loaded DC Bead (DEBDOX): technical recommendations. *Cardiovasc Intervent Radiol*, 2012. **35**(5): 980–5.
115. Constantin, M., Fundueanu, G., Bortolotti, F., Cortesi, R., Ascenzi, P., Menegatti E., Preparation and characterisation of poly(vinyl alcohol)/cyclodextrin microspheres as matrix for inclusion and separation of drugs. *Internat J Pharmaceutics*, 2004. **285**(1–2): 87–96.
116. Gonzalez, M.V., Tang, Y., Phillips, G.J., Lloyd, A.W., Hall, B., Stratford, P.W. *et al.*, Doxorubicin eluting beads-2: methods for evaluating drug elution and *in-vitro*: *in-vivo* correlation. *J Mater Sci Mater Med*, 2008. **19**(2): 767–75.
117. Lammer, J., Malagari, K., Vogl, T., Pilleul, F., Denys, A., Watkinson, A. *et al.*, Prospective randomized study of doxorubicin-eluting-bead embolization in the treatment of hepatocellular carcinoma: results of the PRECISION V study. *Cardiovas Interv Radiol*, 2010. **33**(1): 41–52.
118. Dhanasekaran, R.M., Comparison of conventional transarterial chemoembolization (TACE) and chemoembolization with doxorubicin drug eluting beads (DEB) for unresectable hepatocelluar carcinoma (HCC). *J Surg Oncol*, 2010. **101**(6): 476–80.
119. Kalva, S.P., Pectasides, M., Yeddula, K., Ganguli, S., Blaszkowsky, L.S., Zhu, A.X., Factors affecting survival following chemoembolization with doxorubicin-eluting microspheres for inoperable hepatocellular carcinoma. *J Vasc Interv Radiol*, 2013. **24**(2): 257–65.
120. Prajapati, H.J., Dhanasekaran, R., El-Rayes, B.F., Kauh, J.S., Maithel, S.K., Chen, Z. *et al.*, Safety and efficacy of doxorubicin drug-eluting bead

transarterial chemoembolization in patients with advanced hepatocellular carcinoma. *J Vasc Interv Radiol*, 2013. **24**(3): 307–15.

121. Kalva, S.P., Pectasides, M., Liu, R., Rachamreddy, N., Surakanti, S., Yeddula, K. *et al.*, Safety and effectiveness of chemoembolization with drug-eluting beads for advanced-stage hepatocellular carcinoma. *Cardiovasc Intervent Radiol*, 2014. **37**(2): 381–7.
122. Burrel, M., Reig, M., Forner, A., Barrufet, M., de Lope, C.R., Tremosini, S. *et al.*, Survival of patients with hepatocellular carcinoma treated by transarterial chemoembolisation (TACE) using Drug Eluting Beads. Implications for clinical practice and trial design. *J Hepatol*, 2012. **56**(6): 1330–5.
123. Malagari, K., Pomoni, M., Kelekis, A., Pomoni, A., Dourakis, S., Spyridopoulos, T. *et al.*, Prospective randomized comparison of chemoembolization with doxorubicin-eluting beads and bland embolization with BeadBlock for hepatocellular carcinoma. *Cardiovas Interv Radiol*, 2010. **33**(3): 541–51.
124. Malagari, K., Pomoni, M., Moschouris, H., Bouma, E., Koskinas, J., Stefaniotou, A. *et al.*, Chemoembolization with Doxorubicin-eluting beads for unresectable hepatocellular carcinoma: five-year survival analysis. *Cardiovas Interv Radiol*, 2012. **35**(5): 1119–28.
125. Jordan, O., Denys, A., De Baere, T., Boulens, N., Doelker E., Comparative study of chemoembolization loadable beads: *in vitro* drug release and physical properties of DC bead and hepasphere loaded with doxorubicin and irinotecan. *J Vasc Interv Radiol*, 2010. **21**(7): 1084–90.
126. Martin, R.C., Joshi, J., Robbins, K., Tomalty, D., Bosnjakovik, P., Derner, M. *et al.*, Hepatic intra-arterial injection of drug-eluting bead, irinotecan (DEBIRI) in unresectable colorectal liver metastases refractory to systemic chemotherapy: results of multi-institutional study. *Ann Surg Oncol*, 2011. **18**(1): 192–8.
127. Bower, M., Metzger, T., Robbins, K., Tomalty, D., Valek, V., Boudny, J. *et al.*, Surgical downstaging and neo-adjuvant therapy in metastatic colorectal carcinoma with irinotecan drug-eluting beads: a multi-institutional study. *HPB (Oxford)*, 2010. **12**(1): 31–6.
128. Fiorentini, G., Aliberti, C., Tilli, M., Mulazzani, L., Graziano, F., Giordani, P. *et al.*, Intra-arterial infusion of irinotecan-loaded drug-eluting beads (DEBIRI) versus intravenous therapy (FOLFIRI) for hepatic metastases

from colorectal cancer: final results of a phase III study. *Anticancer Res*, 2012. **32**(4): 1387–95.

129. Riaz, A., Gates, V.L., Atassi, B., Lewandowski, R.J., Mulcahy, M.F., Ryu, R.K. *et al.*, Radiation segmentectomy: a novel approach to increase safety and efficacy of radioembolization. *Int J Radiat Oncol Biol Phys*, 2011. **79**(1): 163–71.
130. Ingold, J.A., Reed, G.B., Kaplan, H.S., Bagshaw, M.A. Radiation Hepatitis. *Am J Roentgenol Radium Ther Nucl Med*, 1965. **93**: 200–8.
131. Geschwind, J.F., Salem, R., Carr, B.I., Soulen, M.C., Thurston, K.G., Goin, K.A. *et al.*, Yttrium-90 microspheres for the treatment of hepatocellular carcinoma. *Gastroenterology*, 2004. **127**(5 Suppl 1): S194–205.
132. Hilgard, P., Hamami, M., Fouly, A.E., Scherag, A., Muller, S., Ertle, J. *et al.*, Radioembolization with yttrium-90 glass microspheres in hepatocellular carcinoma: European experience on safety and long-term survival. *Hepatology*, 2010. **52**(5): 1741–9.
133. Sangro, B., Carpanese, L., Cianni, R., Golfieri, R., Gasparini, D., Ezziddin, S. *et al.*, Survival after yttrium-90 resin microsphere radioembolization of hepatocellular carcinoma across Barcelona clinic liver cancer stages: A European evaluation. *Hepatology*, 2011. **54**(3): 868–78.
134. Mazzaferro, V., Sposito, C., Bhoori, S., Romito, R., Chiesa, C., Morosi, C. *et al.*, Yttrium-90 radioembolization for intermediate-advanced hepatocellular carcinoma: a phase 2 study. *Hepatology*, 2013. **57**(5): 1826–37.
135. Lewandowski, R.J., Kulik, L.M., Riaz, A., Senthilnathan, S., Mulcahy, M.F., Ryu, R.K. *et al.*, A comparative analysis of transarterial downstaging for hepatocellular carcinoma: chemoembolization versus radioembolization. *Am J Transplant*, 2009. **9**(8): 1920–8.
136. Salem, R., Gilbertsen, M., Butt, Z., Memon, K., Vouche, M., Hickey, R. *et al.*, Increased quality of life among hepatocellular carcinoma patients treated with radioembolization, compared with chemoembolization. *Clin Gastroenterol Hepatol*, 2013. **11**(10): 1358–65 e1.
137. Vouche, M., Habib, A., Ward, T.J., Kim, E., Kulik, L., Ganger, D. *et al.*, Unresectable solitary HCC not amenable to RFA: Multicenter radiology-pathology correlation and survival of radiation segmentectomy. *Hepatology*, 2014.
138. Vouche, M., Lewandowski, R.J., Atassi, R., Memon, K., Gates, V.L., Ryu, R.K. *et al.*, Radiation lobectomy: time-dependent analysis of future liver

remnant volume in unresectable liver cancer as a bridge to resection. *J Hepatol*, 2013. **59**(5): 1029–36.

139. Mulcahy, M.F., Lewandowski, R.J., Ibrahim, S.M., Sato, K.T., Ryu, R.K., Atassi, B. *et al.*, Radioembolization of colorectal hepatic metastases using yttrium-90 microspheres. *Cancer*, 2009. **115**(9): 1849–58.
140. Kennedy, A.S., Coldwell, D., Nutting, C., Murthy, R., Wertman, D.E., Jr., Loehr, S.P. *et al.*, Resin (90)Y-microsphere brachytherapy for unresectable colorectal liver metastases: Modern USA experience. *Int J Radiat Oncol Biol Phys*, 2006. **65**(2): 412–25.
141. Jakobs, T.F., Hoffmann, R.T., Dehm, K., Trumm, C., Stemmler, H.J., Tatsch, K. *et al.*, Hepatic yttrium-90 radioembolization of chemotherapy-refractory colorectal cancer liver metastases. *J Vasc Interv Radiol*, 2008. **19**(8): 1187–95.
142. Abi-Jaoudeh, N., Kobeiter, H., Xu, S., Wood, B.J. Image fusion during vascular and nonvascular image-guided procedures. *Tech Vasc Interv Radiol*, 2013. **16**(3): 168–76.
143. Rhee, T.K., Omary, R.A., Gates, V., Mounajjed, T., Larson, A.C., Barakat, O. *et al.*, The effect of catheter-directed CT angiography on yttrium-90 radioembolization treatment of hepatocellular carcinoma. *J Vasc Interv Radiol*, 2005. **16**(8): 1085–91.
144. Virmani, S., Ryu, R.K., Sato, K.T., Lewandowski, R.J., Kulik, L., Mulcahy, M.F. *et al.*, Effect of C-arm angiographic CT on transcatheter arterial chemoembolization of liver tumors. *J Vasc Interv Radiol*, 2007. **18**(10): 1305–9.
145. Meyer, B.C., Frericks, B.B., Albrecht, T., Wolf, K.J., Wacker, F.K., Contrast-enhanced abdominal angiographic CT for intra-abdominal tumor embolization: a new tool for vessel and soft tissue visualization. *Cardiovasc Interv Radiol*, 2007. **30**(4): 743–9.
146. Wallace, M.J., Murthy, R., Kamat, P.P., Moore, T., Rao, S.H., Ensor, J. *et al.*, Impact of C-arm CT on hepatic arterial interventions for hepatic malignancies. *J Vasc Interv Radiol*, 2007. **18**(12): 1500–7.
147. Wilson, M.W., Kerlan, R.K., Jr., Fidelman, N.A., Venook, A.P., LaBerge, J.M., Koda, J. *et al.*, Hepatocellular carcinoma: regional therapy with a magnetic targeted carrier bound to doxorubicin in a dual MR imaging/conventional angiography suite — initial experience with four patients. *Radiology*, 2004. **230**(1): 287–93.

148. Vogl, T.J., Balzer, J.O., Mack, M.G., Bett, G., Oppelt, A., Hybrid, M.R., interventional imaging system: combined MR and angiography suites with single interactive table. Feasibility study in vascular liver tumor procedures. *Eur Radiol*, 2002. **12**(6): 1394–400.
149. Gray, B., Van Hazel, G., Hope, M., Burton, M., Moroz, P., Anderson, J. *et al.*, Randomised trial of SIR-Spheres plus chemotherapy vs. chemotherapy alone for treating patients with liver metastases from primary large bowel cancer. *Ann Oncol*, 2001. **12**(12): 1711–20.
150. Van Hazel, G., Blackwell, A., Anderson, J., Price, D., Moroz, P., Bower, G. *et al.*, Randomised phase 2 trial of SIR-Spheres plus fluorouracil/leucovorin chemotherapy versus fluorouracil/leucovorin chemotherapy alone in advanced colorectal cancer. *J Surg Oncol*, 2004. **88**(2): 78–85.
151. Hendlisz, A., Van den Eynde, M., Peeters, M., Maleux, G., Lambert, B., Vannoote, J. *et al.*, Phase III trial comparing protracted intravenous fluorouracil infusion alone or with yttrium-90 resin microspheres radioembolization for liver-limited metastatic colorectal cancer refractory to standard chemotherapy. *J Clin Oncol*, 2010. **28**(23): 3687–94.
152. Hickey, R., Mulcahy, M.F., Lewandowski, R.J., Gates, V.L., Vouche, M., Habib, A. *et al.*, Chemoradiation of hepatic malignancies: prospective, phase 1 study of full-dose capecitabine with escalating doses of yttrium-90 radioembolization. *Int J Radiat Oncol Biol Phys*, 2014. **88**(5): 1025–31.
153. Sergio, A., Cristofori, C., Cardin, R., Pivetta, G., Ragazzi, R., Baldan, A. *et al.*, Transcatheter arterial chemoembolization (TACE) in hepatocellular carcinoma (HCC): the role of angiogenesis and invasiveness. *Am J Gastroenterol*, 2008. **103**(4): 914–21.
154. Llovet, J.M., Ricci, S., Mazzaferro, V., Hilgard, P., Gane, E., Blanc J.-F. *et al.*, Sorafenib in advanced hepatocellular carcinoma. *N Engl J Med*, 2008. **359**(4): 378–90.
155. Buijs, M., Reyes, D.K., Pawlik, T.M., Blackford, A.L., Salem, R., Messersmith, W.A. *et al.*, Phase 2 trial of concurrent bevacizumab and transhepatic arterial chemoembolization in patients with unresectable hepatocellular carcinoma. *Cancer*, 2013. **119**(5): 1042–9.
156. Hu, H., Duan, Z., Long, X., Hertzanu, Y., Shi, H., Liu, S. *et al.*, Sorafenib combined with transarterial chemoembolization versus transarterial chemoembolization alone for advanced-stage hepatocellular carcinoma: a propensity score matching study. *PLoS ONE*, 2014. **9**(5): e96620.

157. Chow, P.K., Poon, D.Y., Khin, M.W., Singh, H., Han, H.S., Goh, A.S. *et al.*, Multicenter phase II study of sequential radioembolization-sorafenib therapy for inoperable hepatocellular carcinoma. *PLoS ONE*, 2014. **9**(3): e90909.
158. Kulik, L., Vouche, M., Koppe, S., Lewandowski, R.J., Mulcahy, M.F., Ganger, D. *et al.*, Prospective randomized pilot study of Y90 +/- sorafenib as bridge to transplantation in hepatocellular carcinoma. *J Hepatol*, 2014.
159. EASL-EORTC clinical practice guidelines: management of hepatocellular carcinoma. *J Hepatol*, 2012. **56**(4): 908–43.

Chapter 21

Rare Gastrointestinal Malignancies

Walid Shaib, Daniel Goldstein, Vinicus Ernani,
Maria C. Russell and Kenneth Cardona

What is New

- Rare gastrointestinal malignancies include small bowel tumors, neuroendocrine tumors, and also gastrointestinal stromal tumors.

Small Bowel Tumors

Malignant small bowel tumors (SBT) are diseases with variations in histology, clinical presentation, and outcome. These tumors account for approximately 2% of all gastrointestinal (GI) tumors. The Surveillance, Epidemiology, and End Results (SEER) registry has shown an increase in the incidence of SBT over the past three decades.[1] The estimated number of new SBT cases per year in the United States is approximately 8,000 cases. The histologic distribution of SBT includes carcinoid (44%), adenocarcinoma (33%), lymphoma (15%), and sarcoma (8%),[2,3] with a surge in the incidence of small bowel carcinoid tumors in the last decade and a decrease in adenocarcinomas. This marks a notable change in the incidence of SBT where a decade ago the majority of SBT were adenocarcinomas.[3] Although these malignancies may originate in different regions of the small intestine, certain subtypes have a predilection to specific regions: adenocarcinoma commonly affects the duodenum, carcinoids are mostly found in the ileum, and sarcomas and lymphomas can develop throughout the entire small bowel.[4]

Small bowel adenocarcinoma

Epidemiology

Adenocarcinoma of the small bowel tends to occur in older people with a median age at diagnosis of 65. These malignancies are more commonly seen in males and have an equal distribution between Caucasians and African-Americans.[3,5] The distribution of adenocarcinomas affecting the small bowel also varies with location with most of the tumors occurring in the duodenum (65%), followed by the jejunum (16%) and ileum (14%).

Pathogenesis

Although the small intestine constitutes the majority (75%) of intestinal content in the abdominal cavity, the incidence of small bowel adenocarcinoma is 40–60-fold less than that of colon adenocarcinoma. This difference could be attributed to several small bowel factors, such as: (1) high levels of the hydrocarbon, benzopyrene, which metabolizes carcinogens found in cigarettes, smoked and canned foods; (2) high folate receptors; (3) low bacterial loads (bacteria can interact with bile acids and act as a tumor promoter); (4) fast transit time of food leading to less exposure to carcinogens; (5) high cellular turnover; (6) alkaline milieu making carcinogens less active; (7) few stem cells; and (8) the abundance of Peyer's patches as immune protectors, with high levels of IgA in the mucosa.[6]

The pathology of small bowel adenocarcinoma is not well-defined. It is thought to be due to progression from an adenoma to carcinoma. The pathway of this evolution is thought to involve cyclooxygenase (COX) and APC mutations;[7] as well as mutations in the RAS, SMAD4 and p53 pathways.[8–11]

In addition, several genetic and autoimmune factors have been observed to be associated with small bowel adenocarcinoma. Familial adenomatous polyposis (FAP) has the APC tumor suppressor gene germline mutation. FAP primarily affects the colon but can also affect the small intestines, specifically the duodenum.[7] In human non-polyposis colorectal cancer (HNPCC) syndrome, the mutation in the DNA mismatch repair genes leads to the development of tumors in the duodenum and jejunum in 1–4% of HNPCC patients.[12] Peutz-Jeghers syndrome is a disorder caused by a mutation in the tumor suppressor gene STK11 (LKB1) leading to hamartomatous polyps in the small intestines. Patients with this syndrome are at a 15-fold increased risk of developing adenocarcinoma compared to the general population.[11] Cystic fibrosis patients are at increased risk of ileal adenocarcinoma development. Patients with Crohn's disease are at increased risk of developing small bowel adenocarcinoma with 2% of these patients developing adenocarcinoma, mainly in the ileum.

Clinical presentation and diagnosis

Most patients present with non-specific abdominal symptoms, such as nausea, vomiting, abdominal discomfort, GI bleeding and/or weight loss. However, a proportion of patients can present acutely with small bowel obstruction or perforation.

At presentation, adenocarcinomas are usually found at an advanced stage due to an average delay in diagnosis of 8–12 months secondary to the lack of early and specific symptoms. Enhanced computed tomography (CT) is the most frequent imaging modality used to assess small bowel adenocarcinoma at initial presentation. Small bowel adenocarcinomas usually have a distinct annular thickening with discrete and irregular overhanging edges. More specifically, duodenal adenocarcinomas may be seen as polypoid lesions where distal small bowel adenocarcinomas might present as an intussusception and thus have a "target sign," consisting of peripheral enhancement and central low attenuation, on cross sectional imaging. Magnetic resonance imaging (MRI) can have a higher sensitivity and specificity for certain small bowel tumors.[13] Specifically, duodenal tumors can be well-characterized on enhanced-T1 as well as T2-weighted series on MRI scans allowing for detailed characterization of the tumor in relation to essential adjacent structures (mesenteric blood vessels, pancreas, bile duct, and ampulla). Additionally, CT enteroclysis (CTE) and

MR enteroclysis (MRE) are widely used in the examination and diagnosis of small intestinal tumors. In regards to small bowel adenocarcinoma, these studies can provide superior small bowel distention and thus better visualization of tumors. They can reveal the location and appearance of the tumor, assess the degree of mesenteric infiltration, and evaluate for distant tumor metastasis.[14]

Flouroscopy with small bowel follow through (SBFT) technique is able to define abnormalities in the small intestine mucosa but requires high suspicion for SBT and takes a considerable length of time to be performed. This technique has largely been replaced by CTE and MRE as well as advanced endoscopic techniques, such as double-balloon enteroscopy (push enteroscopy) or video capsule endoscopy. Push enteroscopy allows for endoscopic examination of the vast majority of the proximal small bowel with biopsy capabilities of any suspicious mucosal lesions. Video capsule endoscopy has a higher sensitivity and specificity than fluoroscopy with SBFT technique with more precise localization and a missed lesion rate on capsule endoscopy of approximately 10%. The major risk of capsule endoscopy is the retention of the capsule in 1% of the cases.[15–17]

Staging and prognosis

Table 1 summarizes the American Joint Committee on Cancer (AJCC) 7th edition TNM staging for small bowel adenocarcinoma. Most patients with small bowel adenocarcinoma present at a late stage, such that: 32% are stage IV, 27% are stage III, 30% are stage II, and only 10% are stage I at the time of diagnosis. The median overall survival (OS) is reported to range from 20 to 23 months with a five-year disease-free survival (DFS) of 25–30% with worse outcomes for duodenal adenocarcinoma (28% five-year cancer-specific survival) as compared to ileal and jejunal adenocarcinomas (38% five-year cancer-specific survival).[3,5] Furthermore, survival decreases by stage with patients having a: 65% five-year survival for stage I, 48% for stage II, 35% for stage III, and 4% five-year survival for stage IV.[18] When compared to colon cancer, small bowel adenocarcinoma demonstrated worse cancer-specific survival when adjusted by stage of disease.[5] Poor prognostic factors for small bowel adenocarcinoma include advanced

Table 1. Staging of small bowel adenocarcinoma.
American Joint Committee on Cancer (AJCC), Chicago, Illinois. The original source for this material is the AJCC Cancer Staging Manual, Seventh Edition (2010) published by Springer New York, Inc.

T Stage	Description
Tx	Tx Primary tumor cannot be assessed
Tis	Carcinoma in situ
T1a	Tumor invades lamina propria
T1b	Tumor invades submucosa
T2	Tumor invades muscularis propria
T3	Tumor invades through the muscularis propria into the subserosa or into the nonperitonealized perimuscular tissue (mesentery or retroperitoneum) with extension 2 cm or less
T4	Tumor perforates the visceral peritoneum or directly invades other organs or structures (includes other loops of small intestine, mesentery, or retroperitoneum more than 2 cm, and abdominal wall by way of serosa; for the duodenum only, invasion of pancreas or bile duct)
N stage	
NX	Regional lymph nodes cannot be assessed
N0	No regional lymph node metastasis
N1	Metastasis in 1–3 regional lymph nodes
N2	Metastasis in four or more regional lymph nodes
M stage	
M0	No distant metastasis
M1	Distant metastasis

age, African American ethnicity, duodenal tumors, poorly-differentiated tumors, T4 lesions, positive margins, and lymph node involvement.[19] In a SEER analysis, increased nodal sampling demonstrated a marked improvement in outcomes.[20] For cases in which eight or more lymph nodes were sampled, the improvement in five-year cancer-specific survival increased from 65.3% to 80.3% for stage I, 55% to 69.9% for stage II, and 40% to 45.1% for stage III disease.[20] Tumor stage, extent of nodal disease and poorly differentiated histology are independent prognostic factors.[21–23]

Management

Surgery is the mainstay of therapy for patients with locoregional disease and should be performed when technically possible in medically fit patients. The type of surgical resection for duodenal adenocarcinoma will depend on the location of the tumor and may include a segmental resection with 5 cm margin or a pancreaticoduodenectomy with adequate regional lymphadenectomy. Various retrospective studies indicated that pancreaticoduodenectomy was superior to wide segmental resection for tumors that involved the first and second portions of the duodenum.[23,24] However, a series from the Mayo Clinic involving 101 patients where surgery was curative in 68 patients treated with either pancreaticoduodenectomy or segmental resection showed no five-year survival difference between either surgical approaches. The conclusion was that aggressive surgical approach that achieves complete tumor resection with negative margins should be the goal of treatment.

Due to the rarity of this disease, there is a lack of phase III prospective randomized trials evaluating the role of palliative chemotherapy in small bowel adenocarcinoma for advanced stage disease or evaluating the role of adjuvant therapy in resected small bowel adenocarcinomas.

In the advanced setting, many retrospective trials have reported that chemotherapy improves OS (range of 10.7 to 18.6 months) as compared to best supportive care (range of 2 to 13 months) with response rates (RR) to chemotherapy ranging from 5% to as high as 48%.[18,25–28] A retrospective analysis of 80 patients with metastatic small bowel adenocarcinoma compared platinum/5-FU combination to 5-FU alone or 5-FU combined to non-platinum agents. This study reported no OS difference but there was a progression-free survival (PFS) difference of 5 months and a RR difference of 30% for the platinum/5-FU combination chemotherapy group.[29] Irinotecan-based treatment was also studied retrospectively in the second-line setting and showed a RR of 20%.[30] The limitations of these studies are their retrospective nature and thus inherent selection bias and variability in chemotherapy regimens used across the various studies. Nonetheless, two-phase II trials reported a benefit from chemotherapy as palliative treatment for metastatic small bowel adenocarcinoma. One was a multicenter Eastern Cooperative Oncology Group (ECOG) trial utilizing

5-FU, doxorubicin and mitomycin C (FAM regimen) for ampullary and small bowel cancers. This trial enrolled 36 patients. Grade 3 and 4 toxicities were experienced in more than 50% of the patients. The response rate (RR) was 18.4% with a median OS of 8 months.[31] The other phase II trial was conducted by the MD Anderson group in patients with ampullary and small bowel adenocarcinoma. A median OS of 24.4 months with capecitabine in combination with oxaliplatin (CAPOX) was achieved for the entire study group; however a median OS of 15.5 months was achieved in the small bowel adenocarcinoma subgroup. The overall RR seen with CAPOX in this trial was 52% (with 3/25 achieving complete response). The RR in the subgroup of 18 patients with small bowel adenocarcinoma was 61% as compared to 33% with ampullary adenocarcinoma.[32]

In the adjuvant setting, the few retrospective studies that have attempted to shed light on this issue have failed to show a survival benefit to adjuvant chemotherapy. More specifically, the Mayo Clinic reported no survival benefit to adjuvant 5-fluorouracil (5-FU)-based chemotherapy and/or chemo-radiation.[25] However, it is important to note, that historical reports involved 5-FU chemotherapy as a single agent. With the addition of oxaliplatin to 5-FU, an improvement in response rates was appreciated in studies with one study having a 61% response rate.[32]

To this end, based on very limited prospective data, in the current era, we are extrapolating from the colorectal cancer literature and current practices is to treat patients with advanced disease with a FOLFOX-6 regimen without any biologic agents (bevacizumab, cetuximab, panitumumab, ziv-aflibercept) and in the adjuvant setting to offer 5-fluorouracil, leucovorin and oxaliplatin (FOLFOX-6) to patients with lymph node-positive disease[33] and chemo-radiation (with 5-FU as radiosensitizer) to patients with positive margins or T4 disease.

Neuroendocrine Tumors

Based on embryologic origin, neuroendocrine tumors (NETs) were previously classified as foregut (thymus, esophagus, lung, stomach, duodenum, and pancreas), midgut (appendix, ileum, cecum, and ascending colon), and hindgut (distal large bowel and rectum) tumors. This system, however, is now considered outdated because it does not distinguish biologically relevant differences in these tumors. In 2010 the World Health Organization (WHO) updated its classification to describe NETs according to its primary origin (e.g. pancreas, duodenum, small intestine, etc.), clinical syndrome, and differentiation. In this section, well-differentiated small bowel and pancreatic NETs will be discussed.

Clinical presentation

The vast majority (70%) of NETs are *non-functioning* (non-symptomatic, non-secretory) tumors and diagnosed incidentally. The clinical manifestations of NETs are therefore non-specific and can depend on several factors, including location and secretion of specific hormones. Thus, tumors are routinely found incidentally during surgical exploration or cross-sectional imaging of the abdomen for other indications. Of the NETs that are *functional*, the most common clinical manifestations are: (1) flushing, bronchospasm, diarrhea and abdominal pain (VIPoma, carcinoid, gastrinoma); (2) hypoglycemia (insulinoma); (3) dermatitis (glucagonoma); (4) diabetes (glucagonoma); and (5) ulcer and dyspepsia (gastrinoma). The clinical symptoms of functioning NETs generally arise after the tumor has metastasized to the liver. In addition, right-sided heart failure might be a presenting symptom that is seen in patients with carcinoid syndrome. Right-sided heart failure is believed to be the consequence of a fibrotic process affecting the tricuspid valve causing regurgitation and pulmonary stenosis.[34,35] The pathogenesis is not well-defined but thought to be due to endocardial plaque-like deposits likely related to the vasoactive substances secreted by the metastatic tumor cells in the liver that bypass hepatic degradation.[36]

Diagnosis

The diagnosis of NETs can be challenging with an average delay in diagnosis of 5 to 7 years from initial onset of symptoms, with more than 50% of patients diagnosed at an advanced stage of disease. The diagnosis is based on clinical symptoms, hormone levels, cross-sectional and functional imaging, endoscopic ultrasound and pathologic confirmation.

Enhanced, multiphasic cross-sectional imaging, either in the form of a triphasic CT or enhanced MRI scan, will allow for the adequate characterization of the primary tumor as well as possible regional or distant metastasis. More specifically, small bowel and pancreatic NETs have increased enhancement seen primarily during the arterial phase of these studies due to the neovascularity that characterize these tumors. In addition, calcifications can be present in up to 30% of NETs and these calcifications are better seen on CT than MRI. It is important to also note that pancreatic NET can present as cystic pancreatic lesions and should be considered when evaluating a cystic neoplasm of the pancreas. Finally, the typical radiographic presentation seen on cross sectional imaging of small bowel NETs is that of a mesenteric mass. This mass has a stellate pattern with irregular borders and is associated with a desmoplastic reaction that leads to a foreshortening of the small bowel mesentery which can potentially obstruct the small bowel. These mesenteric masses represent regional adenopathy from an underlying small bowel NET that, on many occasions, is not routinely identified on cross sectional imaging. Certain studies suggest that MRI is superior to CT for evaluating disease at follow-up and more importantly for detection of liver metastasis.[37] Dynamic contrast-enhanced MRI sequences help detect small hypervascular, hepatic metastatic lesions.

Nuclear imaging plays a key role in the staging algorithm for suspected or diagnosed NETs.[38–40] Octreotide imaging (^{111}In-Octreoscan), also known as somatostatin receptor scintigraphy (SRS), employs a radiolabeled somatostatin analogue that detects NETs by binding to the somatostatin receptors displayed on the surface of NET cells.[41] Following systemic administration of ^{111}Indium-pentetreotide, whole body scintigraphy is performed to diagnose, localize, and stage neuroendocrine neoplasms. The sensitivity of Octreoscans in identifying the location of the primary tumor, assessing somatostatin avidity, or defining metastatic disease is approximately 90%. However, there is often physiological bowel activity that may produce false-positive results.[42] With the advent of enhanced, multi-phasic, multi-detector cross-sectional axial imaging, the sensitivity of Octreoscans has been put into question.[43] However, consensus guidelines from the North American Neuroendocrine Tumor Society (NANETS) recommend that an Octreoscan be performed as part of the baseline assessment and staging of patients with NET.[44] Finally, positron emission tomography (PET), using [18F]-fluorodeoxyglucose (FDG), is not routinely utilized since it has not been helpful in identifying well-differentiated NETs primarily due to the generally lower proliferative activity seen in these tumors.[45] However, there may be a role for PET in poorly-differentiated NETs which typically have more aggressive tumor biology and thus increased proliferative activity.

Biomarkers

Biomarkers consist of hormones or amines secreted by NETs that can assist clinicians with the diagnosis, treatment, and prognosis of patients with NETs.

Serum chromogranin-A

Chromogranin-A are glycoproteins within secretory vesicles that are found in neuronal and endocrine tissues and its level can be elevated in patients with *functional* and *non-functional* NETs. The sensitivity and specificity of chromogranin A depends on the assay used and the cutoff values. Thus, the sensitivity varies from 77.8% to 84% and the specificity varies from 71.3% to 85.3%.[46] There are conflicting studies about the use of chromogranin A as a diagnostic or prognostic indicator in patients with NETs.[47,48] This is in part due to the fact that elevated chromogranin A levels can also be seen in patients with benign conditions, such as patients with gastritis or reflux who use proton pump inhibitors, renal and hepatic dysfunction, and essential hypertension.[49]

Urine 5-hydroxyindoleacetic acid (*5-HIAA*)

5-HIAA can be used to determine the overproduction of serotonin by carcinoid tumors. 5-HIAA is the main metabolite of serotonin and is most useful in primary midgut NETs. Foregut and hindgut NETs only rarely secrete serotonin (they lack the enzyme dopamine decarboxylase and thus cannot convert 5-hydroxytryptophan to serotonin). 5-HIAA is tested by a 24-hour urine sample. Certain foods (banana, pineapple, kiwi, nut, and avocado) and drugs are known to interfere with this measurement.[50] This assay has a sensitivity of 64% and a specificity of 98% for NETs.

Other hormones

Pancreatic NET (PanNET) can secrete a variety of hormones depending on the PanNET subtype. Examples of these hormones are: gastrin, glucagon, insulin/proinsulin and vasoactive intestinal peptide (VIP). Each of these hormones can cause a specific clinical symptom/syndrome: Zollinger-Ellison syndrome (gastrin), glucagonoma syndrome (glucagon), hypoglycemia (insulin), and diarrhea (VIP).

Carcinoid syndrome

Carcinoid syndrome almost exclusively develops in the setting of midgut primary NETs with liver metastasis and is primarily characterized by the development of flushing, diarrhea, and bronchospasm. Only 5–7% of small bowel NETs develop carcinoid syndrome due to the fact that the liver metabolizes and degrades the biologic secretory amines and/or polypeptides produced by the neuroendocrine tumor cells.[51] Symptoms are usually precipitated by alcohol ingestion, stress, and physical activity.

These symptoms can be controlled by the use of the somatostatin analogue, octreotide, which acts on somatastatin receptors on neuroendocrine cells by inhibiting the secretion of hormones from these tumor cells. For refractory symptoms, cyproheptadine, a non-selective potent anti-histamine, can ameliorate severe diarrhea symptoms.[52] In addition, interferon-alpha has been shown to have some mild activity on symptom alleviation when combined with octreotide.[53] Unfortunately, the vast majority of patients with carcinoid syndrome have extensive unresectable hepatic metastasis and complete surgical resection of all disease is not feasible. However, retrospective studies have shown that cytoreductive (or debulking) surgery can play a role in the treatment of a select cohort of patients.[54] Symptomatic relief may be obtained by cytoreductive surgery; however, the duration of effective relief from these palliative procedures can be short-lived, usually less than 12 months.[51]

Classification

Based on the 2010 World Health Organization (WHO) classification, tumor differentiation and grade are key factors in the staging of NETs. Differentiation refers to the extent to which the neoplastic cells resemble their non-neoplastic counterparts. Most NETs fall into three histologic categories (Table 2): well-differentiated [low grade (G1)], moderately-differentiated [intermediate grade (G2)], and poorly-differentiated [high grade (G3)]. Poorly-differentiated NETs are often associated with a rapid clinical course and poor outcome; as such, the clinical behavior and treatment is similar to that of small cell carcinoma of the lung and will not be further discussed. Grade refers to the inherent biologic aggressiveness of the tumor. Grade is usually defined by mitotic count and/or Ki-67 index. If there is discordance between the mitotic rate and Ki-67 index, the grade will be defined according to the higher index of either test (Table 2).[44]

Small bowel NET

Small bowel NETs are thought to arise from the neuroendocrine cells of Kulchitsky and account for approximately 40% of all GI NETs. The vast majority of these tumors originate in the ileum, followed by the duodenum and jejunum. Carcinoid syndrome occurs in 5–7% of all small bowel NETs.[2,55] Overall, small bowel NETs typically have an indolent course with five-year survival rates ranging between 55% and 78%.[1,3] More specifically, 10-year disease-specific survival rates stratified by AJCC staging

Table 2. NANETS Classification of NETs.

Grade	Gastroenteropancreatic (GEP) NETs	Differentiation
Low Grade (G1)	<2 mitoses/10HPF AND/OR <3% Ki-67 index	Well- differentiated
Intermediate Grade (G2)	2–20 mitoses/10HPF AND/OR 3–20% Ki-67 index	Well-differentiated
High Grade (G3)	>20 mitoses/10HPF AND/OR >20%Ki-67 index	Poorly-differentiated

from a series of 6,792 patients with small intestine NETs ranged from 95% for stage I to 42% for stage IV patients.[56] Predictors of locoregional or metastatic spread in patients with small bowel NETs are size and depth; such that, 10 mm tumors and tumors with transmural invasion have a risk of metastasis of approximately 74% and 68%, respectively.

Treatment for locoregional disease

Surgery is the standard of care for patients with locoregional disease. Surgery should include a wide en bloc resection of the primary small bowel NET with regional lymphadenectomy regardless of tumor size.[57,58] An appropriate oncological operation will allow for an improved local control rate and an improvement in OS.[59] Due to high risk of synchronous lesions within the bowel (approximately 40%), a thorough inspection of the bowel is recommended at time of surgery and all additional sites of disease should be included in the resection, if technically possible.

Treatment for metastatic disease

The liver is the most common site of metastatic spread for small bowel NETs. If metastatic disease is limited to the liver and the disease is technically resectable, a curative-intent hepatic resection should be attempted in medically-fit patients. Data from the Mayo Clinic suggest that there is a role for cytoreductive liver surgery if at least 90% of the liver disease can be removed,[54] such that liver resection of metastatic NET lesions can be associated with a survival advantage. Furthermore, a retrospective study comparing debulking, cytoreductive liver surgery to systemic therapy with octreotide combined with regional therapy [hepatic artery embolization (HAE)] showed improved survival rates for patients undergoing hepatic resection. Hepatic artery embolization (HAE) without chemotherapy (microspheres, polyvinyl alcohol, or gel foam) or with chemotherapy (HACE) has symptom control and potential survival advantages in patients with unresectable NET hepatic metastasis. This is based on the fact that most NET cells derive their primary blood supply from the hepatic arterial system and normal hepatocytes derive their primary blood supply from the portal venous system. A report from MD

Anderson group on 81 patients with hepatic metastasis from small bowel NET treated with HAE showed a 67% response rate, with a >50% reduction in tumor size and a response duration of 17 months.[60] The 1-, 2-, and five-year survival in this series was 93%, 60% and 24%, respectively. Reported common side effects after HAE are: liver failure, abscesses, and post-embolization syndrome (fever, abdominal pain, transient transaminitis, and leukocytosis).[60]

Medical therapy

Somatostatin is an endogenous inhibitor of various hormones secreted from the endocrine system (i.e. serotonin, insulin, glucagon, and gastrin). It binds with high affinity to the five somatostatin receptor subtypes (SST 1–5) on secretory endocrine cells, which have different inhibitory effects in the body. Several studies have highlighted the anti-proliferative effects of the somatostatin analog, octreotide, in patients with NETs. A double-blind, placebo-controlled randomized phase III study (PROMID study) of octreotide LAR or placebo in patients with metastatic well-differentiated (*functioning* or *non-functioning*) midgut NETs, demonstrated that octreotide LAR at 30 mg/month ($n = 42$) more than doubled the time to tumor progression compared to placebo ($n = 43$) from 6.0 months to 14.3 months ($p = 0.000072$).[61] Based on large part on this study, patients who have significant unresectable tumor burden and/or are symptomatic should be considered for treatment with octreotide in the first-line setting. However, there is no clear agreement on the timing of octreotide initiation in the asymptomatic patient with low tumor burden.

Pancreatic NET

Pancreatic NETs (PanNET), previously known as *pancreatic islet cell tumors,* constitute 47% of all GI NETs, the majority (60–90%) of which are *non-functioning*. In addition, although PanNETs are primarily sporadic, they can be part of a hereditary syndrome, such as: Multiple endocrine neoplasia type-1 [inherited via an autosomal-dominant pattern and is associated with neoplasms of the pituitary gland, the parathyroid gland, and the pancreas (the 3 "P"s)] and Von Hippel Lindau syndrome which is a rare, autosomal dominant genetic condition that predisposes individuals to benign and malignant tumors. The most common tumors found in VHL are central nervous system and retinal hemangioblastomas, clear cell renal carcinomas, pheochromocytomas, pancreatic neuroendocrine tumors, pancreatic cysts, end lymphatic sac tumors and epididymal papillary cystadenomas. VHL results from a mutation in the von Hippel–Lindau tumor suppressor gene on chromosome 3p25.3. Finally, approximately half of patients with Pan Nets present with advanced disease which is primarily characterized by the presence of hepatic metastasis at the time of diagnosis.

Treatment for locoregional disease

Surgery has been associated with significant improvements in survival and thus should represent the treatment of choice in medically fit patients with localized PanNETs.[62] Surgery differs according to the location of the tumor within the pancreas, such that head lesions are treated with a pancreaticoduodenectomy while lesions in the body or tail are treated with a left pancreatectomy. These procedures can be undertaken via a minimally-invasive approach (laparoscopic or robotic) or an open laparotomy approach depending on the expertise of the treating surgeon. Furthermore, small lesions may be amendable to enucleation depending on the proximity of the tumor to the pancreatic duct. These resections can be associated with considerable perioperative complications (i.e. pancreatic leak or fistula) in addition to exocrine and endocrine pancreatic insufficiencies.[63,64]

Finally, it is important to note, that advances in cross-sectional imaging techniques have increased the detection of small PanNETs[65] and it is now debated if all small, asymptomatic PanNETs should be routinely resected. More specifically, there is considerable discussion as to whether asymptomatic lesions 1 cm or less in size should be resected or observed. Therapy should therefore be tailored to the individual patient.

Treatment for metastatic disease

In patients with *non-functional* metastatic PanNETs, surgery remains controversial. Whenever a resection leaves no residual disease for low grade

PanNET, a curative intent is recommended.[66,67] Encouraging data have emerged with survival advantage to using chemoembolization, radiofrequency ablation or radioembolization in controlling liver metastasis. These techniques have been limited to small tumors (<5 m) with no extrahepatic metastasis and have been an adjunct to future palliative surgery.[68–71] Liver transplant is another option of treatment in hepatic only metastasis when all other treatments fail.[72–74]

Medical therapy

Although carcinoid tumors and PanNETs are morphologically similar on routine histologic evaluation, they differ in terms of pathogenesis, biology, and response to therapy.[75] Lanreotide was the second somatostatin analogue available. The role of Lanreotide in tumor progression was evaluated in the Controlled study of Lanreotide Antiproliferative Response in patients with gastroenteropancreatic NeuroEndocrine Tumors (CLARINET) study. This study randomized 204 patients with metastatic well-and moderately-differentiated nonfunctioning pancreatic and intestinal NETs to receive either placebo or lanreotide. Preliminary results demonstrated that treatment with lanreotide at two years led to an improvement in PFS over placebo (PFS, not reached versus 18 months; HR, 0.47; 95 % CI, 0.30–0.73; $p = 0.0002$).[76]

Cytotoxic chemotherapy

Patients who are symptomatic from tumor bulk or have rapidly enlarging metastases with well-or moderately-differentiated carcinoid, chemotherapy has shown to have a higher objective RR compared to somatostatin analogues and targeted therapies. Streptozocin combinations have been studied. Streptozocin-doxorubicin showed a RR of 69% in the treatment of advanced islet-cell carcinoma.[77] A retrospective study reported a RR of 39% with the use of 5-FU, streptozocin and doxorubicin for locally-advanced and metastatic PanNET.[78] A phase II trial had a RR of 33% with dacarbazine and temozolomide.[79] Because of the high toxicity rates of both streptozocin and dacarbazine, these agents have fallen out of favor in the management of NET. Temozolomide, an oral alkylating chemotherapy, is a more tolerated agent. It has been studied in combination with different agents (thalidomide, bevacizumab and everolimus) and the reported RR ranged from 25% to 45%.[80–82] In a retrospective series of 30 patients treated with capecitabine (750 mg/m^2 twice daily on days 1 to 14) combined with temozolomide (200 mg/m^2 daily on days 10 to 14), the RR was 70%.[83] A preliminary report of a phase II trial presented at American Society of Clinical Oncology (ASCO) GI Cancers Symposium 2014 showed a partial response rate of 36% in patients with advanced PanNETs.[84] Methylguanine DNA methyltransferase (MGMT) has been shown to play a role in determining response to temozolomide. It is expressed in 50% of PanNET. MGMT expression testing is not routinely performed nor is it a standard of care test and thus has not been widely adopted to assist clinicians in determining treatment or response to temozolomide.[85] Interferon-α has demonstrated an antitumor effect in patients with advanced NET; however, it is not used anymore because of its severe side effects.[86]

Targeted therapy

Sunitinib, a multi-targeted tyrosine kinase inhibitor (TKI), has been studied in the treatment of PanNET. After a phase II trial showing a partial RR of 18% and PFS of 7.7 months using sunitinib (50 mg daily of 4 weeks out of 6 weeks cycle),[87] a phase III trial showed efficacy and safety with a time to tumor progression of 11 months in the sunitinib arm (37.5 mg daily) compared to 5.5 months in the placebo arm for patients with locally-advanced or metastatic well-differentiated PanNET.[88]

Everolimus is an mTOR inhibitor that has shown promising results in the treatment of PanNETs. When compared to placebo, single-agent everolimus (10 mg orally daily) was superior (PFS: 11 vs. 4.6 months) in well- and moderately-differentiated PanNET.[89] A phase III study enrolled 429 patients with advance carcinoid tumors and carcinoid syndrome. Patients were randomized to receive octreotide LAR and everolimus or octreotide and placebo. Patient receiving octreotide and everolimus had a median PFS of 16.4 months compared with 11.3 months for patients receiving octreotide alone ($p = 0.26$).[90] Temsirolimus has also shown activity in NET[91] and is being studied with anti-VEGF combinations.[92] Table 3 summarizes all phase III data in advanced NET disease.

Table 3. Summary of phase III trials in NET.

Study	N	Disease	Grade	Treatment	PFS	RR
PROMID [64]	85	Non-functioning midgut	I	Octreotide LAR vs. Placebo	14.3 vs. 6	
CLARINET [79]	204	NET	I/II	Lanreotide vs. Placebo	Not reached vs. 18	
Raymond *et al.* [90]	171	PanNET	I	Sunitinib vs. placebo	11.4 vs. 5.5 HR = 0.41	9.3 vs. 0
RADIANT III [92]	410	PanNET	1/2	Everolimus vs. placebo	11 vs. 4.6 HR = 0.35	5 vs. 2
Radiant II [93]	429	PanNET	I/II	Everolimus/octreotide vs. octreotide	16.4 vs. 11.3 $p = 0.26$	
CALGB 80701	Accruing	PanNET		Everolimus/Bevacizumab vs. Everolimus	Ongoing	

Sorafenib, a small molecular inhibitor of several tyrosine protein kinases (VEGFR and PDGFR) and Raf kinases (more avidly C-Raf than B-Raf) was studied in a phase II trial of well-differentiated PanNETs and showed a RR of 9%.[93] Pazopanib, a selective multi-targeted tyrosine kinase inhibitor, has a 17% RR in patients with well-differentiated PanNET treated with octreotide.[94]

Gastrointestinal Stromal Tumors (GISTs)

Gastrointestinal stromal tumors (GISTs) represent the most common mesenchymal tumor of the gastrointestinal tract. Yet, GISTs are relatively rare tumors with an annual incidence of approximately 5,000 cases in the United States and comprise less than 1% of all GI tract tumors.[95]

Pathogenesis

GISTs originate from the interstitial cells of Cajal and the molecular hallmarks of GISTs, the mutation of the proto-oncogene *KIT* and tyrosine kinase receptor PDGFR-α, present in the vast majority of tumors.[96] GISTs have since been recognized as a separate pathological entity and have become a model for the targeted treatment of solid tumors.[97] The transmembrane protein, c-*KIT* (CD117), is found on the cell surface and binds to a ligand called stem cell factor. This leads to homo-dimerization of *KIT* and cross-phosphorylation of tyrosine residues in the intracellular domain. There is subsequent activation of the mitogen activated protein kinase (MAPK) and phosphatidylinositol 3-kinase (PI3K) pathways. These signaling pathways ultimately lead to cell proliferation and survival. Thus, mutations in the c-*KIT* proto-oncogene leads to kinase activity causing neoplastic proliferation.[98,99] Ninety percent of GISTs harbor mutations in the *KIT* receptor and 5–7% have PDGFRA activating mutations. The majority of *KIT* mutations are found on exon 11. Other mutations are found on exon 9, 13, 17 and 18.[99]

Clinical presentation

GISTs most commonly originate in the stomach and proximal small intestine with a median age of presentation of 60–65 years of age.[99,100] Small

GISTs can be asymptomatic and may be discovered incidentally, during either endoscopy or CT imaging for other reasons. Larger tumors may present with symptoms such as pain, intestinal obstruction or bleeding. There is further evidence of the high prevalence of asymptomatic GIST by a series of consecutive autopsies performed, where small GISTs (1–10 mm) were found in 22.5% of the autopsies.[101]

Risk assessment

Various risk-stratification models [the National Institute of Health (NIH) consensus criteria, the modified NIH criteria and the Armed Forces Institute of Pathology (AFIP) criteria and Memorial Sloan-Kettering Cancer Center GIST nomogram] have been developed to determine the risk of recurrence for patients with resected GIST.[101,102] The variables most widely identified and incorporated into these risk-stratification models are tumor location, size, and its mitotic index. These risk-stratification models are used to help guide clinicians in determining whether adjuvant therapy with imatinib should be recommended. Additional risk factors such as type of mutation and rupture of tumor have also been shown to be prognostic and have been incorporated in certain models.[103]

Diagnosis

GISTs are usually discovered incidentally. For symptomatic tumors, the most common symptoms at presentation are abdominal pain, bleeding, bowel perforation, and dyspepsia. It is important to note that GISTs are primarily submucosal lesions and therefore routine endoscopic biopsies of intestinal mucosa are normally non-diagnostic unless the tumor has eroded through the mucosa, which typically is the case in patients presenting with gastrointestinal bleeding. Otherwise, these submucosal lesions need to be biopsied with an endoscopic ultrasound guided biopsy — core biopsy being preferred. Endoscopic biopsies are advised as opposed to percutaneous biopsies in order to prevent possible cancer cell spillage into the peritoneal cavity at the time of percutaneous biopsy.[104–106]

On histopathologic assessment, the majority of GISTs display a bland spindle-cell pattern.[95] These show fascicles of fairly uniform spindled neoplastic cells with minimal nuclear atypia and peri-nuclear vacuoles. The remaining 30% of GIST show either an epitheloid cell or a mixed epitheloid and spindle-cell morphology. Although immunohistochemical staining for c-*KIT* (CD117) is positive in 90% of GISTs, it is not an absolute requirement for the diagnosis; CD-34 and DOG-1 are present in 70% and 98% of GISTs, respectively, and can assist with the diagnosis.[95]

Advanced cases of GIST usually present with either liver or peritoneal metastasis and therefore, cross-sectional imaging of the abdomen and pelvis with either CT scan or MRI should be performed to appropriately assess the extent of disease and stage patients prior to surgical intervention. A triphasic, multi-detector CT scan can also be used to assess response to therapy. Size-based response criteria such as the Response Evaluation Criteria in Solid Tumors (RECIST) criteria significantly underestimate the response to therapy. A CT scan can provide subjective evaluation using changes in tumor nodules, density, tumor vascularization and tumor size to assess response, in addition to providing invaluable contrast-enhanced images for surgical planning. Taking these changes into consideration, the Choi criteria for assessing GIST response to therapy were established.[107] The Choi criteria are able to combine morphologic tumor volume response and biologic response from CT scan findings. In addition, positron emission tomography (PET) using 2-[fluorine-18] fluoro-2-deoxy-D-glucose (18FDG) has been shown to be highly sensitive in detecting early response in patients with metastatic GIST due to the increased FDG avidity of GISTs and thus can be used to assess response to therapy in patients with GIST. However, not all GIST tumors are FDG-avid, limiting the applicability of this imaging modality to all patients.[108]

Management

Historically, efforts to treat GIST with conventional chemotherapy have been unsuccessful; however with the arrival of imatinib mesylate, the treatment paradigm was changed. This molecule, also used to treat chronic myeloid leukemia, inhibits the constitutive tyrosine kinase activity of BCR-ABL and was one of the first targeted cancer drugs developed and had excellent outcomes in the management of these patients. It also inhibits the tyrosine kinase activity of c-*KIT* in patients with GIST and has become the mainstay of current therapy. The United States FDA, February 1, 2002, approved Imatinib for metastatic and unresectable GIST. The two-year survival of patients with advanced disease has risen to around 80% following imatinib treatment.[109]

Neoadjuvant

The role of preoperative imatinib for treating primary localized GIST is a matter of surgical and medical discretion.[110] Several studies have evaluated the role of preoperative imatinib followed by surgery.[111–113] However, these trials primarily evaluated the safety and efficacy of imatinib in the preoperative setting and no phase III trials were conducted to evaluate the benefit of neoadjuvant therapy. The report of a phase II trial, RTOG 0132, showed a time to progression (TTP) benefit for patients with 2 cm or larger GISTs who received neoadjuvant imatinib at a dose of 600 mg daily treated for 2 months preoperatively when compared with placebo. Median TTP was not reached in the imatinib arm as compared to 4.4 years in the placebo group. Patients included in this analysis had primary resectable, recurrent, and/or metastatic disease.[114] An additional small trial from MD Anderson randomized 19 patients undergoing surgical resection to receive 3, 5, or 7 days of preoperative imatinib (600 mg/d).[115] Imatinib did not affect surgical morbidity and the response rate was 70%. Median disease-free survival of patients treated with surgery and imatinib was 46 months.

Adjuvant

The role of adjuvant imatinib is well-established; however the optimal duration of treatment is still an area of active investigation. The American College of Surgeons Oncology Group ACOSOG Z9001 trial was the first phase III double-blinded randomized trial to study the benefit of adjuvant therapy. This trial compared imatinib 400 mg daily to placebo for a duration of 12 months after resection of c-*KIT* positive GIST of >3 cm in size. The study closed early because the primary endpoint was met after 19.7 months of follow-up. This study proved a one-year relapse-free survival rate of 97% for patients treated for one year with imatinib compared to 83% in the placebo group (HR:0.325; $p < 0.0001$).[112] A subsequent randomized phase III Scandinavian trial compared patients to one-year and three-year treatment of adjuvant imatinib in high-risk c-*KIT* positive GIST (tumor size > 10 cm and mitotic count > 10/50 HPF, or tumor size > 5 cm and mitotic count > 5/50 HPF, or the presence of tumor rupture) patients. The five-year recurrence free survival was 66% and 48% in the three-year and one-year treatment groups, respectively (HR = 0.46). There was a five-year OS advantage to three-year adjuvant treatment compared to the one year group (92% vs. 82%, HR = 0.45; $p = 0.019$).[116] An ongoing non-randomized study is being conducted to answer the question of five-year adjuvant imatinib treatment in high-risk GIST patients.[117]

Metastatic

Two studies have demonstrated activity of imatinib in metastatic disease and thus imatinib is approved for the treatment of metastatic/recurrent GIST.[118,119] In the U.S.-Finland collaborative study, 147 patients were randomly assigned to receive either 400 mg or 600 mg of imatinib daily. This phase II trial was not powered to distinguish between the efficacies of the two doses. Although there was no statistically significant difference between the doses, there were higher RR for exon 11 mutations compared to those on exon 9 with an objective RR to imatinib therapy of 70% and 40% respectively. Wild type GIST patients had a RR of 30%. Median time to progression was longer for exon 11 mutations compared to other exon mutations.[118] In an European Organization for Research and Treatment of Cancer (EORTC) trial, 27 patients with GIST received 400 mg imatinib twice daily, 4% of patients achieved complete remission, 67% partial response, and 18% had stable disease. PFS at one year was 73%.[119] Correlation of response was improved in tumors harboring exon 9 *KIT* mutation who received higher doses of imatinib.[120,121]

A minority of patients have primary resistance to imatinib (GIST tumor growth within the first 6 months of treatment with imatinib). Secondary resistance occurs at a median of 24 months. The reasons why resistance develops is not well-defined and also continues to be an area of active investigation but theories of acquired *KIT* or PDGFRA mutations affecting the imatinib binding site have been suggested. In addition, other *KIT* independent genotypes might emerge through the course of imatinib

Table 4. Summary of important treatment trials in the neoadjuvant, adjuvant and metastatic GIST.

Neoadjuvant	N	Comparison	TTP/PFS/RR	OS
RTOG 0132-phase 2 [114]	63	Imatinib × 2 months vs. placebo	TTP: not reached vs. 4.4 years	
Adjuvant				
ACOSOG Z9001 [112]	713	Imatinib 400 mg × 1 year vs. placebo	RFS at 1 year: 98% vs. 83% ($p = 0.0001$)	
Scandinavian [116]	400	1 year vs. 3 years of Imatinib	RFS at 1 year: 48% vs. 66% ($p < 0.001$)	82% vs. 92% at 5 years ($p = 0.019$)
Advanced/Metastatic				
US-Finland [118]	147	Imatinib 400 or 600 mg daily	PR: 53.7% Stable: 27.9%	
EORTC [119]	51	Imatinib 400 mg BID	PFS at 1 year: 73%, TTP:58 days	
Demetri *et al.* (second-line)[123]	312	Sunitinib vs. placebo	PFS: 6.3 vs. 1.5 months ($p < 0.001$)	
Demetri *et al.* (Third-line)[125]		Regorafenib vs. placebo	PFS: 4.8 vs. 0.9 months	

treatment.[121] To overcome these resistance mechanisms, higher doses of 600 mg or 800 mg of imatinib has been shown to be beneficial in these circumstances.[122] Second-line therapy with sunitinib [small molecule multi-targeted receptor tyrosine kinase (RTK) inhibitor] was studied in GIST patients progressing on or intolerant to imatinib. Median TTP was 27.3 and 6.4 weeks in patients receiving sunitinib and placebo, respectively. There was no OS benefit however, this may largely be related to the cross-over design of the trial. In a subset analysis, patients with exon 9 mutation and *KIT* wild-type GIST had better RR compared to patients harboring exon 11 mutation.[123]

Further trials have attempted to guide therapy following sunitinib failure. A phase II open-label trial evaluated the use of nilotinib. This molecule inhibits BCR-ABL, PDGFR, KIT, CSF-1R, and DDR and is approved for the treatment of chronic- and accelerated-phase CML in patients resistant or intolerant to prior therapy, including imatinib. The median PFS in the trial was 113 days and the OS was 310 days.[124] A phase III randomized trial demonstrated efficacy of regorafenib (small molecule multi-kinase inhibitor) compared to placebo in the third-line setting for GIST patients who progressed on or were intolerant to imatinib and progressed on sunitinib. Median PFS was 4.8 vs. 0.9 months for regorafenib and placebo, respectively.[125] Table 4 summarizes the important clinical trials in the treatment of GIST patients in the neoadjuvant, adjuvant, and metastatic setting.

Take Home Messages

- The majority of small bowel tumors are adenocarcinomas, which commonly affects the duodenum. Carcinoids are mostly found in the ileum, and sarcomas and lymphomas can develop throughout the entire small bowel.
- The neuroendocrine tumors (NETs) are described according to their primary origins, clinical syndrome, and differentiation. The majority of NETs are non-functioning tumors and diagnosed incidentally.
- Carcinoid syndrome is primarily characterized by the development of flushing, diarrhea, and bronchospasm, which can be controlled by the use of the somatostatin analogue, octreotide, that acts on somatastatin

receptors on neuroendocrine cells by inhibiting the secretion of hormones from these tumor cells.
- Gastrointestinal stromal tumors (GISTs) represent the most common mesenchymal tumor of the gastrointestinal tract. Imatinib has been approved for metastatic and unresectable GIST, with the two-year survival rate of 80%.

References

1. Haselkorn, T., A.S. Whittemore, and Lilienfeld, D.E., Incidence of small bowel cancer in the United States and worldwide: geographic, temporal, and racial differences. *Cancer Causes Control*, 2005. **16**(7): 781–7.
2. Siegel, R., Naishadham, D., and Jemal, A., Cancer statistics, 2013. *CA Cancer J Clin*, 2013. **63**(1): 11–30.
3. Bilimoria, K.Y. *et al.*, Small bowel cancer in the United States: changes in epidemiology, treatment, and survival over the last 20 years. *Ann Surg*, 2009. **249**(1): 63–71.
4. McLaughlin, P.D. and Maher, M.M., Primary malignant diseases of the small intestine. *AJR Am J Roentgenol*, 2013. **201**(1): W9–14.
5. Overman, M.J. *et al.*, A population-based comparison of adenocarcinoma of the large and small intestine: insights into a rare disease. *Ann Surg Oncol*, 2012. **19**(5): 1439–45.
6. Chow, W.H. *et al.*, Risk factors for small intestine cancer. *Cancer Causes Control*, 1993. **4**(2): 163–9.
7. Abrahams, N.A. *et al.*, Adenocarcinoma of the small bowel: a study of 37 cases with emphasis on histologic prognostic factors. *Dis Colon Rectum*, 2002. **45**(11): 1496–502.
8. Sendt, W. *et al.*, Adenocarcinoma of small bowel. An underdiagnosed disease. *Chirurg*, 2012. **83**(4): 374–80.
9. Achour, J. *et al.*, Small bowel tumors: what is the contribution of video capsule endoscopy? *Clin Res Hepatol Gastroenterol*, 2012. **36**(3): 222–6.
10. Neely, D. *et al.*, Small intestinal adenocarcinoma: rarely considered, often missed? *Postgrad Med J*, 2013. **89**(1050): 197–201.
11. Zhang, M.Q., Chen, Z.M., and Wang, H.L., Immunohistochemical investigation of tumorigenic pathways in small intestinal adenocarcinoma: a comparison with colorectal adenocarcinoma. *Mod Pathol*, 2006. **19**(4): 573–80.

12. Rodriguez-Bigas, M.A. *et al.*, Characteristics of small bowel carcinoma in hereditary nonpolyposis colorectal carcinoma. International Collaborative Group on HNPCC. *Cancer*, 1998. **83**(2): 240–4.
13. Masselli, G. *et al.*, Magnetic resonance imaging of small bowel neoplasms. *Cancer Imaging*, 2013. **13**: 92–9.
14. Miao, F., Wang, M.L., and Tang, Y.H., New progress in CT and MRI examination and diagnosis of small intestinal tumors. *World J Gastrointest Oncol*, 2010. **2**(5): 222–8.
15. Lewis, B.S., Eisen, G.M., and Friedman, S., A pooled analysis to evaluate results of capsule endoscopy trials. *Endoscopy*, 2005. **37**(10): 960–5.
16. Mazzarolo, S. and P. Brady, Small bowel capsule endoscopy: a systematic review. *South Med J*, 2007. **100**(3): 274–80.
17. Triester, S.L. *et al.*, A meta-analysis of the yield of capsule endoscopy compared to other diagnostic modalities in patients with non-stricturing small bowel Crohn's disease. *Am J Gastroenterol*, 2006. **101**(5): 954–64.
18. Dabaja, B.S. *et al.*, Adenocarcinoma of the small bowel: presentation, prognostic factors, and outcome of 217 patients. *Cancer*, 2004. **101**(3): 518–26.
19. Howe, J.R. *et al.*, The American College of Surgeons Commission on Cancer and the American Cancer Society. Adenocarcinoma of the small bowel: review of the National Cancer Data Base, 1985–1995. *Cancer*, 1999. **86**(12): 2693–706.
20. Overman, M.J. *et al.*, Prognostic value of lymph node evaluation in small bowel adenocarcinoma: analysis of the surveillance, epidemiology, and end results database. *Cancer*, 2010. **116**(23): 5374–82.
21. Bakaeen, F.G. *et al.*, What prognostic factors are important in duodenal adenocarcinoma? *Arch Surg*, 2000. **135**(6): 635–41; discussion 641–2.
22. Barnes, G., Jr. *et al.*, Primary adenocarcinoma of the duodenum: management and survival in 67 patients. *Ann Surg Oncol*, 1994. **1**(1): 73–8.
23. Sohn, T.A. *et al.*, Adenocarcinoma of the duodenum: factors influencing long-term survival. *J Gastrointest Surg*, 1998. **2**(1): 79–87.
24. Kaklamanos, I.G. *et al.*, Extent of resection in the management of duodenal adenocarcinoma. *Am J Surg*, 2000. **179**(1): 37–41.
25. Halfdanarson, T.R. *et al.*, A single-institution experience with 491 cases of small bowel adenocarcinoma. *Am J Surg*, 2010. **199**(6): 797–803.
26. Ouriel, K. and Adams, J.T., Adenocarcinoma of the small intestine. *Am J Surg*, 1984. **147**(1): 66–71.

27. Czaykowski, P. and Hui, D., Chemotherapy in small bowel adenocarcinoma: 10-year experience of the British Columbia Cancer Agency. *Clin Oncol (R Coll Radiol)*, 2007. **19**(2): 143–9.
28. Fishman, P.N. *et al.*, Natural history and chemotherapy effectiveness for advanced adenocarcinoma of the small bowel: a retrospective review of 113 cases. *Am J Clin Oncol*, 2006. **29**(3): 225–31.
29. Overman, M.J. *et al.*, Chemotherapy with 5-fluorouracil and a platinum compound improves outcomes in metastatic small bowel adenocarcinoma. *Cancer*, 2008. **113**(8): 2038–45.
30. Zaanan, A. *et al.*, Second-line chemotherapy with fluorouracil, leucovorin, and irinotecan (FOLFIRI regimen) in patients with advanced small bowel adenocarcinoma after failure of first-line platinum-based chemotherapy: a multicenter AGEO study. *Cancer*, 2011. **117**(7): 1422–8.
31. Gibson, M.K. *et al.*, Phase II study of 5-fluorouracil, doxorubicin, and mitomycin C for metastatic small bowel adenocarcinoma. *Oncologist*, 2005. **10**(2): 132–7.
32. Overman, M.J. *et al.*, Phase II study of capecitabine and oxaliplatin for advanced adenocarcinoma of the small bowel and ampulla of Vater. *J Clin Oncol*, 2009. **27**(16): 2598–603.
33. Andre, T. *et al.*, Oxaliplatin, fluorouracil, and leucovorin as adjuvant treatment for colon cancer. *N Engl J Med*, 2004. **350**(23): 2343–51.
34. Rossignol, B. *et al.*, Carcinoid heart disease secondary to a tumor of the small intestine. Apropos of a case with associated tricuspid and pulmonary insufficiency. *Arch Mal Coeur Vaiss*, 1977. **70**(11): 1221–6.
35. Thorson, A. *et al.*, Malignant carcinoid of the small intestine with metastases to the liver, valvular disease of the right side of the heart (pulmonary stenosis and tricuspid regurgitation without septal defects), peripheral vasomotor symptoms, bronchoconstriction, and an unusual type of cyanosis; a clinical and pathologic syndrome. *Am Heart J*, 1954. **47**(5): 795–817.
36. Bhattacharyya, S. *et al.*, Risk factors for the development and progression of carcinoid heart disease. *Am J Cardiol*, 2011. **107**(8): 1221–6.
37. Pavel, M. *et al.*, ENETS Consensus Guidelines for the management of patients with liver and other distant metastases from neuroendocrine neoplasms of foregut, midgut, hindgut, and unknown primary. *Neuroendocrinology*, 2012. **95**(2): 157–76.

38. Oberg, K. and Eriksson, B., Nuclear medicine in the detection, staging and treatment of gastrointestinal carcinoid tumours. *Best Pract Res Clin Endocrinol Metab*, 2005. **19**(2): 265–76.
39. Rufini, V., Calcagni, M.L., and Baum, R.P., Imaging of neuroendocrine tumors. *Semin Nucl Med*, 2006. **36**(3): 228–47.
40. Turaga, K.K. and Kvols, L.K., Recent progress in the understanding, diagnosis, and treatment of gastroenteropancreatic neuroendocrine tumors. *CA Cancer J Clin*, 2011. **61**(2): 113–32.
41. Krenning, E.P. *et al.*, Somatostatin receptor scintigraphy with [111In-DTPA-D-Phe1]- and [123I-Tyr3]-octreotide: the Rotterdam experience with more than 1000 patients. *Eur J Nucl Med*, 1993. **20**(8): 716–31.
42. Kvols, L.K. *et al.*, Evaluation of a radiolabeled somatostatin analog (I-123 octreotide) in the detection and localization of carcinoid and islet cell tumors. *Radiology*, 1993. **187**(1): 129–33.
43. Reidy-Lagunes, D.L., Gollub, M.J., and Saltz, L.B., Addition of octreotide functional imaging to cross-sectional computed tomography or magnetic resonance imaging for the detection of neuroendocrine tumors: added value or an anachronism? *J Clin Oncol*, 2011. **29**(3): e74–5.
44. Kulke, M.H. *et al.*, NANETS treatment guidelines: well-differentiated neuroendocrine tumors of the stomach and pancreas. *Pancreas*, 2010. **39**(6): 735–52.
45. Orlefors, H. *et al.*, Whole-body (11)C-5-hydroxytryptophan positron emission tomography as a universal imaging technique for neuroendocrine tumors: comparison with somatostatin receptor scintigraphy and computed tomography. *J Clin Endocrinol Metab*, 2005. **90**(6): 3392–400.
46. Zatelli, M.C. *et al.*, Chromogranin A as a marker of neuroendocrine neoplasia: an Italian Multicenter Study. *Endocr Relat Cancer*, 2007. **14**(2): 473–82.
47. Eriksson, B., Oberg, K., and Stridsberg, M., Tumor markers in neuroendocrine tumors. *Digestion*, 2000. **62** (Suppl 1): 33–8.
48. Nobels, F.R. *et al.*, Chromogranin A: its clinical value as marker of neuroendocrine tumours. *Eur J Clin Invest*, 1998. **28**(6): 431–40.
49. Arnold, R. *et al.*, Plasma chromogranin A as marker for survival in patients with metastatic endocrine gastroenteropancreatic tumors. *Clin Gastroenterol Hepatol*, 2008. **6**(7): 820–7.

50. Feldman, J.M. and O'Dorisio, T.M., Role of neuropeptides and serotonin in the diagnosis of carcinoid tumors. *Am J Med*, 1986. **81**(6B): 41–8.
51. Gu, P. *et al.*, Treatment of liver metastases in patients with neuroendocrine tumors of gastroesophageal and pancreatic origin. *Int J Hepatol*, 2012. 2012: 131659.
52. Moertel, C.G., Kvols, L.K., and Rubin, J., A study of cyproheptadine in the treatment of metastatic carcinoid tumor and the malignant carcinoid syndrome. *Cancer*, 1991. **67**(1): 33–6.
53. Fabian, E., Kump, P., and Krejs, G.J., Diarrhea caused by circulating agents. *Gastroenterol Clin North Am*, 2012. **41**(3): 603–10.
54. Sarmiento, J.M. and Que, F.G., Hepatic surgery for metastases from neuroendocrine tumors. *Surg Oncol Clin N Am*, 2003. **12**(1): 231–42.
55. Maggard, M.A., O'Connell, J.B., and Ko, C.Y., Updated population-based review of carcinoid tumors. *Ann Surg*, 2004. **240**(1): 117–22.
56. Kim, M.K. *et al.*, Revised staging classification improves outcome prediction for small intestinal neuroendocrine tumors. *J Clin Oncol*, 2013. **31**(30): 3776–81.
57. Stinner, B. *et al.*, Surgical management for carcinoid tumors of small bowel, appendix, colon, and rectum. *World J Surg*, 1996. **20**(2): 183–8.
58. Ito, H. *et al.*, Surgical treatment of small bowel cancer: a 20-year single institution experience. *J Gastrointest Surg*, 2003. **7**(7): 925–30.
59. Landerholm, K. *et al.*, Survival and prognostic factors in patients with small bowel carcinoid tumour. *Br J Surg*, 2011. **98**(11): 1617–24.
60. Gupta, S. *et al.*, Hepatic artery embolization and chemoembolization for treatment of patients with metastatic carcinoid tumors: the M.D. Anderson experience. *Cancer J*, 2003. **9**(4): 261–7.
61. Rinke, A. *et al.*, Placebo-controlled, double-blind, prospective, randomized study on the effect of octreotide LAR in the control of tumor growth in patients with metastatic neuroendocrine midgut tumors: a report from the PROMID Study Group. *J Clin Oncol*, 2009. **27**(28): 4656–63.
62. Hill, J.S. *et al.*, Pancreatic neuroendocrine tumors: the impact of surgical resection on survival. *Cancer*, 2009. **115**(4): 741–51.
63. Smith, J.K. *et al.*, Complications after pancreatectomy for neuroendocrine tumors: a national study. *J Surg Res*, 2010. **163**(1): 63–8.
64. Falconi, M. *et al.*, Pancreatic insufficiency after different resections for benign tumours. *Br J Surg*, 2008. **95**(1): 85–91.

65. Bettini, R. *et al.*, Tumor size correlates with malignancy in nonfunctioning pancreatic endocrine tumor. *Surgery*, 2011. **150**(1): 75–82.
66. Aranha, G.V. and Shoup, M., Nonstandard pancreatic resections for unusual lesions. *Am J Surg*, 2005. **189**(2): 223–8.
67. Bettini, R. *et al.*, Primary tumour resection in metastatic nonfunctioning pancreatic endocrine carcinomas. *Dig Liver Dis*, 2009. **41**(1): 49–55.
68. Gupta, S. *et al.*, Hepatic arterial embolization and chemoembolization for the treatment of patients with metastatic neuroendocrine tumors: variables affecting response rates and survival. *Cancer*, 2005. **104**(8): 1590–602.
69. Drougas, J.G. *et al.*, Hepatic artery chemoembolization for management of patients with advanced metastatic carcinoid tumors. *Am J Surg*, 1998. **175**(5): 408–12.
70. Henn, A.R. *et al.*, Percutaneous radiofrequency ablation of hepatic metastases for symptomatic relief of neuroendocrine syndromes. *AJR Am J Roentgenol*, 2003. **181**(4): 1005–10.
71. Dhabuwala, A., Lamerton, P., and Stubbs, R.S., Relationship of 99mtechnetium labelled macroaggregated albumin (99mTc-MAA) uptake by colorectal liver metastases to response following Selective Internal Radiation Therapy (SIRT). *BMC Nucl Med*, 2005. **5**: 7.
72. Rossi, R.E., Burroughs, A.K., and Caplin, M.E., Liver transplantation for unresectable neuroendocrine tumor liver metastases. *Ann Surg Oncol*, 2014. **21**(7): 2398–405.
73. Anthuber, M. *et al.*, Results of liver transplantation for gastroenteropancreatic tumor metastases. *World J Surg*, 1996. **20**(1): 73–6.
74. Jaeck, D. *et al.*, Hepatic metastases of gastroenteropancreatic neuroendocrine tumors: safe hepatic surgery. *World J Surg*, 2001. **25**(6): 689–92.
75. Duerr, E.M. and D.C. Chung, Molecular genetics of neuroendocrine tumors. *Best Pract Res Clin Endocrinol Metab*, 2007. **21**(1): 1–14.
76. Caplin, M., Data presented at the 2013 European Cancer Congress, Amsterdam, the Nethelands, September 28, 2013. Abstract available online at http://eccamsterdam2013.ecco-org.eu/Scientific-Programme/Searchable-Programme.aspx — anchorScpr (Accessed on November 22, 2013). A randomized, double-blind, placebo-Controlled study of Lanreotide Antiproliferative Response in patients with gastroenteropancreatic NeuroEndocrine Tumors (CLARINET) (abstract). .

77. Moertel, C.G. *et al.*, Streptozocin-doxorubicin, streptozocin-fluorouracil or chlorozotocin in the treatment of advanced islet-cell carcinoma. *N Engl J Med*, 1992. **326**(8): 519–23.
78. Kouvaraki, M.A. *et al.*, Fluorouracil, doxorubicin, and streptozocin in the treatment of patients with locally advanced and metastatic pancreatic endocrine carcinomas. *J Clin Oncol*, 2004. **22**(23): 4762–71.
79. Ramanathan, R.K. *et al.*, Phase II trial of dacarbazine (DTIC) in advanced pancreatic islet cell carcinoma. Study of the Eastern Cooperative Oncology Group-E6282. *Ann Oncol*, 2001. **12**(8): 1139–43.
80. Kulke, M.H. *et al.*, Phase II study of temozolomide and thalidomide in patients with metastatic neuroendocrine tumors. *J Clin Oncol*, 2006. **24**(3): 401–6.
81. Chan, J.A. *et al.*, Prospective study of bevacizumab plus temozolomide in patients with advanced neuroendocrine tumors. *J Clin Oncol*, 2012. **30**(24): 2963–8.
82. Chan, J.A. *et al.*, A prospective, phase 1/2 study of everolimus and temozolomide in patients with advanced pancreatic neuroendocrine tumor. *Cancer*, 2013. **119**(17): 3212–8.
83. Strosberg, J.R. *et al.*, First-line chemotherapy with capecitabine and temozolomide in patients with metastatic pancreatic endocrine carcinomas. *Cancer*, 2011. **117**(2): 268–75.
84. Fine, R., Gulati, A.P., Tsushima, D. *et al.*, Prospective phase II study of capecitabine and temozolomide (CAPTEM) for progressive, moderately, and well-differentiated metastatic neuroendocrine tumor (abstract 179). *J Clin Oncol*, 32, 2014 (suppl 3; abstr 179). http://meetinglibrary.asco.org/content/122616–143 (Accessed on March 02, 2014). 2014.
85. Hammel, P. *et al.*, New treatment options with cytotoxic agents in neuroendocrine tumours. *Target Oncol*, 2012. **7**(3): 169–72.
86. Riccardi, F. *et al.*, Therapy innovation for the treatment of pancreatic neuroendocrine tumors. *Expert Opin Ther Targets*, 2012. **16** (Suppl 2): S91–102.
87. Kulke, M.H. *et al.*, Activity of sunitinib in patients with advanced neuroendocrine tumors. *J Clin Oncol*, 2008. **26**(20): 3403–10.
88. Raymond, E. *et al.*, Sunitinib malate for the treatment of pancreatic neuroendocrine tumors. *N Engl J Med*, 2011. **364**(6): 501–13.
89. Yao, J.C. *et al.*, Everolimus for advanced pancreatic neuroendocrine tumors. *N Engl J Med*, 2011. **364**(6): 514–23.

90. Pavel, M.E. *et al.*, Everolimus plus octreotide long-acting repeatable for the treatment of advanced neuroendocrine tumours associated with carcinoid syndrome (RADIANT-2): a randomised, placebo-controlled, phase 3 study. *Lancet*, 2011. **378**(9808): 2005–12.
91. Duran, I. *et al.*, A phase II clinical and pharmacodynamic study of temsirolimus in advanced neuroendocrine carcinomas. *Br J Cancer*, 2006. **95**(9): 1148–54.
92. Hobday, T.J., Q.R., Moore, M.J. *et al.*, Multicenter phase II trial of temsirolimus (TEM) and bevacizumab (BEV) in pancreatic neuroendocrine tumor (PNET) (abstract). *J Clin Oncol*, 2013. **31** (suppl; abstr 4032). http://meeting library.asco.org/content/111832–132 (Accessed on June 18, 2013).
93. Raymond, E. *et al.*, Therapy innovations: tyrosine kinase inhibitors for the treatment of pancreatic neuroendocrine tumors. *Cancer Metastasis Rev*, 2011. 30 Suppl 1: 19–26.
94. Phan, A., Yao, J.C., Fogelman, D.R. *et al.*, A prospective, multi-institutional phase II study of GW786034 (pazopanib) and depot octreotide (sandostatin LAR) in advanced low-grade neuroendocrine carcinoma (LGNEC) (abstract 4001). *J Clin Oncol* 2010; 28:301s. Abstract available online at http://www.asco.org/ASCOv2/Meetings/Abstracts?&vmview=abst_detail_view&confID=74&abstractID=47809 (Accessed on February 11, 2011). (Accessed on February 11, 2011).
95. Asija, A.P. *et al.*, Gastrointestinal stromal tumors: a review. *Am J Ther*, 2013.
96. Hirota, S. *et al.*, Gain-of-function mutations of c-kit in human gastrointestinal stromal tumors. *Science*, 1998. **279**(5350): 577–80.
97. Cassier, P.A. *et al.*, Imatinib mesilate for the treatment of gastrointestinal stromal tumour. *Expert Opin Pharmacother*, 2008. **9**(7): 1211–22.
98. Kim, K.H. *et al.*, Diagnostic relevance of overexpressions of PKC-theta and DOG-1 and KIT/PDGFRA gene mutations in extragastrointestinal stromal tumors: a Korean six-centers study of 28 cases. *Anticancer Res*, 2012. **32**(3): 923–37.
99. Corless, C.L., Barnett, C.M., and Heinrich, M.C., Gastrointestinal stromal tumours: origin and molecular oncology. *Nat Rev Cancer*, 2011. **11**(12): 865–78.
100. Joensuu, H. *et al.*, Risk of recurrence of gastrointestinal stromal tumour after surgery: an analysis of pooled population-based cohorts. *Lancet Oncol*, 2012. **13**(3): 265–74.

101. Agaimy, A. *et al.*, Minute gastric sclerosing stromal tumors (GIST tumorlets) are common in adults and frequently show c-KIT mutations. *Am J Surg Pathol*, 2007. **31**(1): 113–20.
102. Gold, J.S. *et al.*, Development and validation of a prognostic nomogram for recurrence-free survival after complete surgical resection of localised primary gastrointestinal stromal tumour: a retrospective analysis. *Lancet Oncol*, 2009. **10**(11): 1045–52.
103. Seidal, T. and Edvardsson, H., Expression of c-kit (CD117) and Ki67 provides information about the possible cell of origin and clinical course of gastrointestinal stromal tumours. *Histopathology*, 1999. **34**(5): 416–24.
104. Mucciarini, C. *et al.*, Incidence and clinicopathologic features of gastrointestinal stromal tumors. A population-based study. *BMC Cancer*, 2007. **7**: 230.
105. Caterino, S. *et al.*, Gastrointestinal stromal tumors: correlation between symptoms at presentation, tumor location and prognostic factors in 47 consecutive patients. *World J Surg Oncol*, 2011. **9**: 13.
106. Bumming, P. *et al.*, Population-based study of the diagnosis and treatment of gastrointestinal stromal tumours. *Br J Surg*, 2006. **93**(7): 836–43.
107. Choi, H. *et al.*, Correlation of computed tomography and positron emission tomography in patients with metastatic gastrointestinal stromal tumor treated at a single institution with imatinib mesylate: proposal of new computed tomography response criteria. *J Clin Oncol*, 2007. **25**(13): 1753–9.
108. Holdsworth, C.H. *et al.*, CT and PET: early prognostic indicators of response to imatinib mesylate in patients with gastrointestinal stromal tumor. *AJR Am J Roentgenol*, 2007. **189**(6): W324–30.
109. Cohen, M.H. *et al.*, Approval summary: imatinib mesylate for one or three years in the adjuvant treatment of gastrointestinal stromal tumors. *Oncologist*, 2012. **17**(7): 992–7.
110. Demetri, G.D. *et al.*, NCCN Task Force report: update on the management of patients with gastrointestinal stromal tumors. *J Natl Compr Canc Netw*, 2010. 8 Suppl 2: S1–41; quiz S42–4.
111. Cananzi, F.C. *et al.*, Multidisciplinary care of gastrointestinal stromal tumour: a review and a proposal for a pre-treatment classification. *Eur J Surg Oncol*, 2013. **39**(11): 1171–8.
112. Dematteo, R.P. *et al.*, Adjuvant imatinib mesylate after resection of localised, primary gastrointestinal stromal tumour: a randomised, double-blind, placebo-controlled trial. *Lancet*, 2009. **373**(9669): 1097–104.

113. Doyon, C. *et al.*, Prolonged therapy with imatinib mesylate before surgery for advanced gastrointestinal stromal tumor results of a phase II trial. *Int J Surg Oncol*, 2012. 2012: 761576.
114. Wang, D. *et al.*, Phase II trial of neoadjuvant/adjuvant imatinib mesylate for advanced primary and metastatic/recurrent operable gastrointestinal stromal tumors: long-term follow-up results of Radiation Therapy Oncology Group 0132. *Ann Surg Oncol*, 2012. **19**(4): 1074–80.
115. McAuliffe, J.C. *et al.*, A randomized, phase II study of preoperative plus postoperative imatinib in GIST: evidence of rapid radiographic response and temporal induction of tumor cell apoptosis. *Ann Surg Oncol*, 2009. **16**(4): 910–9.
116. Joensuu, H. *et al.*, One vs three years of adjuvant imatinib for operable gastrointestinal stromal tumor: a randomized trial. *JAMA*, 2012. **307**(12): 1265–72.
117. http://clinicaltrials.gov/ct2/show/NCT00867113.
118. Demetri, G.D. *et al.*, Efficacy and safety of imatinib mesylate in advanced gastrointestinal stromal tumors. *N Engl J Med*, 2002. **347**(7): 472–80.
119. Verweij, J. *et al.*, Imatinib mesylate (STI-571 Glivec, Gleevec) is an active agent for gastrointestinal stromal tumours, but does not yield responses in other soft-tissue sarcomas that are unselected for a molecular target. Results from an EORTC Soft Tissue and Bone Sarcoma Group phase II study. *Eur J Cancer*, 2003. **39**(14): 2006–11.
120. Heinrich, M.C. *et al.*, Correlation of kinase genotype and clinical outcome in the North American Intergroup Phase III Trial of imatinib mesylate for treatment of advanced gastrointestinal stromal tumor: CALGB 150105 Study by Cancer and Leukemia Group B and Southwest Oncology Group. *J Clin Oncol*, 2008. **26**(33): 5360–7.
121. Gastrointestinal Stromal Tumor Meta-Analysis, G., Comparison of two doses of imatinib for the treatment of unresectable or metastatic gastrointestinal stromal tumors: a meta-analysis of 1,640 patients. *J Clin Oncol*, 2010. **28**(7): 1247–53.
122. Hislop, J. *et al.*, Systematic review of escalated imatinib doses compared with sunitinib or best supportive care, for the treatment of people with unresectable/metastatic gastrointestinal stromal tumours whose disease has progressed on the standard imatinib dose. *J Gastrointest Cancer*, 2012. **43**(2): 168–76.

123. Demetri, G.D. *et al.*, Efficacy and safety of sunitinib in patients with advanced gastrointestinal stromal tumour after failure of imatinib: a randomised controlled trial. *Lancet*, 2006. **368**(9544): 1329–38.
124. Sawaki, A. *et al.*, Phase 2 study of nilotinib as third-line therapy for patients with gastrointestinal stromal tumor. *Cancer*, 2011. **117**(20): 4633–41.
125. Demetri, G.D. *et al.*, Efficacy and safety of regorafenib for advanced gastrointestinal stromal tumours after failure of imatinib and sunitinib (GRID): an international, multicentre, randomised, placebo-controlled, phase 3 trial. *Lancet*, 2013. **381**(9863): 295–302.

Chapter 22

The Essentials of the Gastrointestinal and Pancreaticobiliary Malignancies Pathology

Yue Xue

What is New

- The practice of gastrointestinal pathology, in particular, oncologic pathology, has undergone a dramatic transformation in the past decade. The increasing integration of molecular biology with gastrointestinal pathology is occurring at a fast pace.
- It is essential for clinicians to remain informed about the changes to provide better patient care.

Gastrointestinal malignancies are some of the most prevalent and important malignancies throughout the world. Within this group of neoplasms is a wide range of organ involvement and histologic variability, and this chapter will focus on the most common examples.

Esophageal Carcinoma

Esophageal carcinoma can be divided into two main histological types: squamous cell carcinomas and adenocarcinomas. These differ markedly in their etiology and epidemiology.

Worldwide, squamous cell carcinoma is the most common neoplasm of the esophagus, but in the United States it is considered a "low-risk" entity with most cases occurring in African-Americans over 50 years of age. There are multiple established risk factors associated with squamous cell carcinoma including smoking, alcohol, consumption of food rich in nitrates and nitrosamines, achalasia, Tylosis, and Plummer-Vinson syndrome.[1] This carcinoma most commonly occurs in the middle and lower thirds of the esophagus. Microscopically, it develops from squamous epithelium often preceded by dysplastic changes. The malignant cells show enlarged, often vesicular nuclei, densely eosinophilic cytoplasm, and intercellular bridges with varying degrees of keratinization, pleomorphism and mitotic rates (Fig. 1). Adenocarcinoma, the more common histological pattern in the United States, has a predilection toward Caucasian males with Barrett esophagus as the only recognized precursor. Most adenocarcinomas are mucin-producing exhibiting intestinal-type features (Fig. 2). They are commonly situated in the lower third of the esophagus.

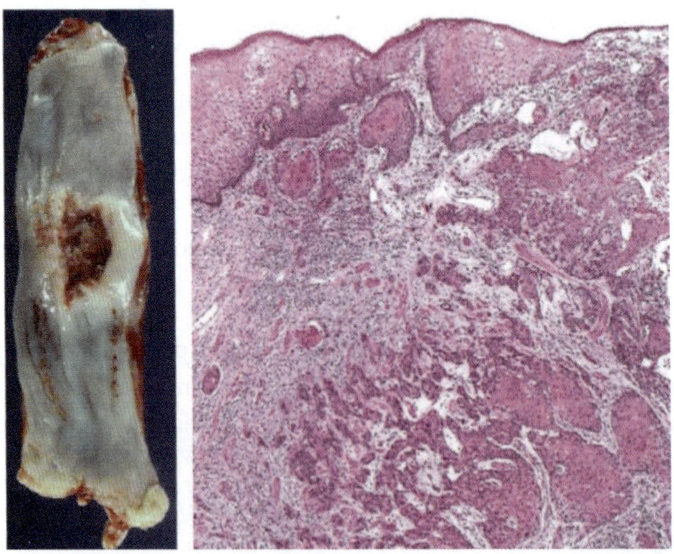

(a) (b)

Fig. 1. Esophageal squamous cell carcinoma. (a) Carcinoma presents as an ulcer. (b) Microscopically, it shows infiltrative keratinizing squamous cell carcinoma (H&E 40x).

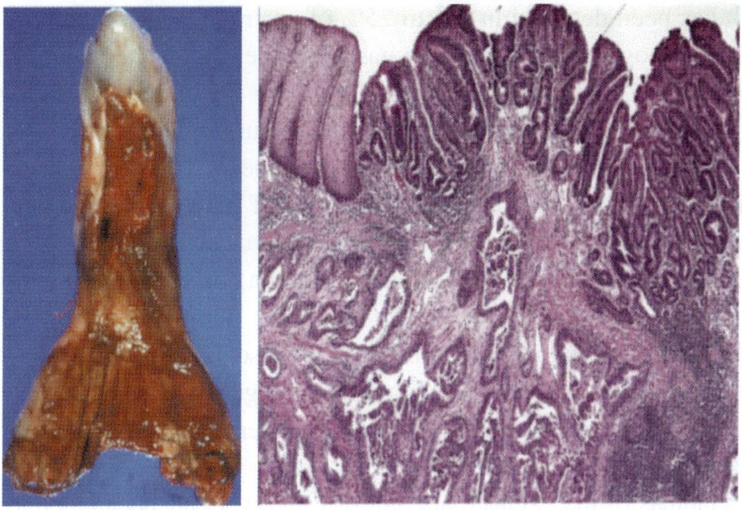

(a) (b)

Fig. 2. Esophageal adenocarcinoma. (a) Adenocarcinoma presents as an ulcer. (b) Microscopically, it shows infiltrative glandular structure (H&E 40x).

Carcinoma of the esophagus usually begins as an ulcer and forms an annular constriction causing dysphasia. Patient prognosis is dependent on the disease stage at presentation. Five-year survival for cancers confined to the mucosa with no lymph node metastases is greater than 90%. However, 70% of patients have widespread local disease or metastatic disease at presentation and can no longer be cured by surgical resection.[2] These patients may receive palliative chemotherapy or chemoradiation with five-year survival less than 10%.[2]

Gastric Carcinoma

Gastric cancer is the fourth most common cancer and the second leading cause of cancer death worldwide.[3] Ten percent of gastric cancer show familial clustering, but only 1–3% of gastric cancer are related to an inherited gastric cancer syndrome, such as hereditary diffuse gastric cancer, a CDH1 (E-cadherin) germline mutation.[4]

Helicobacter pylori have been identified as the most important environmental risk factor for gastric cancer. Additionally, Epstein–Barr virus

(EBV) has been detected in 5% to 25% of gastric adenocarcinoma.[4] The prominent geographic variation in gastric cancer incidence suggests that environmental factors such as diet might play an important etiological role. Smoking, obesity and previous gastric surgery for benign disease have all been implicated in gastric carcinogenesis.[4] Gastric cancers are classified as either "early" or "locally advanced" based upon the depth of invasion into the stomach wall. Early gastric cancer is defined as cancer limited to the mucosa (intramucosal carcinoma) or submucosa irrespective of the lymph node status, tumor size or duration of the disease. Locally advanced gastric cancer invades the muscularis propria or beyond. Ninety percent of patients with intramucosal gastric cancer survive for more than five years, whereas only 16% of patients with locally advanced cancers survive greater than five years.[5]

Carcinomas of the stomach are almost exclusively adenocarcinomas and usually arise in individuals over 50 years of age. Their gross appearance varies from fungating and exophytic to flat, ulcerated, and deeply invasive. Morphologically, they are most commonly classified as either "tubular" or "diffuse" types according to the classification devised by Laurén (Fig. 3). Histologically, they are graded according to their degree of differentiation into well-, moderately-, and poorly-differentiated carcinomas. Sixty to seventy

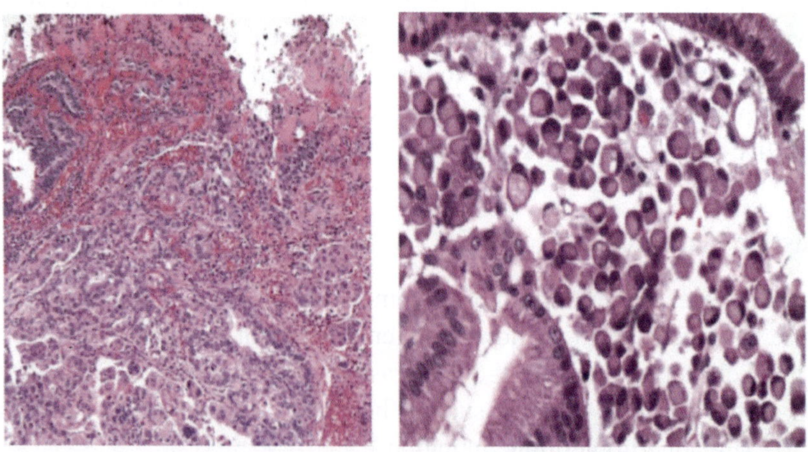

(a) (b)

Fig. 3. Gastric adenocarcinoma. (a) Tubular type (H&E 100x). (b) Diffuse type (H&E 100x).

percent are intestinal-type carcinomas, which are thought to arise from gastric mucous cells that have undergone intestinal metaplasia in the setting of chronic gastritis. The intestinal type resembles colonic adenocarcinoma and is composed of glandular to solid columnar mucus-secreting cells that tend to be more differentiated. The diffuse variant is thought to arise from native gastric mucous cells and tends to be poorly differentiated. This morphology is not associated with chronic gastritis and risk factors are largely unknown, although germ-line mutations in E-cadherin leading to an autosomal dominant inheritance of diffuse gastric carcinoma have been reported. The diffuse-type is characterized by the growth of individual signet-ring cells, marked desmoplasia, and inflammation.

Colorectal and Small Intestinal Carcinoma

Cancer of the colon and rectum is one of the most common forms of malignancy in developed countries with a 20-fold difference in incidence between high-risk areas (Europe, Americas, Australia) and low-risk regions (Asia, Africa) reported.[6] A great majority of all large intestine cancers are adenocarcinomas, and most arise from adenomatous polyps that are generally curable by resection. Most of the cancers are located in the rectosigmoid region, but the incidence of right-sided tumor is rising. Although rare, within the small bowel the tumor favors the duodenum, including the ampulla of Vater.

The peak incidence for colorectal cancer is in the seventh and eighth decade but 20% occurs under the age of 50. In these younger patients, carcinoma is frequently associated with predispositions such as ulcerative colitis, familiar adenomatous polyposis (FAP), or hereditary nonpolyposis colorectal carcinoma (HNPCC).

Although all colorectal carcinomas begin as in situ lesions, they progress into different morphologic patterns. Tumors in the proximal colon tend to grow as polypoid, exophytic masses that extend along one wall of the capacious cecum and ascending colon. When discovered in the distal colon, lesions tend to be annular and encircling, producing the so-called napkin-ring constrictions of the bowel lumen. Regardless of gross appearance, all colon carcinomas are microscopically similar and show varying degrees of mucin production and glandular differentiation ranging from well-differentiated to poorly-undifferentiated, frankly anaplastic masses (Fig. 4). The role of the pathologist is paramount for determination of proper tumor excision and the extent of spread. If microscopic examination of the resection margins establishes that the entire tumor has been removed and the operation has potentially been curative, then the extent of spread through the bowel wall and the presence of lymph node metastases are the major prognostic determinants. Seventy percent of patients with colorectal cancer undergo a potentially curative operation; conversely, about 15–25% of patients have widespread peritoneal deposits or liver metastases.[7] With preoperative radio/chemotherapy, the proportion of potentially curative operations is on the rise. Patients formerly considered inoperable because of liver metastases are now undergoing partial liver resections following treatment. Overall, the outlook for patients with colorectal cancer has improved remarkably in recent years.

Neuroendocrine Tumors

Neuroendocrine tumors of the gastrointestinal tract originate from the diffuse neuroendocrine system. There are two main microscopic types: the "neuroendocrine tumor" which is composed of solid nests of regular

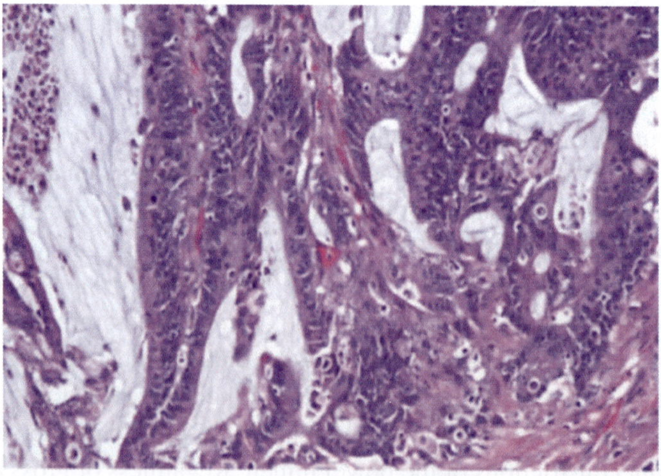

Fig. 4. Colorectal adenocarcinoma. Adenocarcinoma shows glandular differentiation (H&E 100x).

cells with lightly staining nuclei that express neuroendocrine markers by immunohistochemistry; the second type, the "neuroendocrine carcinoma," is rare in the gastrointestinal tract and is composed of undifferentiated small or large tumor cells indistinguishable from its counterpart in the lung.

Gastric neuroendocrine tumors are relatively frequent, comprising up to 30% of all gastrointestinal neuroendocrine tumors.[8] Three forms are encountered. Most common are the multiple, small, polypoid tumors found in association with autoimmune chronic gastritis. A second form is a solitary, usually, larger polyp which is a sporadic finding with no associated disease, and the third form is associated with a familial syndrome, such as MEN II. In the autoimmune associated form, the glandular atrophy leads to achlorhydria, which stimulates antral G cells to produce gastrin. Persistent hypergastrinemia leads to hyperplasia of the enterochromaffin-like (ECL) cells in the body of the stomach which give rise to multiple tumors (Fig. 5). This clinicopathological distinction is important in terms of behavior. Neuroendocrine tumors associated with autoimmune gastritis do not metastasize and can be considered benign. In contrast, the sporadic tumors carry a definite risk of metastasis and require complete removal regardless of their size.[8]

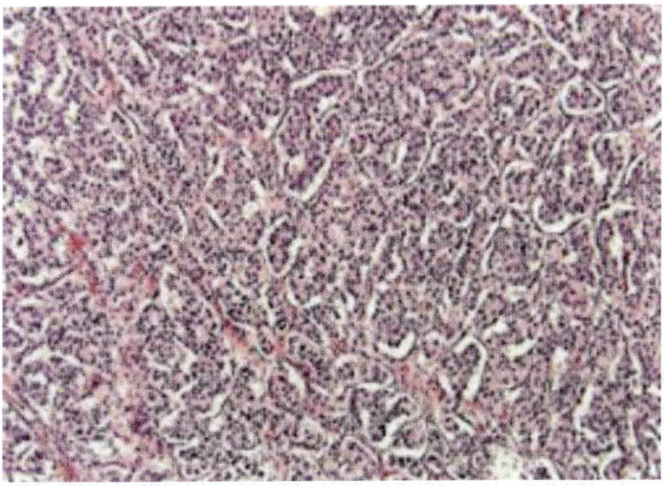

Fig. 5. Well-differentiated neuroendocrine tumor (H&E 100x).

Most duodenal neuroendocrine tumors are gastrinomas, i.e. gastrin-producing tumors, and are associated with the Zollinger–Ellison syndrome. However, there are several other varieties including somatostatinomas, calcitonin-producing tumors, non-functioning tumors, or poorly differentiated neuroendocrine carcinomas.

The distal jejunum and ileum account for about 25% of neuroendocrine tumors, and at the time of diagnosis frequently spread to the mesenteric lymph nodes is present. Additionally, approximately 20% of patients will have liver metastases at presentation. These tumors contain serotonin (5-hydroxytryptamine; 5-HT), substance P, kallikrein and catecholamines. 5-HT released by the tumor is inactivated in the liver by monoamine oxidases to form 5-hydroxyindole acetic acid (5-HIAA), which is excreted in the urine. Once metastases have formed in the liver, the tumor products (5-HT and kinins) are released directly into the hepatic veins resulting in the carcinoid syndrome.

Neuroendocrine tumors in the appendix are generally small (less than 2 cm in diameter), incidental findings situated at or near the tip. Such small tumors can be considered benign, and no further treatment is necessary; however, larger tumors do occasionally metastasize.

Hepatocellular Carcinoma

Hepatocellular carcinoma (HCC) has a high incidence worldwide, accounting for approximately 5.4% of all cancers,[3] but its incidence varies widely in different parts of the world. It is the most common type of cancer in parts of East Asia and central Africa, where it is associated with hepatitis B infection. Aflatoxin, a mycotoxin found in grain stores contaminated by the fungus *Aspergillus flavus*, is an additional synergistic factor in HCC oncogenesis. In Western countries, cirrhosis, especially secondary to alcohol and/or viral hepatitis (particularly hepatitis C), is the most important risk factor. Non-alcoholic fatty liver disease is also emerging as an often synergistic factor in disease development.

Macroscopically, most HCC develop in the setting of cirrhosis, as a result of progression of pre-malignant lesions to dysplastic nodules. The appearance is frequently a round, soft, bulging tumor which can be tan-colored, green or hemorrhagic. In cirrhosis, there are often multiple tumor nodules (Fig. 6). Histologically, the most characteristic pattern recapitulates normal liver architecture with trabeculae and intervening sinusoidal vascular channels (Fig. 6). The tumor cells are large with abundant cytoplasm, high nucleocytoplasmic ratio, and large nucleoli. Though the liver is the site for both primary and metastatic tumors, presence of bile within the tumor cells is diagnostic of a hepatocellular origin.

Pancreatic Cancer

Infiltrating ductal adenocarcinoma of the pancreas (more commonly referred to as "pancreatic cancer") is more common in developed countries and is the fourth leading cause of cancer death in the United States.[3] The most important risk factor for developing pancreatic cancer is cigarette smoking, though an increased risk is also observed with type II diabetes mellitus, hereditary pancreatitis, chronic pancreatitis and a strong family history which could be related to cancer syndromes such as Lynch syndrome or Peutz–Jeghers syndrome.[9]

Approximately 60% of pancreatic cancers arise in the head of the organ.[9] Carcinomas of the pancreas are usually hard, gray-white, stellate, poorly defined masses. Histologically, the tumors recapitulate to some degree the normal duct epithelium with formation of glands and secretion

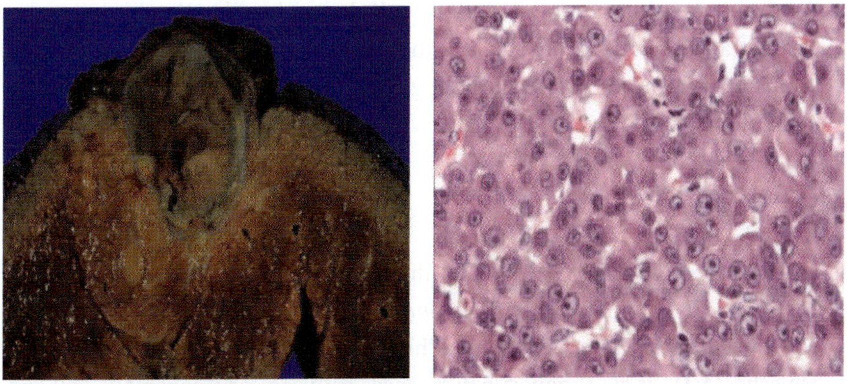

(a) (b)

Fig. 6. Hepatocellular carcinoma. (a) Grossly, it represents as a mass lesion. (b) Microscopically, the carcinoma shows trabecular pattern (H&E 100x).

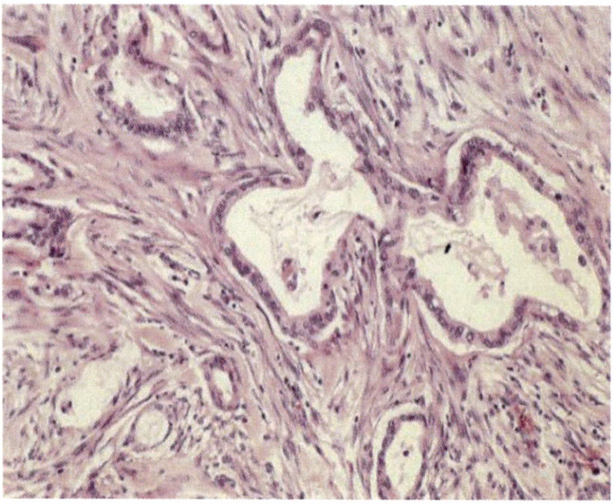

Fig. 7. Pancreatic adenocarcinoma (H&E 200x).

of mucin, but the tumor cells are surrounded by a prominent desmoplastic stroma (Fig. 7).

Take Home Messages

- With the developments of modern cellular and molecular biology, the understanding of the basic pathology underlying common neoplasms plays an important role in the diagnosis and subsequent management of patients with these neoplasms.

References

1. Glickman, J.N., Odze, R.D., Epithelial neoplasms of the esophagus. In: Odze R.D., Goldblum J.R., eds. *Surgical Pathology of the GI Tract, Liver, Biliary Tract and Pancreas. 3rd ed.* Philadelphia; Saunders, 2015.
2. Holscher, A.H. *et al.*, Prognostic differences between early squamous-cell and adenocarcinoma of the esophagus. *Dis Esophagus*, 1997. **10**(3): 179–84.
3. Aarnio, M. *et al.*, Features of gastric cancer in hereditary non-polyposis colorectal cancer syndrome. *Int J Cancer*, 1997. **74**(5): 551–5.

4. Antonioli, D.A., Precursors of gastric carcinoma: a critical review with a brief description of early (curable) gastric cancer. *Hum Pathol*, 1994. **25**(10): 994–1005.
5. Park, J.Y. *et al.*, Epithelial neoplasms of the stomach. In Iacobuzio-Donahue and Montgomery E. *Gastrointestinal and liver pathology 2nd ed.* Philadelphia; Saunders, 2012.
6. Fares, A., Global patterns of seasonal variation in gastrointestinal disease. *J Postgrad Med*, 2013. **59**(3): 203–7.
7. Washington, M.K., Colorectal carcinoma: selected issues in pathologic examination and staging and determination of prognostic factors. *Arch Pathol Lab Med*, 2008. **132**(10): 1600–7.
8. Hirabayashi, K. *et al.*, Histopathology of gastrointestinal neuroendocrine neoplasms. *Front Oncol*, 2013. **3**.
9. Esposito, I. *et al.*, Pathology of pancreatic ductal adenocarcinoma: facts, challenges and future developments. *World J Gastroenterol*, 2014. **20**(38): 13833–41.

Chapter 23

Proton Therapy: A New Dawn for Gastrointestinal Cancer Treatment

Gary Y. Yang and Jerome C. Landry

What is New

- Improvements in radiation delivery techniques have resulted in methods to improve beam conformity around treatment targets.
- Protons have an inherent dosimetric advantage over photons due to their absence of exit dose, resulting in a reduction in the volume of normal structures receiving doses of radiation when compared with IMRT (intensity-modulated radiation therapy) and three-dimensional conformal radiation therapy (3D-CRT) plans.

Introduction

Proton radiation therapy has gained popularity over the past few decades as a means of optimizing radiation treatment. There is still a paucity of data involving the use of proton therapy in gastrointestinal malignancy due to a relative lack of clinically available proton treatment facilities worldwide.

Most of the radiation given with conventional X-ray, or photon, therapy is deposited along the entrance and exit of the beam path. In contrast, protons are small charged particles that travel only a finite distance in tissue. Most of an accelerated proton's energy is deposited as a Bragg peak at the end of the beam path. The depth of this Bragg peak can be modulated by either varying the proton beam energy or adding compensators to the treatment gantry. Therefore, the integral dose is greatly reduced since there is no exit dose and the entrance dose is greatly reduced relative to the Bragg peak.

The ability to dose-escalate at the tumor while maintaining low toxicity in normal tissues may improve the therapeutic ratio of radiation treatment. The kidneys, for example, are often involved in the radiation fields when treating gastric or pancreatic cancer. There is evidence of decline in relative renal function following kidney irradiation.[1] The degree of dysfunction correlates with the amount of radiation received. These adverse outcomes emphasize the importance of sparing normal tissue from dose during radiation therapy.

Proton Beam Therapy

Physical properties of proton beams

Proton beams have limited range, sharp lateral penumbra, without any increased dose effect on beam entry and practically without dose on beam exit as well. Due to the physical properties as mentioned above, proton beams can achieve a homogeneous distribution of a large dose in a limited space (tumor with margin) while simultaneously protect healthy tissues and the vital organs by limiting the dose and irradiated volume.[2]

Mechanisms

Unlike a photon, a proton is a heavy particle (approximately 1800 times the mass of an electron) with a positive elementary charge, which confers certain dosimetric advantages. As opposed to photons, heavy particles will stop within a target.

A proton beam is produced by an accelerating device (generally a cyclotron or synchrotron) which separates the proton from a hydrogen molecule and accelerates it. The accelerated protons then enter the body with a high momentum which carries them to a specific depth.

After traveling a certain distance, the velocity is slowed by interactions with surrounding tissue, and then stopped very abruptly at a very specific area. In contrast, photons do not stop and travel through the entire body from the entrance to the exit sites. These differences can be used to produce potentially safer radiation treatment plans.

Shortly before the entire energy of the proton is lost, the energy loss rate reaches a sharp peak. Once the kinetic energy of the proton is entirely dissipated into the tissue, the proton comes to rest within the body. This is the point at which the energy of the proton is dissipated in collisions with the electrons of the neighboring atoms in the surrounding tissues causing ionization of molecules and radiation damage within the DNA of the target cell.

This unique property allows protons to be targeted so that they have their most therapeutic effects on the tumor, with less radiation delivered in front of the target, and no radiation delivered beyond it. This sharp, well defined peak of maximal dose from charged particles is commonly referred to as the "Bragg peak." The Bragg peak is very narrow and there is no radiation energy imparted upon surrounding tissues as the protons have stopped traveling. Therefore, spread-out Bragg peak (SOBP) is applied to maximize the radiation damage to the cancerous organ to ensure that the range of peak radiation energy encompasses the entire target.

Administrations

Protons can be delivered with two different radiation techniques: passive scattering proton therapy (PSPT) or pencil beam scanning (PBS). In PSPT, the tumor volume is irradiated as a whole. Compensators are employed within the beam to alter the beam profile to better conform the SOBP to the actual tumor. With PBS, the target volume is scanned spot-by-spot with a very narrow, pencil thin proton beam. No blocks or compensators are needed. The pencil beam is swept in a raster pattern back and forth across a target guided out of the nozzle by magnets, which allows the delivery of intensity-modulated proton beam therapy (IMPT) with a greater ability to conform the dose to an irregularly shaped target.

Proton Therapy for Treating Gastrointestinal Malignancy

The use of proton therapy for treating gastrointestinal malignancy is still a topic of many ongoing studies. Nonetheless, the opportunity to improve dose distribution to highly critical organs within the abdominal cavity presents itself as a major topic of interest.

Esophageal cancer

Neoadjuvant chemoradiation followed by surgery, also called as trimodality therapy, is the current standard treatment for nonmetastatic esophageal cancer.[3]

Advanced radiation technologies using either intensity modulated RT (IMRT) or proton beam therapy (PBT) could improve clinical outcomes, while significantly reduced postoperative pulmonary and gastrointestinal complication rates compared to three-dimensional conformal radiation therapy (3D-CRT) in esophageal cancer patients.[4]

Proton beam delivery may enable dose escalation in the primary tumor without a corresponding dose increase in surrounding tissues. Investigators at MD Anderson Cancer Center examined theoretical distal esophageal intensity modulated proton therapy (IMPT) plans using AP/PA, LPO/RPO, or AP/LPO/RPO beam arrangements, and the results showed that all three of the IMPT plan types were advantageous over IMRT.[5]

Hepatocellular carcinoma

As the main cause of the deaths in hepatocellular carcinoma (HCC) population is loco-regional progression,[6] a strong rationale exists for the improvement of loco-regional therapies in HCC patients. Surgery, including resection and liver transplantation, can achieve the best outcomes in the treatment of HCC. However, a certain percentage of HCC patients are unsuitable for surgery due to the unresectable tumor or the patients' co-mobility. Alternative approaches for localized HCC consist of ablation with percutaneous ethanol injection (PEI), transarterial chemoembolization (TACE), and radiotherapy. In the context of HCC, radiotherapy has a narrow therapeutic window due to the low-radio-tolerance of the liver and the need for high doses of radiation for disease control. Irreversible hepatic failure may occur as a consequence of radiation-induced liver disease (RILD).[7]

Proton therapy (PT), due to its unique dosimetric characteristics, could be an excellent option for the treatment of this disease. Many studies proved that PBT is safe and effective in treatment of HCC.[8,9] A five-year survival rate could reach 53.5% in the patients with solitary HCC and Child-A liver function,[9] which was comparable to the results of surgical resection.[10] Since PBT is safe and has limited effects on liver function,[11] it is especially recommended to aged HCC patients[12] or to patients with limited treatment options due to various extrahepatic complications or poor liver function.[13]

Cholangiocarcinoma

At the present time, surgery is the only potentially curative treatment for cholangiocarcinoma. However, only 10% to 30% patients are candidates for surgery, as most patients present with either locally advanced or distant metastatic disease.[14]

Makita C *et al.*[15] applied PBT on 28 patients with advanced cholangiocarcinoma (18 patients with unresectable cholangiocarcinoma and 10 with recurrent tumor after surgery). The results showed that relatively high local control (LC) rates after PBT could be achieved by delivery of a biologically equivalent dose of 10 (BED10) > 70 Gy. The gastrointestinal tract complications may occur due to the irradiation, hereby the irradiated volume of duodenal irradiation should be decreased in PBT to minimize toxicity in patients with cholangiocarcinoma adjacent to the gastrointestinal tract, especially the duodenum.[15]

Pancreatic cancer

The pancreas is located in the retroperitoneum, closely abutting several critical organs. A proton beam's unique qualities would seem to lend itself well to such a situation (Figs. 1–4). Studies from Loma Linda University and MD Anderson compared target coverage and dose-volume histograms of proton therapy plans to various 3D conformal and IMRT photon

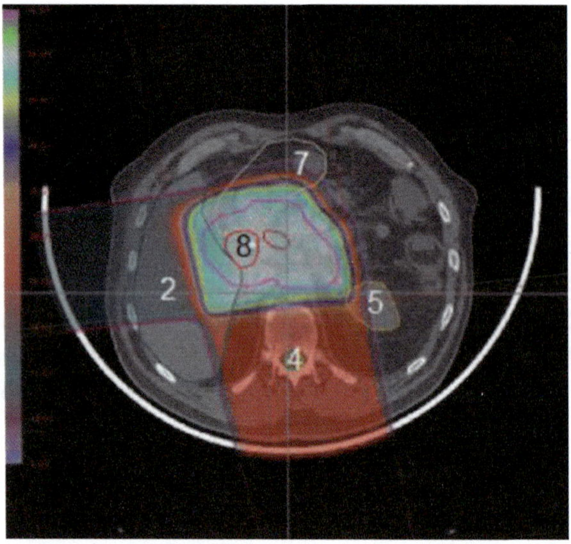

Fig. 1. Axial view of right oblique and posterior oblique proton beam entering the body to treat the postoperative pancreatic bed. The posterior beam is more heavily weighed and the dose from both beams drop off after the postoperative bed is reached; 2. liver; 4. spinal cord; 5. left kidney; 7. duodenum; 8. surgical clips.

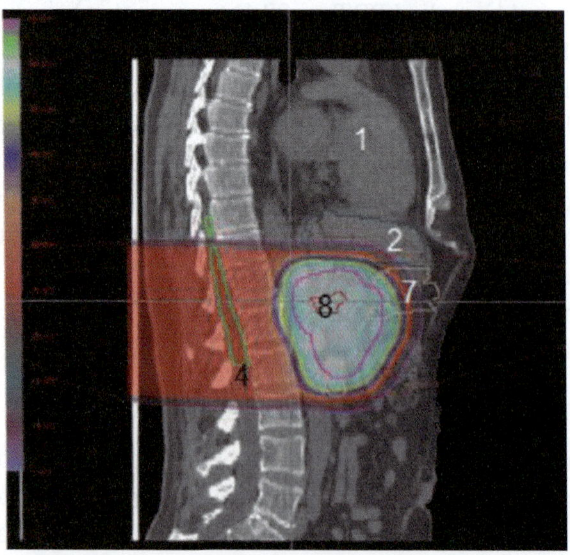

Fig. 2. Sagittal view of posterior oblique proton beam targeting postoperative pancreatic bed. This minimizes radiation dose to the liver, stomach, and bowel; 1. heart; 2. liver; 4. spinal cord; 7. duodenum; 8. surgical clips.

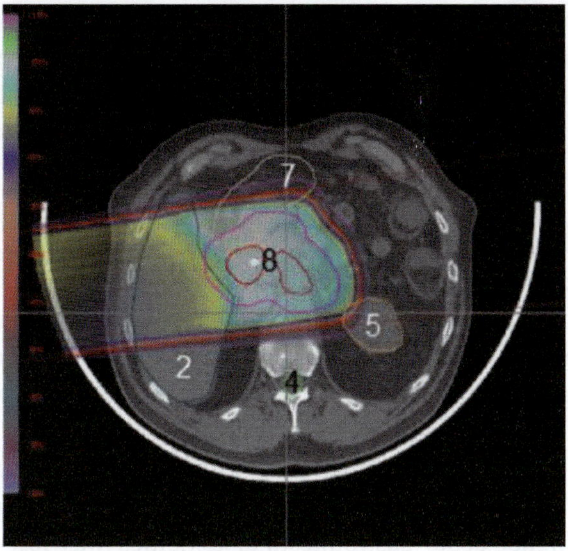

Fig. 3. Axial view of right oblique proton beam targeting postoperative pancreatic bed; 2. liver; 4. spinal cord; 5. left kidney; 7. duodenum; 8. surgical clips.

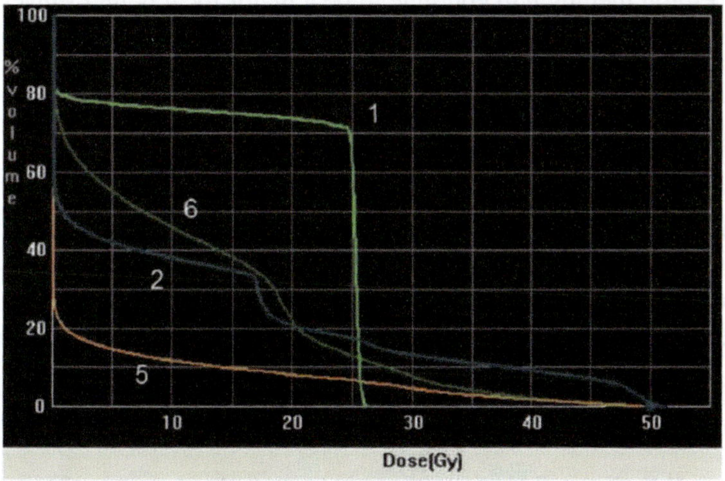

Fig. 4. Dose-volume histogram for treatment plan seen in figures showing the amount of dose received by each organ; 1. heart; 2. liver; 5. left kidney; 6. right kidney.

plans.[16,17] The proton therapy plans demonstrated significantly lower integral doses. In particular, the rapid downstream falloff of dose for tumors near the ligament of Treitz enabled complete coverage of the planning target volume while staying within acceptable normal-tissue toxicity limits.

At the 2014 Gastrointestinal Cancers Symposium, University of Florida reported that proton dose to 59.4 CGE with concomitant capecitabine was well-tolerated with no grade 2 or greater gastrointestinal toxicities. Four of 11 patients achieved a radiographic response allowing for attempted surgical resection. The lack of any meaningful gastrointestinal toxicity suggests significant opportunities for treatment intensification when proton therapy is used in this setting.[18]

In Japan concurrent proton therapy with high-dose gemcitabine has been studied, showing high feasibility and tolerability.[19] The frequency of grade 3 or higher acute gastrointestinal toxicities was low even when using doses as high as 70.2 GyE. Major late toxicities varied, depending on pancreatic tumor position relative to organ anatomy. Nonetheless, they were significantly reduced when using a field-in-field technique, as in this study. Proton therapy will continue to be a major focal point of investigation in future pancreatic cancer dose-escalation studies.

Take Home Messages

- Clinical studies demonstrate a significant tissue-sparing benefit and superior target coverage of proton plans over the IMRT and 3D-CRT plans.
- It appears that proton radiotherapy warrants further investigation as a means of improving the therapeutic ratio for gastrointestinal cancers.

References

1. May, K.S., Yang, G.Y., Khushalani, N.I. *et al.*, Association of Technetium (99m) MAG-3 renal scintigraphy with change in creatinine clearance following chemoradiation to the abdomen in patients with gastrointestinal malignancies. *J Gastrointest Oncol*, 2010. **1**(1): 7–15.

2. Engelsman, M., Schwarz, M., Dong, L., Physics controversies in proton therapy. *Semin Radiat Oncol*, 2013. **23**(2): 88–96.
3. Tepper, J., Krasna, M.J., Niedzwiecki, D. *et al.*, Phase III trial of trimodality therapy with cisplatin, fluorouracil, radiotherapy, and surgery compared with surgery alone for esophageal cancer: CALGB 9781. *J Clin Oncol*, 2008. **26**(7): 1086–92.
4. Wang, J., Wei, C., Tucker, S.L. *et al.*, Predictors of postoperative complications after trimodality therapy for esophageal cancer. *Int J Radiat Oncol Biol Phys*, 2013. **86**(5): 885–91.
5. Welsh, J., Gomez, D., Palmer, M.B. *et al.*, Intensity-modulated proton therapy further reduces normal tissue exposure during definitive therapy for locally advanced distal esophageal tumors: a dosimetric study. *Int J Radiat Oncol Biol Phys*, 2011. **81**(5): 1336–42.
6. Trevisani, F., Cantarini, M.C., Wands, J.R., and Bernardi, M., Recent advances in the natural history of hepatocellular carcinoma. *Carcinogenesis*, 2008. **29**(7): 1299–305.
7. Pan, C.C., Kavanagh, B.D., Dawson, L.A. *et al.*, Radiation-associated liver injury. *Int J Radiat Oncol Biol Phys*, 2010. **76**(3 Suppl): S94–S100.
8. Bush, D.A., Kayali, Z., Grove, R. *et al.*, The safety and efficacy of high-dose proton beam radiotherapy for hepatocellular carcinoma: a phase 2 prospective trial. *Cancer,* 2011. **117**(13): 3053–9.
9. Chiba, T., Tokuuye, K., Matsuzaki, Y. *et al.*, Proton beam therapy for hepatocellular carcinoma: a retrospective review of 162 patients. *Clin Cancer Res*, 2005. **11**(10): 3799–805.
10. Ikai, I., Arii, S., Okazaki, M. *et al.*, Report of the 17th nationwide follow-up survey of primary liver cancer in Japan. *Hepatol Res*, 2007. **37**(9): 676–91.
11. Mizumoto, M., Okumura, T., Hashimoto, T. *et al.*, Evaluation of liver function after proton beam therapy for hepatocellular carcinoma. *Int J Radiat Oncol Biol Phys*, 2012. **82**(3): e529–35.
12. Hata, M., Tokuuye, K., Sugahara, S. *et al.*, Proton beam therapy for aged patients with hepatocellular carcinoma. *Int J Radiat Oncol Biol Phys*, 2007. **69**(3): 805–12.
13. Hata, M., Tokuuye, K., Sugahara, S. *et al.*, Proton beam therapy for hepatocellular carcinoma patients with severe cirrhosis. *Strahlenther Onkol*, 2006. **182**(12): 713–20.

14. Erickson, B.A., Nag, S., Biliary tree malignancies. *J Surg Oncol*, 1998. **67**(3): 203–10.
15. Makita, C., Nakamura, T., Takada, A. *et al.*, Clinical outcomes and toxicity of proton beam therapy for advanced cholangiocarcinoma, *Radiat Oncol*, 2014. **9**: 26.
16. Slater, J.E., Ling, T.C., Nookala, P. *et al.*, A treatment planning evaluation of protons versus IMRT in pancreatic cancer: A comparative study, *J Clin Oncol*, 2014. **32**(Suppl 3): 369.
17. Bouchard, M., Amos, R.A., Briere, T.M. *et al.*, Dose escalation with proton or photon radiation treatment for pancreatic cancer. *Radiother Oncol*, 2009. **92**(2): 238–43.
18. Nichols, R.C., Morris, C.G., George, T.J. *et al.*, First report of a prospective trial of proton therapy and concomittant capecitabine for patients with non-metastatic unresectable pancreatic adenocarcinoma. *J Clin Oncol*, 2014. **32**(Suppl 3): 326.
19. Terashima, K., Demizu, Y., Hashimoto, N. *et al.*, A phase I/II study of gemcitabine-concurrent proton radiotherapy for locally advanced pancreatic cancer without distant metastasis. *Radiother Oncol*, 2012. **103**(1): 25–31.

Chapter 24

Radiotherapy for Rectal Cancer

Jordan Torok, Manisha Palta, Christopher Willett and Brian Czito

What's New

- Current studies are investigating a short course radiotherapy approach neoadjuvantly for rectal cancer as opposed to a more traditional protracted course.
- These short course studies may confer lower cost, increased compliance, and potentially reduced toxicities.

Overview

In the treatment of rectal cancer, the role of radiation therapy (RT) has been rigorously investigated over the past several decades. There have been advancements in imaging, radiation therapy strategies, surgical techniques and the use of chemotherapeutic agents during this time. The introduction of total mesorectal excision (TME) has dramatically reduced the number and altered the patterns of recurrences. Radiation therapy, with or without chemotherapy, reduces local recurrences (LR) in advanced rectal cancers, particularly in the neoadjuvant setting. This section will review the pertinent data of RT for rectal cancer with an emphasis on paradigm shifts, current standards of care, and future directions.

Early Stage Disease

While TME is considered the standard surgical approach for most rectal cancers, transanal excision may be considered for a subset of favorable early stage tumors. This technique has been studied primarily in distal rectal tumors in an effort to conserve the anal sphincter and avoid the morbidity of an abdominoperineal resection (APR). The Radiation Therapy Oncology Group (RTOG)[1] and Cancer and Leukemia Group B (CALGB)[2] both conducted prospective evaluations of this technique in distal rectal tumors with adjuvant radiation therapy reserved for high-risk features. Local recurrence rates were low for T1 tumors, while rates of recurrence increased significantly for T2/T3 tumors despite adjuvant therapy. Local excision alone may be appropriate for small (<3 cm), T1N0 tumors involving <30% of the rectal circumference and within 8 cm of the anal verge. Pathologic factors in the excised specimen supporting this approach include negative margins (>3 mm), well to moderately differentiated histology, no lymphovascular invasion and confinement to the upper 2/3rds of the submucosa.[3] If the tumor does not meet these criteria, either a complete resection by TME and/or adjuvant chemoradiotherapy should be considered.

An alternative approach to early stage disease was investigated by the American College of Surgeons Oncology Group (ACOSOG Z6041).[4] In a prospective phase II trial, patients with T2N0 rectal cancer, as defined by pretreatment endoscopic ultrasound or pelvic MRI, received neoadjuvant chemoradiation therapy (CRT) including capecitabine and oxaliplatin, followed by either transanal excision or transanal endoscopic microsurgery. Among 77 eligible patients who underwent LE, 34 patients achieved a pathologic complete response (44%) and 49 (64%) tumors were downstaged (ypT0-1), although 4 patients (5%) had ypT3 tumors. CRT-related grade ≥3 complications occurred in 39% of patients, prompting chemotherapy dose reduction during the study. The authors concluded CRT before local excision for T2N0 tumors results in a high pathologic complete response rate and negative resection margins, although complication rates were high.

Adjuvant Radiation Therapy

In considering indications for adjuvant therapy, it is first helpful to categorize patients by risk of recurrence based on pre-treatment and/or pathologic factors. Patients generally not requiring additional therapy include those with early stage disease, typically T1-2N0 tumors without high-risk features treated by TME. In addition, highly selected patients with T3N0 tumors may have acceptable outcomes with surgery alone.[5] More advanced rectal cancers (T3-T4 and/or N+) are associated with higher rates of local recurrence and are better suited for radiation or combined modality therapy (CMT).

The historical approach to pathological stage II and III rectal cancers has been the delivery of post-operative pelvic radiation therapy with fluoropyrimidine-based chemotherapy. The advantage to this approach is the ability to select patients at high risk of LR based on pathologic criteria. Disadvantages include devascularization of the tumor bed, which may limit the delivery of chemotherapy and reduced oxygenation, potentially making radiation less effective. In addition, this approach may result in higher acute and late toxicity rates. This is attributable, in part, to increased portions of small bowel receiving radiation therapy as well as the higher rates of anastomotic stenosis.

Early reports from the National Surgical Adjuvant Breast and Bowel Project (NSABP) and the Medical Research Council (MRC) comparing surgery alone to surgery and adjuvant radiation therapy for locally advanced rectal cancer demonstrated improved local control but no impact on overall survival (OS).[6,7] Investigators from the Gastrointestinal Tumor Study Group (GITSG) conducted a four-arm study comparing surgery alone to adjuvant chemotherapy, radiation therapy or combined modality therapy. The combination of radiation therapy and 5-FU chemotherapy significantly reduced LR (10% versus 25%) and improved OS (10-yr, 45% versus 27%) versus surgery alone.[8] In a separate study directly comparing adjuvant radiation therapy versus radiation with bolus 5-FU, the combined modality arm reduced LR by 46%, cancer-related deaths by 36% and overall death by 29%.[9] Additionally, the mode of delivering 5-FU with radiation therapy was found to be important, with an Intergroup study demonstrating improved LR, DFS and OS with continuous infusion versus bolus administration of 5-FU.[10]

Neoadjuvant Radiation Therapy

There are potential advantages in delivering radiation therapy pre- versus post-resection. From a treatment planning perspective, there is much greater certainty in the location of the tumor and normal tissue anatomy. This allows for potentially smaller treatment volumes in some cases and therefore less normal tissue toxicity, particularly for small bowel. Biological advantages include an intact vasculature allowing for improved delivery of chemotherapeutic agents and better oxygenation to tumoral tissues, both of which are felt to enhance the effectiveness of radiotherapy. There is also potential for downstaging, higher rates of complete resection, and enhanced sphincter preservation. Neoadjuvant therapy also allows for early assessment of treatment response. Additionally, from a logistical standpoint, patients are more likely to complete all components of their therapy and without significant delay. The major challenge with preoperative therapy is the uncertainty in pathologic stage, despite use of MRI and rectal endoscopic ultrasonography (EUS), and potential for over-treatment of early stage patients.

The Swedish Rectal Cancer Trial was designed to evaluate preoperative radiotherapy in 1,168 patients with resectable rectal cancer. Randomization in this study was to 5 Gy × 5 delivered in one week followed by surgery a week later or surgery alone. The long-term results at a median follow-up of 13 years demonstrated significant reduction in LR (9% versus 26%).[11] LR rates with surgery alone were 14%, 22% and 46% in stage I, II and III patients, respectively. Overall survival was significantly increased in the preoperative radiotherapy group (38% versus 30%). There was no difference in the incidence of distant metastases (DM) development. The investigators concluded that the marked reduction in local recurrence after radiotherapy improved overall survival. However, this gain was associated with higher rates of bowel frequency, urgency and incontinence in the radiotherapy group. It is important to note that this study was conducted in the era before the routine adoption of TME, likely contributing to the higher local failure rates observed in the surgery alone arm.

With the adoption of TME, LR was reduced significantly[12] and the value of radiation therapy in reducing LR was questioned. To define the role of neoadjuvant radiation therapy in the TME-era, the Dutch Colorectal Cancer Group conducted a multicenter randomized comparison of preoperative radiation therapy (similar regimen to the Swedish trial) and TME or TME alone in 1,861 patients with resectable rectal cancer. The primary endpoint for this study was LR. Long-term results at a median follow-up of 12 years found that radiotherapy significantly reduced the 10-year cumulative incidence of LR (5% versus 11%).[13] Subset analyses of local recurrence by TNM stage and uninvolved circumferential margins showed a benefit across all groups, particularly those with negative margins and node positive disease, in which a survival benefit was seen. The absolute benefit in early-stage patients was low, with no statistically significant differences in 10-year DM rates or OS seen. Similar to the radiation arm in the Swedish trial, the radiation arm demonstrated detriments in bowel function and quality of life.[14,15]

Both of these trials primarily relied on physical examination to determine resectability and were conducted prior to the widespread use of MRI and/or EUS for preoperative staging and surgical planning. The inclusion of early stage patients, particularly stage I patients, would be expected to only minimally improve rates of local recurrence with the potential for long-term morbidity. Additionally, the short interval from neoadjuvant radiation therapy to surgery does not allow any potential downstaging effect. It is important to note the difference in LR between the Dutch and Swedish trials, with TME significantly reducing the overall LR and absolute benefit of neoadjuvant radiation. However, even in the Dutch trial, patients with node-positive disease had local recurrence rates >20% with TME alone. In the era of improved surgical technique (with TME), preoperative staging, and histological assessment, the MRC CR07 trial re-evaluated the role of RT. The MRC attempted to determine if a selective postoperative approach would be comparable to preoperative therapy in terms of local control. Similar to the Swedish and Dutch trials, all resectable rectal cancers, including early stage patients, were included and treated with a short course preoperative radiation-alone regimen or up-front surgery followed by conventional post-operative chemoradiation only for positive surgical margins. Local recurrence was significantly reduced in the preoperative arm (4% versus 11%) as was DFS, with no significant difference in OS.[16]

Adjuvant versus Neoadjuvant Radiation Therapy Comparisons

In order to directly compare neoadjuvant and adjuvant approaches, German investigators initiated a randomized comparison of preoperative versus postoperative chemoradiotherapy (CRT) in EUS/CT-staged cT3-4 or node-positive rectal cancer. TME was mandated in the trial, with radiation delivered concurrently with continuous infusion 5-FU in both arms with total doses of 50.4 Gy and 55.8 Gy in the pre- and postoperative arms, respectively. In contrast to the short-course trials above, surgery was delayed by six weeks following preoperative CRT. Compliance was worse in the adjuvant group, with only (54% versus 92%) completing the entire course of radiation therapy. The effect of downstaging was evident; pathologic complete response (pCR) rate was 8% with neoadjuvant CRT and significantly fewer patients had node positive disease at resection (25% versus 40%).[17] Importantly, higher rates of sphincter-preserving surgery for low-lying tumors initially deemed to require APR were seen in the preoperative group (39% versus 19%), with significant reductions in acute and late toxicities in the preoperative group. Long-term follow-up at 10 years continued to show a small, but significant, reduction in LR with the preoperative approach (7% versus 10%).[18] There was no significant difference in DM rates, DFS or OS. It is important to note that 18% of patients staged as cT3-4 or N+ randomized to the postoperative group were found to have pT1-2N0 disease, highlighting the risk of overtreatment even with modern staging.

The NSABP conducted a trial of similar design that closed early due to poor accrual. A pCR rate of 15% was noted in this trial with significantly higher DFS and a trend toward improved OS in the preoperative arm.[19] A smaller randomized trial from Korea similarly demonstrated higher rates of sphincter-sparing surgery among low-lying tumors with the preoperative approach.[20] Collectively, these trials suggest that in patients with indications for adjuvant radiation therapy, a neoadjuvant approach significantly reduces LR rates as well as treatment-related toxicities and should be considered the standard of care.

Chemotherapy Regimens with Neoadjuvant Radiation Therapy

As in the adjuvant setting, the concurrent administration of chemotherapy to radiation has shown benefit in the neoadjuvant setting. 5-FU has been the most well-studied chemotherapeutic agent to date. The European Organisation for Research and Treatment of Cancer (EORTC) 22921 trial randomized patients with cT3-4 resectable rectal cancers to receive 45 Gy preoperative RT alone versus the same RT regimen with 5-FU, with a second randomization of adjuvant 5-FU. The addition of 5-FU significantly improved the pCR rate (14% versus 5%), reduced node positivity and LR (9% versus 17%) without any effect on overall survival.[21] Similar to the EORTC study, the Fêdêration Francophone de Cancêrologie Digestive (FFCD) 9203 trial compared preoperative radiation with or without concurrent bolus 5-FU. Higher rates of pCR and reduced local recurrence (8% versus 16%) were again noted.[22] In patients with locally unresectable disease, a randomized comparison found that the addition of 5-FU chemotherapy to neoadjuvant radiation therapy significantly improved R0 resection rates (84% versus 68%), local control (82% versus 67%) and cancer-specific survival (72% versus 55%).[23] Capecitabine, an oral 5-FU prodrug, was compared with continuous infusion 5-FU, both of which were given concurrently with long course preoperative radiotherapy. Compared to 5-FU, capecitabine improved downstaging and the number of patients with negative lymph nodes.[24] Although local recurrence rates were not statistically significant, there were less DM and improved OS/DFS with capecitabine. All of these studies consistently demonstrate higher rates of acute toxicity with addition of chemotherapy.

Additional chemotherapeutic agents have since been evaluated in combination with radiation therapy in the neoadjuvant regimen, many of which have shown benefit in the metastatic setting. The addition of oxaliplatin has been studied in the ACCORD and STAR 01 trials, which used capecitabine or continuous infusion 5-FU as the backbone chemotherapeutic, respectively.[25,26] The primary endpoint of these studies was pCR rate, which was not significantly improved with the addition of oxaliplatin. However, the rates of grade 3/4 toxicity were significantly increased with oxaliplatin use. Many other agents are currently being evaluated with the use of pCR as a rapid clinical endpoint. With the available data, capecitabine or continuous-infusion 5-FU-based chemoradiotherapy is considered the standard of care.

Long versus Short Course Neoadjuvant Radiation Therapy

Many of the preoperative studies including the Swedish, Dutch and UK trials discussed above utilized short course (5 Gy × 5) of radiotherapy alone followed by surgery one week later. Potential advantages of this approach include convenience, cost, improved compliance, and reduced acute side effects given the short interval between delivery of therapy and surgical removal of disease. A disadvantage of this sequence, however, is that the opportunity for downstaging is lost and systemic chemotherapy is not utilized. Long course CRT followed by resection 4–8 weeks after is associated with tumor regression and possibly enhanced sphincter preservation.

Two published studies have prospectively compared short course radiation-alone regimen to a long course of 50.4 Gy in daily 1.8 Gy fractions concurrent with 5-FU.[27,28] The Polish study utilized bolus 5-FU concurrent with radiotherapy, while the Australian study used continuous-infusion 5-FU. Long course CMT demonstrated improved pCR (15–16%) and fewer positive radial margins (Polish study), but no significant differences were observed in terms of sphincter preservation, LR, DM, or OS between the two regimens. There was a trend for improved local control with long course CRT for distal tumors. Not unexpectedly, acute toxicity rates were higher with long course therapy, although no differences in late toxicity were apparent. Further updates, especially in terms of late toxicity, are eagerly anticipated from these as well as other ongoing trials, including a prospective randomized German trial. Long-term follow-up from the previously described Swedish Rectal Cancer trial suggest a persistent risk of small bowel obstruction in the radiotherapy arm.[29] Similarly, long-term results from the Dutch TME trial demonstrate higher rates of small bowel obstruction, fecal incontinence, rectal bleeding, and sexual dysfunction with the short course regimen.[13] Although the German Rectal Cancer Study reported grade 3–4 late toxicity rates of 14% in patients in the long course preoperative arm,[17] it is difficult to compare toxicities across the trials given differences in surgical technique and methods of reporting of adverse events, while late toxicities may take many years to manifest.

By increasing the interval from short course radiotherapy to surgery, it is possible that enhanced downstaging would be apparent. This is currently under investigation in the Stockholm III trial, a three-arm comparison of surgery one week after short course RT versus delayed surgery (4–8 weeks) after short course versus long course RT alone. A preliminary report described higher rates of sphincter preservation with long course RT, increased acute toxicity with both delayed arms but a higher rate of surgical complications with the early surgery arm.[30] Several trials comparing short course RT followed by systemic chemotherapy to long course CMT are ongoing.

Recurrent Rectal Cancer

In patients who were not previously irradiated, a neoadjuvant CRT regimen similar to locally advanced tumors is employed, with or without the inclusion of intraoperative radiation therapy (IORT) at the time of resection. Despite aggressive treatment, long-term survival is relatively poor in this population.[31] One randomized control trial compared outcomes of preoperative CRT or radiotherapy alone prior to surgical resection in patients with locally advanced or recurrent rectal cancer who had not received prior radiotherapy. This series included 25 patients with recurrent disease. Higher rates of R0 resection, LC, time to treatment failure, and cancer-specific survival were seen in the chemoradiation arm.[23] Five-year OS in patients with recurrent rectal cancer was 37%. There is little evidence to standardize an approach in patients who have received prior radiation. Of the published studies, many institutions use alternative radiation techniques "neoadjuvantly" (e.g. BID fractionation, intensity modulated radiation therapy, etc.) to low total doses (30–36 Gy) in combination with chemotherapy with a goal of R0 resection,[32–34] with the use of IORT frequently employed. With these techniques, treatment is generally well tolerated acutely, although moderate rates of late toxicity are reported. Patients that are unable to undergo an R0 resection have poor local control and overall survival rates. In terms of quality of life, CRT was particularly helpful in relieving pain and bleeding lesions in many of these studies.

Treatment Planning Techniques

Most patients are simulated in the prone-position and immobilized with a belly board. This device has a cut-out for the abdomen such that the small bowel gravitates away from the low pelvis. Patients are often instructed to have a full bladder, which serves a similar purpose. A radiopaque anal marker is placed to define the anal verge. Intravenous, small bowel, and rectal contrast are often utilized to better define target and normal structure anatomy. It is our institutional preference to utilize thin section CT for planning, using pertinent physical exam/proctoscopy findings, EUS and any other diagnostic imaging to assist in target volume delineation.

CT-based planning is limited by lack of contrast resolution between soft-tissue structures. Compared to CT, MRI tumor volumes are frequently smaller and further from the anal sphincter.[35] MRI also allows for more accurate delineation of the mesorectal fascia. Use of 18-F fluorodeoxyglucose positron emission tomography (FDG-PET) may further refine the target volume and differentiate benign/reactive tissues and detect occult lymphatic involvement, particularly in locally advanced tumors.[36] There is significant variation in target volume based on visual assessment and auto-segmentation algorithms of the FDG signal, with no optimal approach consistently defined.[37] These techniques may reduce treatment volumes and thus permit reduced normal tissue toxicity and/or dose escalation. Further prospective trials on how to integrate these techniques into current practice are warranted.

Treatment fields encompass sites of known and potential occult disease, including the presacral space, mesorectum, internal and distal common iliac lymphatics. In general, patients are treated with a three-field (posteroanterior, right/left lateral) or four-field (anteroposterior, posteroanterior, right/left lateral) conformal technique. Intensity modulated radiation therapy (IMRT) is typically reserved for scenarios where the risk of toxicity is high, particularly in the setting of re-irradiation. Dose volume histograms (DVH) are calculated to ensure adequate target coverage and normal tissue tolerances are respected. Usual doses at our institution are 45 Gy in 25 daily 1.8 Gy fractions to an initial pelvic field, with a tumor boost to a total of 50.4 Gy.

Take Home Messages

- Radiotherapy plays a crucial role in the management of rectal cancer, both neoadjuvantly to get patient's definitive surgical management, and adjuvantly to improve locoregional control of disease.
- Radiotherapy can also be an option for recurrent rectal cancer for those who are inoperable.
- Future studies will explore the validity of short course neoadjuvant regimens of radiotherapy, and ensure its efficacy and safety.

References

1. Russell, A.H., *et al.*, Anal sphincter conservation for patients with adenocarcinoma of the distal rectum: long-term results of radiation therapy oncology group protocol 89–02. Int *J Radiat Oncol Biol Phys*, 2000. **46**(2): 313–22.
2. Greenberg, J.A., *et al.*, Local excision of distal rectal cancer: an update of cancer and leukemia group B 8984. *Dis Colon Rectum*, 2008. **51**(8): 1185–91; discussion 1191–4.
3. National Comprehensive Cancer Network. Rectal Cancer (Version 2.2014) Accessed 1/13/14. http://www.nccn.org/professionals/physician_gls/pdf/rectal.pdf.
4. Garcia-Aguilar, J., *et al.*, A phase II trial of neoadjuvant chemoradiation and local excision for T2N0 rectal cancer: preliminary results of the ACOSOG Z6041 trial. *Ann Surg Oncol*, 2012. **19**(2): 384–91.
5. Gunderson, L.L., *et al.*, Impact of T and N stage and treatment on survival and relapse in adjuvant rectal cancer: a pooled analysis. *J Clin Oncol*, 2004. **22**(10): 1785–96.
6. Fisher, B., *et al.*, Postoperative adjuvant chemotherapy or radiation therapy for rectal cancer: results from NSABP protocol R-01. *J Natl Cancer Inst*, 1988. **80**(1): 21–9.
7. Randomised trial of surgery alone versus surgery followed by radiotherapy for mobile cancer of the rectum. Medical Research Council Rectal Cancer Working Party. *Lancet*, 1996. **348**(9042): 1610–4.
8. Douglass, H.O., Jr., *et al.*, Survival after postoperative combination treatment of rectal cancer. *N Engl J Med*, 1986. **315**(20): 1294–5.

9. Krook, J.E., *et al.*, Effective surgical adjuvant therapy for high-risk rectal carcinoma. *N Engl J Med*, 1991. **324**(11): 709–15.
10. O'Connell, M.J., *et al.*, Improving adjuvant therapy for rectal cancer by combining protracted-infusion fluorouracil with radiation therapy after curative surgery. *N Engl J Med*, 1994. **331**(8): 502–7.
11. Folkesson, J., *et al.*, Swedish Rectal Cancer Trial: long lasting benefits from radiotherapy on survival and local recurrence rate. *J Clin Oncol*, 2005. **23**(24): 5644–50.
12. Carlsen, E., *et al.*, Effect of the introduction of total mesorectal excision for the treatment of rectal cancer. *Br J Surg*, 1998. **85**(4): 526–9.
13. van Gijn, W., *et al.*, Preoperative radiotherapy combined with total mesorectal excision for resectable rectal cancer: 12-year follow-up of the multicentre, randomised controlled TME trial. *Lancet Oncol*, 2011. **12**(6): 575–582.
14. Peeters, K.C., *et al.*, Late side effects of short-course preoperative radiotherapy combined with total mesorectal excision for rectal cancer: increased bowel dysfunction in irradiated patients — a Dutch colorectal cancer group study. *J Clin Oncol*, 2005. **23**(25): 6199–206.
15. Marijnen, C.A., *et al.*, Impact of short-term preoperative radiotherapy on health-related quality of life and sexual functioning in primary rectal cancer: report of a multicenter randomized trial. *J Clin Oncol*, 2005. **23**(9): 1847–58.
16. Sebag-Montefiore, D., *et al.*, Preoperative radiotherapy versus selective postoperative chemoradiotherapy in patients with rectal cancer (MRC CR07 and NCIC-CTG C016): a multicentre, randomised trial. *Lancet*, 2009. **373**(9666): 811–20.
17. Sauer, R., *et al.*, Preoperative versus postoperative chemoradiotherapy for rectal cancer. *N Engl J Med*, 2004. **351**(17): 1731–40.
18. Sauer, R., *et al.*, Preoperative versus postoperative chemoradiotherapy for locally advanced rectal cancer: results of the German CAO/ARO/AIO-94 randomized phase III trial after a median follow-up of 11 years. *J Clin Oncol*, 2012. **30**(16): 1926–33.
19. Roh, M.S., *et al.*, Preoperative multimodality therapy improves disease-free survival in patients with carcinoma of the rectum: NSABP R-03. *J Clin Oncol*, 2009. **27**(31): 5124–30.
20. Park, J.H., *et al.*, Randomized phase 3 trial comparing preoperative and postoperative chemoradiotherapy with capecitabine for locally advanced rectal cancer. *Cancer*, 2011. **117**(16): 3703–12.

21. Bosset, J.F., *et al.*, Chemotherapy with preoperative radiotherapy in rectal cancer. *N Engl J Med*, 2006. **355**(11): 1114–23.
22. Gerard, J.P., *et al.*, Preoperative radiotherapy with or without concurrent fluorouracil and leucovorin in T3–4 rectal cancers: results of FFCD 9203. *J Clin Oncol*, 2006. **24**(28): 4620–5.
23. Braendengen, M., *et al.*, Randomized phase III study comparing preoperative radiotherapy with chemoradiotherapy in nonresectable rectal cancer. *J Clin Oncol*, 2008. **26**(22): 3687–94.
24. Hofheinz, R.-D., *et al.*, Chemoradiotherapy with capecitabine versus fluorouracil for locally advanced rectal cancer: a randomised, multicentre, non-inferiority, phase 3 trial. *The Lancet Oncol*, 2012. **13**(6): 579–588.
25. Gerard, J.P., *et al.*, Clinical outcome of the ACCORD 12/0405 PRODIGE 2 randomized trial in rectal cancer. *J Clin Oncol*, 2012. **30**(36): 4558–65.
26. Aschele, C., *et al.*, Primary tumor response to preoperative chemoradiation with or without oxaliplatin in locally advanced rectal cancer: pathologic results of the STAR-01 randomized phase III trial. *J Clin Oncol*, 2011. **29**(20): 2773–80.
27. Ngan, S.Y., *et al.*, Randomized trial of short-course radiotherapy versus long-course chemoradiation comparing rates of local recurrence in patients with T3 rectal cancer: Trans-Tasman Radiation Oncology Group trial 01.04. *J Clin Oncol*, 2012. **30**(31): 3827–33.
28. Bujko, K., *et al.*, Long-term results of a randomized trial comparing preoperative short-course radiotherapy with preoperative conventionally fractionated chemoradiation for rectal cancer. *Br J Surg*, 2006. **93**(10): 1215–23.
29. Birgisson, H., *et al.*, Late gastrointestinal disorders after rectal cancer surgery with and without preoperative radiation therapy. *Br J Surg*, 2008. **95**(2): 206–13.
30. Pettersson, D., *et al.*, Interim analysis of the Stockholm III trial of preoperative radiotherapy regimens for rectal cancer. *Br J Surg*, 2010. **97**(4): 580–7.
31. Gunderson, L.L., *et al.*, Intraoperative electron and external beam irradiation with or without 5-fluorouracil and maximum surgical resection for previously unirradiated, locally recurrent colorectal cancer. *Dis Colon Rectum*, 1996. **39**(12): 1379–95.
32. Mohiuddin, M., Marks, G., and Marks, J., Long-term results of reirradiation for patients with recurrent rectal carcinoma. *Cancer*, 2002. **95**(5): 1144–50.

33. Valentini, V., *et al.*, Preoperative hyperfractionated chemoradiation for locally recurrent rectal cancer in patients previously irradiated to the pelvis: A multicentric phase II study. *Int J Radiat Oncol Biol Phys*, 2006. **64**(4): 1129–39.
34. Das, P., *et al.*, Hyperfractionated accelerated radiotherapy for rectal cancer in patients with prior pelvic irradiation. *Int J Radiat Oncol Biol Phys*, 2010. **77**(1): 60–5.
35. O'Neill, B.D., *et al.*, MR vs CT imaging: low rectal cancer tumour delineation for three-dimensional conformal radiotherapy. *Br J Radiol*, 2009. **82**(978): 509–13.
36. Braendengen, M., *et al.*, Delineation of gross tumor volume (GTV) for radiation treatment planning of locally advanced rectal cancer using information from MRI or FDG-PET/CT: a prospective study. *Int J Radiat Oncol Biol Phys*, 2011. **81**(4): e439–45.
37. Lee, J.A., Segmentation of positron emission tomography images: some recommendations for target delineation in radiation oncology. *Radiother Oncol*, 2010. **96**(3): 302–7.

Chapter 25

Radiotherapy for Pancreatic Cancer

Lauren Colbert, Richard J. Cassidy and David Marcus

What's New

- Stereotactic body radiotherapy (SBRT) for pancreas cancer offers potentially ablative dose therapy, with dosimetric advantage and lower risk of adverse effects.
- SBRT may potentially improve local control of pancreatic cancer due to the ability to achieve higher dose to cancer cells.

Introduction

Radiation therapy plays an important role in the management of patients with adenocarcinoma of the pancreas. In patients with resectable disease, radiation is often delivered as adjuvant therapy, typically with concurrent chemotherapy. Additionally, radiation may be used in the intact setting, including for patients with either unresectable or borderline resectable disease. In patients with unresectable disease, radiation therapy makes up a component of definitive therapy, along with concurrent chemotherapy. In patients with borderline resectable disease, radiation is used (typically with chemotherapy) in an attempt to achieve resectability by shrinking the tumor and reducing the tumor's proximity to critical structures such as the celiac axis, superior mesenteric artery, and superior mesenteric vein.

Although distant metastasis is undoubtedly a major problem, local control plays an important role in the optimal management of patients with pancreatic cancer. This chapter will review the current standards of radiation therapy for adenocarcinoma of the pancreas and will highlight recent developments and future directions in the delivery of radiation therapy for this aggressive malignancy.

Radiation Therapy for Resectable Pancreatic Cancer

Despite several clinical trials that have attempted to clarify the role of adjuvant radiation therapy in the management of resectable pancreatic cancer, the use of radiation in this setting remains controversial. The primary goal of adjuvant radiotherapy after definitive surgical resection is to eliminate any residual microscopic disease that may remain in the surgical bed. However, this benefit must be weighed against the potential toxicities of therapy, particularly given the close proximity between the pancreas and radiosensitive normal tissues, most notably including the small bowel.

The first clinical trial to evaluate the utility of radiation therapy in this setting was the Gastrointestinal Tumor Study Group (GITSG) 9173 trial, which randomized 43 patients to postoperative 5-fluorouracil (5-FU) based chemoradiation followed by two years of adjuvant 5-FU ($n = 21$) versus no adjuvant treatment ($n = 22$). The study was closed prematurely, partially as a result of poor accrual but also due to a significant survival difference between the treatment arms, with median survival of 20 months in patients receiving adjuvant therapy compared to 11 months in patients undergoing surgery alone ($p = 0.03$).[1] While this study was criticized for poor accrual and non-standard radiation technique (40 Gy split course), it established adjuvant chemoradiation as the standard of care in the United States upon publication of the results in 1985.

Following publication of the GITSG study in 1985, the European Organization for the Research and Treatment of Cancer (EORTC) developed a phase III study to randomize patients with resected pancreatic cancer to adjuvant concurrent 5-FU and radiation (40 Gy split course) versus observation. In contrast to the GITSG study, the EORTC study failed to demonstrate a difference in overall survival between the arms, with five-year overall survival of 25% for patients undergoing adjuvant chemoradiation and 22% for patients undergoing observation.[2] This study, in addition to being underpowered, was also subject to several criticisms, including the fact that 48% of patients had favorable periampullary cancers were included (which may have diluted the impact of adjuvant therapy), the inclusion of patients with positive surgical margins, and the use of non-standard split course radiation with a low total dose.

Finally, the European Study Group for Pancreatic Cancer-1 (ESPAC-1) study examined the roles of both adjuvant chemotherapy and chemoradiation in an international trial involving 289 patients from 11 European countries and 61 treatment centers. All patients underwent R0 or R1 resection and were subsequently randomized to either adjuvant chemotherapy, adjuvant chemoradiation, adjuvant chemoradiation plus maintenance chemotherapy, or observation. Outcome comparisons were made for chemoradiation versus no chemoradiation and chemotherapy versus no chemotherapy. The results demonstrated improved five-year overall survival associated with the use of adjuvant chemotherapy (21% versus 8%, $p = 0.009$). However, the use of adjuvant chemoradiation was associated with a detriment in overall survival, with five-year overall survival of 10% in patients receiving chemoradiation versus 20% in patients not receiving chemoradiation ($p = 0.05$).[3] Despite these discouraging findings, however, the ESPAC-1 study has been criticized heavily for several shortcomings, and the results are highly controversial. Similarly to the GITSG and EORTC studies, limitations of the ESPAC-1 study include the use of split course of radiation and the low total radiation dose. Secondly, the authors failed to provide details of radiation delivery, including the radiation fields used, the machine and dosimetry specifications, and a description of the overall process of radiotherapy quality assurance. Furthermore, despite the recommended dose of 40 Gy in a split course, 30% of patients in the chemoradiation arm received either a different dose of radiation or no radiation at all.[4] Given these limitations and the fact that radiation techniques have evolved significantly since publication of this study, it is difficult to apply the results of ESPAC-1 to modern patients with resected pancreatic cancer.

Currently, the Radiation Therapy Oncology Group (RTOG) is accruing patients on a randomized phase III trial, RTOG 0848, which will help to elucidate the impact of adjuvant chemoradiation on overall survival in patients with resected pancreatic cancer. In this study, patients are randomized to adjuvant gemcitabine alone versus gemcitabine plus erlotinib. Patients who do not progress on chemotherapy subsequently undergo a second randomization between chemotherapy versus chemoradiation with either capecitabine or infusional 5-FU. As of March 2014, the study had accrued 336 patients, with a final accrual goal of 950. The results of this study will be informative regarding the optimal adjuvant treatment for patients with resected pancreatic cancer and are eagerly anticipated.

Management of Borderline Resectable Disease

Borderline resectable pancreatic cancer refers to non-metastatic tumors of the pancreas that would carry a high risk of positive surgical margins if resected immediately without any preoperative therapy. These tumors often involve the mesenteric vessels, but generally not in a manner that would preclude vascular reconstruction. Although several studies have evaluated the use of neoadjuvant chemoradiation for pancreatic cancer,[5–8] the extent to which this treatment may facilitate an R0 resection is currently unknown. Additionally, a number of studies have evaluated the feasibility and efficacy of neoadjuvant chemotherapy alone (without radiation).[9–11] At this time, neoadjuvant therapy prior to surgery is considered the standard of care for borderline resectable disease; however, the optimal combination of preoperative therapies is not well established.

Management of Locally Advanced/Unresectable Disease

For patients with unresectable, non-metastatic pancreatic cancer, the standard of care is concurrent chemotherapy and radiation therapy. Several studies have demonstrated superior overall survival with the combination of chemotherapy and radiation compared to either modality alone. An early report from The Mayo Clinic demonstrated a four-month survival advantage for patients with unresectable pancreatic cancer receiving chemoradiation compared to radiation alone.[12] Similarly, a trial from the GITSG comparing chemoradiation to chemotherapy alone in patients with unresectable tumors demonstrated a significant survival advantage to combined modality therapy (one-year survival 41% vs. 19%).[13] Although several other studies have shown similar results, and in contrast to the aforementioned trials, a trial from the Eastern Cooperative Oncology Group (ECOG) failed to demonstrate a benefit to chemoradiation compared to chemotherapy alone in patients with unresectable pancreatic cancer (median survival 8.2 vs. 8.3 months).[14] Furthermore, the optimal systemic therapy is unknown, whether given alone or in combination with radiation therapy. Nonetheless, combined modality therapy with chemotherapy and radiation therapy is currently considered the standard of care for the treatment of locally advanced/unresectable pancreatic adenocarcinoma, despite several yet unanswered questions.

Radiation Therapy Techniques

Over the past several decades, the technical aspects of radiation therapy have evolved substantially, and this evolution has had important implications for the management of pancreatic cancer. In the past, radiation for pancreatic cancer was delivered with opposed parallel beams (generally in AP/PA configuration), utilizing two-dimensional imaging and bony anatomy to establish a target. Because this system involved substantial inherent uncertainties in the location of the target and daily setup, radiation fields were necessarily large, with minimal sparing of adjacent normal tissues. Due to these limitations, radiation dose escalation was not feasible, as the risk of normal tissue toxicity would be too great. Moreover, even with relatively low doses of radiation, breaks of a week or more were often introduced into a radiation treatment course in order to mitigate acute toxicity. For example, in the GITSG, EORTC, and ESPAC-1 trials, radiation therapy was prescribed to a dose of 40 Gy, delivered in two separate blocks of 20 Gy with a two-week break in between. From a radiobiologic perspective, the presence of a prolonged treatment break is far from ideal, as it allows tumor cells a window of opportunity for repopulation, which is potentially quite detrimental to tumor control. With older techniques, therefore, radiation therapy was limited in its ability to provide tumor control, and toxicity was frequently an issue.

In the modern era, optimization of tumor control and avoidance of normal tissue toxicity remain critical challenges in the delivery of radiation therapy for pancreatic cancer. Nevertheless, improvements in the delivery of highly conformal radiation have led to a greatly enhanced ability to effectively target and treat pancreatic tumors in comparison to older techniques. In particular, these advances have the potential to optimize local control by allowing higher dose delivery to the target volume than would have previously been possible with more antiquated techniques. One important such advance has been the development of three-dimensional conformal radiation therapy (3DCRT), in which computed tomography (CT) simulation allows the radiation oncologist to delineate a three-dimensional radiotherapy target volume. With the utilization of multi-leaf collimators (MLCs) that block selected parts of the radiation portal, the field can be shaped to fit the contour of the target volume while avoiding excess radiation dose to organs at risk (OARs), such as the small intestine, stomach, liver, kidneys, and spinal cord. A further step in the evolution of conformal radiation therapy, called intensity modulated radiation therapy (IMRT), involves the separation of a radiation beam into "beamlets" that can be independently modulated at multiple beam angles to deliver a non-uniform radiation dose and an even more conformal radiation dose distribution. Finally, the use of heavy ion therapy, most notably including proton therapy, offers the potential for the highest degree of conformality currently available by exploiting a property of heavy ions known as the "Bragg Peak," which refers to the rapid fall-off of radiation dose after delivery of the particle's energy at depth.

The currently accepted dose range for treatment of resected pancreatic cancer is 45.0 – 50.4 Gy in 1.8 Gy fractions, with higher doses of up to 60.0 Gy in patients with locally advanced/unresectable disease. In patients with resected disease, the clinical target volume includes the surgical bed (including all surgical clips), lymph node areas at risk, and any residual gross disease left over after surgery. For intact tumors, the target generally includes the entire tumor and lymph node areas at risk, although the inclusion of clinically involved lymph node basins is currently an area of controversy. There is a growing body of evidence suggesting a benefit to radiation dose escalation in pancreatic cancer; however, the benefits of dose escalation must be balanced against the toxicities associated with delivery of higher radiation doses. A recent analysis of the National Cancer Database by Hall *et al.* demonstrated that radiation doses between

50–55 Gy were associated with improved overall survival compared to doses of <50 Gy or >55 Gy in patients with resected pancreatic adenocarcinoma.[15] As radiation techniques continue to evolve, however, dose escalation is gaining traction as potential mechanism for improved local tumor control.

IMRT For Pancreatic Cancer

Currently, the most widely accepted technique for dose escalation to pancreatic tumors is IMRT. Several studies comparing 3DCRT to IMRT have demonstrated that IMRT allows delivery of higher radiation dose without added toxicity. A dosimetric study by Milano *et al.* compared IMRT plans with four-field 3DCRT plans and found that the use of IMRT was associated with decreased mean radiation dose to the liver, kidneys, stomach, and small bowel.[16] A phase I trial from the University of Michigan and William Beaumont Hospital sought to identify the maximum tolerated radiation dose to unresectable or partially resected pancreatic tumors with concurrent weekly gemcitabine using 3DCRT. The study found that dose escalation beyond 42 Gy at 2.8 Gy per fraction (roughly biologically equivalent to 50.4 Gy at 1.8 Gy per fraction with regard to late effects) was not feasible due to unacceptable gastrointestinal toxicity.[17] By contrast, a phase I study from the University of Michigan using IMRT for unresectable pancreatic cancer found that dose limiting toxicities were acceptable at doses up to 55 Gy in 25 fractions.[18] Similarly, a study from the San Raffaele Scientific Institute in Milan, Italy demonstrated the feasibility and safety of using IMRT with simultaneous infield boost technique to deliver doses of 58 Gy in 15 fractions to small subvolumes within the overall clinical target volume.[19] The results of these studies support the hypothesis that the use of IMRT facilitates radiation dose escalation in pancreatic cancer.

As the use of dose-escalated IMRT necessitates more conformal margins, concerns have been raised regarding the risk of geographic miss and subsequent local failure with smaller treatment volumes. To address these concerns, investigators at Johns Hopkins and the University of Maryland published a study describing patterns of failure in patients receiving IMRT for resected pancreatic cancer. The results of this demonstrated that IMRT was not associated with an increase in local recurrences compared to historical controls, suggesting that the risk of geographic miss is minimal.[20]

At present, IMRT is considered within the standard of care for the treatment of pancreatic cancer, both in the postoperative and intact settings. In 2011, a panel of experts from RTOG and the Groupe Cooperateur Multidisciplinaire en Oncologie (GERCOR) published consensus guidelines which endorsed the use of IMRT in the treatment of locally advanced pancreatic cancer.[21] Additionally, the current open RTOG trial, RTOG 0848, in which radiation is delivered as postoperative treatment, allows either 3DCRT or IMRT, with specific guidelines for target volume coverage and constraints for organs at risk. The RTOG has also published consensus guidelines for delineation of the clinical target volume in resected pancreatic cancer.[22]

Stereotactic Body Radiation Therapy for Pancreatic Cancer

For dose escalation beyond what is achievable with IMRT alone, stereotactic body radiation therapy (SBRT) has emerged as a method by which ablative doses of radiation can be delivered to pancreatic tumors in five or fewer fractions. As SBRT is a fairly novel treatment modality, there is little prospective data describing outcomes associated with SBRT in the treatment of pancreatic cancer. A phase I study from Stanford University demonstrated the feasibility and safety of SBRT for patients with locally advanced pancreatic cancer using a dose of 25 Gy in a single fraction.[23] A subsequent phase II study evaluated the use of SBRT boost after 45 Gy IMRT with concurrent 5-FU, demonstrating excellent local control (15 of 16 patients), but higher rates of toxicity compared to SRS alone and no improvement in overall survival.[24] A retrospective study by Chuong *et al.* evaluated the use of SBRT with a dose-painting technique delivering 7–10 Gy per fraction to regions of vascular involvement and 5–6 Gy per fraction to the remainder of the tumor for five consecutive fractions, demonstrating that 96.9% of patients were able to undergo R0 resection with no acute grade ≥3 toxicity and minimal late grade ≥3 toxicity.[25] While these findings are promising, further study is needed to elucidate the role of SBRT in the treatment of pancreatic cancer.

Take Home Messages

- Radiotherapy remains an important mainstay for the locoregional management of pancreatic cancer, either adjuvantly after resection or with concurrent chemotherapy in unresectable disease.
- Several advances, including IMRT and SBRT, allow for higher doses to be delivered to disease while keeping normal tissues safer.
- Further prospective randomized studies are needed to validate the possible advantages to these more modern techniques.

References

1. Kalser, M.H., and Ellenberg, S.S., Pancreatic cancer. Adjuvant combined radiation and chemotherapy following curative resection. *Archi Surg*, 1985. **120**(8):899–903.
2. Klinkenbijl, J.H., Jeekel, J., Sahmoud, T., van Pel, R., Couvreur, M.L., Veenhof, C.H., *et al.*, Adjuvant radiotherapy and 5-fluorouracil after curative resection of cancer of the pancreas and periampullary region: phase III trial of the EORTC gastrointestinal tract cancer cooperative group. *Ann Surg*, 1999. **230**(6):776–82; discussion 82–4.
3. Neoptolemos, J.P., Dunn, J.A., Stocken, D.D., Almond, J., Link, K., Beger, H., *et al.*, Adjuvant chemoradiotherapy and chemotherapy in resectable pancreatic cancer: a randomised controlled trial. *Lancet,* 2001. **358**(9293):1576–85.
4. Koshy, M.C., Landry, J.C., Cavanaugh, S.X., Fuller, C.D., Willett, C.G., Abrams, R.A., *et al.*, A challenge to the therapeutic nihilism of ESPAC-1. *Int J Radiation Oncol Biol Physics*, 2005. **61**(4):965–6.
5. Landry, J., Catalano, P.J., Staley, C., Harris, W., Hoffman, J., Talamonti, M., *et al.*, Randomized phase II study of gemcitabine plus radiotherapy versus gemcitabine, 5-fluorouracil, and cisplatin followed by radiotherapy and 5-fluorouracil for patients with locally advanced, potentially resectable pancreatic adenocarcinoma. *J Surg Oncol*, 2010. **101**(7):587–92.
6. Hoffman, J.P., Lipsitz, S., Pisansky, T., Weese, J.L., Solin, L., and Benson, A.B., 3rd., Phase II trial of preoperative radiation therapy and chemotherapy for patients with localized, resectable adenocarcinoma of the pancreas: an Eastern Cooperative Oncology Group Study. *J Clin Oncol*, 1998. **16**(1):317–23.

7. Hoffman, J.P., Weese, J.L., Solin, L.J., Engstrom, P., Agarwal, P., Barber, L.W., *et al.*, A pilot study of preoperative chemoradiation for patients with localized adenocarcinoma of the pancreas. Am J Surg, 1995. **169**(1):71–7; discussion 7–8.
8. Massucco, P., Capussotti, L., Magnino, A., Sperti, E., Gatti, M., Muratore, A., *et al.*, Pancreatic resections after chemoradiotherapy for locally advanced ductal adenocarcinoma: analysis of perioperative outcome and survival. *Ann Surg Oncol*, 2006. **13**(9):1201–8.
9. Palmer, D.H., Stocken, D.D., Hewitt, H., Markham, C.E., Hassan, A.B., Johnson, P.J., *et al.*, A randomized phase 2 trial of neoadjuvant chemotherapy in resectable pancreatic cancer: gemcitabine alone versus gemcitabine combined with cisplatin. *Ann Surgi Oncol*, 2007. **14**(7):2088–96.
10. Evans, D.B., Varadhachary, G.R., Crane, C.H., Sun, C.C., Lee, J.E., Pisters, P.W., *et al.*, Preoperative gemcitabine-based chemoradiation for patients with resectable adenocarcinoma of the pancreatic head. *J Clini Oncol*, 2008. **26**(21):3496–502.
11. Varadhachary, G.R., Wolff, R.A., Crane, C.H., Sun, C.C., Lee, J.E., Pisters, P.W., *et al.*, Preoperative gemcitabine and cisplatin followed by gemcitabine-based chemoradiation for resectable adenocarcinoma of the pancreatic head. *J Clini Oncol*, 2008. **26**(21):3487–95.
12. Moertel, C.G., Childs, D.S., Jr., Reitemeier, R.J., Colby, M.Y., Jr., and Holbrook, M.A., Combined 5-fluorouracil and supervoltage radiation therapy of locally unresectable gastrointestinal cancer. *Lancet*, 1969. **2**(7626):865–7.
13. Treatment of locally unresectable carcinoma of the pancreas: comparison of combined-modality therapy (chemotherapy plus radiotherapy) to chemotherapy alone. Gastrointestinal Tumor Study Group. *J Nati Cancer Inst*, 1988. **80**(10):751–5.
14. Klaassen, D.J., MacIntyre, J.M., Catton, G.E., Engstrom, P.F., and Moertel, C.G., Treatment of locally unresectable cancer of the stomach and pancreas: a randomized comparison of 5-fluorouracil alone with radiation plus concurrent and maintenance 5-fluorouracil — an Eastern Cooperative Oncology Group study. *J Clin Oncol*, 1985. **3**(3):373–8.
15. Hall, W.A., Colbert, L.E., Liu, Y., Gillespie, T., Lipscomb, J., Hardy, C., *et al.*, The influence of adjuvant radiotherapy dose on overall survival in patients with resected pancreatic adenocarcinoma. *Cancer*, 2013. **119**(12):2350–7.

16. Milano, M.T., Chmura, S.J., Garofalo, M.C., Rash, C., Roeske, J.C., Connell, P.P., *et al.*, Intensity-modulated radiotherapy in treatment of pancreatic and bile duct malignancies: toxicity and clinical outcome. *Int J Radiation Oncol, Biol, Physics*, 2004.**59**(2):445–53.
17. McGinn, C.J., Zalupski, M.M., Shureiqi, I., Robertson, J.M., Eckhauser, F.E., Smith, D.C., *et al.*, Phase I trial of radiation dose escalation with concurrent weekly full-dose gemcitabine in patients with advanced pancreatic cancer. *J Clini Oncol*, 2001. **19**(22):4202–8.
18. Ben-Josef, E., Schipper, M., Francis, I.R., Hadley, S., Ten-Haken, R., Lawrence, T., *et al.*, A phase I/II trial of intensity modulated radiation (IMRT) dose escalation with concurrent fixed-dose rate gemcitabine (FDR-G) in patients with unresectable pancreatic cancer. *Int J Radiation Oncol Biol Physics*, 2012. **84**(5):1166–71.
19. Passoni, P., Reni, M., Cattaneo, G.M., Slim, N., Cereda, S., Balzano, G., *et al.*, Hypofractionated image-guided IMRT in advanced pancreatic cancer with simultaneous integrated boost to infiltrated vessels concomitant with capecitabine: a phase I study. *Int J Radiation Oncol Biol Physics*, 2013. **87**(5):1000–6.
20. Yovino, S., Maidment, B.W., 3rd, Herman, J.M., Pandya, N., Goloubeva, O., Wolfgang, C., *et al.*, Analysis of local control in patients receiving IMRT for resected pancreatic cancers. *Int J Radiation Oncol Biol Physics*, 2012. **83**(3):916–20.
21. Huguet, F., Goodman, K.A., Azria, D., Racadot, S., and Abrams, R.A., Radiotherapy technical considerations in the management of locally advanced pancreatic cancer: American-French consensus recommendations. *Int J Radiation Oncol Biol Physics*, 2012. **83**(5):1355–64.
22. Goodman, K.A., Regine, W.F., Dawson, L.A., Ben-Josef, E., Haustermans, K., Bosch, W.R., *et al.*, Radiation Therapy Oncology Group consensus panel guidelines for the delineation of the clinical target volume in the postoperative treatment of pancreatic head cancer. *Int J Radiation Oncol Biol Physics*, 2012. **83**(3):901–8.
23. Koong, A.C., Le, Q.T., Ho, A., Fong, B., Fisher, G., Cho, C., *et al.*, Phase I study of stereotactic radiosurgery in patients with locally advanced pancreatic cancer. *Int J Radiation Oncol Biol Physics*, 2004. **58**(4):1017–21.
24. Koong, A.C., Christofferson, E., Le, Q.T., Goodman, K.A., Ho, A., Kuo, T., *et al.*, Phase II study to assess the efficacy of conventionally fractionated

radiotherapy followed by a stereotactic radiosurgery boost in patients with locally advanced pancreatic cancer. *Int J Radiation Oncol Biol Physics*, 2005. **63**(2):320–3.

25. Chuong, M.D., Springett, G.M., Freilich, J.M., Park, C.K., Weber, J.M., Mellon, E.A., *et al.*, Stereotactic body radiation therapy for locally advanced and borderline resectable pancreatic cancer is effective and well tolerated. *Int J Radiation Oncol Biol Physics*, 2013. **86**(3):516–22.

Index

ablation, 188, 311, 321
ablative therapies, 552
adenocarcinomas, 625
adjuvant chemoradiotherapy, 221
adjuvant radiation, 220
advanced gastrointestinal malignancies, 141
alpha-fetoprotein (AFP), 474
APC gene, 47
argon laser, 224
arterial stimulation venous sampling (ASVS), 386
associating liver partition and portal vein ligation for staged hepatectomy (ALPPS), 317
autofluorescence imaging (AFI), 281

biomarkers, 42
borderline resectable, 415
borderline resectable pancreas adenocarcinoma (BRPAC), 416

cancer, 45
cancer prevention, 63
CD117, 607
capecitabine, 460, 519
capsule endoscopy, 282
carbohydrate antigen (CA) 19-9, 358, 488
carboplatin, 255
carcinoembryonic antigen (CEA), 358, 488
carcinoid syndrome, 599
celiac axis (CA), 417
chemoprevention, 57
chemoradiotherapy, 216, 297
chemotherapy, 213, 254, 293
cholangiocarcinoma, 485, 507
chromoendoscopy, 172
chromogranin A (CgA), 383, 598
cirrhosis, 632
colorectal cancer, 291, 311, 629
colorectal carcinomas, 279
colorectal liver metastasis (CRLM), 311
colorectal stenting, 286
common hepatic artery (CHA), 417
computed tomography (CT), 72
confocal laser endomicroscopy (CLE), 176, 244, 281
contrast-enhanced, 76

conventional transarterial chemoembolization (cTACE), 558
corticotropinoma (ACTHoma), 382
cryoablation, 147, 556
cryotherapy, 186, 224
CT colonography, 292

diagnostic laparoscopy (DL), 429
dietary factors, 62
digital subtraction angiography (DSA), 558
docetaxel, cisplatin, 255
doxorubicin, 519
drug-eluting bead transarterial chemoembolization (DEB-TACE), 558
ductal pancreatic adenocarcinoma (PDAC), 452

embolization techniques, 311
emerging treatment regimens in pancreatic cancer, 461
endocytoscopy (EC), 175
endoscopic dilation, 146
endoscopic mucosal resection (EMR), 183, 246, 284
endoscopic retrograde cholangiopancreatography (ERCP), 368, 490
endoscopic submucocal dissection (ESD), 185, 247, 285
endoscopic submucosal tunnel dissection (ESTD), 186
endoscopic ultrasonography (EUS), 72, 179, 491
epidemiology, 1
epidermal growth factor, 261
epidermal growth factor receptors (EGFR), 261, 324
epirubicin, 257
erlotinib, 454
esophageal cancer, 171, 199
esophageal carcinoma, 625
esophageal dilation, 190
esophageal prostheses, 191
esophagectomy, 208
EUS guided fine needle aspiration (EUS-FNA), 284, 363
external beam radiation therapy (EBRT), 328
extra-hepatic cholangiocarcinomas (eCCA), 535

5-flourouracil (5-FU), 255, 294, 323, 506, 507
5-FU-based chemotherapy, 459
5-FU, Leucovorin, 459
fine needle aspiration (FNA), 180
five-year relative survival rates, 3
five-year survival rates, 11
floxuridine (FUDR), 326
future liver remnant (FLR), 313

gallbladder carcinoma, 492, 505
gastric cancer, 241, 254, 627
gastrinoma, 377
gastroesophageal junction (GEJ), 254
gastrointestinal malignancy, 1, 123, 640
gastrointestinal stromal tumors (GISTs), 607
gemcitabine, 453
gemcitabine-based chemotherapy, 454
geographic location, 3

glucagonoma, 381
glutamine synthetase, 483
glypican-3, 482

5-hydroxyindoleacetic acid (5-HIAA), 598
heat-shock protein-70, 483
Helicobacter pylori (*H. pylori*), 59
hepatic artery digital subtraction angiography (DSA), 481
hepatitis B virus (HBV), 472
hepatitis C virus (HCV), 472
hepatocellular carcinoma (HCC), 472, 514, 528, 551, 632
HER family, 49
histologic type,, 3

IGF-R (insulin-like growth factor receptors), 261
imatinib, 610
immune-enhancing nutritional supplement, 128
incidence rates, 2
individualized therapy, 208
insulinoma, 377
intensity-modulated radiation therapy (IMRT), 637
intestinal metaplasia, 629
intra-arterial (HIA) infusion of chemotherapy, 326
intra-hepatic cholangiocarcinomas (iCCA), 535
irinotecan, 257, 261, 459
irreversible electroporation, 557

laparoscopic liver resections, 533
laser therapy, 224
liver biopsy, 482

magnetic resonance cholangiopancreatography (MRCP), 79
magnetic resonance imaging (MRI), 71
malignant transformation, 42
malnutrition, 123
medical imaging, 71
mesorectum, 296
metal stents, 150
microwave (MW) ablation, 555
mitomycin C, 506
moderately-differentiated carcinomas, 628
mortality rates, 2
multikinase inhibitor, 514
multimodality therapy, 208

nab-paclitaxel, 454
narrow band imaging (NBI), 172, 280
neoadjuvant chemoradiotherapy, 213, 216
neoadjuvant chemotherapy versus chemoradiotherapy, 220
neoadjuvant radiation, 213
neuroendocrine tumors (NETs), 595, 630
neuron specific enolase (NSE), 384
nonsteroidal anti-inflammatory drugs (NSAIDs), 59
nutritional risk index (NRI), 125
nutritional support, 123

oligometastatic disease, 311
oncogene, 42
optic coherence tomography (OCT), 174
oral nutritional support, 127

orthotopic liver transplantation (OLT), 531
oxaliplatin, 459, 519

p53 genes, 43
paclitaxel, 255
palliative care, 141
palliative local therapy, 224
pancreatic adenocarcinoma (PAC), 415
pancreatic cancer, 352, 633
pancreatic neuroendocrine tumors (PNETs), 373, 599
pancreatic polypeptide (PP), 384
pancreatic VIPoma, 380
parathyroid hormone related peptide producing NET (PTHrPoma), 383
parenteral nutrition. Enteral nutrition, 148
passive scattering proton therapy (PSPT), 639
pencil beam scanning (PBS), 639
percutaneous endoscopic gastrostomy (PEG), 249
percutaneous ethanol injection (PEI), 553
percutaneous transhepatic cholangiography (PTC), 490
photodynamic therapy, 224
photon, 638
plastic biliary stents, 150
platelet derived growth factor (PDGFR), 47
poorly-differentiated carcinomas, 628
portal vein, 417
portal vein embolization (PVE), 318
positron emission tomography (PET)-CT, 74
predictive, 42
prognostic, 42
prognostic nutrition index (PNI), 126
proton, 638
proton beams, 638
proton pump inhibitors (PPIs), 58
proton radiation therapy, 637

race, 3
radiation, 220
radioembolization, 564
radiofrequency ablation (RFA), 321, 553
radiotherapy, 297
Ras G protein, 45, 47
receptor tyrosine kinase KIT (CD 117) gene, 50
resection, 314
resonance imaging, 75
retinoblastoma (Rb), 43
risk factors, 57
robotic hepatic resections, 534
role of surgery, 222

screening, 56
self-expandable metal stents (SEMS), 143
small bowel adenocarcinoma, 590
small bowel tumors (SBT), 589
SMV-PV resection, 432
somatostain-receptor scintigraphy (SRS), 386
somatostatin, 382, 602
sorafenib, 514, 607
spread-out Bragg peak (SOBP), 639
SpyGlass, 491
squamous cell carcinomas, 625
stenting, 224

stricture dilation, 286
sunitinib, 605
superior mesenteric artery (SMA), 417
supportive treatment in advanced pancreatic ductal adenocarcinoma, 464
surgery, 293
surgical resection, 429, 531
surveillance epidemiology and end results (SEER), 2
systemic chemotherapy, 323, 453

targeted therapy, 261, 324, 605
three-dimensional conformal radiation therapy (3D-CRT), 637
tobacco, 61
total mesorectal excision (TME), 296
total parenteral nutrition (TPN), 132
transcatheter arterial chemoembolization, 517
tumor ablation, 146
tumor node metastasis (TNM) system, 371
tumor stage, 245
tumor suppressor genes, 43
tyrosine kinase inhibitor (TKI), 605

ultrasonography (US), 72, 179, 204, 241, 283, 301, 360, 365, 422, 453, 471, 479, 553
United States, 2–7, 9–18, 20–26, 30, 31, 41, 45–47, 49, 61, 62, 208, 311, 452, 505, 610

vaccination, 60
vascular endothelial growth factors (VEGF), 47, 261, 324
vasoactive intestinal peptide (VIP), 380, 599

well-differentiated carcinomas, 628